*The Macrobiotic Path
to Total Health*

The Macrobiotic Path to Total Health

A COMPLETE GUIDE TO PREVENTING AND RELIEVING MORE THAN 200 CHRONIC CONDITIONS AND DISORDERS *NATURALLY*

MICHIO KUSHI and ALEX JACK

BALLANTINE BOOKS · NEW YORK

A Ballantine Book
Published by The Random House Publishing Group
Copyright © 2003 by Michio Kushi

www.ballantinebooks.com

Library of Congress Cataloging-in-Publication Data
Kushi, Michio.
    The macrobiotic path to total health : a complete guide to preventing and relieving more than 200
chronic conditions and disorders naturally / Michio Kushi and Alex Jack.— 1st ed.
        p.   cm.
    Includes bibliographical references.
    1. Macrobiotic diet.   2. Chronic diseases—Diet therapy.   I. Jack, Alex, 1945–   II. Title.
RM235.K855 2003
613.2'64—dc21

                                                                                        2003051844

ISBN 0-345-43987-2

Book design by Helene Berinsky

Manufactured in the United States of America

First Edition: September 2003

10 9 8 7 6 5 4 3 2

CONTENTS

PART III

INTRODUCTION

The use of beneficial food is the only cause of growth of a person, while the use of food that is injurious is the cause of disease. It is in consequence of this deterioration that there took place a corresponding deterioration in the sap, purity, taste, potency, post-digestive effect and quality of seeds and plants. In this manner, righteousness dwindles in each succeeding age by one quarter . . . until eventually the world comes to dissolution [and is reborn].
—Charaka Samhita, Indian medical encyclopedia, first century A.D.

A great health revolution is sweeping the planet. Alternative medicine, holistic healing, plant-based diets, and indigenous home remedies are moving into the mainstream. According to recent surveys, nearly one-half of the American people are using alternative therapies, the vast majority of the population is trying to eat a healthier diet, and every year an estimated 1 million Americans are becoming vegetarian or semivegetarian. Several years ago, the U.S. government established the Office of Alternative Medicine, and it has recently been upgraded to the National Center for Complementary and Alternative Medicine. Natural foods are served regularly in many schools, hospitals, and nursing homes, as well as in restaurants, in hotels, and on airplanes. The U.S. Department of Agri-culture recently approved the unrestricted use of tofu, tempeh, and other soy products in federally subsidized school lunch programs. The Bureau of Prisons similarly approved soy burgers and other meatless entrées at every meal in federal prisons. The White House is encouraging staff and employees to use soy milk instead of dairy milk in their beverages and practice yoga. Even NASA is developing a special all-plant diet for astronauts, featuring brown rice, lentils, seitan, whole-wheat tortillas, garden vegetables, and desserts made with amasake, a rice-based sweetener. Insurance companies are starting to offer reimbursements for dietary therapies and other mind-body approaches.

During the last generation, macrobiotics has been the catalyst for many of the dramatic dietary and lifestyle changes now taking place. Rooted in the traditional teachings of East and West, the term *macrobiotics* derives from the Greek root words *macro*, meaning "long" or "great" and *bios*, meaning "life." It was coined by Hippocrates, the father of medicine, nearly 2,500 years ago, whose approach to health and healing was based on his famous proverb "Let food be thy medicine, and thy medicine be food." As the foundation of a great or long life, modern macrobiotics has introduced and popularized a way of eating based on brown rice, millet, sushi, mochi (sweet rice cubes or dumplings), seitan (wheat-meat cutlets), whole-wheat sourdough bread, vegetable sushi, pasta salads, rice cakes, and other whole grains and grain products; tofu, miso, tempeh, and other soy foods; a cornucopia of fresh garden vegetables; nori, wakame, and other sea vegetables; and a variety of seasonings, condiments, snacks, and other foods and beverages. Macrobiotic-quality foods are organically grown as much as possible, traditionally or naturally processed, and contain no sugar, dairy, white flour, chemicals, or other harmful ingredients.

From the communes and counterculture of the 1960s and 1970s to the spas and wellness centers of the 1980s and 1990s, macrobiotics is now moving into the cultural mainstream. The Ritz-Carlton and Prince Hotel chains are serving gourmet macrobiotic food to their international guests, the Kellogg School of Management at Northwestern University has established a dining room with macrobiotic food for busy executives taking seminars, and macrobiotic teachers and cooks have been invited to the White House, Capitol Hill, and the United Nations. According to a recent profile in *Vogue* and other magazines, Barbra Streisand, John Travolta, Sarah Jessica Parker, Madonna, Gwyneth Paltrow, Steven Seagal, Andie MacDowell, Nicole Kidman, Tom Cruise, and other Hollywood stars have their own personal macrobiotic cooks. Past notables who followed a macrobiotic way of life and attributed a balanced diet to improving their health and well-being were Gloria Swanson, John Lennon, John Denver, and Dr. Benjamin Spock.

The Smithsonian Institution opened a permanent collection on macrobiotics and alternative health care at the National Museum of American History in Washington, D.C., several years ago, and announced plans for periodic public exhibitions, publications, history-oriented symposia, research fellowships, and internships. Recognizing macrobiotics as the spearhead for the natural foods movement, holistic health, and alternative medicine in America, the Smithsonian's Division of Science, Medicine, and Society stated:

> The National Museum of American History at the Smithsonian Institution is honored to present the Michio Kushi Family Collection on Macrobiotics and Alternative Health Care. This collection of health, nutrition, and personal family materials and artifacts documents important and little studied aspects of American life and culture.... The significance of macrobiotics in American life is little understood although it relates to such broad historical issues as the postwar move toward a more healthy diet, our increasingly global culture, alternative healing, peace studies, and traditions of grassroots activism.

Over the last half century, hundreds of thousands of individuals and families have recovered their health using macrobiotic principles. Based on studies of the macrobiotic way of eating, medical research at Harvard Medical School and other leading medical schools and scientific institutions has established high blood pressure and high cholesterol as major risk factors for heart disease, the number one cause of death in modern society. People following a macrobiotic way of life actually have stronger hearts than conditioned athletes, as Dr. Castelli, the director of the Framingham Heart Study, the nation's largest cardiovascular study, observed:

> What a person eats every day is a very important aspect of how his or her health will be in every day as well as later life. Supporting this view is the fact that macrobiotic people studied had a ratio of [total cholesterol to HDL cholesterol of] 2.5 and Boston marathon runners were at 3.4, ratios at which rarely, if ever, is coronary heart disease seen. Studies and observations such as these are a clear indicator that people need to take a critical look at their diet with the intention of making changes now.

On the medical front, the Lemuel Shattack Hospital in Boston served macrobiotic food to its physicians, staff, and longtime geriatric and psychiatric patients, and the Second International Conference on Dietary Assessment Methods, a large conference of six hundred medical researchers sponsored by the Harvard School of Public Health and the World Health Organization, recently featured a macrobiotic banquet at the John F. Kennedy Library in Boston. In

Africa, the World Health Organization convened a regional conference on a macrobiotic dietary approach to AIDS, which was attended by several hundred physicians and medical professionals.

Today, an international network of nearly 1,000 macrobiotic educational centers around the world is providing instruction in cooking, health care, shiatsu massage, and the meeting of East and West. The organic natural foods movement, which the macrobiotic community spearheaded a generation ago, is the most rapidly growing segment of the national food industry, increasing at an annual rate of 20 percent.

In Washington, D.C., the U.S. House of Representatives Government Reform Committee recently heard testimony on the macrobiotic approach to cancer from a half dozen men and women who had overcome incurable cancer with the help of a healthy diet and a natural way of life. The National Institutes of Health will soon issue its report on the macrobiotic approach to preventing and relieving this disorder, the number two overall cause of death in modern society. It is expected to release about 77 medically documented case histories of individuals with incurable cancer who recovered with the help of macrobiotics. In a case-control study of about 100 women at high risk for breast cancer published in 2001, the National Tumor Institute of Milan, Italy, found that a macrobiotic way of eating could reduce the risk of this malignancy by about 25 to 30 percent within several months. Meanwhile, the American Cancer Society says, "Today's most popular anticancer diet is probably macrobiotics." On its Internet site, the American Cancer Society declares:

Macrobiotics may help prevent some cancers. It may reduce the risk of developing cancers that appear related to higher fat intake, such as colon cancer and possibly some breast cancers. The macrobiotic diet, like other fat-free diets, can lower blood pressure and perhaps reduce the chance of heart disease. Taking part in a macrobiotics program may provide some sense of balance with nature and harmony with the total universe and as such promote a sense of calmness and reduced stress.

The U.S. Centers for Disease Control and Prevention (CDC) has awarded a new grant to the University of South Carolina to study the macrobiotic approach to cancer. A special committee of oncologists from the National Cancer Institute (NCI) recently met with a group of individuals who had recovered from terminal cancer solely through the application of the macrobiotic approach and reviewed their biopsies, CT scans, and other supporting medical documentation. These included a businessman who recovered from pancreatic cancer over 20 years ago, a nurse who healed herself of stage IV lung cancer that had spread to multiple organs, a stockbroker with malignant melanoma, a housewife with a rare, inoperable uterine tumor, a mother with the same type of invasive lymphoma as Jackie Onassis, and a physicist with inflammatory breast cancer who was given 3 months to live. As a result of the meeting, the NCI approved clinical trials of the macrobiotic approach to cancer. Dr. George Yu, a surgeon at the Georgetown University Medical School in Washington, D.C., is overseeing this project on behalf of the Kushi Institute.

Over the last generation, many medical associations and centers, including Harvard Medical School, the Framingham Heart Study, and Tulane University, have published research showing the benefits of macrobiotics in helping to reduce blood pressure, lower cholesterol, prevent heart disease, treat sensitivity to chemicals, improve immune function, lower weight, regulate the female hormone cycle, and prolong life span. These articles have appeared in major medical journals, including the *New England Journal of Medicine, Journal of the American Medical Association, American Journal of Epidemiology, Pediatrics, Journal of the American Dietetic Association, Cancer Research, International Journal of Biosocial Research, Lancet, Journal of the American College of Nutrition,* and *Journal of Applied Nutrition.*

As the new century began, the U.S. government issued newly revised dietary guidelines moving broadly in a macrobiotic direction. Calling on Americans to "use plant foods as the foundation of [their] meals," the newly released 2000 edition of *Dietary Guidelines for Americans* establishes whole grains as the base for a healthy diet. "There are many ways to create a healthy eating pattern, but they all start with the three food groups at the base of the Pyramid: grains, fruits, and vegetables," state the official dietary recommendations of the U.S. government. The guidelines call for whole grains to be "the center of the plate," list 10 major whole grains and whole-grain products to select from, and recommend that all healthy adults and children over age 2 "eat foods made from a variety of whole grains—such as whole wheat, brown rice, oats, and whole grain corn—every day."

Recognizing the role that whole foods play

in preventing heart disease, cancer, and many other afflictions, the guidelines go on to note, "Eating plenty of whole grains . . . may help protect you against many chronic diseases." The report explains that vegetarian diets that do not include any animal food can meet all the nutritional requirements for a healthy life, for the first time implicitly endorsing macrobiotics, the vegan diet, and other plant-centered ways of eating.

The American Heart Association (AHA) also issued new guidelines in 2000 calling for people to eat whole grains and grain products as the major portion of their daily diet, eat fresh vegetables and fruits as the second major portion, and reduce animal foods. To lower cholesterol and reduce the risk of heart disease, it recommends that the American people eat soy products daily in natural form, as opposed to capsules or supplements. The AHA has also endorsed balanced vegetarian diets that include no animal food as healthful and nutritionally adequate, and it included recipes using brown rice, tofu, miso, and other wholesome foods in its cookbook. The nation's largest cardiovascular association notes:

> You don't need to eat animal products to have enough protein in your diet. Plant proteins alone can provide enough of the essential and non-essential amino acids, as long as sources of dietary protein are varied and caloric intake is high enough to meet energy needs. Whole grains, legumes, vegetables, seeds and nuts all contain both essential and non-essential amino acids. You do not need to consciously combine these foods ("complementary proteins") within a

given meal. Soy protein has been shown to be equal to proteins of animal origin. It can be the sole protein source if desired.

The U.S. Food and Drug Administration (FDA) has also recognized that whole grains are fundamental to health, and it recently approved food labels stating: "Eating a diet high in whole-grain foods that is low in fat may reduce the risk of heart disease and certain cancers."

Dietary recommendations such as these are now national policy and will be used in planning millions of meals in American schools, hospitals, nursing homes, the military, and other institutions. National organic standards went into effect in 2002, backed by the U.S. government, making certified organic food available in almost every food store and supermarket in the country. The next revision of the U.S. dietary guidelines in 2005 or 2010 may further reduce the importance of dairy food in the Food Guide Pyramid, or even eliminate it completely, and make further restrictions on foods high in fat and sugar. It could take a decade for these changes to trickle down to the local and regional levels, but the diet and health revolution is now spreading rapidly around the world, creating a healthier, more peaceful planet.

◎ The Macrobiotic Path

The Macrobiotic Path to Total Health is intended to help people prevent or relieve more than 200 chronic conditions and disorders. Part I introduces an overview of the macrobiotic way of eating, an introduction to principles of balance, the energetics of food, and a natural approach to health and sickness. In Part II, the conditions and disorders are grouped under nearly thirty broad subject headings, such as "Digestive Problems," "Liver Problems," and "Eye and Vision Problems," touching on body systems, organs, and functions or other subjects. For example, "Digestive Problems" includes specific guidelines for appendicitis, colitis, constipation, Crohn's disease, diarrhea, diverticular disease, enteritis, gas and gas pain, hemorrhoids, hernia, irritable bowel syndrome, motion sickness, and other intestinal ills. Cross references are provided for related conditions. Some classifications are arbitrary, especially those under "Bone and Joint Disorders," "Nervous Conditions and Disorders," and "Muscle Problems," since all these systems and functions are commonly involved in complex conditions such as multiple sclerosis or muscular dystrophy. Major diseases such as cancer, arthritis, and AIDS have their own separate sections. Mad cow disease, repetitive stress injuries, and several other subjects of contemporary health or environmental interest also stand by themselves. Conditions relating specifically to women's health, men's health, and children's health will be presented in a future volume on a macrobiotic approach to family health, including pregnancy and infant care; depression and mood swings; immune disorders; fatigue; shoulder and neck problems; problems related to hair, skin, nails, the mouth, and lips; sexually transmitted diseases; weight problems; sleeping problems; substance abuse; teeth problems; and first aid and emergencies.

Those who have read some of our previous books, such as *The Cancer Prevention Diet* and *Diet for a Strong Heart*, or attended lectures at the Kushi Institute or elsewhere will recognize the general approach in this book. However, many of the specific dietary recommendations have been modified to take into account new insights and understanding, evolving practice within the macrobiotic community, and ever-changing environmental and climatic conditions. There is important new material, including revised classifications, new home remedies, and special dishes for many individual types of cancer, infectious diseases, nervous disorders, bone and joint problems, muscle problems, and other categories of disease. Nearly 100 conditions and disorders are presented comprehensively for the first time in this book.

The specific dietary and way-of-life guidelines for each condition or disorder will differ slightly for each person according to his or her health, age, sex, activity level, and personal needs. The use of salt, oil, and other seasonings, the proportion of grain, the flavor and taste of soup, the balance of vegetables, the strength of condiments, and other factors differ subtly from person to person. Chapter 6 explains how to classify each condition or disorder and combine specific dietary and lifestyle recommendations in the text or section with the standard macrobiotic dietary guidelines for people in general good health or one of the three comprehensive healing diets. Since many similar foods and types of home remedies are recommended, the overall dietary guidelines, menus, recipes, and instructions for home remedies have been gathered together in Part III for easy access.

Our associate Christine Akbar (the scientist mentioned above who healed herself of inflammatory breast cancer 15 years ago) coordinated the gathering of data for many sections of this book, including the menus, recipes, and home remedies, and transcribed many lectures, counseling notes, and other materials. We appreciate her hard work and devotion. We are grateful for the support of our families, including Norio, Lawrence, Phiya, and Hisao Kushi and their families; Gale, Masha, and Esther Jack; Henry and Hanz Genki Swindell; Lucy Williams; and our agent, Susan Cohen. Aveline Kushi, Gale Jack, and our associates Wendy and Edward Esko contributed recipes, home remedies, and other important material. Kazuo and Tony Roberts provided valuable secretarial assistance. We would like to dedicate this book to the memory and spirit of Aveline Kushi, who devoted her life to the modern diet and health revolution, training a generation of macrobiotic cooks and teachers, and who passed away during the last year.

The Macrobiotic Path to Total Health focuses on diet as the foundation for a healthy, happy life and offers comprehensive dietary guidelines for the temperate regions of the world, encompassing most of North America, Europe, Russia, China, Japan, and milder parts of Africa, South America, and Australia. In the future, we hope that the material in this book on lifestyle, environment, physiognomy, and complementary healing methods, such as do-in and shiatsu massage, palm healing, meditation, chanting, and other practices mentioned in the text, can be expanded and integrated in a comprehensive encyclopedia of natural healing, including dietary guidelines for all of the major regions, climates, and environments of the world.

The Charaka Samhita, the great healing text of ancient India, ran to seven volumes and could fit conveniently today on one compact disk. We hope that this book, combining traditional dietary wisdom and healing remedies with modern insights and applications, will serve as a new medicine for humanity in the century ahead until that larger multivolume project can be completed or—even better—becomes unnecessary.

Michio Kushi and Alex Jack
Becket, Massachusetts
March 1, 2002

PART **1**

LIVING A LONG,
HAPPY LIFE

The Macrobiotic Way of Eating

As the 21st century begins, the world faces an unprecedented health and environmental crisis. New diseases and epidemics have emerged, family and social conflicts have increased, and ecological threats have multiplied and spread, imperiling humanity's biological and spiritual evolution, as well as the future of other life on this planet. At the heart of this escalating crisis is the integrity of the world's food supply. Genetic engineering, cloning, food irradiation, microwave cooking, and other new technologies are radically changing the way humans have eaten, fed their families, and managed their health for thousands of years, violating millions of years of natural order.

Personal and planetary health are inseparable. World hunger and poverty cannot be divorced from eating beef, chicken, and other animal foods that require up to ten times more grain to produce than growing grain directly for human consumption. SARS, AIDS, mad cow disease, and other new epidemics are connected with a widespread decline in natural immune function as a result of the modern way of eating

and overmedicalization. Violence and war are intimately related to liver, kidney, and pancreatic imbalances that give rise to anger, fear, and greed on a personal, family, or societal level.

The macrobiotic way of eating is very broad and comprehensive. It has been observed by millions of human beings for thousands of years, contributing to health, happiness, and peace for endless generations and our species' overall biological and spiritual evolution. For the most part, it is based on whole cereal grains (the traditional staff of life), vegetables from land and sea, beans, and other fresh foods, with a minimum of animal products. With the advent of the modern era about 400 years ago, this way of eating steadily declined around the world, as meat, poultry, eggs, and dairy became the center of the diet; white flour and white rice displaced whole-wheat flour and brown rice; and canned and frozen foods, highly processed foods, and foods grown with or containing chemicals largely replaced fresh, local produce grown organically and consumed in season.

Today the modern supermarket and natural

foods store contain a cornucopia of foods from all over the world. Bananas, mangoes, and other tropical foods are eaten by people living in the Arctic, while dwellers in the rain forest have access to hamburgers, french fries, and soft drinks. Watermelon, strawberries, and other perishable fruits are consumed in winter, and steak, fried chicken, and other heavy animal foods are consumed in summer. The typical family today rarely eats home-cooked food together, and electric or microwave ovens are found in the vast majority of households. The end result has been a wave of epidemic and degenerative disease, including heart disease, cancer, AIDS, new multiple-drug-resistant strains of tuberculosis, and other afflictions. The advent of cloning and genetic modification of foods and medicines; the rise in organ transplants and implants, especially from animals to humans; the spread of artificial electromagnetic fields from computers, cell phones, and other technology; and the destruction of the environment, including desertification, the thinning of the ozone layer, and the onset of global warming, have contributed to a further decrease in natural immunity to disease. The biological degeneration of human beings, reflected in a sharp rise in infertility and the use of new artificial birth technologies, as well as the spread of infectious, degenerative, and immune-deficiency diseases, threatens the continued existence of our species. The modern evolutionary crisis encompasses all of the nearly 200 conditions and disorders dealt with in this book.

The world is now splitting into two directions. The first is respecting nature, traditional wisdom, and natural order. The second is oriented toward artificial intervention into natural processes. Our natural evolution on this planet will end if the second way prevails. The present situation is similar to that described in the story of Noah and the great flood. Unless we awaken to the spreading chaos around us, the earth will be engulfed by a biological catastrophe of its own making.

Our species and the planet as a whole are in urgent need of healing. For many years, the macrobiotic community has warned that the outer environment is a reflection of the inner environment and that the key to the health and environmental crisis is a return to a more natural way of life centered on a natural way of eating. Personal and planetary health are indivisible. When one person is nourished, the whole planet benefits. When the earth prospers, each person is energized and refreshed. Modern macrobiotics is devoted to creating a world of universal health, happiness, and peace in harmony with natural order for endless generations.

Despite the lack of a leading philosophy and its practical application to every dimension of the crisis, modern society is beginning to take positive steps to redress the balance. First, the health revolution, as noted in the introduction, is now spreading. This includes organic farming, the environmental movement, and the macrobiotic community. Modern science and medicine has rediscovered the central importance of whole grains, as reflected in the Food Guide Pyramid and other dietary and nutritional guidelines. Second, communications networks are elevating consciousness. Through the Internet, information on health and diet is easily exchanged, and there is the potential to reach every home or community directly through this new technology. Third, new alternative approaches to health and well-being have emerged that emphasize a balanced diet, healing with energy and vibration, and living a natural way of life.

◎ The Macrobiotic Diet

The macrobiotic way of eating has been practiced widely throughout history. Each culture and civilization has applied principles of balance to the proper selection and preparation of food and developed a unique cuisine in harmony with its natural environment. The macrobiotic approach is based not only on meeting optimal nutritional needs but also on a deep understanding of the earth's relation to the sun, moon, and other celestial bodies; the evolution of life on the planet; ancestral tradition and heritage; ever-changing environmental and climatic conditions; humidity, pressure, and other atmospheric influences; local availability, affordability, and other economic factors; natural storability and other practical considerations; and the effects of different foods and beverages on our mind, body, and spirit.

The macrobiotic way of eating is not a set diet that applies rigidly to everyone, but a flexible *dietary approach* that differs according to climate, environment, condition of health, sex, age, activity level, and personal need. Macrobiotics is the collective wisdom and universal heritage of humanity. It is not the manifestation, property, or exclusive possession of a single era, culture, society, nation, religion, school, family, or individual. The goal of macrobiotics is *freedom*—the ability to create and realize our dream in life as part of our endless spiritual journal in the infinite universe. Standard macrobiotic dietary practice provides almost limitless variety and choice to prepare healthful, delicious food suited to our unique requirements, needs, and goals. No food is prohibited in the macrobiotic way of eating, and no food will heal all diseases. The standard macrobiotic diet is based on a comprehensive approach that takes into account the overall balance of energy and nutrients of food and looks at multiple causes and effects. Table 1 summarizes the major approaches to healing.

In comparison with the modern way of eating, the standard macrobiotic way of eating has the following general nutritional characteristics:

- More complex carbohydrates, fewer simple sugars
- More vegetable-quality protein, less animal-quality protein
- Less overall fat consumption, more polyunsaturated fat, and less saturated fat
- A balance of various naturally occurring vitamins, minerals, and other nutrients and less supplementation
- Use of more organically grown, natural food and more traditional food processing techniques and less chemically grown, artificially produced, or chemically processed foods
- Consumption of food primarily in whole form as much as possible and less refined, partial, or processed food
- Greater consumption of food that is high in natural fiber and less food that has been devitalized by overprocessing

The standard macrobiotic way of eating is not designed for any particular person nor for

TABLE I. APPROACHES TO HEALING

	1. Modern and Artificial Medicine	2. Alternative and Holistic Medicine	3. Traditional and Future Medicine
	Complementary or Integrated Medicine		
		Present-Day Macrobiotic Healing	
Aim	Remove symptom, manipulate the genes, or create artificial organs and functions	Reestablish balance within body	Harmonize with larger forces of nature
Approach	Sees mind and body as separate; believes nature can be improved; analytic, specialized	Sees mind and body as a unit; intuitive, holistic	Sees mind, body, and spirit in relation to the order of nature and the universe; comprehensive
Attitude	Defensive, fearful, violent, invasive	Harmonious, balanced	Faith based on understanding
Practitioner's task	Relieve pain, suppress symptoms, or create new organism	Stimulate body's healing ability	Allow forces of nature to heal
Diagnosis	Specialized, complicated, high-tech procedures	Simple observation and techniques	Intuitive
Cause of disease	External factors (germs, genes, stress, toxins)	Energy imbalances caused by diet, lifestyle, lack of exercise, relationships	Ignorance of the principles of life
Treatment	Drugs, chemicals, surgery, transplants, vitamins, supplements, gene therapies	Diet, herbs, natural substances, massage, body work, meditation, and other simple treatments	Education and self-reflection, freely using energy directly or any of the methods in columns 1 and 2
Personal participation or responsibility	Little or none	Client receives consultation, treatment, or advice; self-healing; group therapy	Total responsibility and participation of individual, family, and community
Time frame	Seeks instant results or as quickly as possible	Gradual recovery as balance is restored	Instantaneous recovery through awakening to cause and little concern with how long symptoms will take to disappear
Cost	Expensive, often catastrophic	Some extra cost	Little or no cost

	1. Modern and Artificial Medicine	2. Alternative and Holistic Medicine	3. Traditional and Future Medicine
	Complementary or Integrated Medicine		
		Present-Day Macrobiotic Healing	
Equipment	Specialized and sophisticated high-tech equipment	Simple, low-tech equipment	No special equipment
Result	Temporary relief, as imbalance is driven deeper into body, where it manifests later; creation of new artificial species	Dietary, lifestyle, and environmental causes of imbalance corrected; creation of personal and planetary health	Change in view of life and harmony with nature, the universe, God; continuation of humanity's biological and spiritual evolution

any special condition of health. It serves to maintain physical and psychological health and well-being and contribute to the health and safety of society in general. It further serves, in many instances, to prevent many common ailments and chronic conditions, as well as promote possible recovery from serious diseases and disorders. The dietary guidelines that follow have been practiced daily over the last generation by millions of macrobiotic individuals and families around the world. The guidelines presented in this book are designed primarily for a temperate climate. This includes most of North America, Europe (including most of Russia), China, Japan, and temperate parts of Africa, Latin America, and Australia. The standard macrobiotic diet will differ slightly for other regions, including tropical climates in South Asia, Southeast Asia, the Middle East, Africa, and Latin America; semipolar regions in Siberia, Mongolia, and the Arctic; and other distinctive habitats, including Oceania and other island societies.

Comprehensive guidelines for each of these regions are currently being developed. In the meantime, Table 2 summarizes some of the principal differences in the traditional diet in each of these areas. For example, in the tropics, the standard macrobiotic diet would include a wide variety of tropical fruits and vegetables that are not part of the standard diet in the temperate regions. Similarly, in colder latitudes, animal food would be eaten in larger proportion and more frequently than in a four-season climate. It is important to keep this in mind when the guidelines in this book say to avoid or minimize tropical foods or avoid or minimize animal foods. As part of a balanced diet, these foods may be part of a healthy way of eating in their native habitat. However, in most of the temperate world these foods produce strong energetic effects, can lead to imbalance, and are not suitable for ordinary consumption.

The accompanying chart, the Great Life Pyramid, illustrates the main categories of food that may be taken daily or regularly (5 to 7 times a week), as well as the kinds of foods that may be taken weekly or occasionally (1 to 3 times a week), by persons in usual good health. At the top of the pyramid is a small

TABLE 2. ADJUSTMENTS FOR ENVIRONMENT AND CLIMATE

Cold, Northern Climate	Temperate Climate	Hot, Tropical Climate
Northern grains such as buckwheat, northern winter wheat, northern millet	Short-grain rice, wheat, barley, oats, adzuki beans, lentils	Southern grains such as medium and long-grain rice, cassava, sago, and other roots and tubers; larger beans such as pinto, lima
Local vegetables prepared with longer cooking	Local vegetables, mostly cooked, and a small amount of fruit	Local vegetables with more salads, more fruit, and more raw food
More animal food	A little fish or seafood	Little or no animal food
Heavier cooking, with stronger seasoning	Cooking adjusted according to the season	Light cooking, with more oil and spices

triangle consisting of several food groups that are not generally suitable in a temperate climate but which may be eaten infrequently (once or twice a month) by those in transition to the macrobiotic way of eating or those who eat in a broadly more healthful direction.

The Great Life Pyramid is designed as a graphic depiction of the relative importance and proportions of the different food groups. It shares the same basic orientation as the U.S. Food Guide Pyramid, the Mediterranean Diet Pyramid, the Asian Diet Pyramid, and the Vegetarian Diet Pyramid but is more comprehensive. The Great Life or Macrobiotic Food Pyramid is based on a universal eating pattern found throughout the temperate regions of the world, not just one civilization or culture, and is more in line with current nutritional and medical studies than the other guidelines. Please study this illustration carefully. Smaller pyramids for approximately a dozen different geographical regions of the world are also in preparation, as well as an all-vegetarian macro-

biotic pyramid for those who wish to avoid animal food altogether.

◎ Dietary Guidelines

The following guidelines represent a standard average for persons in usual good health. Those with one of the conditions described in this book may need to limit some types of foods, especially fish and seafood, fruit, juices, seeds and nuts, snacks, and desserts, as well as the amount of salt, oil, or other seasoning used in cooking, until their health improves. Please refer to the specific conditions and disorders in Part II for dietary advice and Part III for one of three comprehensive healing diets that can be individually tailored to your condition and needs. Part III also includes a comprehensive list of the major foods used in the modern macrobiotic diet in a temperate climate as well as a list of foods that are generally avoided or minimized.

Table 3.

Great Life Pyramid
Macrobiotic Dietary Guidelines
for a Temperate Climate

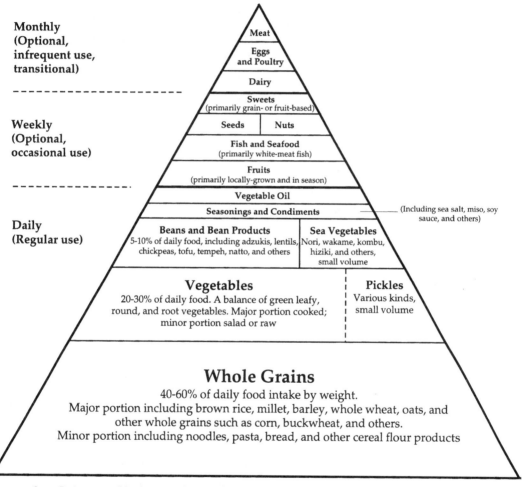

Soup: Grains, vegetables, beans, and sea vegetables may be consumed in the form of soup, 1-2 times daily or several times a week, in addition to the usual styles of preparing these foods

Water: Non-stimulant beverages and natural, clean water, including spring, well, or filtered water for drinking and cooking

Quality: Food to be natural quality (non-genetically engineered), organically grown as much as possible, traditionally or naturally processed, and prepared using gas, wood fire, or other natural fuel

Note: These are standard averages that may be adjusted for climate and environment, cultural or ethnic heritage, gender, age, activity level, individual condition of health and personal needs, and other considerations

DAILY FOOD FOR THOSE IN GOOD HEALTH

WHOLE GRAINS

The principal food is cooked whole cereal grains, comprising from 40 to 60 percent of the daily food intake (average 50 percent by weight). Whole grains include brown rice, whole wheat berries, barley, millet, and rye, as well as corn, buckwheat, and other cereal grasses cooked in a variety of styles. Short-grain or medium-grain brown rice is the staple today in most macrobiotic homes around the world, generally pressure-cooked or occasionally boiled, and is eaten at least once a day. It may be cooked plain or together with about 10 to 20 percent millet, barley, whole wheat berries, fresh corn kernels, or other grain. It may also be cooked together with a small volume of adzuki beans, lentils, chickpeas, or other beans. The majority of whole grains are to be eaten in whole form, and ideally constitute the center of every meal. Occasionally, several times a week, whole-grain products, such as cracked wheat, rolled oats, noodles, pasta, unyeasted sourdough wheat or rye bread, and other unrefined whole-flour products may be taken as part of this category. White flour and other highly refined and polished grains are avoided or minimized. From time to time, organic white rice may be taken for relaxation, enjoyment, or medicinal benefits. Whole grains should be freshly prepared at least once a day and may be used for leftovers the same day or the next day.

SOUP

One to 2 servings of fresh soup are consumed each day, either a cup or bowl, making up about 5 to 10 percent of daily food intake. The soup is frequently seasoned with miso (naturally fermented soybean paste) or shoyu (naturally fermented soy sauce), to which wakame (a sea vegetable) and carrots, onions, or seasonal land vegetables are added during cooking. The taste of miso or shoyu should be mild, not too salty or too bland. Barley miso, rice miso, or hatcho (all-soybean) miso, aged for two to three years naturally, are recommended for regular use. A wide selection of sweet vegetable soups, bean soups, and grain soups may also be prepared. Soup is to be prepared with fresh ingredients each day and not be canned, packaged, or precooked.

VEGETABLES

About 20 to 30 percent of daily food includes fresh vegetables prepared in a variety of ways, including steaming, boiling, and nishime-style (long simmering). Vegetables are also occasionally sautéed, stir-fried, baked, deep-fried, or prepared tempura style. Further, salads are boiled, pressed, or occasionally eaten fresh. The vegetables include a wide variety of leafy green and white vegetables such as kale, collard greens, broccoli, and watercress; round and ground vegetables such as cabbage, onions, and fall-and winter-season squashes and pumpkins; and root vegetables such as carrots, daikon, and burdock. Shiitake and other mushrooms are also used occasionally. The major portion of vegetables is cooked and a minor portion is pickled or eaten raw. When preparing root vegetables, the root and leaf portions may be cooked together to achieve a balance of energy and nutrients. Tropical and semitropical vegetables are best avoided, including eggplants, potatoes, tomatoes, asparagus, spinach, sweet potatoes, yams, avocados, peppers, and others, unless you live in a hot and humid climate. Mayonnaise and commercial salad dressings should also be reduced or minimized. Vegetables are to be prepared as freshly as possible and not canned, frozen, or bottled, which reduces their energy and nutrients. As much as possible, vegetables are to be eaten the same day they are prepared.

BEANS

A small portion, about 5 to 10 percent of daily food, consists of cooked beans or bean products. Beans for regular use include adzukis, lentils, chickpeas, and black soybeans, while all other beans may be used on occasion. Bean products such as tofu, tempeh, and natto may also be used daily. Beans will keep for about 24 hours and may be reheated or added to soups, stews, and other dishes.

SEA VEGETABLES

A small volume of sea vegetables, about 2 percent, is taken daily, including nori sheets, wakame, and kombu. Nori, the thin sheets used to wrap sushi, is eaten as a condiment, while wakame is used daily in miso soup, and kombu is frequently cooked with grains, beans, and vegetables as a seasoning to supply minerals. Hijiki or arame may be taken as a small side dish about twice a week, while all other sea vegetables such as dulse, sea palm, and Irish moss are optional. Sea vegetables are very strong and after cooking will usually keep for a day or two.

SEASONING

Naturally processed white sea salt is used as a regular seasoning, along with miso (soybean paste) and shoyu (naturally fermented soy sauce). Daily meals, however, should not have an overly salty flavor, and seasonings are generally added during cooking and not at the table. Other seasonings may be used occasionally such as umeboshi plums, umeboshi vinegar, rice vinegar, lemon, ginger, horseradish, mirin, garlic, mustard, black or red pepper, and orange. Naturally processed, unrefined vegetable oil is used in cooking, especially light or dark sesame oil. Kuzu is the principal thickener used for gravies and sauces. Commercial seasonings, herbs, spices, and other sugary, hot, pungent, aromatic, or stimulant seasonings are avoided or minimized.

CONDIMENTS

Condiments are placed on the table for use, if desired, to balance the meal. Condiments for daily use include gomashio (toasted sesame seed salt), made usually from 16 to 18 parts roasted sesame seeds to 1 part roasted sea salt, half ground together in a small earthenware bowl called a *suribachi*; roasted wakame or kombu powder, made from baking these sea vegetables in the oven until black and crushing them in a suribachi and sometimes adding toasted sesame seeds and storing in a small container or jar; umeboshi plums, small salted plums that have been dried and pickled for many months with sea salt and flavored with shiso (beefsteak) leaves; tekka, a root vegetable combination of carrot, burdock, and lotus root chopped finely and sautéed in sesame oil and miso for many hours; and green nori flakes. Other condiments may be used from time to time.

PICKLES

A small volume of homemade pickles is eaten each day to aid in digestion of grains and vegetables. A variety of vegetables may be used to make pickles, including daikon, red radish, turnip, carrot, cabbage, cauliflower, and turnip. These are made with bran, brine, miso, shoyu, or umeboshi and are aged from several hours to weeks, months, and even years. Lighter pickles (pickled for a shorter time) are recommended in spring or summer or for persons who need to reduce their salt intake. Saltier pickles (pickled for a longer time) can be eaten during colder weather or by those who need to strengthen their condition. Sauerkraut is a traditional pickle and may be eaten regularly. Commercial pickles made with spices, sugar, and vinegar are avoided or minimized.

GARNISHES

To balance various dishes and make the meal more beautiful, garnishes may be used frequently. These include grated fresh ginger root, chopped scallions, grated daikon, grated radish, grated horseradish, green mustard, lemon slices, orange slices, red pepper, black pepper, and others.

BEVERAGES

Natural water is used for drinking, cooking, and preparing teas. Spring water, well water, or filtered water are most suitable. Bancha twig tea is the principal beverage, while roasted barley tea, brown rice tea, and other grain-based teas or any traditional, nonstimulant, nonaromatic beverage may be used occasionally.

SUPPLEMENTAL FOODS FOR PEOPLE IN USUAL GOOD HEALTH

ANIMAL FOOD

A small volume of fish or seafood may be eaten a few times per week. White-meat fish is less fatty and oily than red-meat and blue-skin varieties. This includes cod, haddock, flounder, trout, and many others. It should be taken with grated daikon, lemon, or horseradish as a garnish and plenty of fresh vegetables at the meal. Infrequently, other types of fish, seafood, or shellfish may be taken. All other animal food is customarily avoided in the modern macrobiotic community, including meat, poultry, eggs, and dairy foods of all kinds.

FRUIT AND JUICE

Fruit may be taken several times a week, preferably temperate-climate fruit such as apples, pears, apricots, berries, or melons. It may be taken stewed or cooked, naturally dried, or fresh in season with a pinch of sea salt. Tropical fruits such as bananas, pineapples, mangoes, papayas, figs, dates, and kiwis are avoided or minimized. Citrus fruits such as orange, tangerine, and grapefruit may be taken in small volume, especially in season or in warmer weather. Juice is very concentrated and has more expansive effects than fruit. A small volume of cider or temperate-climate juice may be taken, preferably in season and at room temperature or warmer.

NUTS AND SEEDS

A small volume of nuts and seeds may be taken, about 1 cup a week. Almonds, walnuts, pecans, and other smaller nuts are preferred over large or tropical varieties of nuts, such as cashew, macadamia, and Brazil nuts. Sesame, sunflower, pumpkin, and other seeds may be eaten lightly blanched or roasted as an occasional snack. Nut and seed butters are highly concentrated and may be taken in small volume.

SNACKS AND DESSERTS

Delicious snacks and desserts may be taken in moderate volume two or three times a week and may include a wide array of sweet dishes prepared with natural ingredients. Often desserts can be prepared with sweet vegetables such as squash, pumpkin, and parsnip; fruits such as apples, berries, or melon; chestnuts; adzuki beans; and other naturally sweet foods without a concentrated sweetener. However, for dishes that need a strong taste, a grain-based sweetener is recommended, including amasake (a fermented sweet rice beverage), barley malt, or brown rice syrup. Soft snacks such as mochi, sushi, noodles, puddings, kanten, and chestnuts are preferred over hard baked snacks and desserts. Cookies, cakes, pies, pastries, rice cakes, popcorn, and puffed grains, however, may be taken in small volume. For custards, whipped toppings, and frosting, agar-agar, tofu, tahini (roasted sesame butter), or kuzu (a white root that is used to thicken dishes) may be used instead of eggs, cream, milk, and other animal products. In macrobiotic households today, sugar, chocolate, brown sugar, honey, molasses, fructose, saccharin, and other highly refined or artificial sweeteners are strictly avoided. Maple syrup is used sparingly for special occasions.

BEVERAGES

Recommended daily beverages include bancha twig tea, roasted brown rice tea, roasted barley tea, and other traditional nonstimulant, nonaromatic teas. Spring water, well water, or filtered water is used for daily drinking, cooking, or preparing teas. Occasional-use beverages include kombu tea, umeboshi tea, mu tea, and grain coffee (made without figs, dates, or tropical sweeteners). Carrot or other vegetable juice may be taken several times a week. Infrequent-use beverages include green tea, soy milk, beer, sake, and other light to moderate alcoholic beverages. Stimulants such as coffee, decaf, black tea, and aromatic herbal teas such as peppermint, rose hips, and chamomile are avoided or minimized. Chlorinated, fluoridated, and other chemically treated water is avoided, as are distilled water, carbonated and bubbling waters, soft drinks, very cold beverages, and hard liquor.

◎ Way of Eating

The standard way of eating provides a complete balance of energy and nutrients. There is no need to count calories or calculate individual nutrients. You may eat regularly 2 to 3 times a day, as much as is comfortable, provided the proportion of each category of food is generally observed. Thorough chewing is essential to digestion, and it is recommended that each mouthful of food be chewed 50 times or more until it becomes liquid in the mouth. As Gandhi wryly observed, drink your food, and chew your liquids. Eat when you are hungry, but it is better not to overeat. Leaving the table satisfied but not full is recommended. Similarly, drink only when thirsty, but do not unnecessarily restrict liquid. Avoid eating for three hours before sleeping, as this can cause stagnation in the intestines and throughout the body, overburden the pancreas and contribute to hypoglycemia, and disturb the kidneys and bladder.

Before and after the meal, express your appreciation to God, the universe, or nature for the food you have received, and reflect on the health and happiness it is dedicated to creating. Appreciation may take the form of grace, prayer, chanting, or a moment of silence. Express your gratitude to parents, grandparents, and past generations who nourished us and whose dream we carry on, to the plants and animals that gave their lives so we may live, and to the farmers, manufacturers, distributors, retailers, and cooks who contributed their energies to making the food available. Every day it is also helpful to reflect on your physical, mental, and spiritual condition. Take just a few minutes to review the events of the day, including thoughts, feelings, and behavior. Try to connect them with your way of eating, especially foods consumed in the last 24 hours. Soon a clear pattern will emerge, and you will know intuitively what kind of effects different foods and beverages have on your daily health and happiness.

Balancing Opposites

Eternal change is the fundamental law of the universe. From the appearance of galaxies to subatomic particles, from the rise and fall of civilizations to the lives of individuals and families, from the structure of body organs and systems to the functioning of tissues and cells, everything unfolds in an orderly pattern of change. The order of the universe was discovered, understood, and celebrated by all traditional cultures and societies throughout history, forming the universal foundation for all great religious, spiritual, philosophical, social, and healing traditions. The way to harmonize with this eternal order in daily life was taught by ancient sages in the East, including Buddha, Lao Tzu, and Confucius, and by great teachers of humanity in the West, including Moses, Jesus, and Muhammad. Under many names and forms, it has been rediscovered, applied, and taught for thousands of years.

Everything changes. Nothing remains the same. Everything is in motion. Nothing remains in one place. Electrons spin around the central nucleus in the atom; the earth rotates on its axis while orbiting the sun; the solar system revolves around the center of the galaxy; and clusters of galaxies move away from one another with enormous velocity, as the universe continues to cycle and expand. Opposites attract each other to achieve harmony; similars repel each other to avoid disharmony. One tendency changes into its opposite, which shall return to the previous state.

In the Far East, the two complementary opposite tendencies that govern all phenomena were known as yin and yang (traditionally pronounced "een" and "eeyong"). On the earth, we experience yang as centripetal energy coming from the sun, the planets, the stars, distant galaxies, and finally cosmic space. This incoming, downward-moving force pushes everything toward the core of the earth and causes the planet to spin on its axis and orbit around the sun. In traditional cultures, this energy was known as the force of heaven. Modern science calls this primary force gravity, mistaking it for a universal force of attraction that pulls things toward the center.

At the same time, the earth generates an opposite, upward, expanding force because of the rotation on its axis. The rising, centrifugal energy from the center of the planet was known as earth's force. The interplay between these two forces creates all manifestations on our planet and throughout the cosmos (see Table 4).

TABLE 4. EXAMPLES OF YIN AND YANG

	More Yin	More Yang
Attribute	Centrifugal Force	Centripetal Force
Tendency	Expansion	Contraction
Function	Diffusion	Fusion
	Dispersion	Assimilation
	Separation	Gathering
	Decomposition	Organization
Movement	Inactive, slower	Active, faster
Vibration	Shorter wave and higher frequency	Longer wave and lower frequency
Direction	Ascent and vertical	Descent and horizontal
Position	More outward and peripheral	More inward and central
Weight	Lighter	Heavier
Temperature	Colder	Hotter
Light	Darker	Lighter
Humidity	Wetter	Drier
Density	Thinner	Thicker
Size	Larger	Smaller
Shape	More expansive and fragile	More contractive and harder
Form	Longer	Shorter
Texture	Softer	Harder
Atomic particle	Electron	Proton
Elements	N, O, P, Ca, etc.	H, C, Na, As, Mg, etc.
Environment	Vibration, Air, Water	Earth
Climatic effects	Tropical climate	Colder climate
Biological	Vegetable-quality	Animal-quality
Sex	Female	Male
Organ structure	More hollow and expansive	More compacted and condensed

	More Yin	More Yang
Nerves	More peripheral, orthosympathetic	More central, parasympathetic
Attitude, emotion	Gentle, negative, defensive	Active, positive, aggressive
Work	More aesthetic and mental	More physical and social
Consciousness	More universal	More specific
Mental function	Future-oriented	Past-oriented
Culture	Spiritually oriented	Materially oriented
Dimension	Space	Time

The thread running through creation is yin and yang, the endless dance of opposites. Each movement creates respective tendencies. Yang force creates contraction, density, heaviness, rapid motion, and high temperature. Yin force creates expansion, diffusion, lightness, slower motion, and lower temperature. At their extremes each force changes into its opposite. For example, high temperature (fire) causes expansion and low temperature (ice) causes contraction.

Yin and yang are not static, fixed conditions or elements, but tendencies that cycle continuously, each changing into the other. At the biological level, yang is identified with masculine energy, while yin is associated with feminine energy. However, nothing is completely one or the other, and the ratio between the two forces is subject to constant fluctuation and change. Man is physically stronger, heavier, and more active than woman, but woman is often spiritually higher and more intuitive than man. Similarly, woman is outwardly more gentle, kind, and loving than man, but inside man is often shyer, more sentimental, and more accepting than woman. Originating from God or the infinite universe, yin and yang manifest in count-

less forms, ultimately merging and returning to their common source. The laws of yin and yang govern all phenomena, from the movements of subatomic particles to the composition of blood and tissue, from the formation of planets and moons to the relationship between the sexes. By knowing how to balance these forces in our own lives, we can turn sickness into health, conflict into peace, and sadness into joy.

◎ The Human Constitution

Human beings, the culmination of billions of years of natural evolution, are formed from the dynamic interaction of heaven's and earth's forces. The ovum, or egg, in a woman forms as a result of the inward spiral motion of follicles in the ovaries, while the sperm in a man is due to the outward differentiation of reproductive cells. These processes are, respectively, yang and yin; fusing, they create new life.

In the womb, the embryo constantly receives heaven's centripetal force, spiraling counterclockwise through the center of the hair spiral on the mother's head, and earth's centrifugal

TABLE 5. THE CHAKRAS AND CORRESPONDING ORGANS AND GLANDS

Chakra	Governs	Organs and Glands
Seventh or crown chakra	Higher consciousness	Pituitary, hypothalamus, brain, central nervous system
Sixth or midbrain chakra	Intuition	Pineal gland, brain, central nervous system
Fifth or throat chakra	Speech and breathing	Thyroid, parathyroid, adenoids, tonsils
Fourth or heart chakra	Love, compassion	Heart, lungs, thymus
Third or solar plexus chakra	Intellect, courage, sympathy, patience, will, perseverance	Pancreas, stomach, spleen, liver, gallbladder, duodenum, adrenals, kidneys
Second or abdominal chakra	Body equilibrium and overall balance	Uterus, small intestine, large intestine, adrenals, kidneys, bladder
First or base chakra	Reproduction and regeneration	Testes, ovaries

force, spiraling up clockwise through the mother's uterus. Both energies charge the developing baby from above and below, generating forces of vital electromagnetic energy. Traditionally, this energy was known as *ki* in Japan, *chi* in China, *prana* in India, *ruach* in Israel, and the Holy Spirit among early Christians. The union of heaven's and earth's forces in the womb creates the fetus's physical, mental, and spiritual constitution. From a single fertilized cell, a complex new being is born with trillions of cells arranged according to a blueprint drawn up by evolution.

In this highly charged environment, a channel of vertical energy appears as the two forces meet. In addition to the two entrance points, from above and below, heaven's and earth's forces collide and charge five major areas in the energy channel, producing seven major centers of activated natural electromagnetic energy. In ancient India, these energy centers were called chakras, or wheels (see Table 5).

Together with the rotational movement of the embryo in the womb, these two highly charged forces produce energy that radiates out from the center of the embryo toward the surrounding atmosphere, forming an invisible layer of energy around the baby. Invisible currents are generated within this field that form a series of inward-moving and outward-moving spirals of energy. The primary inward-moving spiral develops into the digestive and respiratory systems, while the outward-moving spiral develops into the nervous and skeletal systems. In between, the circulatory system develops. Further differentiation leads to the formation of compacted organs, which are slower in movement, and expanded organs, which are faster in movement. The primitive heart, for example, begins to beat on about the 24th day after conception in response to the rhythmic pulsations of heaven's and earth's forces, causing blood to circulate throughout the embryonic disc and primitive placenta. Altogether, seven separate branches of the body's spirallic system develop, unifying digestive, nervous, circulatory, respiratory, skeletal, endocrine, and reproductive systems and functions in one comprehensive whole.

After the heart and other major organs and functions are formed, electromagnetic energy begins to discharge in both upward and downward directions, leading to the development of the arms and legs. Electromagnetic currents or streams of energy branching off the chakras, known as *meridians*, terminate in the formation of arms, hands, and fingers and legs, feet, and toes. The meridians themselves are actually spirals of streaming energy, not lines, channels, or tubes. They represent the entire process of energy flow, entering the body, creating and activating the organs, and then discharging upward or downward to form and activate the limbs. From this view, the organs, glands, and functions of the body are not distinct from the meridians, but the most physicalized, condensed part of the entire meridian system. In turn, each meridian differentiates into numerous smaller branches, streams, and rivulets that transport blood, ki, and consciousness to each of trillions of cells. The human body is an intricate combination of visible and invisible structures and functions. Organs, glands, tissues, and cells are the outward manifestation of an underlying energetic network of meridians and chakras charged by spiraling energy. Together these make up the natural electromagnetic constitution of human beings.

◎ Yin and Yang in the Human Body

The organs of the human body exist in a complementary/antagonistic relationship. Overall, heaven's force creates more compact, solid structures and moves in a downward, inward direction. Earth's force creates expanded, hollow structures and moves in an upward, outward direction. Thus the heart, lungs, kidney, pancreas-spleen, and liver are classified as more yang, while the small intestine, large intestine, bladder, stomach, and gallbladder are classified as more yin. However, the yang organs are nourished by proportionately lighter, slower yin energy, while the yin organs are nourished by a stronger, faster yang energy. Table 6 summarizes this dynamic relationship that contributes to overall balance and harmony among the body's organs and systems.

In general, the left side of the body is influenced more by heaven's force, while the right side is governed more by earth's force. Hence, in paired organs such as the breasts, lungs, ovaries, testicles, and kidneys, the one on the left side is usually slightly smaller and more compact, while the one on the right side is slightly larger and more expanded. Organs located more to the center of the body are affected in a similar manner. The left side of the heart is charged more by heaven's force, while the right side is charged by earth's force. The descending colon and rectum are nourished more by yang energy, while the ascending colon is nourished more by yin energy. In the middle, the transverse colon is governed by heaven's and earth's forces more or less equally.

The upper part of the body is influenced more by earth's force, which rises and spirals

TABLE 6. COMPLEMENTARY RELATIONSHIP AMONG MAJOR ORGANS

Yin Structure and Yang Function	Yang Structure and Yin Function
Colon	Lungs
Gallbladder	Liver
Bladder	Kidney
Small intestine	Heart
Stomach	Spleen-pancreas
Uterus/prostate	Brain

outwardly. In women, who have proportionately more earth's force, it causes the breasts to swell. It also causes the hair to grow profusely at the top of the head, and mental processing activities and functions to be concentrated in the brain. By the same token, the lower part of the body is governed more by heaven's force, which moves downward and spirals inwardly, causing the body's center of gravity to be rooted deep in the intestines, the sex organs to be small and compact, and motor activities to be coordinated largely by the legs and feet. The middle part of the body, containing the heart, lungs, liver, pancreas, and spleen, is charged by both forces more evenly.

In terms of back and front, heaven's force predominately creates the hard, compact spine and condensed central nervous system, while earth's force forms the soft, expanded digestive and respiratory systems. To make balance, the more yang brain and nervous system digest primarily vibrational food in the form of waves and vibrations, while the more yin digestive system processes primarily physical food in the form of material foods and beverages. In between, the circulatory system, representing a balance of heaven and earth, differentiates into complementary/opposite branches, the slightly more compact bloodstream governed by the liver and the slightly more expanded lymphatic system regulated by the spleen.

In terms of periphery and center, heaven's force governs more inward, deep vital functions, while earth's force influences more outward, superficial ones. Yang energy, therefore, tends to gather in the innermost regions of the brain; the liver, heart, and other deep, vital organs; the ovaries and testicles; the bones and nerves; and other interior structures and functions. Yin energy, conversely tends to gather in the outermost regions, including the skin, the mouth, the lips, the breasts, the intestines, and the extremities, including the arms and legs, fingers and toes. Table 7 presents a convenient chart summarizing yin and yang in human structure and function.

Overall, energy moves in a spiral. Phases of contraction alternate with phases of expansion. Expanding spirals reach a limit and turn into contracting spirals and vice versa. Up and down, in and out, right and left, back and front, and other polarities are actually all manifestations of one continuous flow of energy. Created and nourished by heaven's and earth's forces, the

TABLE 7. YIN AND YANG IN HUMAN STRUCTURE AND FUNCTION

More Yin	More Yang
Structures	
Upper body	Lower body
Right side	Left side
Front	Back
Outside (periphery)	Inside (center)
Soft parts	Hard parts
Expanded parts	Contracted parts
Digestive system, respiratory system	Nervous system, skeletal system
Lymph stream	Bloodstream
White blood cells	Red blood cells
B cells	T cells
Suppressor T cells	Helper T cells
Anti-insulin	Insulin
Head hair	Body hair
Growth-enhancing genes	Growth-suppressing genes
Cell membranes	Cell nucleus
Elastin	Collagen
Estrogen	Testosterone
Inhibiting neurotransmitters	Activating neurotransmitters
RNA	DNA
Potassium ions	Sodium ions
Hollow organs	Solid organs
Functions	
Bioenergetic	Biochemical
Breathing in	Breathing out
Inhibition	Activation
Dilation	Contraction
Hydration	Dehydration
Discharging	Taking in
Divergence	Convergence

More Yin	More Yang
Functions	
Relaxation	Tension
Decay	Genesis
Response	Stimulus
Oxygenation	Deoxygenation
Catabolism	Anabolism
Ascending movement	Descending movement
Mental activities	Physical activities
Slower movement	Rapid movement

human constitution is a wondrous replica of the entire universe. Balance and equilibrium are its natural state.

At a very practical level, especially for those for whom yin and yang are new concepts, we can reflect on how expansion and contraction are ever-present realities in our daily lives. The doors and windows of our homes shrink or expand according to the seasons. Our cars, office machines, and other appliances also respond to subtle changes in temperature, humidity, and pressure. These are something like our organs and glands. Outside, the road itself may develop heaves, bumps, ridges, or potholes depending on the elements, especially in response to salt and water. This is something like our skin or the lining of tissues and organs. Through simple analogies and metaphors, almost everyone can begin to understand how yin and yang—expansion and contraction—govern the workings of our bodies.

◎ Food, Health, and Consciousness

In the womb, the fetus receives nourishment from the mother's blood and other nutrients through the placenta. Beyond the original strength and quality of the sperm and ovum, the mother's way of eating during pregnancy has the greatest influence on the developing baby's constitution and future health. After birth, the newborn is nourished by colostrum and breast milk, representing the condensed energy of the animal kingdom. After the teeth come in and the child is weaned, the principal food is predominantly vegetable-quality to ensure proper growth and development.

As we grow up and mature, the main source of ki, or life energy, is the foods that we eat daily. Food transmutes directly into mind, body, and spirit. Through proper food selection and preparation, we take in the condensed essence of heaven's and earth's forces to create our day-to-day health and happiness. The quality and functioning of our organs and tissues depend largely on our diet. Of course, we continue to receive ki directly from nature and the cosmos, but this energy serves to activate and charge the organs and functions, cells and tissues. Relative to each other, the ki energy we receive from the outside world is more yin, while that coming from inside as a result of our daily way of eating is more yang. Food changes directly into blood, lymph, and other bodily fluids that nourish our systems and functions. It keeps the energy channels open to receive the full force of the waves and vibrations coming from the celestial and terrestrial cycles and rhythms around us.

In addition to physical health and vitality, food creates our mind and spirit, determining the quality of our consciousness. Waves from the universe are channeled through the brain and nervous system, which are constructed in the form of a spiral. Each of the trillions of cells is also a receptor and attracts vibrations from the atmosphere and our surrounding environment. Our intellectuality and spirituality are determined by the degree to which our cells are charged with energy. Waves with lower frequencies and longer wavelengths create our bodily activity. Higher-frequency, shorter waves create our thoughts, images, and dreams. By eating predominantly whole grains and cooked vegetables as the center of our diet we are able to receive the higher, shorter impulses and vibrations as well as the lower, longer ones. The scope of our consciousness is broad, and we can deal with both the practicalities of daily life and the music of the spheres. If we take strong yin foods such as sugar, spices, alcohol, or drugs, the spirals within our midbrain, nervous system, and each cell become overexpanded and cannot

catch short waves. If we take strong yang foods such as meat, eggs, poultry, or fatty fish, the spirals become overactive, and we receive and interpret chaotically. Our high spirit and refined consciousness are lost. We start to think erratically, violently, or in a small, fragmented way. The power of food should not be underestimated. As the Upanishads, the traditional wisdom teachings of India, observed: "From food are born all creatures. They live upon food, they are dissolved in food. Food is the chief of all things, the universal medicine. . . . I am this world, I eat this world. Who knows this, knows."

Whole grains have represented the center of the spiral of human evolution on this planet for millions of years. Our species developed its unique upright form and posture, highly developed intellect, and spiritual orientation as a result of eating wild and domesticated grains and other, predominantly plant-quality foods. Whole grains constituted the principal food in all traditional cultures and civilizations: millet and rice in Asia; barley and wheat in southern Europe, northern Africa, and the Middle East; oats and rye in northern Europe; sorghum, teff, millet, and rice in Africa; wild rice and corn in North America; amaranth and quinoa in South America.

The main supplementary foods were vegetables from land and sea, beans, fruits, seeds, nuts, roots, tubers, fungi, and other plant foods. Day to day, meal to meal, people around the world have eaten a balance of foods and beverages derived from the vegetable kingdom.

The third major food constituted animal-quality food, including wild game, small mammals, fish and seafood, domesticated livestock, and in some cultures insects and larvae. According to scientists, people ate animal food on average about two or three times a month during most of human existence on this planet. The exceptions to this pattern were in special climates and environments where grains and vegetables could not be foraged or grown or where the growing season was short. These include hot desert areas, mountainous regions, and cold, northern or southern semipolar regions. In these places, proportionately more animal food was eaten throughout the year. It helped to balance the harsh natural environment or an active, nomadic lifestyle. Under these circumstances, an animal-based diet can be part of a healthy, traditional way of living. However, in most of the temperate and tropical parts of the world, where the vast majority of human beings have lived, a plant-centered way of eating prevailed for countless generations up until the dawn of the modern era about four hundred years ago. A new generation of scientists today is beginning to challenge the view that human ancestors ate primarily meat and developed their unique capabilities as a result of consuming more animal protein than other species. For example, several anthropologists at Harvard University recently proposed that cooking was the main force in early human evolution. Reviewing the archaeological evidence, they explain that humanity's characteristic jaw and skeletal structure, intellect and higher reasoning abilities, and social structure resulted from harnessing fire and learning to cook wild plants.

◎ Classifying Food

To classify food, we need to determine the predominant factors, as all foods have yin and yang qualities. Observing the seasonal cycle is one of the most useful methods of evaluation. In spring, the vegetal energy ascends with the return of warm weather. Buds, sprouts, and green shoots appear as the ground unthaws and the atmospheric energy rises. Tender young greens and other spring vegetables take the chill off the long, cold winter, provide light, fresh energy, and are classified as mildly yin. In summer, the energy rising from the earth reaches a peak of expansion and activity. Cucumbers, zucchinis, and watermelon provide a cooling effect as the weather turns hotter (more yang). In late summer, the energy reaches its zenith and many fruits and vegetables become ripe. They contain plenty of liquid, develop higher above the ground than in spring or early summer, and are very sweet and juicy to the taste. We can classify these foods as very yin. In autumn, the energy of the plant kingdom and atmosphere begins to recede. Wheat, rice, barley, and other grains are harvested, along with pumpkins, squash, onions, apples, and other round vegetables and fruits. Plants harvested at this time and used through the late autumn and winter are more compact and drier, and give stronger energy. They are classified as yang. In winter, the climate turns colder (more yin), and the vegetal energy descends into the root system. Trees lose the last of their leaves as the sap descends to the roots, and the vitality of the plant becomes dormant. Deep snow blankets the ground for much of the winter, the lakes freeze over, and many animals hibernate or migrate south. The energy at this time of the year is frozen, condensed (very yin). About halfway between the winter solstice and the spring equinox, the energy of the earth begins to unthaw, the first buds appear, and the cycle begins anew.

The annual course of the seasons shows the alternation between phases of expansion and contraction, hot and cold, dry and moist, and other complementary opposites. The same principles can be applied to classifying foods according to the region or climate in which they originate. Foods that come from colder or more northerly regions, where the vegetation is sparse and contracted, are more yang. Foods that originate in tropical climates, which are teeming with life and where the plants and animals are more expanded, are more yin. Foods may also be classified according to color, which is another type of energy. Violet, green, blue, and white tend to be more yin, while red and black are more yang, and yellow, orange, and brown are in between. Hence, wine-colored fruits and green leafy vegetables give lighter, more yin effects; animal food containing dark or red blood gives strong yang effects; and beige whole grains and orange and dark yellow vegetables such as squash and pumpkin produce more overall harmony. In addition, the ratio of chemical components can be taken into account. Sodium, the principal element in salt, is very yang, while potassium, a major constituent in potatoes, tomatoes, and eggplants, is very yin. The following summarizes some of these tendencies.

Yin Energy Creates:
Growth in a hot climate
More rapid growth
Foods containing more fluid

Fruits and leaves that are nurtured primarily by expanding energies
Growth upward high above the ground
Sour, bitter, sharply sweet, hot, and aromatic foods
Foods with more potassium and other expansive elements

Yang Energy Creates:
Growth in a cold climate
Slower growth
Drier foods
Stems, roots, and seeds that are nurtured primarily by contracting energies
Growth downward below ground
Salty, plainly sweet, and pungent foods
Foods with more sodium and other contractive elements

All foods can be classified according to their predominant yin and yang qualities. However, practically speaking, we commonly divide the entire spectrum of foods and beverages available in the modern world into three broad categories: (1) *moderate foods*, suitable for regular, occasional, or infrequent use as a part of a balanced daily way of eating; (2) *extreme yang foods*, which create tightness, hardness, and other strong contractive effects and are generally to be avoided or minimized in a temperate climate; and (3) *extreme yin foods*, which create looseness, softness, and other strong expansive effects and are generally to be avoided or minimized in a four-season region.

The first category of moderate foods, consisting of a relatively harmonious blend of yin and yang qualities, includes whole grains, beans and bean products, a wide variety of vegetables from land and sea that are suitable for daily consumption, and an assortment of fruits, seeds, nuts, seasonings, condiments, pickles, garnishes, and nonstimulant, nonaromatic beverages, as well as fish and seafood, especially white-meat fish, that may be used occasionally or infrequently. The second group, strong yang items, consists of meat, poultry, eggs, salted cheese, red-meat and blue-skin fish and shellfish, and other animal products, as well as excessive volume or intake of bread, cookies, crackers, and other baked flour products and too much salt, especially ordinary table salt. Tobacco, ginseng, insulin, thyroxin, and other selected roots, herbs, chemicals, and drugs also produce strong yang effects. The third group, strong yin items, consists of white flour, white rice, and other polished or refined grains; tropical fruits and vegetables, including tomatoes, potatoes, peppers, and other nightshades that originated in the tropics and are now grown in northern latitudes; milk, ice cream, yogurt, and other light dairy foods; soy milk, soy cheese, and other highly processed soy foods; sugar, honey,

and other refined sweeteners; refined oils, margarine, and mayonnaise; spices and herbs; coffee, black tea, and other stimulants; processed foods, including canned, frozen, sprayed, chemicalized, irradiated, or genetically altered foods; and many chemicals and drugs, including amphetamines, antibiotics, aspirin, marijuana, and cocaine. See Table 8 for a summary of these divisions.

Within each category, foods may further be classified as relatively yin or yang depending on their size, shape, growth, color, taste, or other qualities. Different cooking methods, time, pressure, and seasonings can also change the quality of the meals we eat.

In practicing our daily way of eating, we need to select our foods carefully according to their balance of yin and yang. As a rule, we select from foods in the moderate category. However, if certain foods are taken in large volume or too frequently, imbalance can also result. Similarly, not taking certain foods or taking an improper combination of foods can lead to health problems. In the next chapter, we will look at specific foods and their energy.

TABLE 8. GENERAL CLASSIFICATION OF FOOD GROUPS*

Extreme Yang	Moderate	Extreme Yin
Medications (some), refined salt or high-mineral salt	Sea salt	Medications (many)
Eggs, caviar	Sea vegetables	Drugs such as marijuana, LSD, and cocaine
Meat	Whole grains	Chemically grown, processed, or treated foods and water; gene-altered foods; irradiated foods
Hard cheese	Beans and bean products	Vitamin pills and supplements (most)
Poultry	Vegetables	Alcohol
Ginseng, shark fin, and some roots, herbs, and supplements	Temperate seeds and nuts	Sugar, honey, and other refined sweeteners
Tobacco	Temperate fruit and juices such as apple cider and carrot juice	Coffee, decaf, black tea, mint tea, soft drinks, and other stimulant or aromatic beverages
Seafood, shellfish, and red-meat and blue-skin fish	Unrefined vegetable oils	Tropical vegetables, fruits, and nuts; spices and herbs
White-meat fish	Grain-based sweeteners such as amasake, barley malt, and rice syrup	Saturated and refined vegetable oils, mayonnaise, and margarine
Salted, smoked, baked, grilled, roasted, or crunchy foods and salty foods such as chips	Bancha tea, barley tea, and other traditional, nonstimulant nonaromatic beverages	Milk, butter, soft cheese, yogurt, ice cream, and soft dairy foods
Bread, crackers, cookies, and other hard baked flour products	Spring, well, or filtered water	White rice, white flour, and other polished grains

*Foods are classified in each column from strongest at the top to the weakest at the bottom. For example, in column 1, refined salt is more yang than eggs and meat, while in column 3 medications and drugs are more yin than white rice or flour.

The Energy of Food

The energy of food is based on many factors, including: (1) *quality* (animal, vegetable, or mineral; wild or domesticated; heirloom, hybrid, or genetically altered seed; natural, organically, or chemically grown; traditionally, naturally, or chemically processed; naturally or artificially aged; and other considerations), (2) *motion and direction* (rising, expanded motion; very expanded, active motion; condensing, downward motion; inward, solidifying motion; or melting, floating motion), (3) *effect on body temperature* (cooling, warming, cold, hot, or neutral), and (4) *taste* (sour, bitter, sweet, pungent, or salty). Shape, size, color, texture, and other characteristics, including the nutritional and material composition of food, are also forms of energy. When we eat a specific food, we absorb all of these qualities in the form of waves and vibrations that influence the quality of our blood, organs, tissues, cells, and consciousness. The way that food is harvested, transported, processed, stored, cooked, and eaten will further modify its energy and its effects on our health and consciousness. A brief summary of the energetic effects of some of the principal foods in the macrobiotic way of eating follows.

Whole Grains

Whole cereal grains are the foundation of human development and give strong, peaceful energy. The grain stalk corresponds with the brain and spine, contributing to our upright posture and advanced intellect. Firmly rooted in the soil, whole grains grow vertically toward heaven, unifying the energies of earth and sky. The tiny antennae-like endings on the outside of each grain absorb heaven's force, while the rising energy of the earth nourishes the endosperm, bran, and other layers inside the husk. Like grains bending in the wind, our bodies grow strong and flexible the more we eat grains, and we are able to withstand all kinds of weather, challenges, and difficulties.

Grains are the most abundant crop on earth. They demonstrate the greatest flexibility by growing in different climates, ranging from very hot to very cold. They are used to create the widest variety of foods, including cracked, rolled, flaked, and puffed products; bread, crackers, muffins, biscuits, pastries, and other hard baked flour products; tortillas, chapatis, pita, pancakes, and other soft flour products; and miso, shoyu, beer, whiskey, sake, and other fermented foods and beverages. Grain stores easily and retains its energy for a very long time; grains found in ancient tombs have sprouted after thousands of years. Traditionally the longevity of grains served to protect the community when the harvest was lower or when famine threatened.

In the Far East, the ideogram for peace (pronounced *wa*) was made of the characters for "cooked grain" and "mouth," signifying that people who ate whole grains developed a calm, peaceful mind and spirit. Grains have figured prominently in the festivals of all traditional societies and were used in religious and healing ceremonies in shrines, temples, and medicine lodges. Whole cereal grains open us up to higher realms of consciousness, at the same time creating the foundation of day-to-day energy and vitality.

At a nutritional level, whole grains are high in complex carbohydrates and fiber, which contribute to smooth digestive and eliminatory functions; B vitamins, which stimulate the nervous system and ensure smooth mental functioning; high-quality protein, which contributes to improved body growth and maintenance and better hormonal functioning; calcium and other minerals that make strong bones and teeth; and iron and other minerals and vitamins that make strong blood and circulation.

At an environmental level, grains do not require excessive use of the earth's resources to be grown and eaten. They use minimal energy to harvest, store, process, and transport.

Eating whole grains every day is the single most important way to prevent the development of heart disease, cancer, diabetes, and other chronic diseases. In addition to daily food and special dishes, grains are used to make teas, compresses, and other medicinal applications. *Nuka,* or rice bran, for example, is traditionally used to make a poultice that is effective for treating many skin ailments. Major grains and their energetic effects are as follows:

- Brown rice contains a nearly perfect balance of energy and nutrients. It nourishes all organs and functions, particularly the brain, spine, lungs, intestines, kidneys, bladder, and reproductive organs, giving strong day-to-day energy, a tranquil mind, and sound judgment. Rice has traditionally been eaten to develop feelings of oneness and unity with others and for spiritual development. Sweet rice is warm and energizing. In the form of mochi, made by pounding sweet rice into small sticky cakes, it has traditionally been eaten to promote breast milk in mothers and to help keep lovers together.

- Barley has a lighter, cooling energy. It nourishes the liver and gallbladder functions and is used medicinally to help dissolve animal protein and excess fat in the body.

- Millet gives strong, harmonious energy and contributes to practical, creative thinking, inventiveness, and sympathy with others. It nourishes the pancreas, spleen, and stomach and is especially recommended for diabetes, hypoglycemia, lymphoma, and other disorders associated with these organs.

- Whole wheat gives strength, courage, and vision, particularly when eaten in the form of whole wheat berries. In flour form, whole wheat contributes to an analytic mentality as the energy of milled flour, broken down into its component parts and reconstituted into food, is absorbed. Noodles, pasta, pancakes, crepes, and other soft varieties give quick, warming energy and have a rich, satisfying taste. Bread, muffins, cookies, crackers, and other baked goods are very satisfying but much harder to digest. They are also mucus-forming and may need to be limited or avoided altogether by those with digestive or eliminatory problems until the condition improves.

- Whole oats contain more fat than other grains and create strong, warming energy. They are good for a hearty breakfast and other dishes but can be mucus-forming and may need to be limited for those with lung or large-intestine problems.

- Corn is the most expanded of the grains and gives strong, upward, expansive energy. It is strengthening for the heart and small intestine. Traditionally ground into whole-corn dough, or *masa*, it is used in tortillas, arepas, empanadas, cornbread, grits, and other traditional dishes.

- Buckwheat is the strongest of the usual cereal grasses. It gives strong, warming energy and is excellent for performing hard physical labor or housework. It particularly nourishes the kidneys, bladder, and reproductive functions, but because of its high energy may need to be limited for those with either extreme yin or yang conditions. In whole

form, it is eaten primarily as *kasha* and in noodle form as *soba*, combined with whole-wheat flour.

◉ Vegetables

Vegetables are the natural complement to whole grains and form the second most important category. Overall, they are more yin, contributing lightness, crispness, and variety to the diet, while grains are more yang, contributing solidity, stability, and vitality. However, many individual vegetables are very strengthening, creating strong blood and ki energy. Vegetables fall into three major categories:

- Green leafy vegetables such as collard greens, kale, and daikon leaves give gentle, upward energy, stimulating the liver, gallbladder, lungs, heart, and mental faculties. They are light, cooling, and calming. High in iron, calcium, and other minerals and vitamins, they create strong blood, strengthen the bones and teeth, and promote healing. In the form of juice, they are used to treat liver disorders and dissolve heavy, stagnated protein, animal fat, and cholesterol. Several large green leaves may be used whole or prepared into a chlorophyll plaster to reduce fever, soothe inflammation, or relieve burns. Daikon leaves are used in a hip bath to alleviate women's reproductive and skin troubles.

- Round vegetables such as fall- and winter-season squashes, cabbage, onions, and other stem and ground varieties give more evenly balanced energy. They are particularly good for the pancreas, spleen, stomach, and lymphatic system. Their mild, sweet taste calms and centers the mind. Onions are particularly soothing for the nerves, the muscles, and connective tissues. In addition to daily food, round vegetables may be used in special dishes, drinks, and occasional compresses (e.g., cabbage plaster) for healing.

- Root vegetables such as carrots, daikon, burdock, and lotus root give strong downward energy. They are especially good for the lungs and large intestine, urinary system, and, depending on the type of vegetable, the liver, heart, and other organs. Daikon has strong dissolving energy and helps to digest fat and oil as well as discharge animal products from the past. Root vegetables are used in an array of teas, plasters, and other medicinal applications.

◎ Beans and Bean Products

Beans are shaped like the kidneys and the ears, which are related in traditional Far Eastern medicine. Beans particularly nourish these organs, which govern overall vitality and balance, and contribute good-quality protein, fat, and carbohydrate to optimal maintenance of many body functions. They are also strengthening for the reproductive system, and the fiber in beans and bean products assists the intestines to function smoothly. Smaller beans such as adzuki beans, lentils, chickpeas, and black soybeans are recommended for daily or regular use. Soybeans are eaten whole but most commonly in the form of tofu, tempeh, natto, and other traditionally made soy products.

- Adzuki, the most condensed or yang of the beans, gives strong energy and is used in many home remedies, teas, and medicinal applications. Its deep red color adds a festive hue to rice and other special dishes.

- Lentils are an excellent source of protein, iron, calcium, complex carbohydrates, and dietary fiber and are strengthening to digestion, circulation, and the nervous system. They are soothing and calming.

- Chickpeas contribute to a rich, dynamic taste and strong energy and go well with many vegetables, corn, and rice. Like other high-fiber foods, they help lower cholesterol and fat in the body, and they are an excellent source of protein, minerals, and B vitamins, which are strengthening to the kidneys, bladder, and sex organs.

- Tofu, or soybean curd, has a soft texture, mild taste, and versatile shape that combines well with many foods. Rich in protein, iron, calcium, and other nutrients, it strengthens the blood and contributes to better circulation, respiration, and nervous system functioning. It is very digestible and high in phytoestrogens that help protect against breast cancer, prostate cancer, and other malignancies. As a plaster, tofu is used to bring down inflammation, swellings, and bruises.

- Tempeh, a fermented soybean product, has a rich, dynamic taste and gives strong energy. It helps reduce cholesterol, strengthen the urinary system, and prevent tumors. One of the highest sources of vegetable protein, it is also rich in iron, calcium, and other minerals and is a primary plant-quality source of vitamin B_{12}.

- Natto, a fermented soy product that resembles baked beans and has long, sticky strands, is beneficial to digestion, strengthening the intestines, kidneys, blood, and lymph. Its funky odor repels some people, while others appreciate its delicate taste, mucilaginous texture, and strong aroma.

◎ Sea Vegetables

Seaweeds, sea moss, and river moss have traditionally been eaten all over the world. They are soft and flexible, yet constantly move and bend to balance life in the water. In comparison, land plants are fixed in the soil, often have rigid stalks, stems, or leaves, and tend to be brittle. As a result of growing in an alkaline environment, sea vegetables are strengthening to the blood and are especially good in helping to maintain or restore suppleness and flexibility to the arteries and other blood vessels. Some contain *sodium alginate*, a compound that can bind and eliminate radioactive particles and other toxins from the body. Sea vegetables are natural detoxifiers and besides being used in daily cooking have a wide range of medicinal applications, including teas and compresses.

- Wakame, a slender, light plant that turns a beautiful, translucent green when cooked, is customarily added to miso soup. Like other sea vegetables, it is rich in protein, iron, calcium, iodine, vitamin A, B vitamins, and other nutrients. It helps protect against high blood pressure, prevent tumors, and safeguard against infection.

- Nori (also known as laver) is used to wrap sushi rolls and rice balls. It is wafer-thin, crispy, and loaded with protein, iron, calcium, and other nutrients. It strengthens the kidneys and urinary function, as well as the reproductive organs, and helps reduce cholesterol and improve circulation. It is added to the carrot-daikon drink for medicinal use and can be applied to minor cuts and nicks to stop bleeding.

- Hiziki, a brown, pine-needle-shaped plant that turns black when cooked, has a strong ocean flavor and nutty aroma. It has the highest concentration of iron and calcium of any food and gives strong energy. It is also an excellent source of vitamins A, C, and B_{12} and helps reduce cholesterol in the bloodstream and prevent heart disease.

- Arame has a sweet, delicate taste and mild texture, and turns dark brown when cooked. It combines well with other vegetables and soy products and makes a delightful addition to soups and salads. Abundant in iron and calcium, it strengthens the teeth and bones, improves circulation, and is used externally in a hip bath for female reproductive problems.

- Kombu, a large, thick, dark green member of the kelp family, is traditionally used to make *dashi*, the broth used as a stock for soup and noodle dishes. Kombu is also used in side dishes, to make several condiments, and as a tea. It strengthens the blood, discharges toxins from the body, and can be used externally as a compress.

◎ Seasonings

Sea salt, miso, and shoyu are the principal seasonings in the macrobiotic way of eating. Unrefined vegetable-quality oil is used in cooking, and among other seasonings and condiments, umeboshi plum is used frequently.

- Salt is essential to life and one of humanity's oldest staples. Unrefined sea salt (evaporated from the ocean) preserves many of the minerals and trace elements refined from ordinary table salt. The most yangizing food, salt aids digestion, strengthens the blood, and stimulates the brain and nervous system. It is traditionally cooked into food rather than added at the table. It gives both hardening and softening effects. It is one of the most powerful foods, but also one of the most difficult to use properly. Constant adjustments need to be made based on ever-changing seasonal, climatic, weather, and personal conditions and needs.

- Miso, a paste made from fermented soybeans, sea salt, and usually fermented barley or rice, gives strong energy and contains enzymes that facilitate digestion and strengthen blood quality. Consumed regularly in miso soup, used occasionally in seasoning other dishes, and added to sauces and dressings, it is one of the principal foods taken to restore the body to balance and maintain basic health. It helps to prevent heart disease, relieve breast cancer and other malignancies, and treat radiation sickness. It is used externally as a plaster for cuts and burns.

- Shoyu, or naturally fermented soy sauce, is used as a seasoning for soups, noodles, stir-fries, and other dishes. Made from a mixture of soybeans, wheat, sea salt, and water that has been fermented and aged in cedar vats, it aids in digesting grains and vegetables. Rich in protein, minerals, and B vitamins, it is used in home remedies to strengthen the blood, relieve fatigue, and neutralize over-acidity.

- Sesame oil is the standard cooking oil in the modern macrobiotic community. It comes from sesame seeds that have been pressed at low temperature to preserve their natural color, taste, and aroma. Dark sesame oil, with a rich, smoky flavor, gives slightly stronger effects than light sesame oil. Corn oil, the main secondary oil, is light, pleasant-tasting, and combines well with many dishes. However, organic corn oil has recently disappeared from the market following the introduction of genetically altered foods and chaos in the conventional supply of corn. Other unsaturated vegetable oils generally give lighter, more yin, dispersing effects. Olive oil, a heavier monounsaturated oil, is suitable for special dishes, especially if you live in the Mediterranean, southern California, or other hot region.

- Umeboshi plum, a salty, pickled plum, has a tangy flavor, a combined sour and salty taste, and is used as a seasoning, condiment, and medicine. Its paste, made from pitted plums, is used for sauces, dressings, and spreads. Shiso, the deep red or purple leaves umeboshi are pickled in, are used as a condiment or garnish for many dishes. Umeboshi gives a balanced, centering energy that neutralizes extreme foods and conditions. It aids digestion, strengthens the blood, and neutralizes acidity. It is used in ume-sho-ban and ume-sho-kuzu to provide energy and relieve fatigue.

◎ Water

Along with grain and salt, water is one of the three most important foods for daily consumption. A natural source of water is essential for daily cooking and drinking. Natural spring water that is alive and moving carries strong ki or natural electromagnetic energy. It facilitates digestion and absorption, balances salt and other minerals in the body, and contributes to the proper functioning of the kidneys and bladder. Well water comes from deeper in the ground and gives slightly stronger, more contractive effects. Many environmental factors will affect the quality of water and its relative hardness, softness, and proportion of trace elements.

◎ Cooking and Way of Eating

The way we prepare and eat food further modifies its energy. It is important to select fresh foods, eat seasonally, and eat in an orderly way. Eating stale foods or too many leftovers contributes to low energy and vitality, as the natural energy of the food declines. As a general rule, food should be prepared as freshly as possible, with whole grains, beans, and vegetables being prepared fresh at least once or twice a day. Grains, beans, and sea vegetables may be kept overnight and used the following morning or lunchtime as leftovers without appreciably af-

fecting daily health. Soups and vegetables should be prepared fresh every day. Other major influences include:

- Food creates life, and a good cook is an artist who uses the different shapes, sizes, tastes, flavors, and other qualities of food as his or her palette to create physical health and raise the consciousness of the family. Cooking can bring out the natural energy in a food or almost totally transform its effects. Learning how to plan menus, combine foods, use salt, oil, and other seasonings, and master fire and water is true alchemy, the supreme art. Varying the style, ingredients, and cooking according to seasonal changes is also important. Otherwise, the food can become monotonous and unappetizing. Color is one of the most dynamic energies. Condiments, garnishes, and arranging the foods artfully and serving them in beautiful dishes can also enhance the enjoyment of the meal and affect how we feel. Sometimes the slightest garnish or sprinkle of a condiment can completely transform the visual energy of the meal.

- Fire creates strong energy, vitalizing physical, mental, and spiritual functions. Fire for cooking created human culture and civilization. A gas flame gives steady, even heat and is used in most macrobiotic households. Wood gives superior taste and strong, peaceful energy but is impractical for most people in modern society. However, any natural fuel, including coal, charcoal, or a butane or propane camp stove, is satisfactory.

- Chewing food thoroughly, fifty times per mouthful and ideally one hundred times or more, has many positive effects. When we chew, *ptyalin*, an enzyme in saliva, alkalinizes the food, contributing to better digestion and absorption and strengthening the blood. Chewing allows more energy and nutrients in food to be utilized, therefore substantially cutting down on the amount of food consumed. Chewing also charges the food with ki, or natural electromagnetic energy, and leads to greater vitality and spiritual awareness.

- The physical health and mind or spirit of the cook have a strong impact on the energy of the food she or he prepares. Food cooked with love and a calm, peaceful mind creates harmonious energy. Food cooked by someone who is angry, upset, or in poor health creates negative energy. As a rule, it is better not to listen to music, watch television, or surf the Internet while preparing or eating food. Paying attention to the delicate sounds of the foods cooking on the stovetop is a cardinal principle of macrobiotic cooking, and these pastimes easily deflect awareness. Occasionally, peaceful, soothing music may be played, especially to accompany thorough chewing, but listening to the sounds of nature is ideal. Expressing appreciation to God or the universe for the foods that we are given also has an impact on the energy of the food. Grace, prayer, meditation, or a moment of silence before or after the meal develops our awareness of the natural world, contributes to family and community harmony, and energizes and spiritualizes the food.

◎ The Effects of Extreme Foods

The consumption of extreme foods can produce an array of physical, mental, and spiritual effects. The energetic effects of selected foods generally avoided or minimized in the standard macrobiotic way of eating are as follows:

MEAT

Meat gives very strong, short-term energy and has traditionally been eaten to perform sustained, hard physical labor and to protect from cold weather. The protein and minerals in meat create extreme yang energy that moves downward and inward in the body, while fat and cholesterol, the more yin factors, gather toward the periphery of the body or in the bloodstream. Overall the body becomes hard, heavy, stiff, and tight from eating meat. Beef, the staple meat in modern society, creates thick, leathery skin, a forceful expression, and aggressive mentality and behavior—very much like a bull. Excessive consumption of hamburgers, steak, and other beef products, especially in combination with sugar, alcohol, or other strong yin, can result in a loud, noisy expression; a domineering, thoughtless mentality; and rough, violent behavior. Pork also gives strong, aggressive energy, especially to the legs and lower body. It commonly results in pushiness, sloppiness, and other swinish qualities. Lamb creates more docile energy but also promotes a whining nature and conforming, sheeplike behavior. Overall, meat contains high amounts of saturated fat and cholesterol, and meat consumption is the main cause of high blood pressure, heart disease, stroke, many forms of cancer, hypoglycemia, and other chronic diseases.

CHICKEN AND EGGS

Chicken makes the body tight, hard, and inflexible, especially the muscles, bones, and nerves. The upper back tends to become round, the shoulder blades tighten and harden, and fat gathers in the throat and neck, causing possible thyroid problems. Stiffness in the extremities, especially swollen and painful joints, leads to arthritis as the fingers and toes begin to take on the clawlike qualities of poultry. Wobbly thin legs, excessive blinking, pointed nose, and tics, twitches, or other jerky motions frequently accompany long-term chicken eating. Mentally, eating chicken contributes to henpecking, obsession with details and trivia, and a small, fragmented view of life.

Eggs are one of the most condensed foods eaten by humans and give extreme, contractive energy. Excessive egg intake creates hardness in the ovaries, prostate, pancreas, liver, and other vital organs, leading to cysts, tumors, and possible cancer. Energetically, people who eat a lot of eggs have a vibrational shell around them that makes it hard to communicate with others. Just as a baby chick breaks out of its shell, egg eating can lead to spontaneous eruptions and outbursts. Eggs give strong analytic and reasoning abilities, charging the left brain. Scientists, mathematicians, and chess players are commonly known as "eggheads."

DAIRY

Dairy food, including milk, cream, butter, ice cream, yogurt, and cheese, creates large bones; thick, insensitive skin; and slow, dull reactions. Dairy creates strong mucus and contributes to sinus, lung, and digestive problems, as well as vaginal discharge and strong body odor. Dairy gives a kind, gentle character, but one that is overly sentimental, childish, and conformist or herdlike. Dairy protein and fat are a major cause of heart disease, cancer (especially breast, prostate, and lung cancer), diabetes, asthma, allergies, colic, and many other chronic diseases, as well as lowered sexual drive and frigidity.

Traditionally, babies whose mothers couldn't breastfeed were given the milk of a gentle animal, such as a sheep or donkey. Goat's or camel's milk was generally believed to lead to a very active, stubborn child.

FISH AND SEAFOOD

Eating fish and seafood creates sharp senses, mental acuity, and a smooth, flowing expression. But the mentality tends to be narrow and one-sided. People who eat a lot of fish are orderly, nonconfrontational, and develop a group or corporate identity, like fish who swim together in schools. Heavy, dense, fatty fish and seafood, including tuna, salmon, and swordfish, can produce aggressive behavior. Seafood and shellfish can lead to many distinctive energetic qualities. For example, eating too many fried clams can cause the jaws to lock or "clam up." Fish and seafood can also cause intestinal and shoulder cramps, scaly skin, and other complications.

BREAD AND BAKED GOODS

A small volume of high-quality whole-grain bread and baked goods can be part of a healthy, balanced diet. However, most people today tend to eat too many flour products, especially those made with white flour and sweetened with sugar. Though very contracted, bread expands when combined with liquid, baking powder, and sugar and leads to puffy skin, bloated cheeks, and pasty skin. When combined with sugar, baked flour causes flatulence. Bread is also mucus-forming and can produce stagnation in the intestines, shoulder aches and pains, and calluses on the feet. Lung, liver, gallbladder, and pancreatic problems are also common, as these organs become stagnated. The strong contractive energy of baking particularly affects the spine and bones, leading to inflexibility. Eating bread on a regular basis contributes to development of an analytic mentality that focuses on parts instead of wholes as well a harder, more rigid view of life.

FRUIT AND JUICE

Fruit is very cooling and relaxing, but in excess fruit can cause coldness in the body and poor circulation; nervous, erratic energy; and loss of sexual vitality. Juice is even more concentrated. Like monkeys and other primates that eat fruit as their main food, overintake of fruit and juice leads to chattering, mugging, and a mischievous nature. Irregular heartbeat, colds, excessive blinking, thinning hair in the front of the head, dandruff, high-pitched voice, weak lungs, rounded shoulders, stooped spine, and long, thin nose are characteristic signs of taking too much fruit and juice. Those who eat a lot of fruit tend to be taken advantage of by others.

SUGAR AND SWEETS

Sugar releases glucose into the blood and causes a burst of energy as blood sugar levels instantly rise. But this euphoria quickly wears off as blood sugar levels drop, leading to moodiness, sentimentality, scattered thinking, confusion, loss of direction, and depression. Overall strength and vitality decline. Signs of frequent sugar consumption include freckles, brown patches on the skin, white dots on the fingernails, dilated pupils, and overall expanded features. Sugar intake can lead to tooth decay, cataracts and other vision problems, irregular heartbeat, cysts, and tumors. In excess, the body converts sugar into fatty acid in the body, and sugar is a leading factor in the development of coronary heart disease, many cancers, diabetes, schizophrenia, and other degenerative disorders.

Brown sugar, molasses, corn fructose, and other highly refined varieties produce comparable effects. Honey can lead to loss of clarity and lazy, dreamlike behavior. Its chronic use can lead to development of mystical, esoteric beliefs revolving around a strong female figure.

SPICES AND STIMULANTS

In a hot, humid climate, spices serve to cool the body, stimulate the mind and nervous system, and contribute to overall harmony with the environment. In a temperate climate, spices and herbs with a stimulant, aromatic effect can produce excitability, hyperactivity, and overall cooling, weakening effects. People living in a four-season climate who indulge in spices tend to make wild gestures with their hands, speak rapidly, get emotionally upset, and easily come down with viral and bacterial infections, allergies, and other ailments. Spices can also cause cancer to spread and metastasize.

Coffee, decaf, black tea, and other stimulants have a strong yin, expansive effect, causing the energy in the body to rise, contributing to wakefulness and stimulating the brain and nervous system. However, they also cause the heart to beat more rapidly, lead to loss of contractive power in the intestines, raise cholesterol, and weaken the reproductive function. Mentally, caffeine stimulates thinking, conversation, and other intellectual and social activity, but most of this superficial discharge is quickly forgotten. Sugar and milk are frequently added to coffee or tea, or they are eaten with doughnuts and pastries. This may indicate hypoglycemia or developing blood sugar imbalances.

DRUGS

Marijuana, LSD, and other hallucinogenic drugs can heighten the senses, distort time and space, and lead to a life of fantasy and illusion. Such mind-expanding substances produce extreme yin effects, not only expanding the brain and central nervous system but leading to loss of strong, contractive energy in the intestines, reproductive system, and other deep, vital organs.

VITAMIN PILLS AND OTHER SUPPLEMENTS

Synthetic vitamins produce a wide range of effects depending on the source of the vitamins, the processing method, and type of capsule used. On the surface, vitamin and mineral supplements can boost vitality and produce a

glowing look, but deep within they can disturb natural digestive, circulatory, and nervous functions. Endocrine functions can easily be disrupted, as hormones are secreted in quantities that are too great or too little.

CHEMICALIZED WATER

Water containing chlorine, fluoride, and other chemicals can produce a wide range of imbalances, affecting circulation, digestion, and nervous function and reducing susceptibility to infection and other disease. Modern dietary guidelines recommend that everyone drink eight or more full glasses of water a day. However, this standard is based on a population eating meat, eggs, poultry, and other animal foods that heat up the body. In this case, large amounts of water serve to cool the body down. For people eating a more balanced way, a much smaller amount of fluid is required. Excessive water contributes to flabby skin, swollen muscles, and an overall bloated, puffy appearance. Fluid can also accumulate in the abdomen, around the ankles, and under the eyes. Frequent urination, wet hands, and a watery, deep voice are other signs of developing imbalance from excessive fluid intake.

REFINED SALT AND OIL

Refined table salt is 99.99 percent sodium chloride; the rest is added iodide and dextrose (a form of sugar). It lacks the trace minerals found in sea salt and creates overall tightness, hardness, and inflexibility in mind and body. Gray sea salt, available in many natural food stores, is high in trace minerals compared to white sea salt and can also produce extreme effects. Too much salt of any kind can cause the skin to dry, contract, and wrinkle. Darkness around and under the eyes, cold feet and poor circulation, prematurely gray hair, and tightness in the kidneys and back are also common symptoms. Excessive thirst, skinny appearance, enormous appetite, sleepiness, and lack of energy further show too much salt intake. Mentally, the personality grows rigid and inflexible. Impatience, short temper, stubbornness, and a tendency to become fanatical frequently follow. Salt should generally be cooked with food, unless it is used for pickling or salting. Adding raw salt to foods at the table, or not allowing it to cook in foods long enough, can also produce imbalances.

Refined oils (such as corn oil or peanut oil), hydrogenated oils (including margarine and hydrogenated soybean oil), and saturated oils (palm and coconut) give extreme effects. About 40 percent of the modern diet consists of fat and oil, and the majority is in the form of cooking oil, mayonnaise, dressings, sauces, and other light forms. Heart disease, many cancers, liver and gallbladder problems, AIDS and immune disorders, and many other diseases are associated with excessive fat and oil consumption. Canola oil, from the rapeseed plant, has recently been introduced. It is very popular in restaurants, schools, and households because it is light, polyunsaturated, and mild-tasting. However, it is traditionally used as an industrial solvent rather than as a cooking oil. No comprehensive studies have been done on canola oil, but preliminary reports associate it with vision problems and hence probable liver toxicity.

MICROWAVE AND ELECTRIC COOKING

About 90 percent of modern households have microwave ovens or electric stoves. Microwave ovens vibrate at over 2 million cycles per second, while electric stoves vibrate at 60 cycles per second. The intense vibration can affect the cellular integrity of the food as well as be absorbed by those who eat it. Medical studies show that microwaved food produces major changes in blood and immune function, including a decrease in hemoglobin, an increase in hemotocrit and leukocytes, higher cholesterol, and a decrease in lymphocytes. These blood and lymph factors are the first line of defense against many diseases and infections. Microwave cooking also produces changes in the food itself, including increased acidity, damaged protein molecules, enlarged fat cells, and decreased folic acid levels. It can also weaken breast milk. Strains of salmonella and other harmful bacteria have been found to survive in cold spots of food that do not fully cook. From an energetic view, these are predominantly extreme yin, dispersing effects, contributing to the damage, deterioration, and decomposition of body cells. Electric cooking is not as chaotic as microwave cooking, but it can also lead to erratic digestive, circulatory, and nervous functions and produce an overall weakening effect, including loss of mental focus and concentration. A recent medical study has also associated exposure to electric fields of 60 cycles per second (similar to electric cooking) with initiating cancerous changes in the cells of laboratory animals.

CHEMICALLY GROWN OR TREATED FOODS

Thousands of chemicals are used in growing, processing, and preserving foods. Overall, they have extreme yin, or dispersing, decomposing, and disintegrating effects. They contribute to weakening blood quality, greater susceptibility to infection, and slower healing. Itching, irritability, and nervous symptoms commonly result from ingesting pesticides, artificial fertilizers, or other chemicals. Irregular heartbeat, hormonal disturbances (especially from a new class of drugs and environmental toxins known as *estrogen disruptors*), allergic reactions, and other moderate to serious reactions may also develop. Scattered thinking, edgy nerves, wild or erratic behavior, and other bizarre mental and physical behavior are often the direct result of chemicals in the food. Learning disabilities, hyperactivity, and other childhood disorders have been linked with specific dyes, pesticides, and chemicals. At a social and cultural level, chaotic music, painting, film, and other arts represent a discharge of chemically grown, processed, or treated foods and beverages.

GENETICALLY MODIFIED FOODS

Overall, genetically modified (GM) food is weak and devitalized because it lacks the strong, health-giving charge that has evolved naturally over millions of years of evolution. Although there have been no long-term comprehensive studies, preliminary research indicates a wide range of effects, including increased allergies, lung problems, stress on the liver, damage to stomach, intestines, and blood, delayed sexu-

ality and reproductive development, increased infertility, and higher risk of birth defects and developmental disorders. Many GM foods have altered or reduced nutrition. For example, GM soybeans contain 12–14 percent less phytoestrogens than natural soybeans. Phytoestrogens protect against heart disease, cancer, and other chronic ills. GM foods may also lead to the emergence of new viral and bacterial diseases, lower resistance to infection (including herpes, AIDS, and other STDs), and introduce foreign proteins in the body whose effect on the reproductive cells may not be known for generations.

There are also energetic effects of consuming new GM foods that may be contributing to the widespread outbreak of violence in society, especially the use of guns by children and teenagers. First, most GM corn, soybeans, and cotton contain Bt, an altered bacterium that is spliced into every cell and serves as a built-in pesticide. This organism produces a toxin that is designed to kill the corn borer. According to recent scientific studies, however, it also kills the larvae of monarch butterflies and other beneficial insects. Researchers have linked ingestion or exposure to pesticides in children with increased irritability, aggression, and violence.

Second, many GM crops are created by shooting a pistol containing the desired gene into a petri dish to disperse the DNA into the cells of ordinary seeds. This method of shooting "microbullets" coated with DNA was developed at the University of California in Davis and originally involved shooting .22 or .45 caliber guns. The conventional seeds in the petri dish that are successfully penetrated with modified organisms are then planted and produce a new GM crop. From an energetic view, consuming foods originating from gun-fired DNA can have an explosive, violent effect on human cells and tissues, thinking, and consciousness. Today, up to 70 percent of all foods in the supermarket and natural foods stores contain gene-modified ingredients. The spread of untested, unlabeled altered foods in the American marketplace may be one of the underlying, unrecognized factors in the recent wave of violence in schools and communities.

From the point of view that you are what you eat, we absorb the energy and vibration of the foods we take in, as well as the nutrients and other material components. The macrobiotic way of eating emphasizes keeping a calm, peaceful mind in every step of the agricultural and food preparation process. High-quality food is not only pure, whole, natural, and free of chemicals, irradiation, and GM organisms—but also grown, processed, and prepared in a harmonious spirit.

Traditional farmers serenaded their crops; people used slow, natural methods of processing; and cooks put strong, healthful energy into their cooking with their thoughts and prayers. Today the opposite prevails. Modern food is produced, refined, and processed through high-energy methods that artificially speed up natural processes of fermentation, ripening, and curing. In the kitchen, microwave ovens, electric ranges, and other high-energy devices create a chaotic vibration that enters the food and directly affects cells and tissues, thoughts and emotions. Homes are often battlegrounds among family members, cooking is avoided as much as possible, and anger, abuse, and neglect often spill over into the kitchen and dining table. A return to a more natural way of eating that respects the life-giving quality and energy of food is essential to recovering and maintaining our health, refined consciousness, and high spirit.

TABLE 9. ACID-FORMING, MUCUS-FORMING, AND FAT-FORMING FOODS*

Acid-Forming Foods	Mucus-Forming Foods	Fat-Forming Foods
Sweets including sugar, honey, chocolate, and other refined sweeteners; products including sugar; artificial sweeteners	Sweets including sugar, honey, chocolate, and other refined sweeteners; products including sugar; artificial sweeteners	Sweets including sugar, honey, chocolate, and other refined sweeteners; products including sugar
Beef, pork, lamb, and other meats	Meat	Beef, pork, lamb, and other meats
Chicken, eggs, and other poultry	Chicken, eggs, and other poultry	Chicken, eggs, and other poultry
Tuna, salmon, swordfish, and other red-meat and blue-skin fish; crab, lobster, shrimp, and other shellfish	Heavy fish and shellfish	Tuna, salmon, swordfish, and other red-meat and blue-skin fish; crab, lobster, shrimp, and other shellfish
Milk, cream, butter, ice cream, cheese, sour cream, whipped cream, yogurt, and other dairy	Milk, cream, butter, ice cream, cheese, sour cream, whipped cream, yogurt, and other dairy	Milk, cream, butter, ice cream, cheese, sour cream, whipped cream, yogurt, and other dairy
Coconut, palm, and other saturated oils; margarine and other hydrogenated oils; lard, shortening, and other animal fats	Coconut, palm, and other saturated oils; margarine and other hydrogenated oils; lard, shortening, and other animal fats; fried foods	Coconut, palm, and other saturated oils; margarine and other hydrogenated oils; lard, shortening, and other animal fats
Mayonnaise, dressings, dips, and other oily preparations	Mayonnaise, dressings, and other oily preparations	Mayonnaise, dressings, and other oily preparations
Deep-fried, sautéed, and stir-fried foods; chips	Deep-fried, sautéed, and stir-fried foods; chips	Deep-fried, sautéed, and stir-fried foods; chips
Baked flour products, including yeasted bread, biscuits, muffins, doughnuts, pastries, pies, cakes, and cookies, especially those with white flour and yeast	Baked flour products, including yeasted bread, biscuits, muffins, doughnuts, pastries, pies, cakes, and cookies, especially those with white flour or yeast	Baked flour products, including yeasted bread, biscuits, muffins, doughnuts, pastries, pies, cakes, and cookies, especially those with white flour and yeast
	Oats, especially rolled oats, and some grains high in gluten such as wheat	Oats, hato mugi
		Soybeans, kidney, lima, and other larger beans

Acid-Forming Foods	Mucus-Forming Foods	Fat-Forming Foods
Soybean oil, soy milk, soy margarine, soy ice cream, and other highly processed soy products	Soybean oil, soy milk, soy margarine, soy ice cream, and other highly processed soy products	Soybean oil, soy milk, soy margarine, soy ice cream, and other highly processed soy products
Tomatoes, potatoes, eggplants, and other tropical vegetables	Potatoes and other tropical vegetables	Potatoes and other tropical starches
Mushrooms and other fungi	Some mushrooms and fungi	
Fruits and fruit juices, especially of tropical origin	Fruits and fruit juices, especially of tropical origin	Fruits and fruit juices, especially of tropical origin
Lemon, orange, and other citrus	Lemon, orange, and other citrus	Citrus fruits
Nuts and nut butters; seeds and seed butters	Nuts, nut butters, seed butters	Nuts and nut butters; seeds and seed butters
Vinegar, some spices and herbs	Vinegar, some spices and herbs	
Coffee, black tea, green tea, and other stimulants		Coffee beans
Soft drinks, spritzers, carbonated waters	Soft drinks, spritzers, carbonated waters	Soft drinks
Beer, wine, and other alcoholic beverages	Beer, wine, and other alcoholic beverages	Beer, wine, and other alcoholic beverages
Some drugs and medications	Some drugs and medications	
Raw foods	Some raw foods	Some raw foods
Electric or microwaved foods	Electric or microwaved foods	
Overeating in general	Overeating in general	Overeating in general
Insufficient chewing	Insufficient chewing	Insufficient chewing
Eating before sleeping	Eating before sleeping	Eating before sleeping

*Normal digestion is capable of processing a small volume of acidic, mucus-forming, and fatty foods. In excess, however, extreme foods can lead to excessive mucus production. Also excess glucose from the intake of simple carbohydrates (especially sugar, white flour, and potatoes), dairy sugar, fruit sugar, or alcohol and excess protein, especially from animal foods, is converted into fatty acid.

Diet and the Development of Disease

As a result of the diet and health revolution, people today are consuming less red meat, eggs, dairy food, and other foods higher in saturated fat and cholesterol. Mortality from heart disease, the number one cause of death in modern society, has dropped by nearly half over the last generation. For the first time, cancer incidence and mortality have also started to fall. Beyond these two major degenerative diseases, scientists are investigating the connection between diet and scores of other conditions and disorders ranging from arthritis to multiple sclerosis, from Alzheimer's disease to osteoporosis. A trickle of nutritional and dietary research has turned into a flood. Alternative and complementary medicine has blossomed in recent years, and the number of visits to holistic practitioners now exceeds that to physicians and other medical practitioners. In recognition of the importance of a more integrated approach, two-thirds of medical schools in the United States are now offering courses on alternative and complementary medicine, including nutrition. The *Journal of the American Medical Association* recently pub-lished an article recommending that all medical students be acquainted with holistic approaches, especially macrobiotics.

The macrobiotic approach to healing is based on the view that health and happiness result from living in harmony with nature, while sickness and unhappiness mirror a disharmony or imbalance between the internal and external worlds. The way back to health is to understand natural order and harmonize with it, beginning with our daily way of eating. The chronic intake of extreme foods and beverages underlies the progressive development of sickness and unhappiness. This process follows a general sequence of seven stages.

◉ Normal Discharge

Normally, the body eliminates excessive nutrients, toxins, and other wastes that come in through food, water, and air through four metabolic processes: (1) *respiration*, or breathing, which releases carbon dioxide and other gaseous wastes into the atmosphere (accounting for about 70 percent of energy exchange); (2) *perspiration*, or sweating, which transports sodium, urea, oils, fluids, and other wastes to the surface of the body (accounting for about 20 percent of excreted wastes); (3) *urination*, which consists primarily of urea, uric acid, and other nitrogenous wastes, sodium chloride, and about 100 other substances suspended in fluid (accounting for about 7 percent of discharge); (4) *bowel movement*, which consists primarily of cellulose and other undigested food remains, bile pigments, mucus, bacteria, and water (accounting for about 3 percent of waste). Normal discharge also takes place through daily physical activity, including motion, conversation, work, play, dance, song, and other ordinary activities. Mental discharge takes place in the form of waves and vibrations that are released in thought, decision making, wishes, prayers, imagination, and other forms of consciousness. Feelings and emotional expression are also accompanied by the release of metabolic energy.

Sexual activity offers another normal avenue of energy release for both sexes. Women are generally able to exchange energy with the environment more harmoniously than men because they have several additional means of natural discharge. These include (1) *menstruation*, the elimination of blood and parts of the lining of the uterus about once a month during the childbearing years; (2) *childbirth*, or having a baby, which is accompanied by the release of accumulated matter and energy; and (3) *lactation*, or breastfeeding, which releases an array of enzymes, hormones, and other factors in breast milk. As a result, women tend to have a more balanced condition than men, adjust more peacefully to their surroundings, and live longer. To redress this imbalance, men commonly go out into society more frequently than women and engage in more active physical, mental, and social pursuits. In this way, men and women make a balance with the natural environment and each other, creating day-to-day health and happiness. By observing a diet centered on whole grains and cooked vegetables, the traditional human way of eating, people naturally enjoy optimal physical health and vitality, mental clarity, and emotional balance. They will also intuitively begin to develop their spiritual potential and experience the realization of their eternal dream in life.

◎ Abnormal Discharge

If we overeat occasionally or take in only a small to moderate amount of extreme foods and beverages, they will normally be discharged through one of the mechanisms described above. For example, eating several apples may lead to diarrhea. However, if the amount of excess exceeds the capacity of the body to discharge it naturally, various abnormal methods of discharge arise. These include colds, fever, sinus congestion, coughing, sneezing, excessive sweating, frequent urination, and bowel irregularities. If we eat a banana split or take two or three desserts in a row, we may experience chills, a fever, and swollen tonsils as the body tries to release this excess. Scratching the head, tapping the feet, and rapid blinking of the eyes also represent the release of imbalanced energy, as do irritability, anxiety, timidity, complaining, and other mild feelings of unease and discomfort. From time to time, more extreme symptoms may arise, including shivering, trembling, vomiting, and nausea, as well as crying, shouting, screaming, anger, fear, and other wild, erratic actions and emotions.

Today nearly everyone in the modern world overeats or takes improper food from time to time and experiences physical and mental tiredness or *general fatigue*, the first stage of imbalance. This is the beginning of sickness and is frequently accompanied by some of the abnormal symptoms listed above, as well as by muscular tension and hardening, short periods of feeling cold or hot, or temporary constipation or diarrhea. Loss of alertness, lack of clarity, forgetfulness, and other mental changes may also begin to take place. To recover balance usually takes several hours to several days. A good night's sleep, proper rest, healthy food, and regular exercise will normally restore equilibrium.

◎ Aches and Pains

If we ignore these initial signs of imbalance and fail to change our diet or way of life, general fatigue will be followed by occasional *aches and pains*, the second stage of developing sickness. These include muscle pain and tension, headaches, backache, menstrual cramps, abdominal ills, numbness and tingling, and other moderate pains and aches. Sleeping problems, breathing difficulties, heart irregularities, chills and fever, and motion and coordination problems also may start to appear. Worry, general insecurity, and light to moderate feelings of sadness or depression may also arise. To restore balance, several days to several weeks are generally necessary, including a healthy diet, active exercise, and necessary rest.

◎ Decline of Blood Quality and Chronic Discharge

If we fail to heed these warning signs and do not make adjustments in our diet and lifestyle, the third stage in the progressive development of sickness will begin. *A change in blood and lymph quality*, including the red blood cells, white blood cells, platelets, and blood plasma, will lead to skin diseases, susceptibility to infection, and other manifestations of chronic imbalance.

As the blood begins to change quality and accumulates excessive nutrients, toxins, and wastes, the kidneys become overburdened and lose their ability to cleanse the bloodstream properly. Skin diseases commonly appear as the body directs excess to the surface of the body and discharges it in the form of freckles, pimples, spots, rashes, moles, warts, bunions, calluses, and other symptoms. These result from various combinations of sugar, chocolate, honey, and other refined carbohydrates; protein and fat from meat, chicken, eggs, and other animal foods; milk, cheese, ice cream, and other dairy foods; white bread and other flour products; tomatoes, potatoes, and other foods of tropical origin; spices; stimulants; alcohol; drugs; and other imbalanced foods and beverages. Continued intake of these substances may eventually lead to eczema, psoriasis, and other more serious skin disorders. In extreme cases, skin cancer may develop. Skin cancer is usually not life-threatening, because it shows that the body is still able to keep itself relatively clean by discharging excess to the surface.

Over time, a layer of fat and oil builds up beneath the skin, blocking the pores, hair follicles, and sweat glands. The skin grows dry as oil and fluid can no longer flow to the surface. Many people today think that dry skin results from not taking enough oil, so they increase their consumption of oily and fatty foods or apply oily conditioners to their skin, which only makes the condition worse. Hair, nail, and lip problems may also arise in a similar way.

As the blood and lymph quality decline, the body loses its natural resistance to infection. Bacteria, viruses, and other microorganisms that ordinarily pose no risk begin to thrive and multiply. The blood and lymph become coated with fat and mucus from acid-producing foods and are no longer able to discharge potentially infectious agents from the body through the urine, bowel movement, and other ordinary channels. Also, the beneficial microbes that normally live in harmony in the intestinal flora, on the skin, and in other regions of the body and help to protect from disease may start to decline as excessive animal protein, acids, and strong chemicals disrupt their normal functioning. Chronic colds and flu; staph, strep, and *E. coli* infections; Lyme disease; parasitic worms; and herpes, AIDS, and other sexually transmitted diseases can easily develop. As natural immune function declines, the risk of getting hepatitis, pneumonia, tuberculosis, malaria, cholera, dysentery, or other infectious disorders rises sharply, especially new multiple drug-resistant strains. Variant Creutzfeldt-Jakob disease, the human form of mad cow disease, may be contracted by eating infected beef or dairy, taking pharmaceuticals or drugs made from cow products, or coming into contact with potting soil that includes bone meal. Chronic fatigue syndrome, fibromyalgia, lupus, mononucleosis, dry throat disease, shingles, and other autoimmune disorders are also apt to develop at this stage.

Susceptibility to nosebleed and other bleeding, scratches, bruises, insect bites, falls, and accidents also rises as blood quality declines, and cuts and wounds take longer to heal. The small intestine, where blood production begins, is especially weakened by exposure to the artificial electromagnetic radiation emitted by high-voltage lines, computers, televisions, cell phones, and other modern electronic equipment and devices. Nuclear energy and fallout, industrial chemicals, pesticides, plastics, and other toxins in the environment all produce overall dispersing, decomposing, and weakening effects on the mind and body, beginning with the blood.

Acidosis, anemia, high blood pressure, low blood pressure, and other circulatory, lymphatic, and respiratory disorders may arise at this stage. Leukemia, lymphoma, and other nonsolid malignancies may also appear in extreme cases. However, relative to other types of cancer, these are usually easier to heal because the blood and lymphatic system respond more quickly to dietary change than other organs, systems, and functions.

Mentally, chronic discharge may take the form of nervousness, oversensitivity, moderate depression, hyperactivity, or loss of general direction in life. The boundary between the inner and outer environment becomes more pronounced, and thinking and behavior begin to become more withdrawn or offensive. Short temper, angry outbursts, frustration, and melancholy or chronic depression may arise. A general feeling of apprehension prevails, and coping with the challenges of daily life becomes a burden. New people and situations are feared, and flexibility of mind and body is gradually lost as rigidity sets in.

To recover from this stage, the blood, lymph, and other bodily fluids need to be strengthened. Depending on the condition, this can take from ten days (to change the blood plasma) to four months (to fully change the red blood cells). In addition to dietary change and lifestyle adjustments, simple home remedies, including special foods, drinks, and compresses, may be necessary to stimulate active energy circulation.

◎ Accumulation

If the underlying cause of chronic symptoms is not corrected through dietary change, or if it is treated only in a symptomatic way, the body will begin to gather and accumulate excess at a deeper level. *Accumulation* is the fourth stage in the progressive development of disease. Eventually the body's ability to discharge to the surface, through normal, abnormal, and chronic channels, will be exhausted. Continued consumption of meat, eggs, chicken, cheese, fatty fish, and other seafood; milk, ice cream, and other dairy products; and oily, greasy foods of all kinds, including sugar and sweets that are converted into fat in the body, will result in the creation of internal deposits of fat and mucus. Initially, these will begin to form in the more peripheral regions of the body and ones that have access to the outside. The sections below discuss the major regions of accumulation.

SINUSES

Sinus congestion is the most common ailment in modern society, affecting from time to time the vast majority of adults and children. The buildup of mucus and fat in the sinuses can block the nasal and air passages, leading to sneezing, respiratory problems, hay fever, allergies, and other problems. Thick, heavy mucus deposits in the sinuses can reduce alertness and clarity, weaken vitality, and increase susceptibility to infection, disease, and accidents.

TONSILS

The tonsils are a frequent site of inflammation as excess gathers in the throat. These tiny organs are part of the lymphatic system and help to neutralize the effects of consuming too much sugar, milk, ice cream, soft drinks, and other extreme foods. However, if these foods continue to be taken in large volume, the tonsils become overworked, leading to swelling, infection, and fever. Instead of recommending dietary change, modern medicine often takes out the tonsils surgically, weakening the lymphatic system and causing excess to gather and accumulate at deeper levels.

EARS

The buildup of fat and mucus inside the ears can cause earaches, diminish hearing, and produce tinnitus (ringing). As the delicate structures of the inner ear become clogged, more serious disorders can arise, including auditory nerve damage and possible deafness. Dairy food is the most frequent cause of ear and hearing problems, but excessive intake of other animal food, sugar, white flour, and other foods that form acid, fat, or mucus can also lead to accumulation.

EYES

The eyes are also the site of gathering excess. Dietary extremes are responsible for astigmatism, nearsightedness, farsightedness, color blindness, conjunctivitis, crossed eyes, and other common vision problems that may require corrective lenses or medical treatment. Over time, more serious disorders may arise as fat and mucus build up in and around the eyeball, leading to cataracts, glaucoma, macular degeneration, or retinitis pigmentosa and eventually blindness or vision loss.

TEETH AND GUMS

The relation between sugar and cavities is well known. Less well known is the relationship between the consumption of many other foods and the development of tooth decay, irregular teeth, the onset of toothache and pain, the formation of abscesses, and other dental problems. Gingivitis, periodontal disease, and other gum problems are also the direct result of long-term dietary excess.

LUNGS

Excess frequently gathers in the lungs. Mucus and fat may coat the alveoli (air sacs), making breathing more difficult, producing chest congestion and pain, and leading to possible asthma, emphysema, bronchitis, or pneumonia. Coughing will sometimes loosen and discharge this sticky material, but once it becomes firmly attached it can harden and remain trapped for years. Then toxins and pollutants in the air that are inhaled can easily adhere to this sticky environment instead of being normally exhaled. Tar and other heavy components of tobacco smoke can become lodged, producing irritation and eventually leading to cysts and tumors. As a main avenue of normal discharge, the lungs also gather excess and toxins from all other regions of the body, including acid wastes from cells and tissues that enter the venous blood circulation and are discharged through breathing.

BREASTS

The buildup of excess fat and mucus deposits in the breasts may produce lumps, hardening, or cysts. The process is similar to the solidification of water into ice, as sticky, heavy liquid from frequent consumption of milk, cream, cottage cheese, yogurt, ice cream, and other dairy foods, as well as soft drinks, juice, mineral water, iced tea, chilled wine, and other foods and beverages that have a cooling effect, freezes and hardens. Breastfeeding reduces the risk of developing cysts or tumors in this region.

INTESTINES

The accumulation of excess in the lower regions of the body is generally produced by heavy animal protein or fat; salted cheese and other denser dairy foods; hard baked flour products, especially those containing white flour, sugar, and oil; and other oily, greasy foods. As the intestinal walls become coated with fat and mucus, they expand, lose their flexibility, and result in an enlarged or swollen abdomen. This is a major cause of overweight or obesity and can lead to colitis, diverticular disease, irritable bowel syndrome, and other digestive disorders.

KIDNEYS AND BLADDER

Accumulations of fat and mucus in the kidneys and bladder produce a variety of urinary, circulatory, and excretory problems. Excessive protein, fat, mucus, and other substances can clog the delicate network of cells in the kidneys that filter the blood, affecting blood quality as well as elevating blood pressure. As water accumulates, the kidneys may become chronically swollen, hampering elimination and causing excess fluid to build up in the legs. Cold and frozen foods may also crystallize into kidney or bladder stones. Stagnation in the urinary tract easily leads to infection, inflammation, and other complications. Insomnia, oversleeping, and nightmares and other disturbing dreams are also related to kidney imbalances.

REPRODUCTIVE ORGANS

The ovaries, the principal organ of female reproduction, are the frequent site of fat and mucus accumulation. Eggs, heavy animal foods, hard baked foods, and excessive salt can all contribute to this buildup, especially in combination with sugar and concentrated sweeteners, dairy food, cold beverages, and other extreme items, leading to ovarian cysts and fibroid tumors. If the Fallopian tubes become blocked, the egg and sperm cannot unite, resulting in a failure to conceive. PMS, menstrual problems, endometriosis, dermoid tumors, vaginal discharges, candida and

other yeast infections, and cervical problems may also develop, though the combinations of foods producing each disorder will differ slightly. In middle-aged women, hot flashes, vaginal dryness, and other menopausal symptoms are also the direct result of dietary excess. In men, prostate enlargement is the most common consequence of excess fat and mucus accumulation in this region. Hard fat deposits and cysts may form in and around this small organ, leading to urinary problems, reproductive problems, and sexual problems. The testicles may also be affected by hard, condensed, or concentrated foods, including nuts and acorns. Excess in the reproductive organs is the main cause of infertility, sexually transmitted diseases, and sexual dysfunction, with many accompanying mental and psychological anxieties and ills.

◎ Storage

As sickness progresses, excess becomes directed deeper into the body and begins to gather around the heart, liver, gallbladder, pancreas, and other vital organs. *Storage* is the fifth stage of sickness. As blood quality declines over a lengthy period, structural and functional changes begin to take place, producing degenerative changes in organs and glands, cells and tissues. Most major diseases, including cardiovascular disease, cancer, diabetes, and multiple sclerosis, fall into this category.

HEART

The accumulation of excess in and around the arteries is known as *atherosclerotic plaque*. It arises primarily from eating foods high in saturated fat and dietary cholesterol, including meats, eggs, chicken, dairy foods, and other animal products, as well as palm oil, coconut oil, and other saturated oils. However, excessive sugar, bread and baked goods, coffee, and many other foods can also elevate serum cholesterol and contribute to this process. Atherosclerosis is the underlying cause of coronary heart disease, including heart attack and angina, stroke, arteriosclerosis, and peripheral artery disease. Other combinations of food can produce cardiovascular problems, ranging from circulatory problems and blood pressure complications to irregular heartbeat, valve disorders, varicose veins, phlebitis, heart failure, and cardiomyopathy (the progressive swelling of the heart muscle that is the leading reason for heart transplants).

LIVER AND GALLBLADDER

The liver is one of the body's most essential organs, governing many digestive, circulatory, and excretory functions. Accumulation of fat, mucus, protein, and other excessive nutrients and wastes can cause the liver to become hard and tight or loose and sluggish and lead to inflammation, jaundice, or cirrhosis. The end result is problems in filtering the blood of toxins, converting carbohydrates, fat, and protein into one another, and impaired manufacturing of hormones and enzymes. The gallbladder stores bile produced in the liver and is the frequent site of cysts and stones. Troubles in the liver and gallbladder are frequently accompanied by eye and vision problems. Anger, irritability, and other explosive emotions are also related to these organs. The intake of combinations of dietary extremes, including meat and alcohol, dairy and sugar, and fried or baked foods high in oil and salt, can lead to violent outbursts, hyperactivity, and other erratic behavior.

PANCREAS

The pancreas is a small feather-shaped organ in the center of the body. It governs sugar metabolism and secretes enzymes that aid in the digestion of protein, fats, and carbohydrates. From an energetic perspective, its importance cannot be overemphasized. A healthy pancreas will contribute to overall well-being and happiness, while an unhealthy pancreas will lead to depression, mood swings, and overall unhappiness. The accumulation of protein and fat will lead to hardening of the pancreas and chronic low blood sugar, as the organ loses its ability to secrete anti-insulin. Cravings for sweets, alcohol, dairy, and fruits follow, particularly in the afternoon when the atmosphere begins to contract and further tightens the pancreas. This can lead to emotional ups and downs and erratic behavior. About 80 percent of all children and adults in America and other affluent countries have hypoglycemia, making it the most pervasive and unrecognized disorder in modern society. Diabetes, or chronic high blood sugar, results when the pancreas loses its ability to secrete insulin and is a major cause of death in this country. Hypoglycemia is primarily caused by taking too much meat, eggs, chicken, cheese, fatty fish, shellfish, and other heavy animal foods, while diabetes is produced by consuming too much sugar, milk and other light dairy, fruits, juices, and other expansive items.

ENDOCRINE GLANDS

The endocrine system consists of specialized glands located mostly along the vertical channel. They release *hormones*, or highly charged fluids, that influence the functioning of the organs and aid in the digestion of food. The accumulation of fat and mucus in these small, vital glands can cause either too little or too much hormone to be secreted. Pituitary malfunctions can lead to dwarfism, giantism, and other growth problems. Addison's disease, Cushing's syndrome, and virilization (overmasculization in either men or women) can be produced by adrenal blockages. Nutritional imbalances can cause simple goiter, Graves' disease, and other thyroid disorders. Hormone imbalances in the pancreas, as we have seen, are related to the over- or undersecretion of insulin and anti-insulin. As blood sugar levels fluctuate, moods and emotions may swing from one extreme to the other. In the reproductive organs, estrogen or testosterone imbalances can cause secondary sexual characteristics to appear and lead to personality changes.

CANCER

When the body loses the ability to create normal cells, tumors may arise, spread, and create a life-threatening condition. This is directly connected with blood production. When the villi of the small intestine become coated with fat and mucus, they lose the ability to assist in the creation of healthy blood. Overworked lungs, kidneys, liver, and spleen will also weaken the blood and lead to the development of tumors. To protect the rest of the body from collapse, excess is localized in an isolated area that can be likened to a storage or toxic waste depot. When a particular storage site is full, another is created. In this way, tumors arise and metastasize throughout the body. Cancer is actually a wonderful self-defense mechanism by which the body protects itself from the effects of longtime dietary imbalance. If the excess were not isolated and contained, it would flood the bloodstream and cause death by blood poisoning (toxemia). Thus cancer is a healthy response to an unhealthy diet and lifestyle. It postpones total collapse by several months or years. Cancer allows the person time to awaken to the underlying cause of his or her disease and, in most cases, to relieve it with proper diet and other natural means.

In modern society, chronic and degenerative diseases are treated primarily with drugs, medications, and other remedies designed to eliminate pain, control symptoms, and prolong life. Surgery, chemotherapy, radiation treatment, hormone injections, transplants, and other invasive procedures are routinely performed. At the preventive level, vaccines, inoculations, vitamin pills, mineral supplements, and other artificial substances are consumed, ingested, or injected to prevent future ills. However, none of these approaches deals with the underlying origin or cause of the imbalance or disorder, which lies in the daily way of life, including the daily way of eating. As a result, excess is not allowed to come out and is driven deeper into the body, where it may manifest in more serious form.

Reliance on drugs and pills is a contributing factor in the spread of substance abuse. Attraction to alcohol, drugs, and tobacco arises largely from dietary imbalance. For example, people who consume too much meat, poultry, eggs, and other high-energy animal foods are usually attracted to beer, wine, or whiskey to relax and unwind. Similarly, young people eating hamburgers, ice cream, pizza, french fries, and other fast foods are often attracted to marijuana, cocaine, and other illicit drugs. A sedentary lifestyle or hypoglycemic condition predisposes many others to seek release in tobacco or stimulants. Cigarettes commonly contain a high volume of added sugar, and many people add sugar to coffee, decaf, black tea, herbal tea, or other beverages. Weight problems, including overweight, obesity, and underweight, frequently accompany substance abuse or the overuse of stimulants. Bulimia, anorexia nervosa, and other eating disorders also arise from chronic consumption of extreme foods.

In addition to physical degeneration and addictive behavior, the storage stage may be accompanied by mental and emotional imbalances, including feelings of chronic stress and pressure, inability to cope, stubbornness, complaining, skepticism, apathy, depression, isolation, prejudice, narrow-mindedness, and loss of will and self-confidence. Delusional thinking, fanatical behavior, or dysfunction at home or work frequently results. Recovery from chronic and degenerative diseases and disorders, including heart disease and cancer, takes longer than blood and skin disorders. Generally four to six months to one year or more is needed, including careful adherence to a healing diet, reorientation of the way of life, and deep self-reflection.

◎ Nervous Disorders

From the accumulation and storage of excess in the organs and glands, the degenerative tendency progresses deeper into the muscles, bones, and nerves. Arthritis, rheumatism, scoliosis, osteoporosis, and other degenerative bone and joint conditions gradually develop after years of dietary excess. Over time, physical and mental coordination gradually declines and a pessimistic, negative view of life prevails. Muscle tissue begins to atrophy and be lost, the bones weaken and grow susceptible to fracture, and nervous impulses are impeded, giving rise to disability, paralysis, and incapacitation of the brain and mental functioning. Multiple sclerosis, muscular dystrophy, Parkinson's disease, Huntington's disease, Alzheimer's disease, amyotrophic lateral sclerosis, and other complex disorders arise. Mental and emotional disorders grow more imbalanced, frequently leading to schizophrenia, paranoia, and other personality disorders. Destruction or self-destructive tendencies frequently develop.

To overcome nervous disorders takes six months to several years, depending on the case. In addition to completely changing the way of life, including the way of eating, a positive view of life needs to be developed. The active support and loving care of friends and families are essential to recovery. Physical activity, relaxation exercises, and spiritual practices may also be helpful.

◎ Self-Justification

The last stage of sickness is self-justification or arrogance, the view that we are separate from nature and the workings of our own body. Through years of improper eating and living, we become detached from the natural world and see ourselves as blameless for our sickness, difficulties, and problems. Instead of taking responsibility and changing ourselves, we blame other people, society, nature, the universe, or God. Selfishness, egocentricity, vanity, pride, exclusivity, and self-righteousness are the hallmarks of this stage. We lose the ability to listen to others and our own intuition. Arrogance is both the last stage of sickness and the origin of all previous stages. It is the underlying cause of all sickness and unhappiness on our planet: ignorance of our universal origin and destiny. Egocentricity can arise from the modern view that we live in a chaotic, random universe without any purpose or meaning—and therefore anything goes. It can also develop from a belief that the rules of life, including the laws of health and sickness, balance and change, don't apply to us and we can get away with anything.

To recover from self-righteousness can take several years to many lifetimes, as appreciation is gradually recovered and a spirit of sympathy and compassion is cultivated. At the same time, arrogance may be dissolved instantaneously through disease, accident, failure, or other shock that awakens one to the order of nature. Great difficulties, suffering, and sorrow can produce a spirit of humility and modesty, leading to a renewed outlook on life and the recovery of health and happiness. Many great saints and prophets awakened to their true nature after lives of arrogance, indulgence, and ease. Paul's journey to Damascus when he was suddenly struck by the Holy Spirit is a good example. Dr. Anthony Sattilaro's recovery from incurable cancer with the help of macrobiotics after picking up two hitchhikers on the road to Philadelphia is another.

Though some of the previous stages are not always visible, all sicknesses, including the hundreds of conditions and disorders described in this book, follow the general pattern outlined in this chapter. Small, insignificant symptoms progressively develop into large, complex disorders. Abnormal discharges to the outside are followed by chronic discharges to the inside. Gathering, accumulation, and storage follow a predictable cycle, affecting ever more vital organs, systems, and functions. All diseases are interrelated and share a common origin: an unnatural way of life, including improper diet, thinking, and behavior.

Health, happiness, and peace are the universal birthright of every person. Harmonizing with the marvelous, eternal order of the universe—or what we may call God—is the essence of *makrobios*, the infinite life.

A Natural Approach to Healing

The roots of macrobiotics stretch back in time. In ancient Greece, Hippocrates coined the term *makrobios* to refer to longevity and health. To understand why he was known as the Father of Medicine, we have to go back and look at the worldview that prevailed in that era. People commonly believed that health and sickness, life and death, fortune and misfortune, were governed by the gods. The gods and goddesses, including Zeus, Hera, Aphrodite, Hermes, Apollo, and many others, were believed to live on Mount Olympus in northern Greece. The common view was that if you went to temple, prayed, and sacrificed, the gods would bestow upon you long life *(makrobios)*, health, wealth, prosperity, many children, and all the blessings of life. Conversely, if you didn't go to church, light incense, burn candles, or carry out the rituals of that time, the gods would send you short life *(mikrobios)*, sickness, accident, plague, sterility, misfortune, and disaster. Throughout the ancient world, people believed that what little influence, if any, we had on health and sickness, life and destiny, was through religious faith and practice.

The early Greek philosophers, embodied by Hippocrates, came along and introduced a revolutionary new view of life, namely, that our health and well-being, our life and destiny, depend upon our relation with nature. Hippocrates defined health as coming into harmony and balance with the natural world. Conversely, sickness or disease was a disharmony or imbalance. The way back to health was to understand and harmonize with nature. This approach inaugurated a revolution in human culture and civilization. It marked the transition from a supernatural view of life to a natural view. It came to be known as the modern view of life. "Modern" means that we live in a world of natural laws that pertain to everyone regardless of their theological belief. This is a very democratic view that we associate with Greece.

Hippocrates and the early Greek physicians taught their followers, patients, and students to observe nature, beginning with the heavens above. They taught them to look at the motions of the sun, the moon, the stars, and the planets, which exert a vibrational influence on the earth.

They also taught them to study the terrestrial cycles and rhythms: the way the waters flow, the way the winds blow, the way the birds and animals migrate, the way the seasons unfold. If we harmonize with all of these natural cadences around us, we will enjoy usual good health. If we violate nature's laws, a disequilibrium will develop between the inner and outer worlds. This produces symptoms that, if not corrected, will become progressively worse and lead to sickness and disease.

According to the ancient Greeks, the most central way to harmonize with nature is through diet, the daily way of eating. If we had to sum up Hippocrates' entire way of healing, it would be with his own famous proverb: "Let food be thy medicine, and thy medicine be food." The principal food in that era, throughout the Mediterranean world, was whole cereal grains, especially barley and wheat. For thousands of years, people ate these foods in whole form, such as whole barley and whole wheat berries; in cracked grains, such as bulgur and couscous; and in bread and baked goods. Jesus, for example, distributed whole-grain barley bread to his disciples. The same pattern prevailed in Greece and throughout the Hellenistic world. In one of his essays on medicine, Hippocrates observed, "How can any physician possibly hope to heal the diseases of mankind who does not know the different grains, how they are planted, harvested, cooked and combined with other foods, and the effects they have on all who eat them?" This is the foundation of the healing art, and in order to prescribe and diagnose, the physician must know the energy of food.

Hippocrates' healing diet consisted of giving the patient whole-grain barley, somewhat softly prepared, every meal, every day, for a period of about ten days. Soup or broth could also be given, as well as a variety of fresh vegetables. But the chief idea was to give grains in whole form consistently until the person got well. This became the main home remedy in the early Western medical tradition and appeared in medical textbooks for many centuries. Hippocrates made many contributions to the art of healing. He was the first physician to observe cancer and gave it the name *karkinos*, which meant "crab." He evidently took it as an image or metaphor for this affliction because tumors resembled a crab in shape, size, or coloration or because cancer spreads slowly and erratically, something like the way a crab shuffles across the beach. As the word *karkinos* moved into English, it lost its second hard *k* and became *karcinos*, from which our words *cancer, carcinoma, and carcinogen* derive. To heal cancer, Hippocrates warned against surgical intervention. He said taking the tumor out does not address the underlying origin or cause of the imbalance; furthermore, it weakens the patient and makes healing more difficult. Rather than intervening into the body's own healing processes, he recommended a natural approach. In addition to dietary change, which was his foundation, he advised environmental adjustments, improving human relations, and simple spiritual practices. Through these methods, he taught, the sick person could completely recover his or her health and lead a normal, happy life again.

This naturalistic approach is enshrined in the Hippocratic oath. The oath enjoins physicians from giving deadly drugs to their patients, assisting with suicide, giving an abortion, performing surgery, or engaging in any unethical conduct. Its central tenet states: "I will apply dietetic measures for the benefit of the sick according to my ability and judgment; I will keep them from harm and injustice." Of course, this is no longer the oath that medical students today take after graduating from medical school. The modern version has been revised and rewritten. The word *dietetic* is usually taken out of all present translations because modern medicine is no longer oriented in this direction and, in good conscience, could not have an oath for which its graduates were not trained. Until recently only 7 percent of all medical schools, for example, had a required course on nutrition. Hippocrates' approach, and early Western medicine, was completely macrobiotic in its orientation. The methods that he proscribed in the oath are now governing modern medicine. This is a good example of how, in the long course of history, a principle, teaching, or institution turns into its opposite.

Hippocrates lived to be over a hundred and became the symbol of health and longevity. From the Aegean Islands, the concept of macrobiotics spread throughout the classical world. Since Greek was the common language of the Middle East, it quickly spread to Israel, Egypt, and other countries. Both the early Jewish and Christian Bible commentators used the term *makrobios* in their translations and commentaries because there are so many stories of healthy, long-lived people in the Bible. Most of the prophets, sages, and saints in the Hebrew scriptures ate very simply, mostly grain and vegetable-quality food.

The Book of Daniel, for example, opens with young Daniel arriving at the palace of the king of Babylon. Israel has been defeated, the Temple has been destroyed, and the Jews have been taken back to Babylon to live in captivity. Daniel and several young companions are selected by the Jewish elders to become administrators like Joseph, who served Pharaoh during an earlier period of oppression. Daniel and his companions are welcomed by the vizier and given a tour of the magnificent palace, whose hanging gardens were one of the seven wonders of the ancient world. On behalf of the Jewish group, Daniel says that they are happy to be here and look forward to serving their people, but they have one small request, namely, could they have permission to eat in their accustomed fashion? The vizier asks what they eat, and Daniel replies that they eat simply, mostly pulses, or small grains, beans, and seeds. The master of the palace becomes irate and explains that such coarse fare is for animals or peasants and that it is a great honor to share the rich food from the king's table. He summarily rejects their request.

Refusing to take no for an answer, Daniel cleverly proposes that they make a wager. He asks that the Jewish young men be allowed to eat and cook their traditional food for ten days and then be compared to the young men eating the palace cuisine, consisting of rich animal foods, sweets, spices, and other exotic fare from across the realm. The aging official, a gambler, is convinced that there is no way that Daniel's group will surpass the strong, well-fed Babylonians, and he agrees to the bet. But when the time comes to evaluate the two groups, he is amazed to discover that Daniel and his associates are healthier, more energetic, and have a more radiant disposition. Fortunately, he is an honest man and gives permission for them to cook their whole grains, beans, vegetables, and seeds. "God was well pleased with Daniel and his companions," the Bible explains, picking up the narrative, "and bestowed upon them the gift of prophecy and the ability to interpret dreams." Daniel went on to become the greatest prophet of his generation. As the principal advisor to the emperor, he beheld the famous "handwriting on the wall," foretelling the destruction of Babylon and the deliverance of his people.

Often called the world's first nutritional study and scientific case control experiment, the story of Daniel illustrates the deep, central importance of a balanced way of eating in the early Judeo-Christian tradition. Jesus continued this legacy, eating a predominantly whole-grain and vegetable diet, supplemented with occasional fish from the Sea of Galilee, and used the energies of heaven and earth to heal many people. His preferred method was palm healing, channeling ki energy directly to the sick, lame, and dying. Afterward, he would put them on a whole-grain diet, as a careful reading of the more than forty healing episodes in the New Testament reveals. In the Gospel of Thomas, the oldest and most authentic account of his teachings, Jesus tells his disciples, "If they ask you what is the sign of the Father [God, the infinite universe] in you, tell them that it is a movement [yang] and a rest [yin]." Jesus was a great prophet of humanity and supreme macrobiotic healer. His parables of eternal truth are as astonishing today as they were nearly two thousand years ago.

In the Far East, the macrobiotic healing tradition goes back to *The Yellow Emperor's Classic*, the world's oldest medical book. Set during the reign of the first Chinese dynasty, about five thousand years ago, the book takes the form of a dialogue between the Yellow Emperor and his chief advisor, a man by the name of Ch'i Po. The Yellow Emperor is portrayed as a dynamic young ruler who has just come to power in China, and Ch'i Po is not a general or military strategist, as we might expect. Nor is he a merchant, wealthy landowner, or some other powerful figure. He is a physician and a healer, and we can remember him as the Hippocrates of the East. But his responsibility is not to serve merely as the personal physician of the ruler, taking his pulses and blood pressure. Rather, he is the right hand of state, charged with advising the emperor on how to run the empire.

The problem appears to be this. The Yellow Emperor's inclination is to rule the empire by force. Through his edicts, commands, the apparatus of state, and the army, he intends to govern with a strong hand. This is a potentially very dangerous way of leading. Ch'i Po, who is older and wiser, must get him to see that a judicious mixture of energies is needed to rule. Peaceful, gentle methods, negotiations, give and take, surrender, setting an example for others, and, as a last resort, the strong exercise of authority are all needed to rule a state, just as they are needed to be the head of a family. But for a headstrong young monarch with little life experience, this is a very difficult lesson.

Ch'i Po goes about this in a fascinating way. He explains to the Yellow Emperor that the same principles that govern health and sickness in an individual govern war and peace in society. The Yellow Emperor learns that if he is to become a great ruler of China and bring peace to the world, he must first be able to govern himself. If he cannot maintain his own health at all levels, including physical and psychological health, keeping a calm, clear mind, and exercising sound judgment, inevitably the kingdom will decline into chaos and disorder. Ch'i Po teaches the ruler that the heart, the liver, the lungs, and all other body organs and functions find their exact counterpart in society. Learning how ki energy flows in the human body (the microcosm) is the key to understanding how it circulates in the world (the macrocosm). Table 10

TABLE 10. CORRESPONDENCE AMONG PERSONAL, SOCIAL, AND PLANETARY HEALTH*

Bodily Organ/ Function	Social Organ/Function	Planetary Organ/ Function
Heart	Emperor; president	Overall air and water circulation; sunshine
Lungs	Prime minister; legislature	Rain forests
Liver	General, army; environmental protection	Mountains, volcanoes, seismic activity
Gallbladder	Upright judge; judiciary	Valleys and lowlands
Heart governor	Messenger; communications; music and the arts	Rainbow; symphony of natural sounds and rhythms
Stomach	Official in charge of food storage; farming, gardening	Forests, orchards, vineyards
Large intestine	Teacher of virtue; history, religion	Oceans, seas
Small intestine	Finance minister; manufacturing	Biodiversity; roots; evolution
Kidney	Labor minister; vitality; sex; human relations	Water table, underground rivers and lakes; salt deposits
Triple heater	Energy czar; transportation; travel	Energy cycles and currents
Bladder	Magistrates: trade, commerce	Underground reservoirs, springs
Ovary/testis	Magistrates: hidden wealth; regeneration; new life	Deep oceans; seeds; the moon and tides
Brain	Storage: intellectual and cultural affairs	Electromagnetic energy; ozone layer; earth's aura
Blood	Storage: physical vitality and strength; life and spirit	Soil quality, air quality, and water quality, especially salt water
Bones	Storage: energy	Mineral deposits

Bodily Organ/ Function	Social Organ/Function	Planetary Organ/ Function
Spleen and lymph	Energy flow; wishes, visions	Lakes, rivers, and streams
Pancreas	Food; cooking; medicine	Grasslands, savannahs, plains, stands of wild grain, groves
Breast	Nourishment; parenting; education; contentment	Hills, gardens, fountains, flowers
Skin and hair	Fashion, beauty; aging, change	Deserts, special habitats; seasonal change
* The harmony of all organs and functions creates universal health, happiness, joy, and peace.		

summarizes these relationships along with planetary correspondences for our contemporary era.

Ch'i Po explains that in China the two universal energies that make up all things are known as yang and yin, or heaven's and earth's forces. Health is defined as bringing together these two energies in balance, while sickness is a disharmony or imbalance between the two. The best way to create and maintain our daily health, he goes on, is through proper food selection and preparation. Through harmonious cooking, we take in a proper balance of energies that create health and happiness, radiating out from the personal level to society and eventually the world as a whole. The foundation of life is whole cereal grains, and for cases of sickness, Ch'i Po instructs the Yellow Emperor to give the sick person softly prepared millet or rice, every day, every meal, for a period of ten days. This is the same teaching we find in Hippocrates and early Greek medicine. The only difference is that the grains vary according to the environment.

The rest of The Yellow Emperor's Classic goes on to introduce the meridian system of energy flow and the complementary healing arts, including acupuncture, moxibustion (burning a dried herb and charging points along a meridian), acupressure massage, and herbal medicine. Ch'i Po explains that in ancient times, when the earth received heaven's force more intensely, people normally lived to be a hundred and twenty years old and could use yin and yang directly to heal. However, today food is the main source of life energy, and a proper diet is the main way to keep healthy and prevent or relieve disease. The other methods are symptomatic, serving to relieve pain, dissolve blockages, and get energy to flow more freely. According to legend, the Yellow Emperor lived to be exactly 100 years old and brought peace and prosperity to China and the ancient world.

Greece and China represent the two poles of healing on our planet. If we had space for another chapter, we could trace comparable healing traditions among native peoples in North and South America, among traditional European societies such as the Celts and in Africa, India, Australia, Japan, and elsewhere. They all had a deep understanding of natural order and developed healing systems based on an energetic view of life, utilizing diet as the primary way to harmonize with nature. In the modern era, this way of life was rediscovered and reintroduced by Christoph von Hufeland, a German physician who wrote *Makrobiotics or the Art of Prolonging Life* at the end of the 18th century; Sagen Ishizuka, a Japanese medical doctor who helped thousands of people recover from infectious diseases with diet at the end of the 19th century; George Ohsawa, a Japanese educator who developed macrobiotics in the early and mid–20th century; and Lima Ohsawa, his wife, who pioneered modern macrobiotic cuisine and lived to be 101 years old. Over the last generation, macrobiotic teachings have spread worldwide, contributing to personal and planetary health and influencing society at many levels.

◎ Healing Strategies

As human beings, we originated from food, and food continues to sustain us throughout our lives. Ancestral and parental influence, especially the mother's way of eating, creates our physical and mental constitution. What we call heredity or genetic influence is simply the accumulated dietary and environmental influences of our parents, grandparents, and ancestors. Our mother's blood was our first food and created our physical body. After birth, we ate food and continued to grow and develop. This food creates our day-to-day *condition* of health and, together with our *constitution*, largely determines our physical, mental, and spiritual development. It is difficult to change constitutional structures, such as the shape and size of our features, bones, and teeth, and our native strength and vitality. However, we can change our condi-

tion day to day, month to month, and year to year through our food and way of life. While people with strong constitutions have native intuition, reservoirs of strength, and recuperate quickly, they often abuse their constitutions. They usually include people who boast they can eat anything and never get sick, but who then die of a sudden heart attack. Meanwhile, someone with a weak constitution and a past history of chronic ills can completely change his condition, recover his health, and live to an advanced age. Thus natural balance is always present. Table 11 classifies some human characteristics according to yin and yang, arising out of a balance of constitutional and conditional factors.

Yin and yang provides a convenient compass to classify disease and return to balance. When a person's symptoms are caused by excessive yang factors (or a deficiency of yin), we say that the condition or disease is a more yang disorder. Generally, the main strategy is to balance the condition by making the person more yin. It is recommended that slightly lighter foods be prepared, milder cooking methods be used, and salt, miso, shoyu, and other seasonings be used in less volume than in ordinary cooking. Similarly, when the person's symptoms are caused by more yin factors (or a deficiency of yang), a slightly more yang approach will help to bring this yin condition back into balance. Slightly stronger foods may be chosen, heavier cooking methods may be used, and salt and other seasonings may be used in greater volume than normally. Conditions caused by a combination of dietary extremes (or a deficiency of both yin and yang) require a standard approach and a moderate selection of foods, cooking styles, and seasoning. For each condition or disease

TABLE 11. HUMAN CHARACTERISTICS CLASSIFIED ACCORDING TO YIN AND YANG

	Yin	Yang
Sex	Female	Male
Climate of origin	Warmer, more equatorial	Colder, more northern or temperate
Diet	Based on plant foods	Based on animal foods
Body type	Tall and thin	Short and stocky
Orientation	Aesthetic or contemplative	Theoretical or active
Living place	South or west	North or east
Facial shape	Longer and thinner	Square or round
Season of birth	Autumn or winter	Spring or summer
Hair color	Darker	Lighter
Thinking	Right-brain-oriented	Left-brain-oriented
Personality type	Type B (calm)	Type A (focused)
Attitude	Cooperative	Competitive
View of life	More spiritual	More material
Technology	Low-tech	High-tech
Environment	Country	City
Pace	Slower and more relaxed	Faster and more stressful
Response	Adaptation	Modification
Politics	More liberal and progressive	More conservative and traditional
Religion	More complex, ceremonial, and polytheistic	Simpler, more personal, and monotheistic
Art	More abstract, associative, symbolic	More realistic, representative, and literal
Music	More abstract, slower, free-flowing	More patterned, orderly, rapid
Architecture	Larger, elaborate, more spacious	Smaller, simpler, more functional
Cooking	Lighter, relaxing, more complex	Heavier, stronger, simpler

discussed in Part II, one of three healing diets is recommended, based on this approach, along with further suggestions and refinements.

Eating in a slightly opposite energetic direction is the main healing strategy in macrobiotic health care, but not the only one. Sometimes eating a small volume of food or drink that is of the same quality as the overall cause of the condition or disorder is effective. For example, orange juice (which is strongly yin) can help counteract a cold (which is strongly yin), because like repels like. In some cases, especially when people start macrobiotics, they take too many home remedies or special dishes, take them in greater amounts than necessary, or take them too often. Soon they are taking other remedies and dishes to balance the remedies as well as the underlying condition. To prevent this, eating toward the center, regardless of one's condition, is sometimes the wisest course. Also, variety is important in cooking and cannot be overemphasized. In order to heal, it is necessary to generate energy flow or blood and fluid circulation in stagnated areas. Eating the same way every day, even good-quality food, can lead to remaining stuck and not discharging. For movement and release of stagnation to occur, dynamic cooking and energy flow is needed. The diet need not be wide, but it should be varied. Within the temporarily narrow scope of a healing diet, there are virtually endless combinations of different grains, beans and bean products, vegetables, and sea vegetables that can be prepared and varied often. Sometimes just a little seasoning, condiment, pickle, or garnish can provide the opposite energy to spark internal movement.

To restore harmony with nature, adjustments may also need to be made in respect to environmental conditions, climatic conditions, and general level of activity. For yang conditions, it is recommended that the surrounding atmosphere be kept slightly moister, dimmer, and stiller than usual, with less circulation of air. For yin conditions, the humidity should be lower than normal, the air should circulate smoothly in the room, and sunshine or other bright conditions will enhance healing. For conditions arising from a combination of extreme energies, the surrounding environment should be kept in a moderate condition, neither too dry nor humid, sunny nor shady, breezy nor still.

In some cases, a change in climate is advisable because when we travel we change our way of eating to adapt to the new climate and environment. For a yang condition that develops in a cold or temperate region, moving to a warmer, more southern region will be helpful because the diet naturally will be more yin. Conversely, for a yin disease arising in a warmer region, moving to a cooler, northern clime will enhance recovery because the way of eating is more yang. After the condition has improved, the person can usually return home and, through dietary adjustments, continue to remain healthy and active. Only in a small number of cases would a major move or permanent change of residence be advised.

Overall, keeping physically active is one of the best ways to stay healthy. Walking, cleaning, working, gardening, dancing, exercise, and other activities contribute to active energy exchange with the environment. The lungs, intestines, heart, kidneys, and other organs and functions generally all benefit from physical activity. It is highly recommended that everyone walk

TABLE 12. ADJUSTMENT FOR ENVIRONMENT AND ACTIVITY

For Yin Disorder	For Yang Disorder	For Disorder Caused by Yin and Yang Combined
Atmospheric Condition Should Be:		
Drier	More moist	In-between, average conditions
Sunnier	Less sunny	
Brighter light	Dimmer light	
Fresh, cool air	Less air circulation	
Activity Should Be:		
More active, physical exercise	Less active physically	Average activity
Less mental activity	More mental activity	
Climate Should Be:		
Colder	Warmer	Average
More northern regions	Sunnier regions	Normal regions

outdoors for at least a half hour every day, rain or shine, or spend as much time as possible in the forest, fields, seashore, or other natural setting. This helps harmonize us with the rhythms and cycles of nature. Light to moderate exercise such as yoga, tai chi, do-in, and sports will also be helpful to facilitate energy discharge. Chanting, singing, and reading out loud are also recommended.

Activity levels will also change according to our condition and health. For yang disorders, it is generally better to engage in active exercise less often and pursue mental activities more often. For more yin disorders, active physical exercise is advisable, unless the person is in pain or suffering from fever, fatigue, or exhaustion. Less mental pursuits are also advised. For those with conditions arising from both extremes, a more in-between level of physical and mental activities is recommended. Table 12 summarizes these factors. See the way-of-life suggestions in Part III for further guidelines.

⑥ Diagnosing Our Health

Physiognomy, the traditional art of judging character and tendencies from the features of the face or body generally, is based on understanding the dynamic relationship between complementary and antagonistic structures and functions within the body and mind. In the embryo, all major systems gather and form the facial structure. As the baby grows, the upper and lower parts of the body undergo parallel development, as do the inner and outer regions, the softer and harder parts, and the more expanded and contracted areas. Each area of the face corresponds with an organ and function, as well as emotions and character traits. When internal imbalance arises, it is mirrored on the face. For example, the nose corresponds with the heart, which form and develop together in the womb. Problems in the heart immediately appear in the nose. A red swollen nose indicates that the heart is swollen and expanded from taking too much sugar, fruits, liquid, or alcohol. A hardened tip at the end of the nose shows that fat and cholesterol are accumulating in the coronary arteries and may lead to a heart attack. In this way, sickness and disease can often be diagnosed before pain, aches, or other symptoms appear. The basic relationships are as follows:

- The cheeks show the condition of the lungs and respiratory functions, as do the breasts.
- The tip of the nose corresponds with the heart and circulatory functions, while the nostrils show the bronchi region of the lungs.
- The middle of the nose correlates with the stomach and the upper part of the nose with the pancreas.
- The eyes show the condition of the kidneys and the testicles in males and the kidneys and ovaries in females. The left eye further corresponds with the spleen and lymphatic functions and the right eye with the liver and circulatory functions.
- The area between the eyebrows shows the condition of the liver and gallbladder.
- The temples show the condition of the spleen.
- The forehead as a whole shows the small in-

testines, and the peripheral region of the forehead shows the large intestine.
- The upper part of the forehead represents the bladder.
- The ears represent the kidneys: the left ear the left kidney, and the right ear the right kidney.
- The mouth shows the entire digestive system. The upper lip corresponds with the esophagus and stomach, the top part of the lower lip shows the small intestine, the lower part of the lower lip shows the large intestine, and the corners of the lip show the duodenum.
- The area around the mouth and the chin shows the sexual organs and their functions.

Spots, blemishes, and discolorations, as well as hardness and looseness, show developing problems in the corresponding organs and functions.

Macrobiotic diagnosis is simple, safe, and effective. Many of the conditions and diseases in Part II include advice on diagnosis. Table 13 presents some common symptoms that will help you evaluate your condition or that of a friend or family member.

There are also several guidelines related to the appearance of symptoms that are helpful in evaluating whether your condition is too yin or yang. These include:

- Symptoms that appear on the right side of the body tend to be caused by excess yang factors, including overconsumption of animal food; salt, miso, or shoyu; condiments; baked flour; or other contractive foods.
- Symptoms that appear on the left side of the body tend to be caused by excess yin factors,

TABLE 13. EVALUATING YOUR CONDITION

Too Yin	Too Yang
Passive	Aggressive
Overly relaxed	Tense
Complaining	Angry, irritable
Disorganized	Overly organized
Negative, retreating	Attacking, intolerant
Self-pity	Self-pride
Voice too soft, timid	Voice too loud, tense
Soft skin, moist skin	Hard skin, dry skin
Light, pale, or red facial color	Sallow or dark facial color
Rapid pulse	Slow pulse
Shallow breathing	Constricted breathing
Loose muscles	Tight muscles
Overly sensitive	Insensitive
Gets up late	Gets up early
Chubby, overweight	Skinny, underweight
Too excitable	Too serious

including overconsumption of sugar and sweets; tropical foods; refined flour; spices; stimulants; alcohol; and drugs.

- Symptoms that appear in the lower body or deep inside the body tend to be caused by excess yang.
- Symptoms that appear in the upper body or on the surface of the body tend to be caused by excess yin.
- Symptoms that appear in the early morning, at midday, and in the early afternoon (until about 2 P.M.) tend to be caused by excess yang.
- Symptoms that appear in the midafternoon, evening, and late night (until 2 A.M.) tend to be caused by excess yin.

- Symptoms that appear in spring and summer tend to be caused by excess yang.
- Symptoms that appear in the autumn and winter tend to be caused by excess yin.
- Symptoms that appear during or right before the full moon tend to be a discharge of extreme yin.
- Symptoms that appear during or just before the new moon tend to be a discharge of extreme yang.
- Sometimes opposite causes give rise to similar symptoms. Hardening, swelling, and inflammation can arise from either extreme yin or extreme yang factors or from a combination of both (see Table 14).

TABLE 14. SYMPTOMS ARISING FROM EITHER EXTREME (TOO MUCH YIN OR TOO MUCH YANG)

Swelling
Inflammation
Tightness
Hardness
Cold, numbness
Hot, sweating
Frequent urination
Constipation
Diarrhea
Coughing
Fever
Tiredness
Fatigue
Depression
Aches
Pain
Paralysis

In a small number of cases, the opposite tendency may prevail because at their extreme, yin changes into yang and yang changes into yin. Also, sometimes multiple factors are involved, and weighing a preponderance of signs and symptoms is necessary to determine the underlying cause. Thus it is important to confirm these tendencies with other diagnostic methods, including facial correspondences, meridian diagnosis, pulse diagnosis, iridology, and others.

◉ Understanding Health

In modern society, health is commonly viewed as an absence of sickness, while sickness is regarded as the absence of health. In contrast to this circular definition, health is regarded in the macrobiotic community in dynamic, positive terms. The seven conditions of health include the following:

- *Endless energy.* Keeping active, alert, and flexible all day; working tirelessly in pursuit of our dream; maintaining a state of physical and mental balance under any circumstances and at all times.

- *Strong appetite.* Having a strong appetite for whatever we engage in or encounter, including food, knowledge, work, experience, and sexual activity, and a passion for freedom, justice, and truth.

- *Deep sleep.* Maintaining the ability to fall asleep immediately, sleep deeply, and never have nightmares or disturbing dreams; occasionally experiencing true dreams of new inventions, communicating with the spirit world, or visions of impending accidents or natural catastrophes; waking renewed and refreshed.

- *Strong memory.* Maintaining strong mental faculties, including day-to-day recall, focus, and concentration, but most important, memory of spiritual destiny and remembrance of our universal oneness.

- *Peaceful mind.* Keeping calm and peaceful under all circumstances; never being angry; seeing all difficulties, sicknesses, and failures as complementary; developing patience and perseverance; changing difficulties into opportunities and turning enemies into friends.

- *Being joyful and alert.* Keeping a bright, optimistic mind; radiating love and happiness to everyone around us; cheerfully greeting everyone we meet; embracing all beings; thinking clearly; expressing ourselves concisely; moving swiftly and gracefully; maintaining order in our behavior.

- *Endless appreciation.* Recognizing all people and all beings as fellow brothers, sisters, and companions on the eternal journey of life; taking responsibility for all of our difficulties and sorrows; appreciating the endless order of the universe and all its manifestations; being grateful for the gift of life.

As you read this book and start practicing macrobiotics, you may be asking yourself the question, "When will I get healthy?"

Health is a dynamic, constantly changing process. It is not fixed, nor is there a firm borderline between health and sickness. Many people who appear in good health, never get sick, and have abundant energy are moving in the direction of sickness because they are not paying attention to their diet, environment, or lifestyle.

Others who have many symptoms, frequently get sick, and have low vitality are moving in the direction of health because they are now paying attention to their way of eating, adjusting to their environment, and altering their way of life. The state of perfect health does not exist. There is only perfect adaptation to ever changing conditions and circumstances.

The answer to the question "When will I get healthy?" is that you are healthy right now, this moment, if you sincerely desire to change and awaken to a larger view of life *(makrobios)*. By taking responsibility for your sickness, embracing your difficulties, and confessing your mistakes, you will immediately begin to realign with the natural order. Your intuition will become strong. Through day-to-day changes in your way of life, especially your way of eating, your condition will steadily improve. Of course, it may take several months or years to completely transform your physical, emotional, and spiritual condition. But you have erased the attachment to the past that is preventing you from changing. You are adapting perfectly to the moment. With yin and yang as your compass, you are starting to realize your endless dream: infinite health, happiness, and peace now and forever.

PART II

BALANCING YOUR CONDITION

Introduction

Macrobiotics classifies all conditions and disorders under three simple headings, emphasizes self-healing, and utilizes common, everyday foods and dietetic applications to bring the person safely back into balance. In contrast, conventional medicine divides sickness into hundreds of categories and thousands of diseases, requires highly trained specialists to diagnose and treat each condition, and utilizes drugs, radiation, and other invasive, potentially harmful procedures that relieve symptoms but do not address the underlying cause of the disease. From an energetic perspective, the three types of imbalance are (1) conditions and disorders arising from predominantly strong yin factors (or lack of yang), (2) those arising from predominantly strong yang factors (or lack of yin), and (3) those due to an excess (or deficiency) of both extreme yin and yang. For the most part, since the diseases and disorders of modern society are the result of overnutrition, this book focuses primarily on excessive conditions. (For an introduction to yin and yang, please review Chapter 2 in Part I and Table 13, "Evaluating Your Condition.")

Part II includes specific advice for some 200 ailments, conditions, and disorders, grouped into 30 comprehensive sections. For each specific disease, you will be directed to one of the three healing diets in Part III. Diet #1 will help relieve conditions caused by predominantly extreme yin factors, Diet #2 will help alleviate conditions caused by predominantly extreme yang factors, and Diet #3 will be beneficial for those resulting from a combination of both extremes. Further adjustments may be suggested in the text accompanying each condition or disease, along with home remedies and other special advice. In each of the major sections, "Solution" will offer further dietary and lifestyle guidelines for the entire group of conditions under discussion.

When properly applied, the macrobiotic way of eating helps to restore an excessively yin or yang condition to one of more natural balance. After the condition improves, the diet may be gradually widened to include many of the foods that were limited in the initial period. The exact time will differ according to the type of disorder, whether it is mild or severe, and the individual's practice and progress on the diet.

Minor symptoms will usually clear up immediately, and no major dietary adjustments may be needed. However, as a general rule, for more moderate to serious diseases, one of the three healing diets should be followed for about three to four months. If followed conscientiously, the blood quality will change completely during this time, allowing deep healing and revitalization of inner organs and tissues to proceed. For advanced cases, six to twelve months may be needed to recover, and for some cases, especially nervous disorders, it may take two to three years. As the condition improves, the standard macrobiotic diet for people in general good health may gradually be followed (see Part III). For minor conditions and complaints, this standard way of eating may be followed from the beginning after making a few dietary adjustments and taking a special drink or remedy.

◎ Causes

The section on cause looks at the underlying origin and cause of the condition or disorder from an energetic view, identifying the principal dietary and environmental factors involved. Note that it is usually the *excessive* intake of a combination of specific foods and beverages over time that creates a condition or disorder, not simply the intake of a specific food or drink. Because combinations of foods are virtually limitless and everyone's personal eating pattern is highly individualistic, only major combinations of foods and beverages are listed for any given condition. If you do not eat some of the foods listed, or if you eat other foods that are not listed, please be aware that these are general

tendencies and your pattern will probably be slightly different.

◎ "Regular Use" and Other Key Terms

In the guidelines, *regular* means suitable for daily use or from 4 to 5 or more times per week. *Occasional* means that the food or beverage may be used 2 to 3 times a week. *Infrequent* means the item may be used a few times a month. *Avoid, limit,* and *minimize* indicate that the articles are not to be used at all, rarely, or only if cravings arise. Capitalization in the text (e.g., TOFU PLASTER, NORI CONDIMENT) signifies that instructions on how to prepare special dishes, drinks, or other home remedies are found in Part III. Note that throughout the text, *1 cup* refers to a 6-ounce serving, not 8 ounces. (It is similar to a small teacup or coffee cup.)

◎ Caution

Specific cautions are included for many conditions and disorders, especially at the bottom of the comprehensive sections. It cannot be emphasized too strongly that the macrobiotic approach is educational, not medical. A physician or other appropriate medical or health care professional should be consulted for any serious, potentially life-threatening disorder or for anything that does not respond promptly to the approach recommended in this book. In healing, it is helpful to get the opinions of friends, families, and experts. But in the final analysis, you must rely on your own deepest intuition.

◎ Counseling

It is strongly recommended that everyone see an experienced macrobiotic teacher or counselor for advice on how to implement the approach recommended in this book and to help tailor the recommendations to his or her unique condition. People who are new to macrobiotics or are in transition will especially benefit, as well as anyone with a moderate to serious disorder. Even people who have been practicing regularly will benefit from an experienced counselor, who may point out simple mistakes they may be making. For information on contacting a counselor, please see "Macrobiotic Resources."

◎ Medical Research

At the end of most of the 30 major sections, a summary of recent scientific and medical research is presented, including macrobiotic studies and other dietary studies. Only a small, representative sampling of research that supports the approach in this book is given.

◎ Case Histories

Case histories of individuals who have recovered with the help of a macrobiotic way of eating are available in many other books and publications. For further information, see "Recommended Reading."

◎ Further Information

Consult the index to locate any condition that is not included in the main list of ailments or diseases. Sometimes related conditions are mentioned in the text. Also, there is more extensive cross-referencing in the index than in the text. In the event that the condition you are looking for is not discussed in this book, use Table 15, "Comprehensive Evaluation of Conditions," and follow one of the three healing diets according to your own evaluation. If you are unsure of your condition, follow Diet #3, which is centrally balanced and safely avoids both extremes.

TABLE 15. COMPREHENSIVE EVALUATION OF CONDITIONS

Balanced	Too Yin	Too Yang	Too Yin and Yang
Adaptable	Passive	Aggressive	Both tendencies
Flexible	Overly relaxed, lazy	Tense, workaholic	Both tendencies
Active	Inactive	Overactive	Hyperactive
Even-minded	Easily excitable	Overly serious	Both tendencies
Calm, peaceful	Complaining	Angry, irritable	Both tendencies
Trustful	Gullible	Suspicious	Mistrustful
Positive, open	Negative, retreating	Attacking, intolerant	Hateful
Self-reflective	Self-pity	Self-pride	Self-righteousness
Clear voice, friendly	Voice too soft, timid	Voice too loud, tense	Both tendencies
Clear, slightly moist skin	Soft skin, moist skin	Hard skin, dry skin	Oily and/or dry skin
Natural facial color	Light, pale, or reddish facial color	Yellow, dark, or drawn facial color	Various, including green and gray shades
Normal pulse	Rapid pulse	Slow pulse	Irregular pulse
Even breathing	Shallow breathing	Constricted breathing	Irregular breathing
Flexible muscles	Loose muscles	Tight muscles	Both tendencies
Sensitive	Overly sensitive	Insensitive	Hypersensitive
Caring	Neglectful	Abusive	Both tendencies
Alert, good memory	Forgetful	Fixated, preoccupied	Attached to old memories
On time	Spaced out	Rushed, in a hurry	Both tendencies
Get up on time	Get up late	Get up early	Irregular sleeping
Accepting	Unhappy, sad	Frustrated	Depressed
Normal weight	Chubby, overweight	Skinny, underweight	Obese or undernourished
Romantic	Feel lack of attraction	Overly passionate	Hot and cold

How to Use This Section

1. Locate the condition or disorder in the topic index that follows. For example, for high blood pressure, go to the section "Heart Disease and Circulatory Problems."

2. Read the introductory material for the section as a whole, as well as the material on symptoms, cause, and the specific condition or disorder you are concerned about under "Forms." Then refer to the solution, home remedies, caution, medical research, and case histories. If you like, you can read about related conditions and disorders under "Forms," but this is not necessary.

3. In the text for each condition or disorder, you will generally be advised to follow one of three healing diets. Follow the dietary guidelines recommended for Healing Diet #1 for conditions arising from more yin factors, Diet #2 for those arising from more yang factors, or Diet #3 for those arising from a combination of factors. (Please read or reread the introduction to yin and yang in Part I and study the charts in Part III so that you have a clear understanding what these terms refer to.) For example, you will discover that there are two main types of

high blood pressure. The first type, *systolic high blood pressure,* arises from more yang factors and can be relieved by following Diet #2. The second type, *diastolic high blood pressure,* arises from a combination of yin and yang factors and can be relieved by following Diet #3. For minor fluctuations in blood pressure or to prevent high blood pressure from developing, follow the standard macrobiotic dietary guidelines in Part III for people in usual good health.

4. The specific conditions and healing diets describe foods in very broad, general terms, such as "take plenty of leafy green vegetables." For a more comprehensive list of specific foods in the macrobiotic way of eating and a list of foods to avoid for better health, see Part III. Here, for example, over a dozen types of leafy greens are listed for you to choose from, including collards, kale, bok choy, napa cabbage, turnip greens, and many others.

5. In addition to one of the healing diets and specific guidelines in the text, refer to "Diet" under the heading "Solution" in each comprehensive section for further suggestions. For example, in "Heart Disease and Circulatory Problems" this section explains that corn is beneficial for the heart and heart conditions, including high blood pressure.

6. Follow the standard way-of-life suggestions in Part III with any further modifications under the specific condition or in the "Lifestyle" section under "Solution."

7. To practice the dietary recommendations, it is important to take macrobiotic cooking classes. This will introduce you to the breadth and scope of the diet and show you how to prepare healthful, delicious foods day after day. If you don't know how to make the food or it is unappetizing or grows monotonous, it will be difficult to follow the recommendations. The standard cookbook is *Aveline Kushi's Complete Guide to Macrobiotic Cooking* by Aveline Kushi with Alex Jack (Time-Warner Books). Other cookbooks are listed in "Recommended Reading." Basic recipes and menus are included in Part III to help you get started.

8. In some cases, special dishes, drinks, compresses, and other home remedies are recommended in the text or under the "Home Remedies" section. The recipes for those that are capitalized (e.g., SWEET VEGETABLE DRINK, GINGER COMPRESS) are grouped together in Part III. For more information on home remedies, see *Basic Home Remedies* by Michio Kushi with Alex Jack.

Conditions and Disorders

AIDS

ALLERGIES
Atopy
Chemical Allergies
Drug Allergies
Food Allergies
Lactose Intolerance
Hay Fever
Hives and Other Skin Allergies
Insect Bites

BLEEDING AND BLOOD DISORDERS
Anemia
Bleeding
Hemophilia
Rh Incompatibility
Sickle Cell Anemia

BONE AND JOINT DISORDERS
Arthritis
 Rheumatoid Arthritis
 Ankylosing Spondylitis
 Osteoarthritis
 Gout

Bone and Joint Infection
 Osteomyelitis
 Infectious Arthritis
Bunion
Bursitis
Osteoporosis
Scoliosis

BRAIN DISORDERS
Hemorrhage
Meningitis, Encephalitis, and Other
 Infections
Seizure
Tumors

CANCER
Bone Cancer
Brain Cancer
Breast Cancer
Colon and Rectal Cancer
Kidney and Bladder Cancer
Leukemia
Liver Cancer
Lung Cancer
Lymphoma and Hodgkin's Disease

Mouth and Upper Digestive Cancers
Ovarian, Uterine, Cervical, and Other
    Female Cancers
Pancreatic Cancer
Prostate and Testicular Cancer
Skin Cancer and Melanoma
Stomach Cancer

DIGESTIVE PROBLEMS
Appendicitis
Colitis
Constipation
Crohn's Disease
Diarrhea
Diverticular Disease
Enteritis
Gas and Gas Pains
Hemorrhoids
Hernia
Irritable Bowel Syndrome
Motion Sickness

EAR AND HEARING PROBLEMS
Auditory Nerve Damage
Earache
Menière's Disease
Presbycusis
Ruptured Eardrum
Tinnitus

ENDOCRINE DISORDERS
Adrenal Disorders
    Addison's Disease
    Virilization
    Cushing's Syndrome
Pituitary Disorders
    Dwarfism, Cachexia
    Diabetes Insipidis
    Giantism, Acromegaly

Thyroid Disorders
    Simple Goiter
    Myxedema or Gull's Disease
    Graves' Disease
    Toxic Goiter
    Tetany
    Osteitis Fibrosa

EYE AND VISION PROBLEMS
Cataracts
Conjunctivitis
Detached Retina
Glaucoma
Macular Degeneration
Retinitis Pigmentosa
Stye

FOOT AND LEG PROBLEMS
Ankle Problems
Athlete's Foot
Corns and Calluses
Knee Problems

GALLBLADDER PROBLEMS
Gallstones

HEADACHES
Tension Headaches
Cluster Headaches
Sinus Headaches
Migraines

HEART DISEASE AND CIRCULATORY PROBLEMS
Aneurysm
Angina
Atherosclerosis
Cardiomyopathy
Congenital Defects
Coronary Disease and Heart Attack

Heart Failure
High Blood Pressure
High Cholesterol
Rheumatic, Pulmonary, and Infectious
    Heart Disease
Stroke
Thrombosis and Embolism
Valve Disorders
Vein Disorders
Varicose Veins
Spider Veins
Phlebitis

INFECTIOUS DISEASES
Anthrax
Influenza
Lyme Disease
Malaria
Tuberculosis
Other Infectious Diseases

KIDNEY AND BLADDER PROBLEMS
Abnormal Urination
    Oliguria
    Dysuria
    Anuria
Kidney or Bladder Infections
Kidney or Bladder Stones
Kidney Disease
    Uremia
Nephritis
Tight Kidneys

LIVER PROBLEMS
Cirrhosis
Hepatitis
Jaundice

LUNG PROBLEMS
Asthma
Bronchitis
Coughing
Cystic Fibrosis
Emphysema
Pleurisy
Pneumonia

MAD COW DISEASE (VARIANT CREUTZFELDT-JAKOB DISEASE)

MENTAL AND EMOTIONAL PROBLEMS
Bipolar Disorder
Phobias, Obsessions, and Compulsions
Post-traumatic Stress Disorder
Schizophrenia
Seasonal Affective Disorder
Stress

MUSCLE PROBLEMS
Backache
Cerebral Palsy
Cramps and Spasms
Muscular Dystrophy
Myasthenia Gravis
Sprains and Strains
Tetanus

NAUSEA AND VOMITING

NERVOUS CONDITIONS AND DISORDERS
Alzheimer's Disease
Amyotrophic Lateral Sclerosis
Dizziness and Vertigo
Epilepsy
Gulf War Syndrome
Huntington's Disease
Multiple Sclerosis
Neuralgia

Numbness and Tingling
Parkinson's Disease
Peripheral Nerve Disorders
Pinched Nerve
Spinal Cord Disorders
Tourette's Syndrome

PANCREATIC PROBLEMS
Diabetes
Hyperinsulinism
Hypoglycemia
Pancreatitis

REPETITIVE STRESS INJURIES
Carpal Tunnel Syndrome
Tarsal Tunnel Syndrome

SINUS PROBLEMS

SPLEEN PROBLEMS
Enlarged Spleen
Ruptured Spleen

STOMACH PROBLEMS
Gastritis
Gastroenteritis
Heartburn
Stomach Ulcers

TMJ AND RELATED PROBLEMS

◎ AIDS

AIDS, or acquired immune deficiency syndrome, is one of the major epidemic diseases of modern times. Transmitted primarily sexually or by contact with contaminated blood or body fluids, it surfaced in the early 1980s, and since then has killed an estimated 20 million persons and infected tens of millions of others. Initially appearing in the male homosexual, Caribbean, or other minority communities, today it affects both males and females, heterosexuals and homosexuals, and has spread around the world. In some African regions, the infection rate has reached one in three, and in some prenatal clinics 70 percent of mothers have tested positive for HIV. With 4 million infections, India has the largest number of HIV carriers in the world today. In the United States AIDS is the leading cause of death in young adults age 25 to 44. The United Nations warns that 65 million people will die of AIDS in the next 20 years. Despite many years of research on a vaccine, there is no medical cure. In some cases, the disease can be controlled by antiretroviral drugs, while in other cases, drugs worsen the condition. In our experience, AIDS can be prevented, controlled, and in some cases relieved through a macrobiotic way of life, including proper food and lifestyle practices.

SYMPTOMS

1. General fatigue, including a decline in mental and physical vitality. The person is unable to meet the challenges of daily life. A negative, pessimistic mind replaces a positive, optimistic one. Passivity and inactivity increase, as the individual seeks more comfortable situations and surroundings.

2. Development of colds and infections. Dietary extremes produce an acidic blood condition and other imbalances that reduce natural immune function. As the internal environment weakens, viruses and bacteria can easily spread. Colds, infections, and light fevers are frequent.

3. Skin problems. Red and white discolorations or shadings from consumption of too much milk, fruit, and other strong yin may appear on the skin. These result from the discharge of infectious material to the body's surface along with excessive oily and fatty substances. In some cases, Kaposi's sarcoma, a rare form of skin cancer, may arise. In other cases, white-yellow patches appear, signifying the discharge of excessive dairy fats.

4. Intestinal weaknesses and disorders. Gas formation, constipation, and chronic diarrhea are frequent. Parasites may arise in the case of diarrhea. Colitis may develop.

5. Feelings of nausea may arise after meals or snacks, though not usually vomiting.

6. The appetite may become irregular. Sometimes an enormous appetite may arise, while at other times the person may not want to eat at all. Cravings for specific foods, especially sweets or fruits, may arise, and these preferences may change suddenly.

7. Abnormal perspiration may occur, especially at night between midnight and early morning. It may be accompanied by a light fever and shivering.

8. Hypoglycemia or chronic low blood sugar may be present. This is commonly experienced as large ups and downs in mood and emotions, including mental depression and irritability, particularly in the afternoon. During sleep, exhaustion may be experienced, and the hands, feet, and other extremities may feel colder than usual. Cravings for simple sugars are also strong, especially in the midafternoon.

9. Liver problems are often present, including jaundice, hepatitis, mononucleosis, and a general tendency to get angry or upset easily.

10. Lymph glands in the groin, armpit, neck, and chest area often grow swollen as they help neutralize excessive viral activity. The spleen may also become swollen and weak. In extreme cases, this can lead to lymphoma.

11. Blood quality begins to weaken, as improper food continues to be consumed. Within the bloodstream, the ratio of red blood cells, white blood cells, platelets, and other formed elements, as well as the quality of the plasma or fluid, may change. Generally, in the case of AIDS, white blood cells decrease, particularly lymphocytes, which are involved in neutralizing infection. The ratio of T4 to T8 cells, involved in immune responses, drops to less than 1.0 and may even reach 0.1 or lower, which is considered by the medical profession a standard benchmark for AIDS.

12. Other symptoms may appear as infection spreads, and these differ according to the individual.

CAUSE

THE HIV HYPOTHESIS

Since 1984, when it was isolated by Dr. Luc Montagnier of the Pasteur Institute and Dr. Robert C. Gallo of the National Institutes of Health, HIV—human immunodeficiency virus— has been associated with AIDS, and almost all the world's medical resources have been devoted to combating the virus. This includes the Centers for Disease Control and Prevention, National Center for HIV, STD, and TB Prevention, Divisions of HIV/AIDS Prevention; the National Institute of Allergy and Infectious Disease (NIAID); the Joint United Nations Programme on HIV/AIDS (UNAIDS); and other national and international bodies.

"By leading to the destruction and/or functional impairment of cells of the immune system, notably CD4+ T cells, HIV progressively destroys the body's ability to fight infections and certain cancers," an NIAID fact sheet updated in 2000 explains. "An HIV-infected person is diagnosed with AIDS when his or her immune system is seriously compromised and manifestations of HIV infection are severe." In persons older than thirteen, AIDS is defined as "the presence of one of 26 conditions indicative of severe immunosuppression associated with HIV infection, such as *Pneumocystis carinii* pneumonia (PCP)." Most other AIDS-related conditions are also "opportunistic infections." AIDS is also diagnosed when T-cell counts fall below 200 cells/cubic millimeter of blood. (Normal is 600–1,500/mm^3.)

According to this model, HIV has clearly been shown to be the cause of AIDS. Tests for HIV antibody in persons with AIDS indicate that they are infected with the virus; HIV has been isolated in persons with AIDS and grown in pure culture; and studies of patients who received blood transfusion before 1985 have documented the transmission of HIV to previously unaffected persons who subsequently developed AIDS. The CDC reports that, through 1999, fifty-six health-care workers in the United

States with no other risk factors have developed occupationally acquired HIV infection; 25 of these workers subsequently developed AIDS in the absence of other risk factors. A Florida dentist accidentally passed on HIV to six patients. The dentist and three of the patients died of AIDS; another is living with AIDS. There have also been repeated cases of HIV transmission (and subsequent infection and death) among infants and adults, either through contaminated blood transfusions, mother-to-child transmission, or IV drug use. A multitude of clinical, epidemiological, and cohort studies in Europe, Africa, and around the world have shown substantially higher infection and death rates from AIDS and related conditions among those who test positive for HIV in comparison to those who test negative for the virus.

Based on this paradigm, most scientific and medical research on the AIDS epidemic has been devoted to developing a vaccine against the disease, promoting safe sex, and preventing contamination of the blood supply. During the last decade, the development of a new generation of anti-HIV drugs known as HAART (highly active antiretroviral therapy) has prolonged survival of many AIDS patients. This may be the reason the death rate from AIDS in the United States has dropped by more than 50 percent in the last several years. Also, aggressive public health campaigns, including the introduction of condoms, clean needles, and other efforts to reduce the spread of the virus, in Uganda and several other African countries has sharply reduced the percentage of people who test positive for HIV and those who have died from the disease.

THE DRUG AND LIFESTYLE HYPOTHESIS

Challenging the conventional view that AIDS is caused by a virus, a small but growing number of medical researchers has proposed that AIDS may be the result of immunosuppressive behavior and lifestyle, especially the abuse of drugs and medications. In his book *Rethinking AIDS: The Tragic Cost of Premature Consensus*, Robert S. Root-Bernstein, a professor of physiology at Michigan State University, contends that the disease is the result of numerous synergistic insults to the immune system, including illicit and prescription drug use and improper diet. "HIV infection may be an epiphenomenon of immune suppression rather than a necessary cause," he explained. "Immune suppression may predispose people to HIV infection (just as it predisposes them to other opportunistic infections) rather than resulting from such an infection."

Based on his study of patients' medical histories, Root-Bernstein showed that probable cases of AIDS long predate the current epidemic and that there are a number of cases without HIV infection. Reviewing current medical research, he argued that it is very difficult for a healthy person to get AIDS, even following sexual contact with someone who tests positive for HIV. "Alternative hypotheses to AIDS provide alternative frameworks for interpreting as valid some otherwise unexplainable treatments or 'cures.' For example, a holistic approach to AIDS focusing on nutrition and behavior modification and emphasizing a positive mental image may bolster the immune system and simultaneously curtail exposure to drugs and infections, leading to improved health. This is a

reasonable prediction of the co-factor and multifactorial theories of AIDS that differentiate
them clearly from the HIV-only theory."

Other researchers have concluded that AIDS
is not a single infectious disease or syndrome
but a set of separate conditions with different
risk factors. They cite the use of amyl nitrite inhalants or "poppers" and other aphrodisiac
drugs, as well as prior use of alcohol, heroin, cocaine, marijuana, Valium, and amphetamines as
chief causes of loss of natural immunity in the
gay community.

THE POLIO VACCINE HYPOTHESIS

Other critics accept the HIV hypothesis but
find evidence that HIV emerged in the 1950s as
the tragic result of mass polio vaccines in
Africa. According to this hypothesis, oral polio
vaccines may have been made with chimpanzee
kidneys contaminated with SIV (simian immunodeficiency virus), from which HIV then
evolved. (SIV is transmitted by chimpanzees
only, not other primates.) In *The River: A Journey to the Source of HIV and AIDS*, Edward
Hooper, a former United Nations official and
BBC correspondent in Africa, theorizes that the
first known cases of AIDS occurred in central
Africa in the late 1950s. The incidence corresponds to the region where an oral polio
vaccine cultured by Dr. Hilary Koprowski, a pioneer American medical researcher, was given
to more than a million people between 1957
and 1960. Hooper's survey found that the
earliest AIDS cases—which were first documented in 1959—commonly occurred in areas
where the polio vaccine had been administered. In a summary of his findings, Hooper
noted:

The most plausible iatrogenic theory of origin, and the one which I came to favor, is
called the oral polio vaccine (OPV) hypothesis. It proposes that the AIDS pandemic was sparked by the vaccination of
approximately 1 million Africans with
an experimental oral polio vaccine called
CHAT. The 27 known African trials of
CHAT vaccine occurred between the years
of 1957 and 1960, in the central African
countries now known as Democratic Re-
public of Congo (DRC), Burundi, and
Rwanda. In the fifties, these countries were
all administered by Belgium. . . . Through
1981, there are 70 instances of African
Group M [HIV-1] infection which can
be linked to a town or village, of which
30% come from Kinshasa [capital of the
Congo]. However, there is a far stronger
correlation, for 76% of these infected sera
come from cities, towns, or villages where
CHAT vaccine was fed in the late fifties.

Of course, during that era, polio vaccines
were not screened for SIV, and the possible risk
of infected animal organs was not known. The
vaccine was given to many infants less than a
month old whose immune function had not yet
fully developed. In some cases, Hooper reported, they were given 15 times the standard
dose to ensure effective immunization.

Dr. Koprowski, now in his eighties, and most
of his surviving American and European staff
denied that chimpanzees were used in making
the serum. Recent DNA testing of a remaining
sample of the polio vaccine was inconclusive.
However, no laboratory records remain, and
some Africans who worked as orderlies in the
Koprowski clinic at the time have stated that

chimpanzee kidneys were used to prepare some batches of vaccine.

THE BIOLOGICAL WEAPON HYPOTHESIS

Other investigators suggest that HIV was the result of genetic engineering or biological warfare experiments that went awry. Investigating the possibility that AIDS, Ebola, and other new diseases are the result of biological weapons experiments, Dr. Leonard G. Horowitz, a dentist and medical researcher who has served on the faculties of Harvard and Tufts universities, investigated the U.S. biological warfare program at Fort Detrick, Maryland, which received a $10 million authorization in the early 1970s to develop a genetically altered retrovirus that would destroy the human immune system as part of the Special Virus Cancer Program.

The secret biological warfare program was overseen by Dr. Henry Kissinger, national security advisor and later secretary of state in the Nixon and Ford administrations; carried out by the National Cancer Institute, Merck Sharp & Dohme, the world's largest pharmaceutical company, and Litton Bionetics, the nation's largest bioweapons contractor; and involved Dr. Robert C. Gallo, the cancer virus researcher who went on to become the codiscoverer of HIV more than a decade later.

Clandestine research, Horowitz theorizes, dated back even further. In 1967, a lethal virus broke out in Germany and Yugoslavia among vaccine researchers. The epidemic, known as Marburg disease, was attributed to infected monkeys that had been brought to Europe from Africa. Horowitz traces the monkeys to a Litton medical research laboratory in Africa. The facility was located in an area of southeast Zaire that was secretly leased until the year 2000 to OTRAG, a German corporation with ties to NATO, the CIA, and Litton. The official purpose of OTRAG's contract was to launch private communication satellites, but biowar experiments and other covert military activities may also have been conducted in this remote area (which is twice the size of England). In 1976, Ebola—the extremely contagious, highly lethal viral disease that is genetically identical to Marburg—broke out in central Africa. It is in this "thinly populated" region—inhabited by 760,000 Africans—over which OTRAG was granted "complete sovereignty and control" that AIDS also may have first emerged.

Horowitz speculates that fear of Communism, Black nationalism, and overpopulation (especially in neighboring Angola, which bordered Zaire and was a center of revolutionary political movements) fueled these medical experiments. (Ebola also broke out in South Africa, whose apartheid-era government was committed to overthrowing Angola.) Through the late 1970s, USAID vaccination teams immunized more than 20 million people in central Africa. Horowitz claims that between 1978 and 1979—several years before AIDS appeared in America—the New York City Blood Center introduced an experimental hepatitis B vaccine, which may have contained HIV or a monkey virus that mutated into HIV, into the gay male community.

The evidence for the bioweapons connection to AIDS is troubling but far from proven. However, in the aftermath of recent terrorist attacks, it cannot be dismissed entirely. Following 9/11, *The New York Times* and other publications reported that the United States has been secretly pursuing genetically engineered bioweapons—including anthrax, smallpox, and the plague—since the early 1970s, in apparent violation of the Biological and Toxin Weapons Convention.

THE ENDOGENOUS HYPOTHESIS

According to this hypothesis, HIV—in some or all cases—may be self-generated or endogenous (produced by our own DNA). The agent that causes AIDS may arise following the decomposition of blood cells, lymph cells, and other normal body cells into bacteria, viruses, DNA, and other more primitive forms of life.

From a macrobiotic perspective, biological degeneration represents a reversal of the evolutionary process. When human beings stop eating food in harmony with nature—predominantly whole cereal grains and cooked vegetables as their main food—they can no longer adapt to their changing environment, and they begin to lose their human condition and quality. Biological degeneration can transform multicellular organisms to single-cell organisms, and single-cell organisms may revert back to bacteria and viruses. In the human body, individual cells that are not properly nourished can degenerate into more primitive stages of life. Such cell degeneration would possibly occur more easily in less-developed cells such as blood cells—especially white-blood cells and reproductive follicles—than in well-developed body cells.

Such degeneration could arise if the body's internal environment reproduced conditions similar to those present in primordial earth, when bacteria and viruses flourished. If the blood, lymph, body fluid, and interior of the intestines, as well as reproductive organs, increase their content of fatty acids, sulfur compounds, uric acid, ammonium compounds, methane, and other gases, and decrease their content of minerals, white-blood cells and other, more primitive, human cells may weaken and degenerate into bacteria and viruses. In short, AIDS may not be transmitted virally from the outside through sexual or other contact with someone who is infected. AIDS may arise internally from the longtime degenerative effects of dietary and environmental imbalance. This hypothesis may explain why AIDS-related symptoms have appeared in some individuals who have not been exposed to HIV through sexual contact or other known means of transmission.

In the late 19th century, Louis Pasteur, the father of microbiology and the germ theory of disease, observed that microorganisms commonly change their properties, including their virulence, within an organism and under varying environmental conditions. Early in this century, medical researchers began to study the fermentative, morphological, and other properties of microorganisms and reported that microbes could transform into one another. In the *Journal of Infectious Diseases* in 1914, Edward C. Rosenow of the Memorial Institute of Infectious Diseases in Chicago reported that in laboratory experiments, *pneumococci* (the microbes associated with pneumonia) could be transmuted into *streptococci* (the microbes associated with strep infections). His conclusion that nutritional and environmental factors may cause microorganisms to change or transmute into pathogenic species within the body without stimulus or entry from outside flew in the face of scientific theory regarding the fixity of species and hence was never seriously considered.

More recently, in his book on AIDS, Dr. Robert C. Gallo, the codiscoverer of HIV, referred to a similar theory: "Some scientists have speculated that in a weird case of reverse evolution, viruses are descended from more complex parasites, adapting by shedding their ingredients to the barest form capable of survival. . . ."

In *The Virus Within: A Coming Epidemic*, Nicholas Regush, a journalist and commentator for ABC News, gathered further evidence that the agents associated with the epidemic may arise internally rather than externally. He observed that some people with AIDS-like symptoms test negative for HIV antibodies or that autopsies on those who have died confirm that they were HIV-free. In a study of alternative approaches to AIDS, he described several cases in which scientists have found evidence of internally generated infection. For example, one woman who consistently tested HIV-negative appeared to have an HIV-like virus several years later. The researchers found evidence for the reshuffling of genetic material. "What is called HIV may be a product of this reshuffling process, which involves genetic material streaming from damaged human cells," concluded Regush. "It may be only a marker associated with AIDS that indicates cell damage has occurred and that a disease process is likely under way." As for cofactors, Regush concluded that HHV-6 (Human herpes virus 6), may be more directly linked to AIDS than HIV, which was relatively harmless.

A PRUDENT NATURAL APPROACH

As the AIDS epidemic continues to spiral out of control, widely divergent views proliferate on what caused it and how best to contain its spread. The AIDS issue has become so highly charged with emotion that there has been little dialogue or effort to find common ground. The global medical community fears that questioning the HIV hypothesis and HAART will expose millions of people to greater risk of infection and is tantamount to denying a medical holocaust. Critics—many with equally impeccable medical credentials—charge that the war on AIDS is an economic boondoggle and has become an end in itself, enriching the pharmaceutical industry, the scientific establishment, and the AIDS support community at the expense of patients and people's general welfare. President Thabo Mbeki of South Africa suggests that it may also be racist and genocidal, targeting Africans and other regions of the Third World for dubious medical treatment and experimentation.

A prudent natural approach to AIDS tries to take into account all of the major theories and come up with a multifactorial model. The evidence for HIV involvement is overwhelming, though the course of AIDS does not follow that of other viral diseases. The critics of the HIV hypothesis have raised embarrassing scientific questions that suggest a rush to judgment in the early 1980s, when the medical profession was under immense pressure to come up with a cause. For example, Dr. Heinz Ludwig Sänger, professor emeritus of molecular biology and virology at the Max Planck Institute of Biochemistry in Munich and Robert Koch Award winner, wrote in 2000, "Up to today there is actually no single scientifically really convincing evidence for the existence of HIV. Not even once such a retrovirus has been isolated and purified by the methods of classical virology." Dr. Bernard Forscher, former managing editor of the

Proceedings of the National Academy of Sciences of the United States of America, was even more blunt, as quoted by the *Sunday Times* of London in 1994: "The HIV hypothesis ranks with the 'bad air' theory for malaria and the 'bacterial infection' theory of beriberi and pellagra [which are caused by nutritional deficiencies.]"

A broader, holistic perspective recognizes that HIV is probably involved in the transmission of AIDS but also holds that environmental, nutritional, and lifestyle factors predispose one's susceptibility and greatly influence the course of the illness. It seeks to understand why HIV emerged when it did and why it became so virulent. It tries to discover why some people remain immune to infection when exposed to the virus, while others contract it. It recognizes that a significant number of HIV-positive people never progress to AIDS, while others who do not test positive for the virus exhibit clinical symptoms. It strives to understand the role that various environmental, chemical, physical, mental, and nutritional factors may play in mediating immune response and the development of AIDS-related diseases.

A balanced approach to AIDS also recognizes that statistics appear to have been exaggerated and manipulated by national and international medical bodies to justify increased budgets and spending. Critics of the HIV hypothesis have also been silenced or attacked so harshly that virtually no research funds are available to explore alternative hypotheses. HAART and other controversial new drug therapies should also be evaluated more rigorously and physicians should conscientiously inform their patients about the risks and benefits. It is not altogether clear whether the

sharp decline in AIDS mortality in America and Europe is due to the new antiviral medication or from changing lifestyles, including decreased drug use. Moreover, in the United States, zealous public health authorities have sometimes required HIV-positive individuals to submit to antiviral therapy against their will. In view of the well-documented side effects of the "drug cocktails"—including stroke, heart attack, and sometimes death—such measures have led to a sort of underground railway for mothers with HIV-positive children fleeing compulsory medical treatment. Such abuses only fuel conspiracy theories and stoke the fears of African leaders like South Africa's President Mbeki, who grew up under apartheid and understandably mistrusts Western institutions. Overall, the medical profession needs to self-reflect, develop humility, and admit how little it really knows about AIDS.

THE ENVIRONMENTAL APPROACH

From a larger, environmental perspective, AIDS follows the general pattern of other infectious diseases. It emerged in Africa following centuries of slavery and colonialism that introduced modern food and agricultural practices, the decline of the traditional way of life and eating, and the spread of hunger, poverty, and disease. Genetic research suggests a connection between HIV and SIV. The microbes' earliest genetic line goes back several centuries, possibly a thousand years, but signs of virulence do not show up until the early twentieth century, and symptoms of illness did not appear until the late 1970s and early 1980s. Based on environmental principles, we may postulate that in a traditional African setting, ancestors of SIV and

HIV were relatively benign organisms that co-existed peacefully with animal and human populations for thousands of years. In any ecosystem, multiple checks and balances create a system of homeostasis, or balance.

Throughout history, epidemics have generally been associated with social, cultural, or environmental factors that upset this delicate balance. For example, yellow fever, which is also associated with simian, or monkey, carriers, was virtually unknown until modern times. It emerged following sweeping social and cultural changes in Latin America and Africa. As a result of colonization, hot tropical lands that had traditionally grown grains, vegetables, tubers, and roots were now used to produce sugar, fruits, and other commodity crops. Those foods attracted monkeys from the surrounding jungles. *Aedes aegypti* mosquitoes, in turn, feasted on the blood of infected monkeys, picked up the yellow fever virus, and passed it on to human beings. This is the ecological chain of transmission.

A similar process appears to underlie the emergence of AIDS. The regions in central and West Africa where strains of HIV are believed to have originated were the site of former European colonies, including Zaire, Ivory Coast, Cameroons, Senegal, and French Equatorial Africa. In addition to being under European political and economic control during the last several hundred years, these areas were also subject to the influx of Western microbiologists, parasitologists, tropical physicians, and other scientists and public health officials who were disciples of the modern germ theory of disease and devoted to the sacred task of eradicating harmful microorganisms from the face of the earth.

From Brazzaville to Dakar, from Kinshasa to Nairobi, doctors and medical researchers served in the vanguard of the European colonial administration. In an article called "The Scientific Mission of the Institute Pasteur and the Colonial Experience" early in the century, Albert Calmette noted, "It is now the turn of the scientific experts to come onto the stage.... Their task is to draw up inventories of the natural resources of the conquered countries and to prepare the way for their expertise. These scientific experts are the geographers, engineers, and naturalists. Among the last, the microbiologists have a considerable role to play in protecting the colonies, their native collaborators, and their domestic animals against their most fearsome, because invisible, enemies."

Their methods of "protection," which resulted in widespread ecological imbalance, included uprooting millions of families, replacing traditional housing and farming practices with modern ones, and constructing mines, dams, highways, and plantations, to support the colonial infrastructure. In particular, traditional African farmlands were converted into vast plantations to produce sugar, cocoa, coffee, bananas, and other single commodity, or monoculture, crops. The result was an environmental catastrophe that set the stage for an endless cycle of drought, desertification, and disease accompanied by poverty, malnutrition, and starvation.

After World War II, colonialism in Africa declined and political independence was attained. However, the economic pattern and effects of social dislocation continued. To deal with recurrent famines and epidemics, the United Nations mounted international relief efforts, and private charities distributed millions of tons of infant formula, powdered milk, white flour, and canned food. Further, people living in Africa—as elsewhere around the world where a similar process was under way—were subjected to mass inoculations and treatment with antibiotics and other drugs, and medical procedures. In the short run, these measures helped save millions of people suffering from acute infection and malnutrition. However, in the long run, they weakened people's natural immunity to disease. In this setting, natural selection favored the evolution of virulent microbes that are resistant to vaccines, antibiotics, and drugs. This has led to a rampage of infectious diseases across Africa, including malaria, sleeping sickness, river blindness, hookworm, and AIDS.

In Africa, modernization created a legacy of unemployment, poverty, hunger, and sprawling urbanization as displaced farmers and their families flocked to cities and slums. "During the 1960s and 1970s extensive migrations occurred from rural areas in central and east Africa because of socioeconomic problems," biologist Paul W. Ewald explains in *Evolution of Infectious Disease.* "This mobility in response to economic forces was partly a legacy of the colonial period, during which a migrant labor force developed in response to centralization of jobs. When agricultural options deteriorated, men left the agricultural areas to obtain industrial jobs. The large populations of men without families created a market for sexual commerce, drawing young women from rural into urban areas. . . ." Amid this ecological and social imbalance, prostitution—both female and male—served as the primary vector for the transmission of the AIDS virus.

Briefly, the emerging ecological theory of infectious disease, including AIDS, is that clearing land for cattle pasture, sugar plantations, mining, logging, or urban development disrupted the local environment, favoring the emergence of microbes that are benign in a natural setting but virulent when natural checks and balances are eliminated or altered. Then, as a result of international jet travel and trade, these microorganisms are swiftly transported to distant climes and environments where they have no natural predators. In this way, new and extremely dangerous microorganisms can quickly spread around the world. In India, for example, Kyasanur Forest disease virus (KFDV), which causes severe hemorrhaging, first appeared in the mid-1950s. Initially affecting monkeys, it then spread into the human population. A generation ago, scientists would have declared KFDV a mutant organism that had arisen randomly and had to be destroyed by any means necessary. Today, the approach is more sophisticated. "Ecological factors, including deforestation, cattle grazing, and an increased opportunity for tick density were probably responsible for the appearance of this disease, which has persisted as an endemic infection since that time," observes Dr. Thomas Monath in *Emerging Viruses: AIDS and Ebola: Nature, Accident or Intentional?*, an anthology of essays by current viral researchers. "The virus was probably circulating silently in ticks and rodent hosts; ecological changes provided an opportunity for amplified transmission, and human encroachment in this altered environment led to the emergence of epidemic disease." Social, cultural, and environmental measures will be more important in reversing this epidemic than medical treatment.

Increasingly ecology is seen as the key to understanding the development of animal and human epidemics. "Introduction of viruses into the human population is often the result of human activities, such as agriculture, that cause changes in natural environment," explains Dr. Stephen S. Morse, a virologist at the Rockefeller University, in *Emerging Viruses*. He showed, for example, that herbicides introduced into the Latin American pampas led to the rise of Argentine hemorrhagic fever beginning in 1960. The chemical sprays altered the ecology and led to the emergence of a new rodent that, in the absence of traditional predators, was the carrier of the deadly virus.

THE NUTRITIONAL APPROACH

Whichever hypothesis ultimately proves to be correct about the origin of AIDS, all of them point to the role that modern civilization—including medicine, agriculture, and changing patterns of food consumption—played in the spread of the epidemic. AIDS is caused fundamentally by an imbalance with nature, brought out by a weakened internal environment produced by a variety of extreme dietary and lifestyle practices. The end result is more fat, mucus, and acidic conditions arising in the blood, lymph, and other bodily fluids, the intestines, and the reproductive organs, making the person more susceptible to infection from viruses either introduced from the outside or those produced from the inside as the result of degenerating cells and tissues.

In recent years, both Montagnier and Gallo, the codiscoverers of HIV, have distanced themselves from the viral hypothesis, stating that there appears to be one or more cofactors involved and that HIV, by itself, will not lead to AIDS. Their search for other infectious agents or predisposing influences suggests that diet and nutrition may play a leading role.

In a review of the nutritional factors that may compromise natural immunity and contribute to AIDS, Dr. Roberto A. Giraldo, president of Rethinking AIDS: The Group for the Scientific Reappraisal of the HIV-AIDS Hypothesis, observes, "Cell division is a very singular characteristic of the functioning of immunocompetent cells. All types of immune cells and their products, such as interleukins, interferons, and complement, are known to depend on metabolic pathways that employ various nutrients as critical co-factors for their actions and activities. Most of the host defense mechanisms are altered in protein-energy malnutrition [PEM], as well as during deficiencies of trace elements and vitamins." In particular, he cited how vitamin A deficiency results in the weight reduction of the thymus, decreased lymphocyte proliferation, impaired natural killer cell and macrophage activities, and increased bacterial adherence to epithelial cells. Vitamin B_6 deficiency results in malfunctioning of cell-mediated and humoral immune responses. Vitamin C deficiency interferes with phagocytosis and cell-mediated immune reactions, while vitamin E deficiency produces lymphoid atrophy, reduces lymphocyte responses and skin delayed hypersensitivity. Low intake of selenium and copper reduce T and B lymphocyte functions, while reduced amino acids such as arginine and glutamine also impair immunity. Finally, excessive lipid and fat intake may create free radicals that harm the immune function by oxidative stress. "There is an uncanny similarity between the immunological findings in nutritional deficiencies and those seen in AIDS," Drs. V. K. Jain and R. K. Chandra observe in an article entitled "Does Nutritional Deficiency Predispose to Acquired Immunodeficiency Syndrome?" that appeared in *Nutrition Research* in 1984 in the early days of the epidemic.

Whether HIV is ultimately found to be harmful or harmless, whether it is natural, the result of a contaminated polio vaccine campaign, or the product of a biological warfare project gone awry, and whether AIDS is related to other cofactors and lifestyle practices, a return to a more balanced way of life, including a diet centered around whole grains and vegetables, will help prevent, stabilize, and in some case relieve AIDS.

The dietary pattern that commonly underlies AIDS includes many of the following elements:

1. Frequent consumption of sugar and sweets, including refined sugar of all varieties, chocolate, honey, carob, mocha, and chemical sweeteners, and foods containing these products

2. Frequent consumption of fruits and fruit juices, especially tropical fruits such as mango, avocado, papaya, banana, kiwi, and others

3. Frequent consumption of dairy products, especially milk, ice cream, yogurt, cream, butter, and other lighter dairy, and foods containing dairy

4. Frequent consumption of refined flour products, especially yeasted bread, crackers, cookies, muffins, bagels, croissants, and other pastries made with white flour, as well as white rice and other polished grains and grain products

5. Frequent consumption of tropical vegetables, especially tomatoes, potatoes, eggplant, peppers, and other nightshade plants

6. Frequent consumption of oily, greasy, and fatty foods, including animal-quality foods, as well as salad dressings, spreads, sauces, nut and seed butters, and deep-fried foods

7. Frequent consumption of soft drinks, carbonated beverages, and mineral waters; aromatic and stimulating beverages, including flavored coffees, herbal teas, and spicy drinks; and wine or other lighter alcoholic beverages

Many aspects of modern life can also weaken natural resistance to disease. See "Solution" for lifestyle influences that may be considered contributing factors to the onset of AIDS.

SOLUTION

DIETARY GUIDELINES

The following recommendations may help prevent infection or slow the spread of viral contamination in a temperate climate. They are similar to those followed by the macrobiotic AIDS group in New York, some of whom are still alive and well today, twenty years after the medical study ended.

1. Avoid all meat, poultry, eggs, dairy food, sugar, chocolate, honey, sweets, spices, herbs, soft drinks, wine, alcohol, fruit, juice, coffee, chemicalized tea, and other stimulants, foods of tropical origin, and oily, greasy foods.

2. Avoid all baked flour products, which are excessively mucus-producing, except for occasional consumption of non-yeasted unleavened whole-wheat or rye bread, if craved.

3. Eliminate all chemicalized and artificially produced and treated foods and beverages.

4. Avoid or minimize vegetable oil in cooking and salad dressings for one to two months.

5. Raw salads are also to be avoided temporarily for one month or more.

6. All ice-cold foods and drinks should be avoided.

7. Fifty to 60 percent of daily food consumption, by weight, should consist of whole-cereal grains. The first day prepare plain pressure-cooked short-grain brown rice. The second day prepare brown rice cooked with 20 to 30 percent millet, the third day prepare brown rice with 20 to 30 percent barley, and the fourth day prepare brown rice with 20 to 30 percent adzuki beans or lentils. Then repeat the cycle starting with plain brown rice. A delicious morning porridge can be made by taking left-over rice, adding a little more water to make it soft, and seasoning with a small volume of miso at the end and simmering for two to three minutes more. Except for morning porridge, which may be soft, the grain should be cooked in a ratio of 2 parts grain to 1 part water. For seasoning, cook with a small postage stamp–size piece of kombu instead of salt—though in some cases sea salt may be substituted, depending on the person's condition. Other grains can be used occasionally, including whole wheat berries, rye, corn, and, after the first month, whole oats. Buckwheat and seitan (wheat gluten) should be minimized. Noodles, either udon or soba, may be eaten two or three times a week. Avoid all hard baked products until the condition improves, including cookies, cake, pie, crackers, muffins, and the like.

8. Five to 10 percent of the daily diet may

consist of soup, one or two servings. Miso soup may be eaten daily or frequently, prepared with wakame (a type of seaweed) and various land vegetables such as onions or kale. Occasionally a small volume of shiitake mushroom may be added to the soup. The miso may be barley miso, brown rice miso, or hatcho miso and should be naturally aged two to three years. To satisfy a desire for something sweet, millet soup with sweet vegetables such as squash, cabbage, onions, and carrots may be prepared often. Soups made from grains or beans may be taken from time to time.

9. Twenty to 30 percent of the daily diet may consist of vegetables, cooked in a variety of ways. Eat plenty of hard, green leafy vegetables, which are good for the liver and detoxification; round vegetables, such as squash, cabbage, and onions, which are good for the spleen and immune system; and root vegetables, such as daikon, carrot, and burdock, which are strengthening to the intestines and the blood and lymph system. As a rule, the following dishes may be prepared, though the frequency may differ from person to person: nishime-style (long-stewed) vegetables three to four times a week; squash-adzuki-kombu dish three times a week; dried daikon, one cup, three times a week; carrots and carrot tops or daikon and daikon tops, three times a week; boiled salad five to seven times a week; pressed salad, five to seven times a week; steamed greens, five to seven times a week; sautéed vegetables, use water instead of oil the first month, then occasionally a small volume of sesame oil may be brushed on the skillet; kinpira-style (matchsticks), sautéed in water, two-thirds of a cup, two times a week, then oil may be used after three weeks; dried tofu, tofu, or tempeh with vegetables, two times a week. As a special dish, vegetable nabe (lightly boiled vegetables and noodles cooked homestyle on the table) may be eaten frequently. Raw salad and salad dressing should be avoided.

10. Five percent small beans such as adzuki beans, lentils, chickpeas, or black soybeans may be used daily, cooked together with sea vegetables such as kombu or with onions and carrots. Other beans may be used altogether two to three times a month. For seasoning, a small volume of unrefined sea salt or shoyu or miso can be used. Bean products, such as tempeh, natto, and dried or cooked tofu may be used occasionally but in moderate volume. Avoid making the tofu too creamy and use firm rather than soft tofu.

11. A small volume of sea vegetable may be eaten daily, including wakame and kombu cooked in miso soup or used as a seasoning in preparing grains or beans. A sheet of toasted nori may also be taken daily. A small dish of hijiki or arame should be prepared two times a week.

12. Condiments to be available on the table are gomashio (sesame salt), on the average made with 1 part salt to 18 parts sesame seeds (reduced to 1:16 after two months), kombu, kelp, or wakame powder, umeboshi plum, and tekka. These condiments may be used daily on grains and vegetables, but the volume should be moderate to suit individual appetite and taste. Umeboshi (½ to 1 plum a day) and tekka (¼ to ⅓ teaspoon a day) are good to neutralize infection and restore digestive ability.

13. Pickles, made at home in a variety of ways, are to be eaten daily, 1 teaspoon in all, though long-time salty pickles should be minimized.

14. Though animal food is to be avoided, a small volume of white-meat ocean fish may be eaten once every week or two weeks. The fish should be prepared steamed, boiled, or poached and be garnished with grated daikon or ginger. After two months, fish may be eaten once or twice a week and may be prepared with other cooking styles such as broiling, grilling, and baking. Strictly avoid blue-meat and red-meat fish and all shellfish. For energy and vitality, *koi koku* (carp and burdock soup) may be taken if desired, 1 bowl for no more than three days in a row. For anemia, small dried fish (*iriko*) may be taken, sautéed in a little water or oil with shoyu at the end, 2 small pieces a day.

15. Avoid fruit as much as possible, including temperate as well as tropical fruit, until the condition improves. If cravings develop, a small volume of cooked fruit, especially apples, with a pinch of salt or dried fruit may be taken. Avoid all fruit juices and cider.

16. Avoid all sweets and desserts, including good-quality desserts, until the condition improves. Just a little sugar, chocolate, carob, honey, maple syrup, or soymilk will increase viral activity and bring out symptoms. To satisfy a sweet taste, use sweet vegetables every day in cooking, drink sweet vegetable drink (see special drinks below), and use sweet vegetable jam. Mochi, rice balls, sushi, and other grain-based snacks may be eaten frequently. Limit rice cakes, popcorn, and other dry or baked snacks as they may cause tightening. In the event of cravings, a small volume of grain-based sweeteners such as barley malt or rice syrup may be taken.

17. Nuts and nut butters are to be avoided due to their high amount of fat and protein, except for chestnuts. Unsalted, roasted seeds such as squash seeds and pumpkin seeds may be consumed as a snack, up to 1 cup altogether per week. Sunflower seeds may be taken only in the summer.

18. Seasonings, such as unrefined sea salt, shoyu, and miso, are to be used moderately to avoid unnecessary thirst. Avoid mirin (a sweet cooking wine) and garlic. If thirst arises after the meal or between meals, cut back on these seasonings until normal thirst returns. Do not add shoyu to food at the table.

19. Drink bancha twig tea as the main beverage. Strictly avoid all aromatic, stimulant beverages, and refrain from grain coffee for the first two to three months. Spring water is ideal for drinking and cooking, followed by well water or filtered tap water. Avoid distilled and mineral waters.

20. The most important thing in connection with dietary practice is chewing very well, until all food becomes liquid in the mouth and well mixed with saliva. Chew very well, at least 50 times, preferably 100 times per mouthful. It is also important to avoid overeating and eating within three hours of sleeping.

21. Persons who have received or who are currently undergoing medical treatment may need to make further dietary modifications. Please consult your medical doctor, nutritionist, or other health-care professional.

CAUTION

1. Many people who have tested positive for HIV and are asymptomatic respond to these nutritional and lifestyle guidelines. In cases where the person has been diagnosed with AIDS and has light to moderate symptoms, this approach is also often helpful, though it may need to be modified. In an official statement on Diet and Nutrition, the Office of Alternative Medicine, a branch of the U.S. National Institutes of Health, observed:

Persons with inadequate nutrition who are HIV infected have an increased susceptibility to opportunistic infections and a more rapid disease progression. Even when nutritional intake is adequate, an HIV-positive person may lose weight long before he or she develops AIDS. This happens because, throughout the progression of HIV infection, the patient's nutritional status is challenged by the manifestations of symptoms such as nausea, vomiting, malabsorption, diarrhea, oral/esophageal problems, and infections that impeded fat storage. People with HIV may also develop lactose intolerance. After HIV infection has progressed to AIDS, malabsorption of nutrients may become severe. Weight loss can cause a vicious cycle of fatigue, muscle-wasting, and loss of appetite. Nutritionists and dietitians work with people with HIV infection to design diets that provide those nutrients that may be lacking. Some practitioners work within mainstream medicine, while others have unique approaches.

In more serious cases, depending on the degree of immune function loss or complications from opportunistic infections, medical attention may be required. In any life-threatening situation, a physician should immediately be contacted.

2. In the case of prior or ongoing medical treatment, the dietary recommendations may need to be adjusted further. AIDS patients suffering from "wasting" symptoms or lipodystrophy syndrome (a clinical condition characterized by poor or uneven distribution of fat cells) may also need to make modifications, such as increased protein, more fat and oil, and other adjustments. Please consult with a medical doctor, nutritionist, or other health-care professional.

3. AZT, HAART, and other drugs used to control AIDS are helpful in some cases and are harmful in others. Very serious side effects have been reported in the medical literature and in personal accounts of AIDS patients, including abortion, miscarriage, stroke, heart attack, kidney and liver damage, diabetes, and death. For example, researchers reported in 1994 (Kumar et al., *J. AIDS*, 7:1034) that in a study of 104 women with HIV treated with AZT, 8 had spontaneous abortions, 8 had to undergo therapeutic abortions, and 8 gave birth to babies with birth defects such as heart defects, extra fingers, misplaced ears, triangular faces, misformed spine, and cavities in the chest.

Lipodystrophy, a common side effect of HAART, results in the storage of large amounts of fat in inappropriate places in the body, which can lead to obesity in the lower abdomen and a buffalo-like hump on the upper back. It is strongly advised that anyone considering the use of such procedures carefully weigh the risks and benefits and consult with his or her physician or other health-care giver.

LIFESTYLE

Observe the standard way-of-life suggestions. The following influences can all lower, weaken, or suppress natural immune function, contributing to increased susceptibility to infection and the spread of viruses associated with AIDS. They should be avoided or minimized as much as possible.

1. Artificial influences at birth, including cesarean section, the use of forceps, drugs, and other emergency measures; and lack of breast-feeding as an infant

2. Overuse or abuse of medication, including over-the-counter and prescription drugs

3. Removal of the tonsils, adenoids, and other glands

4. Exposure to X rays, CAT scans, MRIs, radiation therapy (internal or external), and other strong forms of artificial electromagnetic radiation during medical or dental examinations and procedures

5. Exposure to ELF (extremely low frequency) radiation, from television, computers, cellular phones, and other electronic devices

6. Abuse of drugs, including amphetamines, barbiturates, marijuana, LSD, cocaine, and substances that enhance sexual performance

7. Exposure to or abuse of medical treatments, including surgery, chemotherapy, and mercury amalgam dental fillings

8. Abuse of antibiotics and antivirals to treat infections, especially herpes and other venereal diseases

9. Environmental pollution, including declining air, water, and soil quality; exposure to chemicals and toxins; living in overly insulated modern houses made of synthetic building materials and furnished with synthetic carpets, drapes, and furniture; and the overall weakening effects of global warming and the thinning of the planet's ozone layer

10. Promiscuous sexual activity, including multiple partners, unprotected sex, frequent oral or anal sex, and sexual activity accompanied by drug use

HOME REMEDIES

In addition to the above dietary recommendations, there are several special drinks or foods that may be taken to strengthen the immune function.

1. UMEBOSHI PLUMS may be eaten often, every day or every other day, for several weeks, and then gradually less often or as needed.

2. SWEET VEGETABLE DRINK may be prepared, 1 to 2 small cups every day for the first month, then every other day the second month, and then several times a week after that as desired.

3. Prepare a special condiment of chopped lotus root, carrots, kombu, and adzuki beans (cooked with five times as much water and with a pinch of sea salt). Take 1 to 2 small cups every day for 20 days.

4. BAKED KOMBU CONDIMENT is also helpful for this condition. Take 1 teaspoon daily for ten days, then every other day for ten days, and then occasionally as desired for four to six weeks.

5. For strength and vitality, KOI-KOKU or KINPIRA SOUP may be taken occasionally.

MEDICAL EVIDENCE

AIDS PATIENTS RESPOND TO MACROBIOTIC DIET

A group of men with AIDS in New York City began macrobiotics under the auspices of researchers at Boston University's School of Medicine and the medical director of the Fashion Institute of Technology. The blood and immune functions of men with Kaposi's sarcoma were tested. Most of the men (originally 10 and later expanded to 20) stabilized on the diet, and their lymphocyte number increased steadily over the first two years from diagnosis. The researchers reported significant improvement in their total T cell numbers, notably in T4 counts. "The approach has demonstrated effective in managing their condition while minimizing opportunistic infections and use of toxic drugs," observed principal researcher Martha Cottrell, M.D. "They are all working full time and enjoying a quality of life atypical of most AIDS patients." The results compared favorably with those from any other AIDS study published.

Sources: "Patients with Kaposi Sarcoma Who Opt for No Treatment" (letter), *Lancet,* July 1985; Elinor Levy et al., "Patients with Kaposi's Sarcoma Who Opt for Alternative Therapy," International AIDS Conference, Paris, France, 1986; Elinor M. Levy, letter to the American Cancer Society, March 3, 1988; Martha Cottrell, letter to the American Cancer Society, March 14, 1988.

RICE BRAN INHIBITS HIV

A compound found in rice bran inhibits HIV in laboratory and clinical tests. A scientific team at Drew University of Medicine in Los Angeles reported that MGN-3, isolated from rice bran that had been modified enzymatically, inhibited HIV activity in cultured blood tests. Further studies of ingestion of the rice bran product found that it resulted in significant increase in T and B cell mitogen response two months after treatment. The scientists concluded that the substance "possesses potent anti-HIV activity and in the absence of any notable side effects, MGN-3 shows promise as an agent for treating patients with AIDS."

Source: M. Ghoneum, "Anti-HIV Activity in Vitro of MGN-3, an Activated Arabinoxylane from Rice Bran," *Biochem Biophys Res Commun* 243(1):25–29, 1998.

BEANS CONTAIN STRONG ANTI-HIV FACTORS

Beans contain substances that have strong anti-HIV effects. In Hong Kong, Chinese scientists reported that rice beans contained an antifungal protein that inhibited the activity of HIV-1 reverse transcriptase. Another study found that a variety of leguminous plants, including French bean, cowpea, field bean, peanut, and red kidney bean, contained antifungal proteins that produced the same effect. The legumes also suppressed protease and integrase, enzymes essential to the life cycle of HIV. "The results indicate that nearly all leguminous antifungal proteins examined were able to inhibit HIV-1 reverse transcriptase, protease, and integrase," the researchers concluded.

Sources: Ye Xy and Ng Tb, "Delandin, a Chitinase-like Protein with Antifungal, HIV-1 Reverse Transcriptase Inhibitory and Mitogenic Activities from the Rice Bean Delandia Umbellata," *Protein Expre Purif* 24(3):524–29, 2002, and Ng Tb et al., "Inhibitory Effects of Antifungal Proteins on Human Immunodeficiency Virus Type 1 Reverse Transcriptase, Protease, and Integrase," *Life Sci* 70(8):927–35, 2002.

CASE HISTORY

MACROBIOTICS HELPS CONTROL SYMPTOMS OF AIDS

Frank, a young man in New York, suffered from parasites and AIDS-related complex, including Kaposi's sarcoma. His doctor recommended that he stop eating dairy products and red meat and look into macrobiotics. Frank responded immediately to the diet, losing substantial excess weight and experiencing increased vitality and brighter, clearer skin and eyes. His T cell counts rose to normal levels. He no longer craved meat, ice cream, liquor, marijuana, coffee, and the other foods he was used to. Instead of steaks and martinis, he ate rice balls on frequent business trips around the country. Frank wrote up his experience for the *New York Native*, a gay publication, and raised public awareness about diet and AIDS. "I'm not going to take any chances or be foolish in any way of living. The time to heal, the time to live, is now," he observed.

Source: Michio Kushi and Martha Cottrell, M.D., *AIDS, Macrobiotics, and Natural Immunity* (New York and Tokyo: Japan Publications, 1990).

◎ ALLERGIES

Allergies are abnormal reactions to a food, chemical, drug, or other substance. They may be mild and occasional, serious and troubling, or dangerous and life-threatening. Common allergies include hay fever, asthma, and other respiratory allergies; hives and other skin allergies; food allergies; drug allergies; and allergies to bee stings and other insect bites. In this section, we shall look at the general macrobiotic approach to allergies and several types of allergies. *See also "Asthma" in "Lung Problems."* In most cases, dietary imbalance underlies susceptibility to allergic reactions, and changing the way of eating will eliminate most abnormal reactions to windborne particles, foods, drugs, or environmental irritants.

SYMPTOMS

The following symptoms may accompany allergies:

1. Sneezing, coughing, or nasal congestion
2. Itchy eyes, mouth, or throat
3. Stomachache, indigestion, heartburn
4. Cramps, diarrhea, nausea
5. Inflamed, reddened, itchy skin
6. Stiffness, swelling, and pain in the joints or bones
7. Anaphylactic shock, indicated by sudden skin welts, intense flushing and itching, rapid heartbeat

CAUSES

1. Allergies are usually triggered by contact with specific foods such as milk, nuts, or shellfish; substances such as pollen, dust, or animal dander; drugs and medications; and insect bites. Such reactions usually show that the blood, lymph, and other bodily fluids are imbalanced from consumption of too many acid-producing foods, including animal products, dairy foods, sugar and sweets, stimulants, spices, alcohol, chemically grown or treated foods, and other articles in the modern way of eating as well as lack of whole grains, fresh vegetables, and other high-fiber foods that help discharge toxins from the body.

2. Overall the condition of someone with allergies tends to be more yin—overly expansive, loose, and weak. Most allergens or triggers are also extremely yin, so that yin repels yin and the body attempts to throw off the allergen or trigger by sneezing, itching, or other reaction. The principal foods that cause allergies are milk and all other dairy products, overly oily and greasy foods, animal fat, sugar and other concentrated or artificial sweets and sweeteners, refined foods and flour products, tropical fruits, juices, and vegetables with tropical origins (tomatoes, potatoes, eggplants, avocados, and others), and often various drugs, chemical additives, and similar products. Among these, dairy foods, sugar, and tropical fruits are probably the most common and prevalent causes.

3. In some cases, a person who is imbalanced and rarely eats healthy foods will take something balanced, which triggers a discharge. For example, wheat and rice are very strengthening and when taken by someone whose condition is too acidic may cause the person to rapidly eliminate excess mucus, fat, and other stagnation. The person may think she is allergic to whole grains, when actually the lack of these

foods is causing her problem. In this case, the amount of whole grain or other healthy food needs to be reduced or taken less frequently to avoid an overreaction. Over time, as the condition improves, she will be gradually able to consume more of the healthy foods that she could not eat before.

4. Sometimes reactions to potentially harmful drugs, chemicals, and other toxins are a normal reaction and not an allergic reaction. Penicillin and other strong drugs, for example, will cause strong effects in a generally healthy person because his immune function is strong and immediately reacts to the medication.

FORMS

Atopy. Atopy refers to a type of allergy in which the irritant produces a reaction at a distance from the contact—for example, swallowing a substance that leads to eczema or dermatitis. The underlying cause of atopic reactions is weak blood and acidic conditions brought about by dietary extremes, particularly strong yin in the form of sugar, chocolate, and other refined sweeteners; milk, cream, and other dairy products; white flour in bread, cookies, and pastries; excessive fruit and juice, especially of tropical origin; stimulants; spices; and other overly expansive items.

To help relieve atopy, observe Diet #1 for conditions caused by extreme yin factors. Take SWEET VEGETABLE DRINK, 2 cups a day (1 cup in the morning and 1 cup in the evening) for 3 to 4 weeks. Take UME-SHO KUZU, 1 cup a day or every other day, for 3 weeks when the intestines have a problem. Drink BANCHA TWIG TEA, cooled to room temperature after boiling, in between and after meals. Take a BANCHA TEA BATH every day or every other day. To stop itching, do a BANCHA TEA COMPRESS on the affected region or apply one of the following: pure CAMELLIA OIL; RICE BRAN COMPRESS; KOMBU PLASTER; DRIED DAIKON LEAVES COMPRESS (apply the last for 2 to 3 hours and change the gauze frequently).

Chemical Allergies. There are an estimated 50,000 or more different chemicals in foods, drugs, and the environment. Everyone is exposed to these substances to some extent. Strong reactions may be produced by chemical fertilizers, pesticides, or additives in foods; toxic fumes; factory smoke; aerosol sprays; automobile exhaust; and other pollutants. Allergic reactions to latex, a rubber used in protective gloves, condoms, and many other items, have soared in recent years. In most cases, these have strong yin effects, contributing to forgetfulness, loss of clarity, scattered thinking, lack of coordination, and other dispersing, disintegrating, and weakening effects. Carbon dioxide, heavy metals, and some other elements and compounds can produce heaviness, tightness, rigidity, and other contracting, yang effects. To protect against or relieve chemical allergies, follow the guidelines for Diet #1 or Diet #2 and see the suggestions below, adjusting slightly for yin or yang if the cause is known. Otherwise, centrally balanced Diet #3 may safely be followed. In addition, pay careful attention to getting as much organic food as possible. Eat nishime-style vegetables two or three times a week for two to three months. As part of a varied diet, take brown rice, miso soup, and sea vegetables daily. Miso rice can be included often. Take UME-SHO

KUZU twice a week. Some of the home remedies in "Home Remedies" may be helpful.

Drug Allergies. Over a half million Americans experience allergic reactions to penicillin and other drugs and medications each year. In extreme cases, these can lead to *anaphylaxis*, a severe reaction that can cause death within minutes. Symptoms include closing down of the air passages, a sharp drop in blood pressure, irregular heartbeat, vomiting, cramps, and loss of consciousness. Three-quarters of lethal reactions are caused by penicillin or other antibiotics, but virtually all drugs can cause this reaction, including aspirin, ibuprofen, and other anti-inflammatory medications, sulfa drugs, muscle relaxants, hypertension drugs, and blood products and dyes used in X-ray examinations. Vaccines and inoculations can also cause serious, sometimes lethal reactions, in susceptible children and adults. Physicians treat anaphylaxis with epinephrine (adrenaline), which can be administered by syringe or a self-injecting device.

From a macrobiotic perspective, reactions to drugs, medications, and vaccines are usually a healthy sign. The body is rejecting foreign, potentially dangerous substances. However, in the event of an anaphylactic reaction, immediate medical attention is required. Epinephrine is an artificial form of adrenaline, a strong yang hormone, that relaxes respiratory muscles, constricts blood vessels, stimulates the heart, and reduces swelling. UMEBOSHI PLUM, TEKKA, GOMASHIO, or other yang condiment may also be helpful. To prevent future attacks, a balanced macrobiotic way of eating is essential. Follow the guidelines for Diet #3 until the con-dition improves. Be extremely careful not to eat any meat, poultry, or dairy from animals treated with antibiotics.

Food Allergies. Various foods including dairy products, egg whites, wheat products, corn products, chocolate, peanuts and other legumes or nuts, fruits, mustard, tomatoes, sweets, shellfish, and various meats can trigger allergic reactions. Symptoms include indigestion, nasal irritation and mucus discharge, vomiting, diarrhea, cramps, nausea, swelling of the face and tongue, dizziness, sweating, and faintness. About two-thirds of people with food allergies are under thirty, and the majority are children under six. Tests for food allergies are not always reliable since different combinations of foods, different cooking styles, and the amount of chewing can vary, producing different effects. Allergies to extreme foods, especially dairy products, meat, and shellfish, are actually the body's natural reaction to harmful substances. Monosodium glutamate (MSG), an artificial flavor enhancer used in Oriental cooking, may produce tingling, numbness, headaches, and temporary paralysis. Sulfites, commonly added to foods and wine as a preservative, can also produce allergic reactions that are unhealthy.

In most cases, children and young adults who experience food allergies are too yin and should follow the guidelines for Diet #1 to strengthen their blood quality and reduce their sensitivity to selected foods. In the meantime, they should avoid the food that causes a reaction for three to four months, until their blood quality changes. Every day, miso soup and a small amount of sea vegetables should be taken. Special items to be taken daily or every other day for one month include (1) a small cup of KOMBU TEA, (2) ½ to 1 UMEBOSHI PLUM or an equivalent amount of shiso leaves in BANCHA TWIG TEA as a condiment with rice or other grains, and (3) SHIO-KOMBU, roasted wakame, nori condiment, or other sea vegetable condiment. Thorough chewing is also essential, at least fifty times per mouthful. Some of the remedies at the end of this section may also be beneficial.

Lactose Intolerance. Lactose intolerance, the inability to digest milk and other dairy products, affects the vast majority of the world's people. Except for some people of European origin, after infancy most people lack lactase, the pancreatic enzyme that enables them to digest lactose or milk sugar. As a result, a little milk can produce cramps, nausea, diarrhea, and bloating. Responding to this widespread condition, the dairy industry has introduced lactose-reduced or lactose-free milk that has from 70 to 99 percent of the lactose removed. The 2000 edition of the *U.S. Dietary Guidelines* recognized that many people suffer from this condition and can get sufficient calcium, iron, and other nutrients exclusively from plant sources. To prevent or relieve lactose intolerance, follow the standard macrobiotic diet and avoid dairy products. The home remedies section below has hints on how to discharge accumulated mucus and fat.

Hay Fever. Hay fever is an allergy accompanied by sneezing, itchy eyes or nose, a runny nose, head and nasal congestion, and sometimes fever. The seasonal form is commonly triggered by pollen from trees, grass, weeds, rag-

weed, fungus, or other plants when they come into bloom. The perennial form can take place at any time of the year and be triggered by dust, animal dander, mold, feathers, or household fabrics (linen, bedding, clothing, pillows, carpets). Attacks typically last 15 to 20 minutes and may occur several times a day. An estimated 20 million Americans suffer from hay fever.

Cold milk is a primary cause of hay fever, with fruit, juice, sugar, sweets, soft drinks, and chemically grown or treated food as contributing factors. From the macrobiotic view, pollen is yin—light, expansive, blowing up and out. When it enters the nasal passages or lungs, yin (pollen) repels yin (dairy, fruit, sweets, etc.), causing sneezing, coughing, and discharge of mucus. Extreme yin foods also make the blood, lymph, and internal membranes sticky, so that when pollen is inhaled, it remains and adheres to the surfaces, producing irritation, instead of being discharged smoothly. A balanced macrobiotic way of eating can often relieve hay fever and other allergies without the need for antihistamines, nasal sprays, decongestants, and other medications.

To prevent or relieve hay fever, follow the guidelines for Diet #1 with the following considerations: Avoid or minimize oatmeal, flaked grains, corn grits, and other processed grains in favor of grains in whole form. Take miso soup or miso rice daily. Limit or avoid "occasional-use" vegetables temporarily, emphasizing those for "regular use" until the condition improves. Avoid raw foods except for pickles. Minimize oil, using it only for lightly sautéed vegetables once or twice a week. Reduce the intake of beans and bean products, using smaller portions of the regular-use beans only. Among bean products, dried tofu is the best. Seasonings, including shoyu, miso, and umeboshi, should be light. Avoid nuts and nut or seed butters. Avoid fruit completely, as well as spices and animal foods, except for white-meat fish, if desired, once or twice a week. Do a BODY SCRUB with a hot, damp towel once a day. The home remedies below include several teas and external applications that may be helpful to discharge mucus and relieve discomfort.

Hives and Other Skin Allergies. Hives are raised white welts that are surrounded by a red border and usually itch. Swellings may also appear beneath the skin that burn instead of itch, particularly around the eyes and lips and occasionally on the hands and feet or inside the throat or reproductive organs. Generally, hives are short-lived, lasting several minutes to several days. However, they can cause serious, potentially fatal complications, especially if they appear in the throat, block the air passages, or lead to severe intestinal contractions. Modern medicine considers hives an allergic condition triggered by certain foods, such as dairy products, fish, and nuts; penicillin, aspirin, and other drugs; food additives, flavorings, or preservatives; exposure to temperature extremes; stress; insect bites; and other factors. Antihistamines, oral corticosteroids, and ultraviolet light are common treatments.

From the macrobiotic view, hives and other skin allergies are the result of overly acidic blood and weakened natural immunity. Intestinal weaknesses, an overactive gallbladder, and other organ troubles are often present and generally correspond with the location of the outbreak, for example, hives on the outside of the calves along the gallbladder meridian. A centrally balanced diet will help prevent and relieve hives. Observe the guidelines for Diet #1 with the following modifications: Avoid buckwheat and soba noodles. Take nishime-style vegetables daily or every other day for one month, especially daikon and daikon leaves cooked with kombu, with a little shoyu or miso to taste. Reduce the volume of beans and their products. Avoid salad and fruit. Avoid fish, though a small portion of white-meat fish may be taken occasionally, mixed in with vegetables, if craved. Avoid sunflower seeds and nuts. Sesame and pumpkin seeds are fine. Take 1 cup of ADZUKI BEAN TEA daily for 5 to 7 days and then twice a week. Add a pinch of sea salt to the juice. If the skin is inflamed or irritated, apply either a RICE BRAN PLASTER with green leafy vegetables or a green nori plaster with green leafy vegetables. Wear organic cotton, especially against the skin. Scrub the body with a rice bran wash.

Insect Bites. Mosquito bites, wasp or bee stings, and other insect bites are directly related to a person's blood quality. Overconsumption of sugar, honey, chocolate, and other refined sweeteners, soft drinks, tropical foods, fruit and juice, ice cream and dairy products, and other extreme yin foods, as well as animal foods, create an overly acidic condition. Mosquitoes and other insects like thinner, sweeter-smelling, yin blood and will avoid heavier, yang blood that tends to thicken before it reaches their stomachs. Whole grains, vegetables from land and sea, and other more alkalinizing foods will strengthen the blood and dramatically reduce insect bites.

To relieve simple mosquito bites, slice the white section of a scallion or leek and run it over the affected area. The juice of an onion or ginger root may also be used. For bee or wasp stings, use a similar treatment using a daikon or radish. For a spider bite, mix 1 teaspoon of sesame oil with ¼ teaspoon of salt and apply on the bite. For scorpion or centipede bites, crush and mix a raw egg and cover the affected area. To improve the overall condition, follow Diet #1 for more yin conditions for several days or several weeks. Take UME-SHO KUZU several days in a row to strengthen the blood. In case of severe itching, such as bites from blackflies all over the legs, senna tea is traditionally used in the East to eliminate the pain and reduce swelling. It is available in some Oriental food stores.

SOLUTION

DIET

Follow the guidelines recommended above, focusing on the following:

1. Eat whole cereal grains at every meal, temporarily avoiding all processed grains and grain products.

2. Vegetables can be prepared in a variety of cooking styles, especially iron-rich vegetables such as collards, kale, mustard greens, turnip greens, and other green leafy vegetables. NISHIME-STYLE VEGETABLES, including root vegetables cooked with kombu, are especially recommended to strengthen the blood, and cooked adzuki beans with winter squash and kombu are also indicated. SAUTÉED VEGETABLES may be prepared a few times a week. In this case, you may use a little sesame oil for stir-frying.

3. Slightly reduce the consumption of beans and bean products, focusing on regular-use beans.

4. All types of sea vegetables are helpful and will help strengthen the blood.

5. Choose organic foods for your ingredients as much as possible.

LIFESTYLE

Observe the way-of-life suggestions, emphasizing the following:

1. It is desirable to keep physically active. This will increase the intake of oxygen and strengthen the blood.

2. Avoid taking long baths and showers: make them shorter. It is helpful to add a handful of salt to the hot water of the bathtub when bathing.

3. Try to spend your time as often as possible in a natural environment with many trees and plants.

4. Avoid electrical appliances such as computers, television sets, and cell phones as much as possible.

5. Avoid or limit exposure to chemicals, plastics, and other artificial materials in the environment, including body care products, home furnishings, fabrics, and clothing. Use natural materials as much as possible, especially plant-quality as opposed to animal-quality.

HOME REMEDIES

Some of the following home remedies may be helpful for chronic allergies, especially the accumulation of mucus in the body, or for allergic reactions. The frequency and duration of use will depend on the person's condition and the nature of the symptoms.

1. Take UME-SHO KUZU two to three times a week to strengthen the blood.

2. For strength and vitality, KINPIRA SOUP may be taken occasionally.

3. A daily BODY SCRUB will help improve blood and energy circulation.

4. To relieve coughing and dissolve excess mucus, take LOTUS ROOT JUICE TEA. This is especially helpful for allergic bronchitis, hay fever, or asthma.

5. LOTUS ROOT TEA taken occasionally is also good for eliminating mucus.

6. Lotus seeds cooked with kombu can also help to clear up stagnated mucus. Fresh or dried lotus root may be used instead of the seeds.

7. A GINGER COMPRESS will help soften mucus deposits. Apply two to three times a week for several weeks until the condition improves.

8. A LOTUS ROOT PLASTER will draw out excess mucus from the sinuses, lungs, and bronchi.

9. A BUCKWHEAT PLASTER will draw out excess fluid from swollen areas.

10. A MUSTARD PLASTER will stimulate circulation and loosen stagnation.

11. For female sexual organ troubles, a DAIKON HIP BATH and bancha tea douche are recommended.

12. A rice bran–leafy greens plaster will reduce discomfort from skin irritation or inflammation. Apply on the feverish area and remove it when the paste becomes warm or hot.

13. Greens with nori plaster will also help reduce discomfort from skin irritation or inflammation.

14. A TOFU AND LEAFY GREENS PLASTER will also help bring down inflammation and swelling. When the mixture becomes warm, generally every two to three hours, exchange it for a fresh application.

15. Take a BANCHA TEA BATH every day or every other day to help neutralize acidity and improve energy flow. (Tea stains the bathtub, so it is better not to keep the tea in the tub for a long time. Wash the tub well after using.)

16. To stop itching and irritation, do a BANCHA TEA COMPRESS on the affected region or apply one of the following: pure CAMELLIA OIL; RICE BRAN COMPRESS; KOMBU PLASTER; DRIED DAIKON LEAVES COMPRESS (apply the last for about two to three hours and change the gauze frequently).

CAUTION

1. In rare cases, a person with allergies will experience anaphylactic shock. This is a medical emergency that can be life-threatening, and prompt medical attention is necessary.

2. Read food labels and product labels carefully and avoid those containing chemicals or artificial additives. Avoid genetically altered foods as much as possible (note that many are not labeled as such).

CASE HISTORY

MACROBIOTICS HELPS CONTROL ENVIRONMENTAL ILLNESS

As a child, Vincent Armenio had allergies to eggs, cow's milk, wheat, and nuts. Later he suffered from asthma, frequent colds, and constant lung and head congestion. Though treated by the leading allergy specialist in Boston, he never really improved. Vincent struggled through high school but had to drop out of Georgetown Law School because of his worsening health. The major exams always coincided with the cherry blossoms and pollen season in Washington, D.C.

Moving to New York, Vincent got a job in TV time sales, a high-pressure position, and led an active singles lifestyle. However, his allergic reactions were almost impossible to bear. He could sleep only with Valium and would wake up each morning in a zombielike trance. "It was as if someone had charged my head with an electric shock," he recalled. Even with the support of family and friends, his life became dysfunctional. Moving to California, he took a job in the San Joaquin Valley, which had a year-long growing season and the most chemically intensive agriculture in the country. Taking classes in nutrition and experimenting with vegetarianism, Vincent's quest for health eventually led him to macrobiotics. He realized that he had been eating too much animal food, flour products, oily foods, chips, and a lot of what he called "health food junk food." On a diet centered around whole grains and vegetables, Vincent finally began to get well. His pollen and food allergies dramatically improved, and his hypoglycemia and candida started to clear up. At the Kushi Institute, where he studied and worked in the gardens, he met a young woman from Japan. Today, Vincent is married, a proud father, and free from the allergies and illnesses that plagued him most of his life.

Source: "Diet and Environmental Illness: The Vincent Armenio Story," *One Peaceful World Journal* 10, spring, 1992.

⊚ MEDICAL EVIDENCE

BREAST-FEEDING PROTECTS BABIES FROM ALLERGIES

Several clinical studies in infants at risk for atopic disease found that prolonged breast-feeding reduces the incidence of this disease. "Sensitization to food antigens may occur already in utero because infants whose mothers avoid common allergenic foods during the whole pregnancy and then during the lactation period have a lower incidence of atopic eczema than infants whose mothers are on an unrestricted diet," scientists at the Universitats-Kinderklinic in Wien, Germany, reported. The researchers reported that avoiding common allergenic foods by the mother only during the last three months of pregnancy had no effect.

Source: F. Haschke et al., "Does Breast Feeding Protect from Atopic Diseases?," *Padiatr Padol* 1990; 25(6): 415–20.

DIETARY APPROACH TO INFANT ALLERGIES

Prolonged breast-feeding, avoidance of infant dairy formula, and delayed introduction of dairy food, eggs, fish, nuts, and soybeans may reduce the incidence of allergic symptoms and reactions from infancy and childhood through puberty and the teenage years. A medical researcher at the Memorial University of Newfoundland in St. John's, Canada, reported that the protective effects of these measures could last up to 18 years. "Diet and nutrition in early life are crucial for the development of allergic and infectious disease throughout childhood and into adulthood," the researcher concluded.

Source: R. K. Chandra, "Food Allergy and Nutrition in Early Life: Implications for Health," *Proc Nutr Soc* May 2000: 59(2); 273–7.

DAIRY PRIMARY CAUSE OF CHILDHOOD ALLERGIES

Food causes 82.9 percent of allergic reactions in school-aged children, and among these milk was involved in 32 percent of the cases, the Division of Allergy & Immunology, Department of Pediatrics, Mount Sinai Medical Center in New York City reported. In a study of 132 children with known allergies, 58 percent reported allergic reactions in the past two years. Eighteen percent experienced one or more reactions in school. After milk, the most allergenic foods were peanuts (29 percent of cases), eggs (18 percent), tree nuts (6 percent), and other foods (3 percent).

Source: A. Nowak-Wegrzyn et al., "Food-Allergic Reactions in Schools and Preschools," *Arch Pediatr Adolesc Med* 2001 Jul; 155(7): 790–5.

ALLERGIC TO PIZZA?

Pizza may be a main cause of the rising incidence of allergies in modern society. An Italian researcher states that the increased availability of pizza, number of varieties, and different spices and artificial additives added to pizza may be responsible for this trend. "In the beginning, it was the food of the poor, but was made with natural foods, but nowadays has been enriched by a number of ingredients and flavorings, thus multiplying the risk of allergic reactions," the scientist concluded.

Source: A. Cantani, "Allergy to Pizza," *Eur Rev Med Pharmacol Sci* 1999 Sep–Oct; 3(5):235–6.

MACROBIOTIC DIET EFFECTIVE
FOR CHEMICAL SENSITIVITY

In a study of 160 patients with chemical sensitivity, including multiple allergies, those who observed a macrobiotic dietary approach, high in whole grains, vegetables, beans, and sea vegetables, for at least one year, reported an average decrease in symptoms of 76 percent. A macro-

biotic diet "should be considered for those with persistent symptoms triggered by chemical exposure," the physician concluded.

Source: S. Rogers, M.D., "Improvement in Chemical Sensitivity with the Macrobiotic Diet," *Journal of Applied Nutrition* 48: 85–92, 1996.

GM FOODS MAY PROVE FATAL

Genetically altered soybeans and rapeseed (used in making canola oil), altered with genes from Brazil nuts to boost their low cysteine and methionine content, were withdrawn from development after medical studies showed that they could cause deadly allergic reactions in people sensitive to the nuts. "Since genetic engineers mix genes from a wide variety of species," noted Dr. Rebecca J. Goldburg of the Environmental Defense Fund, "other genetically engineered foods may cause similar health problems. People who are allergic to one type of food may suddenly find they are allergic to many more."

Source: J. Nordlee et al., "Identification of a Brazil-Nut Allergen in Transgenic Soybeans," *New England Journal of Medicine* 334:688–92, 1996.

FARM PESTICIDE PRODUCES ALLERGIES

A medical study found that almost half of farm workers who harvested vegetables sprayed with a common pesticide developed allergies in one month after picking, and 70 percent developed reactions after three months. The study examined Bt, the most common pesticide spliced into genetically engineered food. Mary-Howell Martens, an environmental specialist, expressed concern that "many, many more people will be exposed to the Bt toxin and will likely be sensitized by eating crops engineered with the gene for the toxin."

Source: "Bt Is as Bt Does," *Science News*, Sept. 4, 1999.

◎ BLEEDING AND BLOOD DISORDERS

Blood, the essence of life, includes red blood cells, white blood cells, platelets, and plasma, or the fluid in which the other elements are suspended. The plasma constitutes about 55 percent of the bloodstream, while the formed elements make up the other 45 percent. Blood disorders range from a mild tendency to bleed to severe hemophilia, from Rh incompatibility to leukemia. Modern medicine treats blood primarily as a fuel and has developed many blood products, including artificial substances, to fortify and purify the blood. In macrobiotic healing, blood is directly related to diet, and changes in our daily way of eating can strengthen or weaken the blood. Broadly, all sicknesses and disorders are related to our blood quality. A balanced way of eating, centered on whole grains and vegetables, will create healthy blood and protect against most diseases. *For abnormal blood pressure and other circulatory disorders, see "Heart Disease and Circulatory Problems."*

SYMPTOMS

The following symptoms may accompany blood disorders:

1. Bleeding
2. Pale face
3. Cold hands and feet
4. Irregular heartbeat
5. Low blood sugar level
6. Lack of drive
7. Fatigue of the whole body
8. Headache
9. Nervousness or nerve dullness
10. Anemia
11. Mental and emotional instability, including lack of positive view of life, anxiety, lack of courage and patience, depression, stress

CAUSE

1. Under normal conditions, blood is produced in the intestines. Food molecules are absorbed in the villi of the small intestine and enter the bloodstream, where they change into white blood cells, plasma, and eventually red blood cells and platelets. The iron core of the blood, hemoglobin, has a construction similar to that of chlorophyll, which has magnesium at the center of the molecule instead of iron. Through transmutation, magnesium from plant foods, in combination with oxygen circulating in the cells, changes into iron, contributing to the formation of strong blood. The intestines create white blood cells and plasma, and later with the assistance of the liver and spleen, white blood cells change into red blood cells. This process is not understood by modern science and medicine, which believe blood is created in the bone marrow. The reason for this misunderstanding is that the classic experiments on the origin of the blood were conducted with chickens, mice, and other animals placed on a fasting diet. Due to lack of food, normal blood was no longer being produced in the intestines. Instead, stored elements in the

bone marrow, which is at the very end of the bloodstream, converted back into red blood cells, giving the appearance that they originated at this site. Hence, modern science focuses on healthy bones and bone marrow, rather than diet, as the underlying factor in maintaining healthy blood. Blood and bones are also associated in the popular imagination with red meat, and so sirloin steak, roast beef, and other animal foods are mistakenly considered to be superior sources of iron, protein, and other nutrients.

2. The blood is normally slightly alkaline, with a pH between 7.3 and 7.45. Acidosis results if the pH falls below this level. The body compensates by exhaling more acids during respiration and by buffer mechanisms that neutralize acids in the bloodstream, such as the conversion of hydrochloric acid into water, carbon dioxide, and other byproducts. Many foods in the modern diet are acid-producing, including meat, poultry, eggs, milk and other dairy products, sugar and other refined sweeteners, oil and oily, greasy foods, refined grains, tropical foods, fruit and juice, spices, stimulants, alcohol, and drugs. These foods create weaker, more acid blood, causing the lungs, kidneys, liver, spleen, heart, and other major organs to work harder to maintain an alkaline condition. In addition to chemical reactions, the bloodstream offsets acidosis by drawing upon stored minerals, including sodium, calcium, and phosphorus, in the teeth, bones, and other compact areas of the body, weakening these organs and functions in order to keep the blood slightly alkaline.

3. Extreme yin foods, including sugar, chocolate, honey, and other sweeteners; milk, ice cream, butter, and other dairy foods; oily foods; fruits and juices; nuts and nut butters; herbs and spices;

soft drinks, herbal teas, and mineral water; and alcohol and drugs produce a thinning and weakening of the blood.

4. Extreme yang foods, including meat, eggs, poultry, cheese, fish, seafood, and other animal products, produce a thickening of the blood. In the long run, they have weakening, acid-producing effects, but in the short run they may contribute to alkalosis or elevation of the pH into the higher range. These foods, as well as too much salt and baked flour products, are the principal cause of clotting in the blood and a variety of serious and potentially lethal circulatory disorders such as embolisms.

5. There are four major human blood types: O, A, B, and AB. Some can be mixed together, while others cause clumping (agglutination) of blood cells and result in serious complications, including death. It is important to know your blood type, especially in the event of an accident or illness in which you require a blood transfusion. People with similar blood types share similar tendencies. However, popular books about blood types and personality development, including specific foods for different types, are largely misguided. Type O is the most yang blood type. People with this type can give blood to people with any other type and are classified as universal donors. O people tend to be more physically and socially active. Type B is also relatively yang, but less than O. People with this type are optimistic and outgoing. Type A is the most yin type, and people with this A blood are usually more calm and introverted. Type AB is in between A and B, sharing characteristics of both. While these types are not deterministic, type O and B people should be slightly more careful about overconsuming strong yang foods, such as animal products, salt, and hard, baked flour products. A and AB types, meanwhile, are more susceptible to the effects of strong yin foods, such as sugar and sweets, dairy, oily foods, salad, and an excess of beverages.

FORMS

Anemia. Anemia occurs when the cells and tissues of the body receive an inadequate amount of oxygen. Red blood cells circulating in the bloodstream are generally low, or not enough hemoglobin is available. Several hundred forms of anemia have been classified, including *iron-deficiency anemia* (the most common form), *hemolytic anemias* (associated with inherited defects that cause red blood cells to be destroyed prematurely), *megaloblastic anemias* (associated with folic acid deficiency), and *pernicious anemia* (associated with vitamin B_{12} deficiency). *See also "Sickle Cell Anemia" later in this section.* A balanced way of eating will usually prevent or relieve most cases of anemia.

The following symptoms can accompany anemia: dizziness or staggering, pale face, cold hands and feet, irregular heartbeat, low blood sugar level, lack of drive, general fatigue, headache, nervousness or nerve dullness, and mental instability, including lack of positive view of life, anxiety, lack of courage and patience, depression, persecution complex (paranoia), stress, megalomania, feeling of approaching death, or insanity. In the case of pernicious anemia, a burning tongue, tingling in the arms or legs, coordination problems, depression, scattered mind, or memory loss may be present.

There are several different causes of anemia, including the following: (1) lack of minerals in the diet, especially iron; (2) an excess intake of minerals (for example, an excess intake of salt), which stagnates the flow of blood; (3) a diet that is out of balance in some essential nutrients, includes malnutrition as well as folic acid or vitamin B_{12} deficiencies; (4) excessive bleeding or persistent internal bleeding, such as that due to uterine cancer, cervical cancer, colon cancer, hemorrhoids, and other internal diseases.

Follow the guidelines for Diet #1, for conditions caused by extreme yin factors, with an emphasis on the further dietary suggestions below. Some nutritionists recommend that you should eat a lot of animal food to relieve anemia because it is high in iron. In the macrobiotic way of eating, we avoid meat, poultry, eggs, and other strong animal foods, including dairy foods of all kinds, because they are the principal cause of heart disease, cancer, and other degenerative diseases. If animal food is taken, fish and seafood are preferable. It is all right to take fish or seafood every day until you recover from anemia, so long as the amount is small. White-meat fish is the most recommended, but red-meat fish, which we ordinarily avoid or limit, may be chosen to help overcome this condition. Avoid shellfish, however, until the condition improves.

Follow the standard way-of-life suggestions and home remedies described later in this section.

In case of anemia due to excessive or chronic bleeding, a blood transfusion may be necessary. Discuss with your doctor the need for a blood transfusion. The dietary recommendations noted above may reduce the need for a transfusion and enhance healing.

If the bleeding is due to injury, uterine cancer, colon cancer, hemorrhoids, or other serious condition and continues for some days, seek medical attention, including a diagnosis that makes the cause of bleeding clear.

Anemia is often accompanied by feelings of being cold. Do not use an electric blanket to keep warm, but instead use a HOT-WATER BOTTLE.

Bleeding. Bleeding can occur internally or externally and is referred to as a *hemorrhage.* Internal bleeding can be caused by a bruise, injury, accident, or contusion. Bleeding in the brain is a type of stroke *(see "Hemorrhage" in "Brain Disorders").* External bleeding can be caused by a cut or wound or from an ailment or illness. These include nose bleeding, stomach bleeding, and uterine bleeding *(see below).*

Overall, bleeding or hemorrhaging is classified as yin. In most cases, the person's underlying condition, including blood quality, is overly expanded. Hence bleeding arises or their imbalance results in an accident or injury. In some cases, an overly yang person will also be hurt and suffer loss of blood. In most cases, the tendency to bleed can be relieved through a balanced macrobiotic way of eating, emphasizing slightly more yang factors, such as proportionately more root vegetables and sea vegetables, stronger cooking, and more seasoning. Follow the dietary guidelines for Diet #1 for more yin conditions. The home remedies below list several remedies for cuts and wounds.

Hemophilia. Normally, blood clots when it is exposed to oxygen. Hemophilia is a condition in which the blood does not clot at the usual rate and even small cuts or bruises may result in prolonged bleeding. Large black-and-blue spots commonly appear under the skin following even a slight blow or bruise. Members of many royal and aristocratic families in Europe suffered from hemophilia, but it is not hereditary. It is caused by a rich diet and luxurious lifestyle, which create an excessively yin condition. The blood loses its contractive power to coagulate and ruptured blood vessels are too weak to fuse or close after they have been injured. Milk, butter, ice cream, and other light dairy foods, as well as eggs, other animal fats, and sugar underlie this condition. Men are more susceptible to hemophilia than women because they cannot absorb as much yin without growing imbalanced. Observing a macrobiotic way of eating, focusing slightly on more contractive foods and cooking methods, proportionately more salt and seasonings, and other yang factors, will help relieve this condition. Follow the dietary guidelines for Diet #1, for more expansive conditions. Physical activity, exposure to the elements, and difficulties and challenges will help. Through proper eating and activity, hemophilia can be reversed, though it may take several years to completely change the blood quality and condition of the internal organs.

Rh Incompatibility. Rh refers to an agglutinating agent found in the blood of about 85 percent of the population. It takes its name from the rhesus monkey, used in the first experiments involving this factor. People with Rh are referred to as "Rh-positive," while those who do not have this factor are "Rh-negative." Persons with Rh-negative blood produce an anti-agglutinogen if they receive Rh-positive blood in a transfusion, usually within two weeks. A second transfusion can result in a serious hemolytic reaction, destruction of red blood cells, and even death. In the womb, an Rh-positive baby may die if its mother is Rh-negative. From the macrobiotic perspective, clumping together is a gathering, contractive phenomenon, so compared to each other, "Rh-positive" is yang and "Rh-negative" is yin. Through proper eating, the agglutinating ability can be modified. Rh-negative blood may become positive, and vice versa. A diet centered on whole grains and vegetables will produce blood with an Rh factor that is more in between or balanced. Extreme hemolytic reactions will usually not arise following a blood transfusion or the exchange of blood between mother and fetus in the womb. Those still eating in a modern way or in transition should be very careful.

Sickle Cell Anemia. Several million African-Americans are carriers of sickle cell anemia, a condition in which the red blood cells are shaped like sickles or quarter moons. This disorder commonly arises in the teens and may lead to periodic bouts of paralysis similar to epilepsy, fatigue, and brain seizures. Forgetfulness, pain in the nerves or muscles, and curling up in the fetal position and not moving are also frequent symptoms. A small number of cases result in death. The prevailing medical view is that this disease originated in West Africa, where malaria is endemic, and the sickled cells carry a factor that counteracts the malaria parasite in the blood. In some regions of Africa, sickled cells are present in the population, but illness is rare. According to modern medicine, sickle cell anemia is hereditary and incurable.

From the macrobiotic view, sickled cells are caused primarily by diet, especially consumption of refined, processed foods such as sugar, soft drinks, ice cream, refined flour, chemicals, and drugs. Prior to World War II, sickle cell anemia was rare, and its spread coincides with the introduction of these foods. Compared to ordinary red blood cells, sickled cells are thinner and longer—more yin. Compared to people of European or Asian descent, Africans and African-Americans are constitutionally more yin and are more susceptible to developing sickle cell anemia as a result of their mother's diet during pregnancy or an excess of poor-quality yin foods and beverages after birth. The principal food that contributes to this disorder is plantains, a staple in Africa. Traditionally, plantains are pounded, salted, and cooked to help offset their extreme yin energy and effects. Also in Africa, a predominantly hot, humid, tropical environment, plantains and other tropical fruits are part of the local environment. In temperate parts of North America, bananas are not suitable for ordinary consumption. Raw bananas especially produce strong yin effects. While African-Americans may be more susceptible to abnormal blood changes, consumption of bananas or plantains by those of other backgrounds can also lead to overall weakening and disease. Other foods that contribute to sickle cell anemia are sugar, ice cream, oily and greasy foods, white flour, white rice, stimulants, spices, alcohol, and other overly expansive items. On the standard macrobiotic diet, the formation of sickled cells and anemic symptoms can generally be changed in 4 to 6 months. Follow the dietary guidelines for Diet #1, for more yin factors. Cases with bacterial and intestinal troubles may take 6 to 18 months.

SOLUTION

DIET

Follow the dietary guidelines referred to above, paying special attention to the following.

1. Eat whole cereal grains at every meal; the grain should not be refined or polished. This includes brown rice or semi-refined rice. Take MISO-ZOSUI with scallions often.

2. Take MISO SOUP WITH BROWN RICE MOCHI 2 to 3 times a week. Soup, including miso soup, should also include wakame or other sea vegetable, and other vegetables, beans, and grains from time to time.

3. Avoid baked flour products (for example, bread, crackers, cookies, chips) as much as possible; but it is all right to have sourdough bread and other unrefined breads 2 to 3 times a week.

4. For vitality, a small amount of white-meat fish may be taken 2 to 3 times a week, if desired.

5. Vegetables can be prepared in a variety of cooking styles, especially iron-rich vegetables such as collards, kale, mustard greens, turnip greens, and other green leafy vegetables. NISHIME-STYLE ROOT VEGETABLES and ADZUKI BEANS, SQUASH, AND KOMBU DISH are recommended, as well as sautéed vegetables a few times a week. In this case, you may use a little sesame oil for stir-frying. Avoid vegetables that originated in a tropical region, such as tomatoes, eggplants, potatoes, and peppers.

6. You can take beans and bean products (such as tofu, natto, and tempeh) every day. These contain high-quality protein and will increase vitality.

7. All types of sea vegetables are fine and will help strengthen the blood.

8. Take as little fruit and fruit juices as possible. Eat them with a pinch of sea salt if cravings arise. Avoid fruits that originated in tropical and subtropical regions, such as fig, avocado, and citrus fruits.

9. Take a standard amount of salt.

10. It is best to use vegetable-quality oil, especially sesame oil, for sautéed vegetables, for KINPIRA-STYLE BURDOCK, or for FRIED BROWN RICE. TEMPURA-STYLE VEGETABLES may be taken once or twice a week in small amounts, if desired.

11. Cooked pumpkin, onion, cabbage, and carrots may be taken frequently to supply a sweet taste. For a more concentrated taste, a grain-based sweetener (brown rice syrup, barley malt) is preferable to fruit-based sweeteners. Strictly avoid simple sugars (sugar, honey, chocolate, molasses, corn syrup, fructose, etc.) and food products and beverages that include these ingredients.

12. It is best to use miso and shoyu that have fermented through at least two summers (two to three years of fermentation) and sea salt that includes a small quantity of minerals. Avoid stimulating seasonings (such as mustard, pepper, and curry), and avoid alcohol, even mirin (sweet rice cooking wine). Brown rice vinegar, umeboshi vinegar, and ginger may need to be limited until the condition improves.

13. For other dietary recommendations, follow the standard macrobiotic dietary guidelines. Choose organic foods for your ingredients as much as possible.

LIFESTYLE

1. Do a BODY SCRUB every morning and every evening. This will promote circulation of blood and bodily fluids.

2. Keep physically active. This will increase the intake of oxygen and strengthen the blood.

3. Keep a natural environment in your home, and promote good ventilation. A very humid condition, or one in which the flow of air is stagnated, will reduce oxygen and impair the blood.

4. Avoid environments where artificial electromagnetic radiation is present and where air conditioners or heaters are used in excess, as these can weaken the blood.

5. Avoid taking long baths and showers, which can deplete the body of salt and minerals and weaken the blood. Add a handful of salt to the hot water of the bathtub when bathing.

6. Avoid electric and especially microwave cooking, which creates chaotic energy and can produce precancerous changes in the blood.

HOME REMEDIES

1. MISO-ZOSUI is helpful to improve the quality of the blood and to promote better circulation. Eat this every day for 3 to 10 days.

2. BROWN RICE MOCHI fried in oil will also help strengthen the blood.

3. Take a small cup of UME-SHO KUZU or UME-SHO BANCHA every other day for 10 days.

4. For strength and vitality, KINPIRA SOUP may be taken 2–3 times a week.

5. Prepare TEMPURA-STYLE VEGETABLES 2 to 3 times a week.

6. Prepare SALMON HEAD–SOYBEAN STEW to strengthen the blood. Have a bowl of this dish every day for 2 to 3 days.

7. A hot GINGER COMPRESS applied to the small intestine will help stimulate the production of healthy red-blood cells.

8. LOTUS ROOT TEA made from powdered lotus root is good taken internally for bleeding in the colon and intestine.

CAUTION

1. A physician should be consulted for any condition that does not clear up quickly using the home remedies recommended above. For accident, emergency, or any potentially life-threatening condition accompanied by loss of blood, emergency medical treatment is essential.

2. There is widespread concern about the safety of the national blood supply. Despite the best efforts of the medical profession, HIV, prions, and other potentially lethal substances may go undetected. Even ordinary, uncontaminated blood, by macrobiotic standards, is not ideal, because for the most part it originates from donors eating meat, sugar, and other extreme foods. In the event that a blood transfusion is required, it is preferable to use one's own donated blood (stored at an earlier time in case of emergency) or that of a friend and family member who is eating well and has healthy blood.

MEDICAL EVIDENCE

MACROBIOTIC MEN HAVE OPTIMAL BLOOD VALUES

In a study of the blood values of 20 men working at the Lima Natural Foods Factory in Belgium, a macrobiotic company, researchers reported that all the men were healthy, their blood pressure and body weight were low, their hormone levels were favorable, and they had normal values for all nutrients. The average age of the men was 36 and they had been macrobiotic for about eight years. "In the field of cardiovascular and cancer risk factors, this kind of blood is very favorable," concluded J. P. Deslypere, M.D., one of the experimenters. "It's ideal; we couldn't do better; that's what we've dreamed of. It's really fantastic, like children, whose blood vessels are still completely open and whole. This is a very important matter, deserving our full attention."

Source: Rik Vermuyten, *MacroMuse*, Fall 1984, p. 39.

TABLE 16. BLOOD AND LYMPHATIC DISEASES

1. More Yin Cause	2. More Yang Cause	3. Yin and Yang Combined
Typical Symptoms		
Lack of vitality, fatigue	General fatigue	General fatigue
Dilation, swelling, inflammation	Constriction of vessels	Hardening
Reduction of red blood cells	Reduction of white blood cells (some cases)	Imbalance among blood cell ratios
Some bleeding	Some bleeding	Higher cholesterol and fat in the blood
Weakening of arteries and veins	Thickening of blood, clotting	
Diseases		
Nosebleed		
Anemia	Scurvy	Pernicious anemia
Sickle cell anemia		
Hemophilia		
Purpura		
Leukemia (most cases)	Leukemia (some cases)	
Hodgkin's disease		
Lymphoma (most cases)	Lymphoma (some cases)	

Ⓡ BONE AND JOINT DISORDERS

Common bone and joint disorders include bunion, flat foot, scoliosis, bursitis, arthritis, rheumatism, and osteoporosis. *See also "Bone Cancer" in "Cancer," "Disk Problems" ("Nervous System Conditions and Disorders"), "Foot and Leg Problems," "Muscle Problems," and "Carpal Tunnel Syndrome" in "Repetitive Stress Injuries" for discussion of these associated conditions.* In modern society, stiffness, swelling, and hardening of the bones and joints are considered a natural part of aging, and millions of people are disabled because of degenerative bone or joint conditions. A variety of traction devices, slings, plaster casts, and splints are used to treat dislocations, fractures, and diseases related to these organs. A battery of drugs and medical procedures, including surgery, are used in many cases. In traditional societies, bone and joint problems are rare and do not emerge with age. A more natural approach, centered on a diet of whole grains and vegetables, will contribute to a healthy skeletal structure throughout life.

SYMPTOMS

The following symptoms may accompany bone and joint disorders:

1. Swelling, inflammation, or pain
2. Stiffness, hardness, and tightness
3. Softness, loosening, or redness
4. Protruding features
5. Difficulty walking, stretching, or performing normal physical activities
6. Knee problems
7. Balance problems

CAUSE

1. Overall, the bones, joints, and skeletal system are harder, denser, and more compact than other systems and are classified as relatively yang. Healthy bones and joints are formed by whole grains, beans, vegetables from land and sea, and other strengthening foods, especially those that are high in minerals, including miso, shoyu, sea salt, and sea vegetables. The bones and joints attract strong yin and can be damaged by too much sugar, dairy foods, oily and greasy food, stimulants, spices, alcohol, drugs, and other expansive items. They are also weakened by extreme yang such as meat, eggs, poultry, and other animal foods that produce an overall acidic effect.

2. In traditional Oriental medicine and philosophy, the bones are governed by the kidney and bladder and their related functions, including the bladder meridian, which extends from the top of the head and moves down the entire length of the spine, the legs, and the feet. Dietary items that particularly nourish these organs and functions are whole grains, beans, sea vegetables, dried vegetables and other dried foods, and good-quality sea salt and natural water. Kidney-bladder energy contributes vitality, strength, and flexibility to the bones, joints, and other skeletal structures.

3. Swelling or inflammation of the bones and joints can be caused either by strong yin factors (such as sugar, ice cream, or tomatoes) or by a combination of strong yin and yang factors (also including meat, poultry, eggs, and too much salt or baked goods).

4. Softening or deformation of the bones is caused by extreme yin factors.

5. Stiffness and deformation of the bones is caused by a combination of strong yin and yang factors.

6. Abnormal inward curve of the bones accompanied by deformation is caused by strong yang factors.

7. Infectious conditions of the bones are caused by strong yin factors.

8. Consolidation of joints is caused by strong yang factors.

9. Hardening of the bones or joints is caused by a combination of strong yin and yang factors.

FORMS

Arthritis. Arthritis refers to an inflammation or stiffness of the joints and is one of the most common afflictions in modern society. Modern medicine has identified over 100 different types. However, from a macrobiotic perspective, they can be simplified into (1) those caused by extreme yang factors, which cause the joints to contract and tighten, (2) those caused by extreme yin factors, which cause the joints to become encased in fat, swell, and press against a nerve, or (3) those caused by a combination of extreme yin and yang factors. Overall, arthritis represents a form of premature aging. When healthy, children have soft and flexible joints and muscles. Their bodily flexibility is reflected in their mental condition: resiliency, open-mindedness, enthusiasm, and originality. Arthritis is the opposite: mind and body become progressively more rigid and inflexible. The main types of arthritis include:

Rheumatoid arthritis. Rheumatoid arthritis (RA), also known as *rheumatism* or *synovitis,* primarily occurs in women over 40. Men get RA about a third as often. It may also develop in children, particularly young girls from 2 to 5 years old. Main symptoms are inflammation and intense cyclical pain in the hands, arms, legs, and feet accompanied by general fatigue and insomnia. The knuckles and second joints are particularly affected. Other organs of the body, including the heart, lungs, nerves, muscles, and eyes, may also be damaged. In the elderly, RA can result in gnarled or deformed hands and feet. Modern medicine often treats RA as an autoimmune disease. Aspirin and other anti-inflammatory drugs are given for RA. Corticosteroid injection or surgery is used in advanced cases.

From an energetic view, RA is a more yin disorder, caused by chronic intake of milk, ice cream, yogurt, and other dairy; white flour in bread and pastries; oily and fatty food of all kinds; sugar, chocolate, candy, and other concentrated sweeteners; too much fruit and fruit juice; tropical foods; spices; stimulants; alcohol; or drugs. To relieve RA, observe Diet #1 for more yin disorders, noting the following: Short-grain brown rice should be the primary grain, with millet, whole wheat berries, barley, and others eaten from time to time. Avoid or minimize rolled oats temporarily. Whole oats may be taken once every 10 days. Hard baked products should be avoided, including cookies, crackers, and chips. A small volume of unyeasted sourdough bread may be taken several times per week. Udon noodles may be eaten several times a week, but avoid soba until the condition improves. Similarly, avoid or minimize buckwheat and seitan, as these may accelerate the discharge.

For miso soup, alternate mugi and hatcho miso. Vegetables in soup should frequently include daikon, leafy greens, and sweet vegetables. A variety of vegetables is important every day. However, daikon roots and leaves are especially helpful for this condition and may be taken regularly. Avoid the use of oil in cooking for the first month. Water-sautéed vegetables may be used instead. During the second month, oil may be used once a week for sautéed vegetables, and about twice a week during the third month. Avoid raw salads. KINPIRA-STYLE VEGETABLES and NISHIME-STYLE ROOT VEGETABLES are beneficial for RA and may be eaten several times per week. Daikon, turnip, carrot, and other contracted leafy greens are particularly helpful for this condition.

Avoid the occasional-use beans for the first month, then use them 2–3 times the second month. Sea vegetables can be taken in regular, small volume. GOMASHIO can be made in a 16:1 proportion of sesame seeds to salt. UMEBOSHI PLUM can be eaten 2–3 times a week, as can shiso leaves. NORI CONDIMENT and TEKKA are also good. If pain is present in the joints, avoid umeboshi or brown rice vinegar until the condition improves. Minimize pickles with a sour taste temporarily. A few slices of takuan may be eaten several times a week.

White-meat fish may be consumed 1–2 times per week, steamed, boiled, or cooked in soup. Avoid raw fruit and juice, which can enhance swelling and inflammation. If craved, a small amount of fruit cooked with a pinch of sea salt may be taken. Cooked or dried peaches are especially helpful and can be used most often. In summer, a small amount of fresh peaches may be taken with a pinch of sea salt.

Avoid or limit nuts and nut butters. Seeds may be taken occasionally, blanched or lightly roasted (without seasoning), but avoid sunflower seeds or take only in the summer. Chestnuts may be taken occasionally, especially with rice, sweet rice, or adzuki beans. In general, sweets and desserts are to be minimized, using only high-quality ingredients. A half cup of carrot juice may be taken 1–2 times a week unless there is pain in the joints.

Seasonings are to be moderate. Avoid ginger and horseradish temporarily until the condition improves. The following home remedies are helpful for this condition:

1. Take SWEET VEGETABLE DRINK every morning and every evening for 3 to 4 weeks.

2. Make your circulation better by doing one of the following: Apply a GINGER COMPRESS for about 15 minutes every other day on the stiff muscle area. Continue this for about 2 weeks. If a GINGER COMPRESS is too strong, try just a HOT TOWEL COMPRESS. Or do a SESAME OIL–GINGER RUB on the stiff area for 10 to 15 minutes, and then wipe the oil off with a warm towel. This may be repeated every day or every other day for 2 to 3 weeks.

3. In case of inflammation or redness on the hands, fingers, heels, or other region, directly apply a fresh, raw CABBAGE LEAF PLASTER. Alternatively, a KOMBU PLASTER may be helpful. Wear it for 2 to 3 hours a couple of times a day, or apply it when you go to sleep and keep it on overnight.

4. ROASTED BROWN RICE PORRIDGE is very soothing. Eat this with UMEBOSHI PLUM, shiso leaf powder, or GOMASHIO 3 to 4 times a week.

5. Make ADZUKI BEAN, BROWN RICE, DRIED DAIKON, and SHIITAKE TEA. Drink 1 to 2 cups every day for about 2 weeks. After that, drink it 2 to 3 times per week. This can improve the functioning of the kidneys and indirectly help relieve rheumatoid arthritis.

The treatment for juvenile rheumatoid arthritis is similar to that above for adults. It may be accompanied by chronic fever and anemia, also arising from excessive intake of extreme yin foods and beverages. *See "Anemia" in "Bleeding and Blood Disorders" for further information.* Constitutional influences, especially the mother's diet during pregnancy, may be a factor in the onset of this form of the disease, as well as the diet in infancy and childhood.

Ankylosing spondylitis. Ankylosing spondylitis (AS) is a progressive fusing of the joints, leading to bending and stiffness of the spine. It affects about 1 in 100 people, most commonly young men age 20 to 40. It usually starts in the pelvis or lower back and moves upward. The following symptoms may accompany AS: lower back pain, chest pain when inhaling, weight loss, fatigue, and severe stooping.

While AS appears to be a predominantly yang, contracting condition, it is actually caused by extreme yin foods and beverages. Extreme yin makes bones expand and fuse, and the tissues then become tight. As a result, it can affect vegetarians as well as those eating a diet high in animal foods. AS is usually treated with anti-inflammatory drugs and considered irreversible. With proper diet, it can be controlled without medication and in many cases relieved.

The primary cause is sticky food, especially white flour, honey, oatmeal, mashed potato, avocado, and other foods that create fusing and expansive tendencies. Other foods in the standard modern way of eating, including meat, poultry, eggs, dairy, sugar, and tropical foods, that create acidic conditions in the body are contributing factors.

To relieve AS, follow the guidelines for Diet #1, observing the following: Avoid all sticky foods, even good-quality mochi or natto, until the condition improves. Eat whole grains as primary food in whole form, avoiding even noodles temporarily. Eat grains, vegetables, and other foods prepared separately, i.e., not mixed or cooked together. Prepare primary foods with long cooking and avoid stirring or mixing. Take strong MISO SOUP regularly, prepared with grated ginger and scallions. Miso stew made with brown rice to which miso and occasionally vegetables have been added may also be taken frequently. KINPIRA-STYLE VEGETABLES are helpful, 3 to 4 times a week, and KINPIRA SOUP may be taken occasionally. Daikon or turnip leaves water-sautéed with a little shoyu at the end are very beneficial. Minimize tofu, limiting to about ⅓ cake per week. Limit the use of tempeh to once every 7–10 days. Minimize oil, using sesame oil 3 times a week if craved. Avoid or minimize fruits unless cravings come, in which case a small volume of cooked fruit may be prepared. Avoid all nut and seed butters and nuts (sesame seeds are okay). Helpful condiments include MISO-SCALLION CONDIMENT and UMEBOSHI PLUM (1–2 a day). Kuzu is helpful for this condition, used in a variety of ways. Avoid or minimize desserts and sweets, including those made with barley malt or rice syrup, which are sticky.

As a home remedy, prepare a special drink

consisting of dried daikon, adzuki beans, and a little dried shiitake mushroom cooked together. You may also prepare a special drink of dried daikon, carrots, and burdock, adding 4 times as much water, boiling for about 25 minutes, and adding a pinch of salt at the end. A GINGER COMPRESS on the spine will help reduce stiffness and restore flexibility.

Osteoarthritis. Osteoarthritis is characterized by erosion of cartilage, loss of bone tissue in the joints, and sometimes development of bony growths in the joint. It is the most common form of arthritis, and the elderly are particularly affected. It is most pronounced in the spine and legs and can lead to nerve and muscle damage, deformity, and movement difficulty. From an energetic view, osteoarthritis is caused by predominantly strong yang factors, including meat, eggs, poultry, and other animal protein and fat; dairy products, especially hard, salted cheese; too much hard baked flour, chips, and similar items; excessive salt and salty food; and iced foods and beverages. Though not main causes, sugar and other refined sweeteners, fruits and juice, tropical foods; refined grains, spices, stimulants, alcohol, and drugs may enhance the development of this condition, especially the growth of bone spurs.

To relieve osteoarthritis, follow the general dietary guidelines for Diet #2 for strong yang disorders or, if strong yin factors are also consumed, Diet #3 for conditions arising from a combination of dietary extremes. Note the following: Short-grain brown rice should be the primary grain, with barley, millet, and corn on the cob taken as main secondary grains. Barley may be eaten often; it can be prepared 2–3 times a week with rice or in soup. Avoid or minimize rolled oats and other cracked or flaked grains temporarily. Whole oats may be taken once every 10 days. Hard baked products should be avoided, including cookies, crackers, and chips. A small volume of unyeasted sourdough bread may be taken several times per week, preferably steamed. Udon noodles may be eaten several times a week, but avoid soba until the condition improves. Similarly, avoid or minimize buckwheat and seitan, as these may accelerate the discharge.

Use very light miso or shoyu in seasoning soups, avoiding a salty taste. Miso soup may be taken daily with wakame and a variety of vegetables, especially daikon, shiitake, and leafy greens and garnished with chopped scallions, chives, or parsley. A variety of vegetables is important every day. However, cooked dandelions are especially helpful for this condition and may be taken 2–3 times a week. Avoid the use of oil in cooking for the first month. A small amount of sesame oil may be used in cooking, but avoid all raw oil. Avoid raw salads until the condition improves.

Follow the standard guidelines for beans and bean products. If overweight, avoid larger beans for 1 month and then take only once every 7–10 days. GOMASHIO can be made in a 16:1 proportion of sesame seeds to salt. Umeboshi plums can be eaten 2–3 times a week, as can a small volume of brown rice or umeboshi vinegar. Light, quick pickles or sauerkraut are preferred for regular use. White-meat fish may be consumed 1–2 times per week, steamed, boiled, or cooked in soup, but avoid fatty varieties of fish such as tuna and salmon. Cooked temperate-climate fruit may be enjoyed about 2–3 times per week. Plums are especially helpful and can be prepared more frequently. Minimize raw fruit until the condition improves. Avoid or limit nuts and nut butters. Seeds may be taken occasionally, blanched or lightly roasted (without seasoning), but avoid sunflower seeds or take only in the summer. Chestnuts may be taken occasionally, especially with rice, sweet rice, or adzuki beans. Limit rice cakes, popcorn, and puffed cereals, as these are drying and can have a contractive effect.

Seasonings are to be moderate. Follow the standard beverage guidelines. Roasted barley tea or pearl barley tea are especially beneficial for this condition and can be altered with BANCHA TWIG TEA as the main beverage. Dandelion coffee is also recommended and may be used several times a week as a supplement to other beverages.

The following special home remedies are recommended for osteoarthritis:

1. Oil may be used every day in cooking for osteoarthritis. It is necessary to help get minerals in the bones. Prepare frequently okara sautéed in a little sesame oil with a slight shoyu taste at the end of cooking. Okara is the residue that is left when making tofu. It is not usually available at the natural foods store, but can easily be made at home when making tofu. See one of the macrobiotic cookbooks in the recommended reading list.

2. Another recommended dish using oil is daikon or turnip greens, finely chopped, and sautéed in a little sesame oil with a slight shoyu taste at the end of cooking.

3. KINPIRA SOUP is strengthening for osteoarthritis. Prepare 2–3 times a week.

4. Prepare the special OSTEOARTHRITIS AND OSTEOPOROSIS STEW.

5. For painful joints, apply hot towels or a hot GINGER COMPRESS to improve circulation and reduce hardening, unless there is inflammation in which case a TOFU PLASTER or LEAFY GREENS PLASTER is recommended. A BODY SCRUB should be performed twice daily, with a hot, damp towel, in the morning and evening. A half-hour walk daily, as well as light exercise, is recommended. A short shower or bath may be taken daily.

Gout. Gout is marked by swelling and inflammation and pain in the joints, especially at the base of the large toe, but occasionally in the knees, elbows, thumbs, or fingers. Pain usually occurs suddenly at night and is cyclic. Ninety percent of those with gout are middle-aged men, especially those who are overweight or have high blood pressure. It is commonly treated with nonsteroidal anti-inflammatory drugs or corticosteroid injections. Gout arises from a combination of dietary extremes, including meat and alcohol, cheese and wine, heavy sauces and gravies, sugary baked desserts, and chilled or iced foods and drinks. Combinations of excess yin and yang energy produce uric acid crystals that form in the soft flesh of the hands, feet, or sometimes the earlobes. These are similar to the formation of stones in the kidneys, bladder, or gallbladder.

The most common symptom of gout is pain in the big toe, arising from excess in the spleen and liver meridians that end in this location.

To relieve gout, generally observe the dietary recommendations for Diet #3, arising from a combination of dietary extremes. Note the following: Short-grain brown rice should be the primary grain, with millet as the secondary grain, and barley, fresh corn, and others taken from time to time. Avoid or minimize rolled oats and other cracked or flaked grains temporarily. Whole oats may be taken once every 10 days. Hard baked products should be avoided, including cookies, crackers, and chips. However, unyeasted sourdough bread may be taken 2–3 times per week, preferably steamed. Udon noodles may be eaten several times a week, but avoid soba until the condition improves. Similarly, avoid or minimize buckwheat and seitan, as these may accelerate the discharge too rapidly.

MISO SOUP may be taken daily with wakame and a variety of vegetables, especially daikon, shiitake, and leafy greens. A variety of vegetables is important every day. Cabbage is especially helpful for this condition and may be prepared often, as can other sweet vegetables such as squash and onion. ADZUKI BEAN, SQUASH, AND KOMBU DISH can be taken 2–4 times a week and will provide additional sweetness. Keep the use of oil to a minimum. If swelling and pain are present, avoid oil temporarily. Otherwise, a small amount of sesame oil may be used in sautéing.

Follow the standard guidelines for beans and bean products. If overweight, avoid larger beans for 1 month and then take once a week, if desired. GOMASHIO can be made in a 16:1 proportion of sesame seeds to salt. UMEBOSHI PLUM can be eaten 2–3 times a week. Minimize the use of brown rice and umeboshi vinegar, especially when there is joint pain. Light, quick pickles or sauerkraut are preferred for regular use. Avoid or limit animal protein and fat, which is the underlying cause of this condition. However, if cravings arise, white-meat fish may

be consumed 1–2 times per week, steamed, boiled, or cooked in soup and properly garnished. Temperate-climate fruit may be enjoyed about 2–3 times per week, cooked, dried, or raw. Avoid or limit nuts and nut butters. Seeds may be taken occasionally, blanched or lightly roasted (without seasoning), but avoid sunflower seeds or take only in the summer. Chestnuts may be taken occasionally, especially with rice, sweet rice, or adzuki beans. Limit rice cakes, popcorn, and puffed cereals, as these are drying and can have a contractive effect.

Seasonings are to be moderate. Avoid ginger or horseradish until the condition improves. Follow the standard beverage guidelines. Amasake can be used on occasion. Carrot juice may be enjoyed several times a week. It is especially important to avoid icy and cold beverages and not to drink excessively. SWEET VEGETABLE DRINK may be taken 2–3 times a week for 1 month or longer. A special drink can be made consisting of ⅓ cup of fresh grated daikon, ⅓ cup of grated carrot, and ⅓ cup of water, simmered for 2–3 minutes with a few drops of shoyu added at the end. Take 2–3 times a week for 1 month. KOMBU TEA is also recommended and may be used several times a week until the condition improves.

For painful joints, a TOFU AND LEAFY GREENS PLASTER can be applied directly to the painful area. Raw greens or tofu may also be applied separately. Apply when painful or 2–3 times a week for 1 month. A hot GINGER COMPRESS can be applied to the kidney region twice a month. However, persons experiencing acute attacks of gout or swelling and inflammation in the feet are advised not to do a ginger compress or ginger foot soak until the condition subsides. A BODY SCRUB should be performed twice daily, with a hot, damp towel, in the morning and evening. A half-hour walk daily, as well as light exercise, is recommended. A short shower or bath may be taken daily. It is best not to smoke, as this is very contracting. If the large toe is affected, it is important to wear cotton socks.

Bone and Joint Infections. Infections of the bones and joints include *osteomyelitis* and *infectious arthritis*. Osteomyelitis is associated with a bacterial or fungal infection that causes the inner part of the bone to swell. This expansion can press against blood vessels in the bone marrow, impeding blood supply and in severe cases causing part of the bone to die. Osteomyelitis occurs most frequently in the ends of the large arm or leg bones in children or in the spines of adults. Kidney dialysis patients and drug users are at high risk for infection. The microbes associated with tuberculosis or other infectious condition can also invade adjacent bone tissues. Surgery is also a common route for the spread of bacteria. Antibiotics are usually prescribed to treat the infection, and surgery may be indicated to eliminate abscesses or treat other complications.

An infection in the fluid and tissues of a joint is called infectious arthritis. A wide variety of bacteria, viruses, and fungi can cause joint infections, including staph, strep, parvoviruses, HIV, and the viruses associated with rubella, mumps, and hepatitis B. Infants, children, and adults are all susceptible. Symptoms include red, warm, and swollen joints and fever and chills. The knee, shoulder, wrist, hip, finger, and elbow joints are common sites of infection. Antibiotic treatment is prescribed for infectious arthritis, usually intravenously in order to reach the affected region, and pus is drained with a needle or surgery.

Both osteomyelitis and infectious arthritis are classified as strong yin disorders. Like other infectious conditions, they arise from underlying acidity in the blood, lymph, and other body fluids that provides an environment in which potentially harmful microorganisms can grow and multiply. The main cause is consumption of extreme yin foods and beverages, including sugar, chocolate, and other refined sweeteners; milk, ice cream, cottage cheese, and other light dairy foods; white flour and other refined grains and grain products; excessive fruits and juices; tropical foods; soft drinks, mineral waters, and excessive fluids; stimulants; spices; alcohol; drugs; and other overly expansive substances. Overmedicalization, including exposure to X rays, drugs and medications (especially antibiotics), and other environmental and lifestyle factors can increase the risk of infection or accelerate its spread. Adopting a standard macrobiotic way of eating, with a slight emphasis on good-quality yang factors, will usually relieve infectious bone and joint conditions. Follow the guidelines for Diet #1 for more yin conditions and the recommendations below. *See "Infectious Diseases" for further specific dietary recommendations and home remedies.*

Bunion. A bunion is a bumpy swelling or growth on the big toe. It is usually accompanied by redness, tenderness, and pain, especially while walking. Bunions are treated medically with anti-inflammatory drugs, analgesic cream, orthopedic shoes, and in severe cases surgery.

From an energetic perspective, a bunion forms on the big toe along the spleen/pancreas meridian, which is involved in sugar metabolism. Excessive intake of sugar, chocolate, honey, and other refined sweets, as well as simple sugars from fruit and milk and other dairy products and other overly expansive foods and beverages, is the main cause of swelling in this area. In addition to discontinuing these items and following a balanced diet centered on whole grains and vegetables, a GINGER COMPRESS on the affected region or a FOOT BATH with ginger will help reduce pain and release stagnation. Follow the guidelines for Diet #1 for more yin conditions and the recommendations below.

Bursitis. Bursitis is an inflammation, swelling, or pain in the shoulders, elbows, hips, knees, hands, or feet, especially when physically active or stretching the joints. A network of 150 bursae (sacs filled with fluid) lubricate the bones, tendons, and ligaments of the body, allowing them to move when they come in contact. Excessive pressure on the joint results in fluid buildup, causing symptoms to appear. Athletes, laborers, and other who push their bodies to the limit are especially susceptible. Anti-inflammatory drugs are commonly prescribed, and deep-heat therapy, ultrasound, and surgery are used in some cases. Calcification can result if the bursitis is left untreated, resulting in permanent damage to the joint and diminishment of its range of motion.

From the macrobiotic view, bursitis arises from combinations of both extreme yin and yang dietary factors, including meat and sugar, poultry and spices, and dairy food and excessive fruit, juice, and vegetables of tropical origin.

The metabolic energy from these foods results in both overexpansive and overcontractive reactions that eventually cause the joints to lose their contractive power and fill with excess fluid. Bursitis can be prevented and relieved with a standard macrobiotic way of eating. Follow the guidelines for Diet #3 for conditions caused by a combination of yin and yang factors and the recommendations below. A BODY SCRUB will help relieves soreness and improve energy circulation. HOT TOWELS, a GINGER COMPRESS, or a SALT PACK may help relieve aches and pains. However, in the case of swelling or inflammation, use a cool application instead. See the home remedies below.

Osteoporosis. Osteoporosis, the thinning and loss of bone tissue, leaves the body subject to fracture and falls and loss of supporting structures. In can lead to spinal collapse, recurrent back pain, "dowager's hump," and hip fractures. In the United States an estimated 1.3 million fractures occur each year as a result of this disorder, primarily in the spine, hip, and wrist. Eighty percent of sufferers are women, and about one-third of elderly women who break a hip die from blood clots, pneumonia, or other complications within six months. Men rarely develop osteoporosis before age 70. Symptoms include backache, gradual loss of height, a stooped posture, loss of bone in the jaw, teeth and gum difficulties, and transparent skin. Women are believed to be at greater risk because at menopause, the production of estrogen drops, leading to calcium loss in the bones. Conventional medicine treats osteoporosis with hormone replacement therapy to stimulate bone growth and increase density. Artificial estrogen helps to maintain bone density and results in fewer hip and wrist fractures. Milk and other dairy foods high in calcium, as well as canned seafoods (such as tuna, salmon, shrimp, and sardines) and poultry, are frequently recommended, as are vitamin D supplements and more exposure to the sun.

From a macrobiotic view, the principal cause of osteoporosis is consumption of too much meat, dairy, and other animal protein that leaches calcium, phosphorus, and other minerals from the bones. Too much salt, caffeine, alcohol, and smoking can also increase bone loss. These extreme substances produce an acidic condition in the blood and body, eventually depleting the minerals stored in the bones to maintain an alkaline condition. The result is weak bones, teeth, and gums. Taking dairy food as a source of extra calcium actually depletes this mineral from the bones, as medical studies are now showing. Hormone replacement therapy will reduce the likelihood of bone fracture but carries major risks of contracting other serious diseases. A balanced way of eating can help prevent osteoporosis and even help remineralize the bones in many cases. Some bone loss will naturally accompany aging, but even in advanced cases, bone density can be increased up to 90 percent after one or two years of careful eating.

Follow the standard macrobiotic way of eating, avoiding extreme foods, and using light to moderate cooking, salt, and seasoning. Be careful to avoid vinegar and citrus, including lemon, which will aggravate this condition. Follow the guidelines for Diet #3 for conditions caused by a combination of extreme yin and yang factors and the recommendations below.

Excellent natural sources of calcium include collard greens, kale, turnip greens, watercress and other leafy green vegetables; natto, tofu, kidney beans, and other beans; sea vegetables, especially hiziki and wakame; sesame seeds, almonds, and sunflower seeds; and other plant-quality foods.

The following special home remedies are recommended for osteoporosis:

1. Oil may be used every day in cooking for osteoporosis. It is necessary to help get minerals in the bones. Prepare frequently okara sautéed in a little sesame oil with a slight shoyu taste at the end of cooking. Okara is the residue that is left when making tofu. It is not usually available at natural foods stores but can easily be made at home when making tofu. See one of the macrobiotic cookbooks in the recommended reading list.

2. Another recommended dish using oil is daikon or turnip greens, finely chopped, and sautéed in a little sesame oil with a slight shoyu taste at the end of cooking.

3. KINPIRA SOUP is strengthening for osteoporosis. Prepare 2–3 times a week. For this condition, plenty of daikon greens, turnip greens, collards, kale, or other hard leafy greens can be added directly to the soup.

4. Prepare the special OSTEOARTHRITIS AND OSTEOPOROSIS STEW.

Scoliosis. Scoliosis is a sideways curvature of the spine, producing a characteristic C- or S-shape. While occasionally congenital, scoliosis usually appears in early adolescence. Both boys and girls may develop it, but it is more pronounced in females. Symptoms include tilting of the body to one side, uneven shoulders, one leg longer than the other, hips that shift to one side, a crooked back, and protruding ribs. Scoliosis is not painful in itself but may lead to disk problems, arthritis, sciatica, or other painful complications. Cerebral palsy, polio, or other diseases of the muscles, bones, and nerves can give rise to this disorder, as can a broken back or other serious injury. Medical specialists prescribe exercise, orthopedic braces and splints, and surgery in more advanced cases.

From an energetic perspective, scoliosis is a more yin disorder, arising from loss of strong, yang energy in the spine and central energy channel. Normally, the back is vertically aligned. However, excessive intake of sugar, chocolate, honey, and other sweets; milk, ice cream, yogurt, and other dairy; cookies, crackers, and pastries made with white flour; fruits and juice; tomatoes, potatoes, and other vegetables of tropical origin; spices; stimulating beverages such as herbal teas and carbonated waters; and other overly expansive foods soften and weaken the spine, causing it to curve. To prevent or help reverse scoliosis, a standard macrobiotic way of eating should be observed. Whole grains are to be eaten as the center of each meal, especially brown rice, millet, and barley, with occasional intake of buckwheat groats and soba noodles. Beans and bean products may be taken regularly, as well as fresh vegetables prepared in a variety of ways, and mineral-rich sea vegetables daily in small volume. Slightly more salt, miso, and shoyu may be used in seasoning. Limit flour products, raw foods, fruit and juice, sweets, and oily or greasy foods until the condition improves. Follow the guidelines for Diet #1 for more yin conditions and the recommendations

below. A BODY SCRUB or GINGER BODY SCRUB along the spine and whole body is recommended once or twice a day. A GINGER COMPRESS on the kidneys twice a week will also be helpful.

SOLUTION

DIET

The following general guidelines for bone and joint problems may be helpful, unless modified by more specific suggestions noted above in the text:

1. Eat whole grains, not refined grains, as the main dish of every meal. Buckwheat is particularly strengthening for the bones and joints in young people or generally healthy adults. However, as a general rule, avoid buckwheat or soba if these organs are already too tight and contracted. Black rice and other black or dark-colored grains are also nourishing for the skeletal system but may be too yang for those with arthritis and other contractive conditions.

2. Reduce flour products as much as possible. Noodles may be taken several times a week, especially udon, somen, or whole-wheat spaghetti.

3. Avoid simple sugars (including refined sugar, honey, and chocolate).

4. Avoid animal food; however, fish or seafood, preferably white-meat fish such as perch, trout, or flounder, may be taken once or twice a week.

5. Beans are particularly strengthening for the bones and joints. Select among a variety of beans, particularly the smaller beans such as adzuki beans, lentils, chickpeas, and black soybeans. Bean products may also be eaten regularly, especially dried tofu.

6. Among vegetables, root vegetables and dried vegetables, including dried daikon, dried shiitake mushrooms, and winter vegetables such as kale particularly nourish the bones and skeletal system. For tight, contractive conditions, leafy green vegetables are particularly recommended.

7. While excessive oil is to be avoided, a small volume of sesame oil or good-quality vegetable oil may be used for many bone and joint disorders. Avoid raw oil.

8. Sea vegetables are very nourishing for the bones and joints, especially kombu, but this may be too contractive for overly yang conditions.

9. The amount of salt (miso, shoyu, and sea salt) should be moderate, adjusting slightly for a more expanded or contracted condition.

10. As a rule, fruit and fruit juices should be limited or avoided, except in the case of overly contracted conditions, in which case a small volume may be taken. Dried fruit, dark or black fruits such as blackberries, and watermelon are very relaxing for tight bones and joints.

11. Limit nuts and nut and seed butters until the condition improves. However, chestnuts and dark sesame seeds may be taken.

12. Among condiments, TEKKA, SHIO-KOMBU, shio nori, and dried fish condiment are strengthening

13. Cut down on water consumption to a moderate level, but do not reduce it too much. Besides BANCHA TWIG TEA, teas that nourish the kidney function and skeletal structure, include ADZUKI BEAN TEA, KOMBU TEA, and occasionally MU TEA.

14. Reduce the total volume of food and chew more.

15. Avoid late-night eating.

LIFESTYLE

Observe the way-of-life suggestions, emphasizing the following:

1. Get up early and go to bed early. Lead an active life, both physically and mentally.

2. It is advisable to exercise moderately but not to exhaustion.

3. Avoid or limit exposure to artificial electro-magnetic radiation as much as possible, for example, from computers, television, cell phones, and other electronic devices, as well as X rays and other medical procedures. The bones are particularly susceptible to damage from radiation.

4. Avoid wearing wool and synthetic clothing, especially nylon, which is irritating to the skin, bones, and joints. Wear cotton underwear and use cotton sheets and pillowcases.

5. Keep the lower back and kidneys protected and warm at all times, especially during the winter or when it is cold.

6. Avoid long baths or showers, which can deplete the body of minerals and cause bone loss.

HOME REMEDIES

Some of the following home cares may be helpful for relieving bone and joint conditions and disorders. The frequency and duration of treatment will depend on the person's condition and severity of symptoms.

1. ADZUKI BEAN TEA is beneficial for kidney-bladder function and bone development. Take 1 or 2 cups cooked with a little sea salt or a piece of kombu 2 to 3 times a week to help restore smooth functions.

2. CARROT-DAIKON DRINK will help eliminate fat and oil that accompany stagnated conditions. Take 1 small cup every day for 5 days and then every second or third day for several weeks.

3. SHIITAKE-DAIKON TEA is also good to help eliminate the accumulation of fat. Take 1 small cup every third day for 1 month.

4. RICE JUICE, the liquid that rises to the surface after cooking brown rice, may be taken frequently to harmonize the kidney, bladder, and skeletal functions.

5. For yang disorders, BLACK SOYBEAN TEA may be taken 3 times a day for several days to help relax.

6. For yin disorders, UME-SHO KUZU may be taken once every three days for several weeks to give energy and vitality.

7. The special OSTEOARTHRITIS AND OSTEOPOROSIS STEW may be helpful for other bone conditions.

8. KINPIRA SOUP is very strengthening and may be taken 2 to 3 times a week for many conditions.

9. A BODY SCRUB or GINGER BODY SCRUB every day or twice a day on the whole body, including the spinal region, will promote better circulation and activate physical and mental energies.

10. A HOT TOWEL COMPRESS can be used to relax specific areas of the body and for the relief of aches, pains, and stiffness in the joints. Apply it hot to the area you wish to treat. Hold it in place until it cools, and then reheat the towel and apply again. Continue applying the hot towel for 5–10 minutes or until the area becomes red or warm. Note: Hot towels or other hot applications should not be applied to joints or other parts of the body that are hot, swollen, or inflamed. Cool applications such as a TOFU PLASTER or LEAFY GREENS PLASTER are better for easing discomfort under these conditions.

11. A hot GINGER COMPRESS may be applied over the kidneys, lower back, and spine several times a week to reduce stagnation and improve blood and energy flow. It will help loosen stagnation and dissolve hardening, as in hard, stiff, or tight joints. However, it should not be used on joints or other parts of the body that are hot, swollen, or inflamed. Change every several hours or leave on until the greens become warm or the temperature drops.

12. Apply a raw TOFU PLASTER to draw out a fever or help ease swelling or inflammation in the joints.

13. A LEAFY GREENS PLASTER can also be used to lower fevers or ease swelling and inflammation in the joints. Apply directly to the affected area. Change every several hours or leave on until the greens become warm.

14. A TOFU AND LEAFY GREENS PLASTER combines the effectiveness of raw tofu and leafy greens and will help bring down a fever or ease swelling and inflammation. Apply as above.

15. A SALT PACK may be used to warm and soothe the shoulders, lower back, or other region where aches and pains are experienced. As with other hot applications, it should not be applied in cases of swelling, fever, or inflammation.

16. In case of stiff bones and joints, apply SESAME OIL–GINGER RUB on the stiff area for 10 to 15 minutes, and then wipe the oil off with a warm towel. This may be repeated every day or every other day for 2 to 3 weeks.

CAUTION

1. A physician or other medical professional should be seen promptly for any fractured bone, internal bleeding, or other serious disorder.

2. Radiation treatment or therapy can make the bones expand, contributing to pain, discomfort, and long-term complications. Sometimes radiation treatment may be advisable, but limit its frequency or dosage if possible. At such times, slightly more miso, sea vegetables, GOMASHIO, UMEBOSHI PLUM, and other salt-based seasonings and condiments may be taken to help offset the effects of radiation.

MEDICAL EVIDENCE

EXCESS ANIMAL PROTEIN CAUSES BONE LOSS

Excess protein from meat, dairy foods, and other animal foods can adversely affect the bones. In a study of protein metabolism, scientists at Montefiore Medical Center and the Albert Einstein College of Medicine in New York reported that a diet high in meat and dairy produced a large amount of acid, mainly as sulfates and phosphates, which are offset by buffer reactions involving resorption of calcium from the bones. Vegetables, fruits, and other alkaline plant foods can help reduce acidity and the burden on the kidneys, resulting in less calcium and bone loss.

Source: U. S. Barzel and L. K. Massey, "Excess Dietary Protein Can Adversely Affect Bone," *Journal of Nutrition* 128(6):1051–53, 1998.

MEAT LINKED TO OSTEOPOROSIS

A diet high in meat causes osteoporosis, according to a study of the Inuit, who have the highest rates of osteoporosis in the world. In a study of 217 children, 89 adults, and 107 elderly Inuit living in Alaska, researchers found that they had lower bone mineral content, onset of bone loss at an earlier age, and more bone thinning than other Americans. The high rate of bone degeneration was attributed to adopting a modern diet high in beef, pork, and other animal foods. Traditionally the Inuit eat whale, fish, and other seafood and other wild game, but did not suffer from osteoporosis until hamburgers, sugar, and other highly processed foods entered their diet.

Source: R. Mazess and W. Mather, "Bone Mineral Content of North Alaskan Eskimos," *American Journal of Clinical Nutrition* 27:916–25, 1974.

DAIRY INCREASES RISK OF BONE FRACTURE

Dairy products fail to protect against bone fracture, according to a review of the scientific literature in the field. Researchers at the University of Minnesota found that high dairy intake may actually increase susceptibility to the disease. In contrast, they reported that many studies showed a diet high in whole grains, vegetables, and fruit reduced the risk of degenerative bone disease and resulted in many other health benefits.

Source: L. H. Kushi et al., "Health Implications of Mediterranean Diets in Light of Contemporary Knowledge: Plant Foods and Dairy Products," *American Journal of Clinical Nutrition* 6(6 Suppl): 1407S–1415S, 1995.

FLUORIDATION MAY PRODUCE ADVERSE EFFECTS

Fluoridation of water may be harmful to the bones. In a review of recent studies, Australian researchers reported that fluoridation damages bones, leading to hip fractures, skeletal fluorosis, osteosarcomas, and other disorders.

Source: M. Diesendort et al., "New Evidence on Fluoridation," *Australian and New Zealand Journal of Public Health* 21(2):187–90, 1997.

TABLE 17. BONE AND JOINT CONDITIONS AND DISORDERS

1. More Yin Cause	2. More Yang Cause	3. Yin and Yang Combined
Typical Symptoms		
Swelling	Consolidation of joints	Swelling
Inflammation	Inflammation	Inflammation
Softening or deformity	Immobility	Hardening
Infectious conditions		Stiffness and deformity
Abnormal outward curve	Abnormal inward curve	Irregular curve
Diseases		
Infectious arthritis	Osteoarthritis	Rheumatoid arthritis
Ankylosing spondylitis	Hunchback	Gout
Bunion		Osteoporosis
Flat feet	Club foot	Bursitis
Acromegaly		Paget's disease
Scoliosis		Bone spurs
Rickets	Tarsal tunnel syndrome	Carpal tunnel syndrome
Ruptured spinal disk	Bone cancer	Malignant melanoma
Frequent dislocation		

RHEUMATOID ARTHRITIS IMPROVED BY VEGAN DIET

In a random case-control study of 66 patients with active rheumatoid arthritis, scientists reported overall improvement in 40 percent of the vegan diet group (which avoids meat, poultry, fish, dairy, and other animal products) compared to 4 percent of the group eating a conventional modern diet. "The immunoglobulin G (IgG) antibody levels against gliadin and beta-lactoglobulin decreased in the responder subgroup in the vegan diet-treated patients, but not in the other analysed groups." The scientists concluded that a diet high in whole grains, vegetables, and other plant quality foods may be of benefit to certain RA patients.

Source: I. Hafstraim et al., "A Vegan Diet Free of Gluten Improves the Symptoms of Rheumatoid Arthritis," *Rheumatology* 40(10):1175–79, 2001.

CASE HISTORY

MACROBIOTICS STABILIZES OSTEOPOROSIS

Gale Jack was shocked when her dentist told her, "You have the most advanced case of osteoporosis I've ever seen in a woman your age." For many years, while growing up and teaching school in Texas, she had eaten plenty of cheese, eggs, milk, meat, chicken, or tuna on a daily basis. Later she added calcium supplements. Because of her declining health, including ovarian tumors and other female disorders, she started macrobiotics and gradually recovered her vitality and well-being. Eliminating all animal foods except for occasional white-meat fish and substantially reducing bread and flour products, her bone condition stabilized, her tumors went away, and she went on to become a macrobiotic cooking teacher and counselor. "Osteoporosis is a silent threat only for those who don't understand the order of the universe or who refuse to live in harmony with it," she observed. "For those who understand yin and yang, maintaining healthy bones and teeth may not be 'a piece of cake,' but it may begin with avoiding one."

Source: Gale Jack and Wendy Esko, editors, *Women's Health Guide* (Becket: One Peaceful World Press, 1997), pp. 79–83.

◎ BRAIN DISORDERS

The human brain is the most highly developed organ of its kind on the planet and capable of receiving and processing the widest possible range of waves and vibrations. Human thinking, imagination, awareness, aspiration, intuition, and other forms of consciousness depend on the proper functioning of this principal organ of the central nervous system. The brain can be impaired by injury or disease, including concussion, bleeding, hemorrhage, and tumors. In addition, there are several major degenerative diseases that can affect the brain. *See "Cerebral Hemorrhage" in "Heart Disease and Circulatory Problems"; "Nervous Conditions and Disorders," especially "Alzheimer's Disease,"*

"Amyotrophic Lateral Sclerosis," "Epilepsy," and "Multiple Sclerosis"; and "Mad Cow Disease." A natural way of life, centered on a balanced diet, will maintain proper brain functioning and activity. This section will look at how food gives rise to some of the common brain ailments and disorders and how it affects thinking and consciousness.

SYMPTOMS

The following symptoms may accompany brain disorders:

1. Persistent headaches
2. Memory loss
3. Vision or hearing loss
4. Speech problems such as slurring words
5. Weakness or paralysis on one side of the face or limbs
6. Loss of coordination or balance
7. Seizures
8. Personality changes
9. Impaired mental functioning

CAUSES

1. The brain and the intestines are interrelated. The brain is the upper digestive organ, taking in energy and vibration, producing images and consciousness, while the body takes in solid, liquid, or gaseous food and produces blood. Food affects thinking and imagination, while energy and vibration influence the stomach, intestines, kidneys, and other organs. Intestinal and digestive problems result in corresponding problems in the brain and central nervous system, and vice versa.

2. As a whole, the brain and central nervous system are extremely yang, small, and compact, and serve as a magnet to attract drugs, medications, synthetic vitamins, food and mineral supplements, and other extremely expansive, yin substances.

3. The human brain is commonly divided into three parts: the cerebrum, the midbrain, and the cerebellum. For convenience, these are commonly described as the *forebrain, midbrain,* and *rear brain.* The forebrain governs intellect and is often referred to as the human or primate brain. The midbrain coordinates emotions and sensations and is called the mammalian brain. The rear brain regulates basic, involuntary responses and is known as the reptilian brain. These brain structures evolved during the last 400 million years as life shifted from water to land. As biological life became more complex, the ability to process external stimulation increased, leading to the development of higher levels of consciousness. To maintain our human structure and form, it is essential to eat whole cereal grains as our principal food. Wild grains and grasses, later to be domesticated into cereal crops, have nourished the human species. When we eat fruits, seeds, nuts, or uncooked vegetables as our main food, our thinking, consciousness, and behavior begins to resemble those of earlier primates, including apes and monkeys, as well as the larger herbivores and other mammals and birds that forage largely on raw plants. When we eat large quantities of meat, eggs, poultry, fish and seafood, dairy food, and other animal food, our mind and character begin to resemble those of carnivorous mammals, reptiles, or birds that eat substantial amounts of flesh and flesh products.

4. Whole grains nourish the forebrain, governing reasoning and judgment. Eating too many refined or polished grains will result in a limited, fragmentary, or incomplete view of life.

5. The midbrain governs sensory input and discrimination, including impulses from the eyes, ears, nose, taste buds, and pressure receptors, and regulates communication between the forebrain and rear brain. Good-quality plant foods, including vegetables, sea vegetables, seeds, nuts, fruits, roots, tubers, and fungi, are essential for the proper functioning of the midbrain. Lack of fresh, well-cooked plant foods will impair sensory development.

6. The rear brain governs breathing, heartbeat, and other autonomic responses, as well as the flight-or-fight response and other basic survival mechanisms. Salt, flour products, and other yang items will nourish this region, creating smooth voluntary and involuntary responses. Too little salt will result in physical weakness, confusion, and susceptibility to accident, while too much salt or animal food will lead to an overaggressive mentality and behavior.

7. Strong yin foods such as sugar, ice cream, and soft drinks attract yang vibrations such as loud music, rough activity, and aggressive behavior.

8. The midbrain is the gathering place for perceptions and is easily dulled or leads to hallucinations if improper food is taken.

9. The forebrain is the site of more creative thinking and imagination. Its layers are affected from the bottom to the top by poor-quality food, leading to illusions and delusions. Strong yin foods in particular are attracted to this region and lead to poor judgment and less activity.

10. A balanced diet, including strengthening

whole grains, cooked vegetables from land and sea, and sea salt and other seasonings attract yin vibrations and invisible short waves, including images related to God, life, truth, peace, and other universal values. Lack of these foods and chaotic eating creates a dark, negative view of life as a random event in a meaningless universe.

11. Strong yang foods are attracted to the rear brain, resulting in low, narrow judgment and a tendency toward violent, aggressive behavior.

12. The right hemisphere of the brain is more highly charged by earth's force and governs more associative, spatial, or artistic thinking, leading to more outward, active expression and behavior. The left hemisphere receives proportionately more heaven's force and governs rational, analytic consciousness, leading to more inward, quiet activity and accomplishment. Dietary extremes can damage, block, or limit the energy received by the hemispheres. For example, too much meat, eggs, or salt can stimulate the left hemisphere and produce an overly analytic mentality, while it can create stagnation in the right hemisphere, blocking artistic, creative expression. Conversely, too much sugar, fruits, and alcohol or drugs can cause loss of focus and concentration in the left hemisphere and chaotic, dissociative expression in the right hemisphere.

FORMS

Hemorrhage. Bleeding inside the brain is known as *intracranial hemorrhage*. Bleeding between the brain and the subarachnoid space is *subarachnoid hemorrhage*, bleeding between the brain's layers is *subdural hemorrhage*, and between the skull and the covering of the brain is

epidural hemorrhage. Bleeding destroys brain cells, raises pressure in the skull alarmingly, and can result in other serious complications. The most common cause of a brain hemorrhage in young persons and adults under 50 is injury. Congenital defects and aneurysm can also cause bleeding, especially in subarachnoid hemorrhages. Brain hemorrhaging is treated with hospitalization (including supplies of fresh oxygen and intravenous feeding), analgesics to control severe headaches and pain, and sometimes a drainage tube in the brain to relieve pressure.

From an energetic perspective, hemorrhaging is a more yin condition, resulting from a weak or burst blood vessel. It tends to arise from consumption of extreme yin foods and beverages, including sugar, chocolate, and other sweets; polished or refined grains; excessive fruits and juices; oily and greasy foods; tropical foods; spices; stimulants; and alcohol and drugs. Because of its yin nature, physicians are careful not to treat brain hemorrhaging, especially strokes caused by cerebral hemorrhage, with anticoagulant drugs such as heparin. Blood thinners are used to treat cerebral infarctions, embolisms, or thrombi. These arise from blood clotting or hardening and narrowing of the arteries' yang factors. To help relieve brain hemorrhaging, dietary extremes need to be discontinued and a standard macrobiotic way of eating observed, slightly adjusted in a more yang direction. Follow the dietary guidelines for Diet #1. Strong MISO SOUP, hard leafy vegetables, and sea vegetables in particular will help restore strength and elasticity to damaged arteries and capillaries. Avoid oil, fruits, nuts, raw foods, and even good-quality sweets as much as possible until the condition improves.

Some of the home remedies and external applications described below will also be helpful in recovery.

Meningitis, Encephalitis, and Other Infections. The brain and spinal cord are subject to a variety of infections, including meningitis, encephalitis, and other bacterial, viral, or parasitic diseases. *Meningitis* is a potentially fatal inflammation of the meninges or lining covering the brain and spinal cord. It usually arises from bacterial or viral infection but can also be a reaction to ibuprofen or other drugs. It most frequently occurs in children between 1 month and 2 years old, but outbreaks can occur in college dorms, the military, or other close-knit groups. *Encephalitis* is an infection of the brain itself, usually resulting from viral contact or occasionally an autoimmune reaction. An *abscess* may also form in the brain, producing headaches, nausea, vomiting, fever, and seizures.

Since meningitis can prove deadly within hours of the onset of symptoms, immediate medical attention is required. It is usually treated with intravenous antibiotics or corticosteroids. There is also a chronic form of meningitis that develops more slowly and arises in those with AIDS, cancer, or other chronic diseases. Depending on its cause, it is treated with prednisone, antifungal drugs, antiherpes drugs, or other medication. Encephalitis is associated with a viral infection that takes different forms but commonly causes seizures, weakness in the limbs or body, and sleepiness. Sometimes called "sleeping sickness," it can progress into a coma. Brain abscesses may also be fatal and are treated with antibiotics, usually over the course of 4 to 6 weeks.

From a macrobiotic view, brain infections are primarily the result of acidic blood that weakens the immune function and allows virulent viruses, bacteria, fungi, or other parasites to spread. Acid-producing foods are the underlying cause, especially sugar, sweets, and soft drinks; milk, ice cream, and light dairy food; oily and greasy foods; polished grains and flour products; excessive fruits and juice; tropical foods; stimulants; spices; alcohol; and drugs. While usually not the main cause, animal foods high in protein, fat, and cholesterol are also acid-producing and can contribute to weakening of the blood and susceptibility to infection. A standard macrobiotic way of eating, emphasizing slightly more yang factors such as stronger miso soup, proportionately more root vegetables, sea vegetables, and stronger cooking, seasoning, and condiments, will help strengthen the blood, neutralize microbial activity, and promote healing. Observe the dietary guidelines for Diet #1. *See "Infectious Diseases" for further dietary and lifestyle guidelines, as well as home remedies.*

Seizure. A seizure is any abnormal electrical activity or discharge in the brain. Seizures range in intensity from mild, single episodes affecting a small area or function to severe, chronic attacks leading to convulsions throughout the body. Seizures typically last for two to five minutes and are accompanied by distorted sensations, loss of consciousness, and problems with muscle and bladder coordination. The person usually doesn't remember what happened during the seizure and is confused and disoriented. Seizures have many causes, including high fever; brain infections such as meningitis and rabies;

metabolic disturbances; oxygen insufficiency such as near drowning or carbon monoxide poisoning; destruction of brain tissue from stroke, injury, or tumor; epilepsy and other illnesses; exposure to toxic drugs or substances in the environment; withdrawal from alcohol, tranquilizers, or sleeping pills; or adverse reaction to prescription drugs.

Energetically, seizures generally arise from strong yin dietary and environmental factors, including long-term consumption of too much sugar and sweets, fruits and juices, tropical vegetables, stimulants, spices, alcohol, or drugs, or exposure to electromagnetic radiation, chemicals, and other weakening influences. For acute relief of seizures, give a small cup of SHOYU BANCHA TEA, UME-SHO BANCHA, or UME-SHO KUZU. This will instantly yangize the condition and hopefully stabilize electrical activity. Overall, strong yin foods and beverages should be discontinued to prevent a recurrence, substituting a standard macrobiotic way of eating, slightly adjusted in a more yang direction. Observe the dietary guidelines for Diet #1.

Tumors. Brain tumors can be either benign or malignant *(see "Brain Cancer" in the "Cancer" section).* Though noncancerous, benign tumors can destroy brain cells, press on nerve tissues, and cause serious complications in other parts of the body. The types of brain tumors include *Schwannomas,* in the Schwann cells that wrap around nerves; *ependymomas,* in the cells in the interior surface of the brain; *meningiomas,* in the outer lining of the brain; *adenomas,* in the pineal or pituitary glands; *osteomas,* in the bones of the skull; and *hemangioblastomas* in blood vessels. There are also congenital birth tumors such as *chordomas* that originate in the nerve cells of the spine. In adults, the most common form is meningioma, which occurs frequently in middle-aged women, but may begin in childhood or not appear until old age. Symptoms include weakness, numbness, seizures, bulging eyes, and changes in vision and smell. Children are also liable to brain tumors, though the most common form is a malignant type, *medulloblastoma,* that affects embryonic cells.

Conventional medicine usually removes benign tumors. However, surgery can sometimes lead to partial paralysis, impaired sensory perception, and other brain damage, including impaired thinking and speech. Radiation therapy is then employed to kill remaining tumor cells. Drugs may also be administered to relieve pressure on the skull and prevent a hernia from forming.

From an energetic perspective, brain tumors can arise from a variety of dietary extremes. Tumors in the outer region of the brain such as meningiomas are caused primarily by overconsumption of strong yin foods and beverages, including sugar and sweets, light dairy foods, oily or greasy foods, polished grains and flour products, fruits and juices, tropical foods, stimulants, spices, and alcohol and drugs. They are found most commonly in children or young adults who have grown up on fast food, chemically grown food, and a lack of whole grains and vegetables. Tumors deep in the inner region of the brain tend to be produced by intake of too much meat, eggs, chicken, fish, seafood, cheese, and other yang animal products. To prevent or relieve brain tumors, observe the standard guidelines and strictly avoid all dietary extremes that can accelerate tumor growth. Observe either Diet #1 for more yin conditions or Diet #2 for more yang conditions. SWEET VEGETABLE DRINK, UME-SHO KUZU, and other special dishes and drinks may be taken. A daily BODY SCRUB and FOOT SOAK will also improve circulation and help bring the energy from the head to the lower part of the body. A LOTUS ROOT PLASTER can relieve heavy pressure and pains in the head or brain. Apply directly on the affected region and keep there about three hours.

SOLUTION

DIET

Follow the dietary recommendations described above.

LIFESTYLE

1. Avoid exposure to computers, televisions, cell phones, and other devices that emit radiation toward the face or head.

2. Brain disorders can be aggravated if the intestinal functions are stagnated. Keep the bowels smooth and menstrual function regular. An enema may help chronic constipation. SHIATSU or a GINGER COMPRESS on the abdomen may also be helpful.

3. Avoid synthetic clothing, especially underwear, socks, hats, scarves, and anything that touches the face or head. Avoid wigs and hairpieces, and use natural fabrics and materials in the home as much as possible.

4. To prevent depletion of minerals, avoid long baths or showers.

5. Excitability, hypersensitivity, despondency, and lowered self-esteem frequently accompany brain and nervous disorders. Meditation, prayer, chanting, yoga, or other exercises can help center the thoughts and calm the mind.

6. Reading, music, and the arts can help create a positive mind and spirit, but the subject matter should be peaceful and harmonious.

7. Light exercise is excellent, especially walking. Deep breathing exercises, massage, and other gentle activities are preferable to strenuous activities.

HOME REMEDIES

1. A TOFU PLASTER on the brain or head will help relieve inflammation, swelling, and fever. The cold temperature of the tofu will produce contraction, offsetting heat or swelling. It is more effective than ice. In the case of serious accidents or injuries, apply crushed, cold tofu to the affected area, repeatedly changing the plaster as necessary until medical help arrives and in the hospital. Apply as soon as possible, even if the person is unconscious, as a few hours' delay can mean it is too late to help heal and repair the damage quickly.

2. As an alternative to the tofu plaster, a LEAFY GREENS PLASTER will help reduce a fever and reduce inflammation. In an emergency, just a CABBAGE LEAF COMPRESS or putting large leaves (such as collard leaves, daikon leaves, or turnip leaves) on the head will produce an immediate cooling effect.

3. In the case of brain disorders caused by too much yin, give a small cup of SHOYU BANCHA TEA, UME-SHO BANCHA, or UME-SHO KUZU.

4. A tea made from the stems of lotus root will help strengthen the cells and tissues of the brain.

5. For strength and vitality, KINPIRA SOUP may be taken 2–3 times a week.

6. Intestinal problems such as chronic constipation commonly accompany brain ailments and disorders. An enema of lukewarm water (at body temperature) can help release stagnation, facilitate discharge, and allow expansive, upward energy to move to the brain area. Use salted water if the condition arises from more yin causes, or regular water if from more yang factors.

7. A FOOT SOAK will help stimulate blood and energy flow and bring energy down from the brain, head, and upper body. This will help alleviate swelling, inflammation, and fever.

8. A foot massage especially of the big toe, is helpful for seizures. This will also help warm the body and promote circulation.

CAUTION

1. For accident, emergency, or any potentially life-threatening condition accompanied by loss of blood, emergency medical treatment is essential.

2. A GINGER COMPRESS is not recommended for use on the brain or on the head when high fever is present.

MEDICAL EVIDENCE

CURED MEATS LINKED WITH CHILDHOOD BRAIN TUMORS

In a study of 1,300 children and their mothers, researchers at the University of South California Norris Comprehensive Cancer Center reported that the consumption of meats cured with sodium nitrite during pregnancy increased the risk of brain tumors in the children.

Source: S. Preston-Martin, "Maternal Consumption of Cured Meats and Vitamins in Relation to Pediatric Brain Tumors," *Cancer Epidemiology Biomarkers Prevention* 5(8):599–605, 1996.

◎ CANCER

One in every three women in modern society will get cancer in her lifetime and one in every two men will get this disease. Though the earliest cases of cancer go back thousands of years, it remained a rare disorder until the 20th century. From killing about 1 to 2 percent of the population in 1900, it jumped to 10 percent in the 1920s, 15 percent in the 1940s, 20 percent in the 1950s, and 25 percent in following decades. This sharp rise in cancer incidence and mortality parallels the spread of the modern way of eating, high in saturated fat, cholesterol, sugar, salt, and highly processed foods. It also coincides with the introduction of canned, bottled, and frozen foods; chemical agriculture; electric and microwave cooking; fast foods, irradiated foods, and genetically altered foods; and the ready availability of foods from radically different climates and environments at the local supermarket. Health reformers and pioneer researchers linked cancer with diet back in the early 1800s. However, modern medicine generally ignored this connection until the 1980s, when the U.S. government, the major scientific and medical organizations, and private cancer foundations issued the first dietary guidelines. Since then the modern way of eating has been linked with virtually every major form of cancer. While admitting the role of diet in the origin and development of many malignancies, the medical profession continues to treat cancer largely with chemotherapy, radiation, hormone therapy, or surgery. These methods sometimes can eliminate symptoms but do not address the origin of the disease, which is underlying dietary and environmental imbalance. In many cases, conventional treatments are harmful and make the condition worse. With the rise of alternative and complementary medicine, many physicians and health care professionals have recently adopted an integrated approach, combining nutrition, visualization, and lifestyle changes with conventional therapies. Over the last generation, thousands of people have followed a macrobiotic way of eating to prevent or relieve cancer, including many terminal cases. Researchers at Tulane University, the University of Minnesota, the National Tumor Institute of Milan, Italy, and elsewhere have documented the efficacy of this approach. The National Cancer Institute was so impressed with individual recovery cases that it just approved clinical trials of the macrobiotic approach. This section will present an overview of the macrobiotic perspective, including specific guidelines for the 20 major types of malignancy. *For a comprehensive overview of the subject, please see our book* The Cancer Prevention Diet *(New York: St. Martin's Press, 1993) and seek the guidance of a qualified macrobiotic teacher or counselor (see "Macrobiotic Resources").*

SYMPTOMS

The following symptoms may accompany cancer:

1. Chronic tiredness and fatigue
2. Localized pain or tenderness in an organ

3. Lumps, fat deposits, or other masses in the breasts, testicles, or elsewhere
4. Weight loss
5. Loss of appetite
6. Blood in the stools
7. Change in bowel or bladder habits
8. Abnormal bleeding
9. Persistent fever or infection
10. Lowered resistance to infection
11. Nagging cough or hoarseness
12. Swollen lymph glands in the armpit, groin, or elsewhere
13. Change in size, shape, or color of a mole or wart
14. Persistent bone pain

SIGNS

In traditional Oriental medicine and philosophy, a precancerous or cancerous condition is indicated by a green hue or tint on the skin. This includes:

1. Green on the outside of either hand in the indented area between thumb and forefinger shows developing colon and rectal troubles.
2. Green on the outside of the little finger shows small intestine troubles.
3. Green on the inside of the arm, from the wrist moving up to the inside of the elbow, shows developing breast or lung tumors. Green on one or both cheeks also shows this condition.
4. Green on the outside front of either leg, especially below the knee or in the extended area of the second and third toes, shows developing stomach tumors.

5. Green around either ankle on the outside of the leg shows developing problems in the bladder, uterus, ovaries, or prostate.

6. Green around the top of the foot in the outside central area, with its area extending to the fourth toe, shows liver or gallbladder problems.

7. Green inside the foot from the outer root of the big toe toward the area below the ankle bone shows possible malignancies in the spleen or lymphatic system.

Developing tumors may also be indicated by abnormal colors in the whites of the eyes:

1. Dark spots in the upper portion of the white of the eye show calcified deposits in the sinus.

2. Dark spots in the lower white of the eye indicate kidney stones or ovarian cysts.

3. A blue, green, or brown shade or white patches in the white of the eye on either side of the iris indicate accumulation of mucus and fat in the liver, gallbladder, spleen, or pancreas.

4. A yellow or white coating on the lower part of the eyeball in men shows the buildup of fat and mucus in and around the prostate.

5. A yellow coating on the lower part of the eyeball in women shows accumulation of fat and mucus in the ovaries, uterus, vagina, or cervix.

6. A white or gray coating on the lower part of the eyeball in a woman indicates possible vaginal discharges, ovarian cysts, or fibroid tumors.

CAUSES

1. Cancer is primarily a disease of dietary excess. It is the final stage in the progressive development of illness through which individuals in the modern world tend to pass because they fail to appreciate the beneficial nature of disease symptoms.

2. A healthy person can deal with a limited amount of excess nutrients or toxic materials consumed in his or her daily food. This imbalance can be naturally eliminated through sweating, urination, bowel movement, perspiration, or daily activity that burns off excess metabolic energy. However, if the person continues to take in too much excess, the body resorts to abnormal measures of discharge, including colds, fever, coughing, skin rashes, and other symptoms. Such sickness is a natural adjustment, the result of the body maintaining natural balance. However, in modern society, these symptoms are commonly suppressed by over-the-counter medications, prescription drugs, and other artificial methods that separate people from the natural workings of their own bodies. If minor ailments are treated in this symptomatic way, discharge begins to be directed inwardly rather than externally. Fatty-acid deposits and chronic mucus begin to gather in the form of kidney stones, breast or ovarian cysts, prostate enlargement, vaginal discharge, and other internal disorders. These can be considered precancerous conditions.

3. In this state, the body is still able to localize the excess and toxins ingested. By gathering the superfluous material in local areas, the remainder of the body is maintained in a relatively clean condition and can function smoothly.

Localization of excess is a natural healing mechanism, preventing the body from completely breaking down. However, the modern view regards these manifestations as invasive enemies that have to be removed or destroyed.

4. As long as excessive nutrients and energy from daily food continue to accumulate and exceed the body's normal or abnormal discharge capacity, they will continue to be stored inside the body. These storage areas gradually grow and develop into tumors. When they reach their limit, they spread and overflow into new storage areas (metastasize).

5. As long as the person continues to eat animal protein, saturated fat, dietary cholesterol, simple sugars, refined salt, chemicals, and other dietary extremes, excess will continue to gather, accumulate, and spread in order to continue normal living functions. If tumors did not isolate this excess, it would spread through the bloodstream and entire body, resulting in the total collapse of vital functions and death by toxemia. Cancer is the last stage of a long process. It is the body's healthy effort to isolate extreme foods and toxins consumed and accumulated through years of eating the artificial modern diet and living in an unnatural environment. Cancer serves to prolong life a few more months or years.

6. If the person awakens to the underlying origin and cause of the cancer, this entire process can often be reversed naturally. Through proper food, including special dishes, drinks, and sometimes compresses and other home remedies, the tumor or malignancy can often be discharged gently and peacefully without the need for drugs, chemicals, or surgery that can weaken the body and interfere with its natural healing ability. In some cases, however, medical attention, including chemotherapy, radiation, hormone treatment, or surgery, may be necessary and can be combined with the macrobiotic approach.

7. The rise of cancer in the modern world has accompanied the change from a way of eating based on organic and natural-quality food to chemically grown and artificially processed food. White flour, white rice, and other refined or polished grains replaced whole grains. Beef, pork, chicken, eggs, cheese, and other animal products high in protein and fat became the center of the modern way of eating. Canned, bottled, and frozen vegetables and fruits replaced fresh produce. Tropical foods, oils, spices, and other items from radically different climates and environments became available all year round. Many local and regional foods disappeared with the influx of mass-produced, artificially aged and preserved foods. Hardy heirloom and open-pollinated varieties of seed gave way to new hybrid and genetically modified strains. All of these trends have contributed to the rise of cancer.

8. Through the blood, the lymph, and other bodily fluids, excessive protein, fat, sugar, and other nutrients from high-energy foods enter the cells and tissues of the body. Eventually, the cells' storage capacity reaches a limit and the cells start to divide. Rapidly increasing cell division is the immediate cause of cancer.

9. Cancer develops in different locations in the body according to the person's constitution and condition, the energetic quality of the overall way of eating, and the relative influence of specific foods and combinations of foods.

10. Excessive intake of meat, eggs, poultry,

cheese, fish, seafood, and other animal foods, as well as too much hard baked flour products, salt, and other contractive foods, tends to gather and accumulate downward and deep in the body, leading to tumors in the colon, rectum, prostate, ovary, liver, pancreas, bone, and inner regions of the brain. These include the harder types of tumors, including most carcinomas.

11. Excessive intake of sugar and other concentrated sweeteners; refined or polished grains; oil and dressings; milk, ice cream, and other light dairy products; fruits and juices; raw foods; foods of tropical origin such as potatoes, tomatoes, and bananas; spices; stimulants; alcohol; drugs; and other expansive substances tends to gather and accumulate upward and in the peripheral parts of the body, leading to malignancies in the breast, skin, upper part of the stomach, mouth, esophagus, lymphatic system, outer regions of the brain, and blood (leukemia). These include the softer types of tumors, including most sarcomas.

12. Excessive intake of both extreme yang and yin foods causes excess to be localized in the more central regions, organs, or systems of the body, leading to tumors in the lung, kidney, bladder, uterus, spleen, lower part of the stomach, tongue, and intermediate regions of the skin (melanoma).

13. An array of environmental and lifestyle factors may contribute to the development of cancer. In most cases, these are not the primary cause, but may contribute to an overall decline in natural immune function, reduce the ability to discharge excess, and accelerate the spread of tumor growth. These include many over-the-counter medications, prescription drugs, and treatments; exposure to X rays, mammograms, CT scan, MRIs, and other invasive medical procedures; industrial chemicals, pollutants, and pesticides; exposure to artificial electromagnetic radiation from computers, cell phones, and other electronics equipment; exposure to nuclear energy or fallout; synthetic clothing, household products, and building materials; chemically treated body care products; electric or microwave cooking; and use of tobacco or exposure to cigarette smoke.

14. A lack of physical activity, sedentary jobs, mental and psychological stress, and other lifestyle factors can weaken the body, inhibit discharge of excess, and contribute to the development of disease.

FORMS

Bone Cancer. Bone cancer claims the lives of about 15,000 Americans annually and accounts for 20,000 new cases. The most deadly form is *multiple myeloma*, which affects the bone tissue and the plasma cells of the blood. It appears primarily in adults over 50, is accompanied by spontaneous fracture of the vertebrae, ribs, pelvis, skull, or other bones, and accounts for two-thirds of all bone cancer deaths. Other types include *osteogenic sarcoma*, a tumor that begins in the bone and cartilage, spreads to the bone marrow, muscles, and lungs, and affects primarily children and young adults; *chondrosarcoma*, which originates in the cartilage of the large bones and affects mostly those of middle age; *chordoma*, a rare tumor that is found at the base of the skull or end of the spine; and *rhabdomyosarcoma*, a tumor in the muscles and fatty tissues that affects young children and spreads rapidly. Surgery is performed for many bone tumors, though many myelomas are untreatable. Radiation and chemotherapy are used as complementary treatments. The survival rate for myeloma is about 17 percent and for other bone tumors up to 50 percent.

From an energetic perspective, bone cancer is classified as an extreme yang disorder. The bones are dense, compact structures that attract refined salt and minerals as well as meat, poultry, and other extreme contractive foods. The primary cause is high animal protein and fat, especially beef, pork, chicken, eggs, hard salty cheese, and salted or smoked fish and seafood. Too much hard baked food such as cookies, crackers, and chips and too much salt and salty food may also contribute to an overly contracted condition. Though not a direct cause, strong yin in the form of sugar, dairy, spices, stimulants, and alcohol should be avoided completely, as they can accelerate tumor growth.

To relieve bone cancer, follow the general dietary guidelines for Diet #2. Avoid all animal food, including white-meat fish, unless cravings arise, in which case a small volume may be consumed once every 10–14 days. All hard baked flour products, including good-quality sourdough bread, are to be avoided for several months, as well as all roasted, baked, or crunchy foods.

Prepare brown rice as the main grain, combined or alternated day to day with millet or barley. Use a square of kombu the size of a postage stamp instead of salt. Avoid buckwheat and soba noodles for about 6 months, minimize seitan, and for 1 month avoid whole oats or oatmeal. Whole-grain noodles or pasta may be used a couple times a week in small volume.

One to 2 servings of soup are recommended daily, especially MISO SOUP cooked with wakame and onions, carrots or other vegetables. A little shiitake mushroom may occasionally be added to miso soup or shoyu broth. Overall, the soup should be milder than usual. Green leafy, round, and root vegetables are to be eaten daily, with a slight emphasis on sweet, round varieties. Minimize burdock, which may be too contracting. While oil is not usually recommended for many types of cancer, for bone cancer one dish of sautéed vegetables prepared with sesame oil may be taken daily or every other day. Special vegetable dishes can be prepared according to the dietary guidelines. Among beans, black soybeans are especially beneficial for this type of cancer. Beans may also be cooked with a small volume of sea vegetables from time to time, as well as 30 to 50 percent squash or 10 to 30 percent onions and carrots. Follow the standard recommendations for sea vegetables and pickles. GOMASHIO may be used with a ratio of 1 part salt to 18 to 20 parts sesame seeds. Shiso powder, ½ to 1 teaspoon sprinkled on grain and vegetable dishes, is very helpful for this condition.

Minimize fruits until the condition improves, though a small volume of cooked apples or other temperate-climate fruit may be taken if cravings develop, and it may help reduce swelling. Tree fruits are preferable to ground fruits such as strawberries and watermelons. Avoid raisins, all fruit juice, and cider. Avoid all sweets and desserts, including good-quality macrobiotic desserts, until the condition improves. Use sweet vegetables daily in cooking, SWEET VEGETABLE JAM, occasional AMASAKE, and if cravings arise, a little BARLEY MALT or BROWN RICE SYRUP. Avoid all nuts except chestnuts, and avoid nut butters. Unsalted blanched sunflower or pumpkin seeds may be consumed in small volume, up to 1 cup a week. Limit rice cakes, popcorn, and other dry or baked snacks, as they may harden the tumor. Sea salt, miso, shoyu, and other seasoning is to be moderate. Avoid mirin, garlic, and all herbs and spices. BANCHA TWIG TEA should be the principal beverage. Strictly avoid all mineral or carbonated waters, soft drinks, iced beverages, and for 2 to 3 months grain coffee. Carrot juice several times a week is helpful for this condition.

The following special dishes, drinks, and home remedies may be helpful:

1. Have 1 to 2 cups of SWEET VEGETABLE DRINK every day.

2. Make ZOSUI WITH SWEET VEGETABLES and NORI. Season with a small amount of miso, shoyu, or sea salt. Seasoning is not necessary for 10 days, in the event you need to restrict or have no appetite for salt.

3. For bone pain, make HATO MUGI–CABBAGE PLASTER. Spread it over cotton linen about ¼ inch thick, and apply it directly to the painful part for 3 to 4 hours, twice a day; or sleep with it until the next morning.

4. After having radiotherapy, the muscles sometimes get stiff and pain is experienced when moving. In this case, do a SESAME OIL–GINGER RUB. After 10 minutes, clean the skin with a warm towel. Do it twice a day.

5. For loss of appetite, take BROWN RICE MILK (SWEETENED). Take it as much as possible, up to a couple of bowls a day.

6. Make mild MISO SOUP WITH OKARA and VEGETABLES and have it 3 to 4 times a week for 2 to 3 weeks.

7. A BODY SCRUB, especially on the abdominal and spinal regions, with a hot, wet towel will help activate circulation and energy flow.

Follow the standard way-of-life suggestions, being careful to avoid artificial electromagnetic radiation, which is very weakening to the bones. Avoid activities and exercise that produce exhaustion. Walking, breathing exercises (focusing on long exhalations), relaxation exercises, and other gentle activities are helpful. Avoid damp and humid environments.

Brain Cancer. Brain tumors and cancer of the central nervous system take about 12,000 lives each year in the United States and 17,000 new cases surface. Men age 50 to 60 have the highest risk, but the fatality rate among both sexes has risen sharply, especially among the elderly. Most brain tumors are classified as *gliomas* and affect the brain tissue itself. These include: *glioblastoma multiforme,* a fast-spreading tumor of the cerebrum, cerebellum, brain stem, and spinal cord affecting both children and adults; *astrocytoma,* a childhood malignancy affecting the cerebellum and brain stem; *ependymoma,* another childhood tumor affecting the ventricles of the brain; and *oligodendroglioma,* a tumor in the white matter in the frontal lobe found in children and adults. Other brain tumors include *meningioma,* a tumor in the membrane covering the brain and spinal cord; *pituitary adenoma,* a tumor in the hypothalamus and optic nerve; *neurofibrosarcoma,* a malignancy in the peripheral nervous system, and *ganglioneuroblastoma,* a tumor that spreads quickly through the nerve cells. Though many brain tumors are untreatable, surgery and radiation therapy may be performed. These are risky and may result in brain damage or permanent damage to the spinal cord, especially in children. Hormone therapy, steroids, hypothermia (lowering the temperature of the brain or body), and other treatments are also occasionally employed.

From an energetic perspective, there are two types of brain tumors: those that arise in the outer, peripheral regions of the brain and those that affect the deep, inner regions. The first softer, sarcoma-type affects the more yin, expanded region of the brain and central nervous system and is caused primarily by long-term overconsumption of milk, butter, cream, yogurt, ice cream, and other light dairy foods; sugar, honey, and chocolate; white flour and white rice; oily, greasy food; tropical foods; stimulants; spices; alcohol and drugs; and chemicalized food. The second harder, carcinoma-type occurs in the more yang, contracted part of the brain and is caused primarily by excess protein and fat, especially of animal quality, including eggs, meat, poultry, hard salty cheese, and oily or fatty fish.

To relieve brain tumors, follow the general dietary guidelines for Diet #1 for tumors in the outer region arising from predominantly extreme yin factors. Follow Diet #2 for tumors in the deep, inside region of the brain arising from extreme yang factors. Avoid all hard baked flour products except for good-quality unyeasted sourdough bread, which may be taken 2–3 times a week. Avoid oil for the first month and then use sesame oil two or three times a week, brushed on the skillet, to sauté vegetables. Avoid raw salad and salad dressing for several months.

Prepare brown rice as the main grain, combined or alternated day to day with millet or barley. Generally, use a small square of kombu (the size of a postage stamp) or a pinch of sea salt in seasoning grain. Those with more yang tumors should avoid buckwheat, soba, and seitan, while those with yin tumors may use these occasionally. Both types should avoid whole oats or oatmeal for 1 month. Whole-wheat noodles or pasta may be used a couple of times a week in small volume.

One to 2 servings of soup are recommended daily, especially MISO SOUP cooked with wakame and onions, carrots, or other vegetables. However, those with more yin tumors may need to take soup only once a day, or just 2 small cups and should avoid chickpeas or black soybeans in soup. A small amount of shiitake mushroom may occasionally be added to miso soup or shoyu broth. Lotus root may be added to soup often and is particularly good for brain tumors. MILLET AND SWEET VEGETABLE SOUP is also good and may be prepared frequently. Green leafy, round, and root vegetables are to be eaten daily. Special vegetable dishes can be prepared according to the dietary guidelines. Avoid the use of oil in cooking for 1–2 months, after which a small volume of sesame oil may be used for sautéing vegetables or frying rice or noodles from time to time. For more yin brain tumors, lentils and adzuki beans may be taken in usual amounts, but minimize chickpeas and black soybeans. Use only ½ cake of tofu per week maximum. Dry tofu or natto is all right. Avoid tempeh for the time being. Follow the standard recommendations for sea vegetables, condiments, and pickles. GOMASHIO may be used with a ratio of 1 part salt to 18 parts sesame seeds for two months and 1:16 thereafter.

A small volume of white-meat fish may be eaten once every 2 weeks by those with more yang tumors and once a week by those with more yin tumors. After 2 months, this may be increased to twice a week, if desired. The fish should be steamed, boiled, or poached and garnished with grated daikon, lemon, or ginger. Minimize fruits until the condition improves, though a small volume of cooked apples or other temperate-climate fruit may be taken if cravings develop. Avoid raisins, all fruit juice, and cider. Avoid all sweets and desserts, including good-quality macrobiotic desserts, until the condition improves. Use sweet vegetables daily in cooking, SWEET VEGETABLE JAM, occasional AMASAKE, and, if cravings arise, a little BARLEY MALT or BROWN RICE SYRUP. Avoid all nuts except chestnuts, and avoid nut butters. Unsalted lightly steamed or boiled squash or pumpkin seeds may be consumed in small volume, up to 1 cup a week. Avoid sunflower seeds. Limit rice cakes, popcorn, and other dry or baked snacks, as they may harden the tumor. Sea salt, miso, shoyu, and other seasoning use is to be moderate. Avoid mirin, garlic, and all herbs and spices. BANCHA TWIG TEA should be the principal beverage. Strictly avoid all mineral or carbonated waters, soft drinks, iced beverages, and for 2 to 3 months grain coffee.

The following remedies are helpful to stop a brain tumor from growing and to reduce the tumor:

1. Cook DRIED DAIKON, SHIITAKE, CABBAGE, BURDOCK, AND ROASTED RICE TEA. Drink 1 small cup every morning and every evening for 3 weeks. After that, reduce it to once a day and continue for another 3 weeks.

2. Make SHIO-KOMBU and have 2 to 3 pieces every day at mealtime.

3. Have one small cup of UME-SHO KUZU every other day or once every 3 days for 1 month. Then after that, reduce it to 1 cup every 4 to 5 days, and continue for another 1 month.

4. Apply a CABBAGE LEAF COMPRESS on the diseased part of the head, and keep changing it to cool it down. (In this case, ice cubes cannot be used.)

5. MASSAGE all five toes, especially by pulling the big toes strongly, for 10 to 15 minutes. Do this every day, 2 to 3 times a day.

6. If the patient has a seizure or loses consciousness as in epilepsy, cool the whole head, including the forehead, immediately with a COLD TOWEL COMPRESS. MASSAGE all the toes well (especially the big toes). If conscious, give UME-SHO BANCHA using a spoon. BANCHA TWIG TEA WITH GOMASHIO may be given instead.

7. If some liquid has accumulated around the tumor, eat 1 small cup of GRATED DAIKON WITH CARROT AND SHOYU every day for 5 days. After that, continue it once every other day for 10 days; then after that, 2 to 3 times a week for another 3 to 4 weeks. In this case, home remedy no. 1, above, may also be helpful, to help relieve this condition.

Follow the standard way-of-life suggestions, trying to be positive, happy, and outgoing. Avoid synthetic clothing, including wigs and hairpieces, and refrain from using chemical shampoos and other products, especially on the hair and head. Meditation, prayer, visualization, chanting, yoga, and other peaceful, gentle exercises may help calm the mind and spirit. Harmonious music, arts, and literature may also be beneficial. Avoid long baths or showers that can deplete minerals from the body.

Breast Cancer. Breast cancer is the most common form of cancer in women and accounts for one-third of all malignancies. One of eight women now living in modern society will get this disease, and the overwhelming majority are over 50. Breast cancer is the third leading cause of cancer death in women after lung and colon cancer. The incidence among men is less than 1 percent. Conventional medicine treats breast cancer with *radical mastectomy,* or total removal of the breast; *modified radical mastectomy,* or partial removal of the breast, leaving the muscle on the chest wall intact; *lumpectomy,* or removal of the malignant lump and lymph nodes under the arm; *radiation therapy;* and *chemotherapy,* especially the drug tamoxifen. About 70 percent of women who use conventional therapies survive five years or more, and many cases are considered untreatable.

From an energetic perspective, breast cancer appears in the upper and outer parts of the body and arises as a result of consuming more yin, expansive foods. Primary dietary factors are sugar, honey, chocolate, and other concentrated sweeteners; milk, cream, butter, cottage cheese, and other dairy products; oily and fatty foods, including french fries, salad dressings, and chips; and white flour in the form of white bread, pastries, and other flour products. The day-to-day consumption of ice cream or yogurt accelerates the creation of breast cancer, as does too much fruit and fruit juice, a large amount of vegetable oil, spices, stimulants, and wine and other alcohol. Birth control pills, drugs, medications, and chemically grown, processed, and treated foods may also be contributing factors. Electric or microwave cooking will also further its spread.

There are two main forms of breast cancer: the soft type, which results from extreme yin substances and influences, as described above, and the hard type, which results from strong yin foods in combination with strong yang foods, including meat, eggs, poultry, hard cheese, and too many hard baked flour products. To help alleviate the first type of breast cancer, which includes inflammatory breast cancer, observe the guidelines for Diet #1. For the second type, which includes harder, more compact tumors, observe the guidelines for Diet #3, arising from extremes of both kinds.

All extreme foods are to be discontinued, including flour products, with the exception of occasional consumption of unyeasted, unleavened whole-wheat or whole-rye bread if cravings arise. All oil, including good-quality vegetable oil, is to be avoided or minimized in cooking for at least 1 month (preferably 2 months). Prepare brown rice as the main grain, combined or alternated day to day with millet or barley. Avoid buckwheat, soba noodles, and seitan. One to 2 servings of soup are recommended daily, especially MISO SOUP cooked with wakame and onions, carrots, or other vegetables. A little shiitake mushroom may occasionally be added to miso soup or shoyu broth. MILLET AND SWEET VEGETABLE SOUP may be eaten often. Green leafy, round, and root vegetables are to be eaten daily, with a slight emphasis on carrot, burdock, daikon, and other root varieties. Special dishes can be prepared according to the dietary guidelines. Follow the standard recommendations for beans and bean products, but use firm rather than soft tofu and avoid raw tofu or tofu that is too creamy. Observe the suggestions for sea vegetables, condiments, and pickles, all of which are very important in helping to heal this condition. Avoid all animal food, including fish, for 1 month (preferably 2 months), though a small volume of white-meat fish may be taken once every 2 weeks if craved or for energy. After that time, it may be taken once a week, but strictly avoid tuna, salmon, and other red-meat and blue-skin varieties and all shellfish. Avoid fruits until the condition improves, though a small volume of cooked apples or other temperate-climate fruit may be taken if cravings develop. Avoid raisins, all fruit juice, and cider. Avoid all sweets and desserts, including good-quality macrobiotic desserts, until the condition improves. Use sweet vegetables daily in cooking, SWEET VEGETABLE JAM, occasional AMASAKE, and, if cravings arise, a little BARLEY MALT or BROWN RICE SYRUP. Avoid all nuts except chestnuts, and avoid nut butters. Unsalted blanched sesame or pumpkin seeds may be consumed in small volume, up to 1 cup a week. Sea salt, miso, shoyu, and other seasoning is to be moderate. Avoid mirin, garlic, and all herbs and spices. BANCHA TWIG TEA should be the principal beverage. Strictly avoid all mineral or carbonated waters, soft drinks, iced beverages, and for 2 to 3 months grain coffee.

The following special dishes, drinks, and home remedies may be helpful for breast cancer:

1. Take CABBAGE AND CARROT JUICE. Take 1 to 2 small cups of this juice every day for 2 weeks; after that, every other day for another 2 weeks.

2. Make DRIED DAIKON, SHIITAKE, AND CABBAGE TEA. Drink 1 cup every morning and every evening for 3 weeks; then reduce it to 2 to 3 times a week, and continue for another 1 month.

3. If you have constipation, take UME-SHO KUZU every 3 days for 1 month.

4. For strength and vitality, KINPIRA SOUP may be taken 2 to 3 times a week.

5. Take GRATED DAIKON AND CARROT to help eliminate old fat and oil. Eat this preparation every other day for 2 weeks; after that, twice a week for another 1 month. You may also add a small amount of water and simmer for 2 to 3 minutes.

6. In some cases, a HATO MUGI–CABBAGE PLASTER can be applied externally to help facilitate the discharge of toxic matter. Spread the mixture about 1 inch thick on a cotton cloth. Apply the mixture directly on the breast and tie with a cotton strip or bolt of cheesecloth. Leave the plaster on for 4 hours or more. Use once or twice every day. The plaster may be left on overnight.

7. If you feel pressure on the pancreas, especially in the event of chemotherapy, take 1 to 2 small cups of SWEET VEGETABLE DRINK every day for about 3 weeks.

8. After surgery, a lump of fat sometimes grows on the scar. To prevent a lump from forming, apply a KOMBU-CABBAGE PLASTER. Leave on for about 4 hours or overnight.

9. If you have the lymph nodes removed from the armpit, the arm sometimes swells. In this case, wrap the arm in CABBAGE LEAF COMPRESS, and take CABBAGE AND CARROT

JUICE, as mentioned above. This will clear up many cases, but if the swelling persists, please seek medical attention.

Follow the standard way-of-life suggestions, especially remaining as cheerful and positive as possible and singing a happy song every day. A daily BODY SCRUB is important; avoid wearing synthetic clothes, use cotton sheets and pillowcases, and avoid radiation from computers, television, and other sources, which tends to gather in the chest. Discontinue birth control pills and hormone replacement therapy, which raise the risk of breast cancer. For new mothers with breast cancer, breast-feeding will not transmit the disease and may be safely practiced. Men who work with radar, microwave energy, telephone lines, and other electronics equipment are at high risk for developing breast cancer, and avoidance of artificial electromagnetic energy of all kinds, including electrically cooked and microwaved food, is recommended.

Colon and Rectal Cancer. Colorectal cancer accounts for about 150,000 new cases in the U.S. each year and about 60,000 deaths. Men have slightly more tumors than women, and about 75 percent of malignancies are located in the lower end of the colon (known as the *sigmoid colon*)or in the rectum. This type of cancer primarily affects urban, affluent people and whites more than blacks, Asians, and other groups. Ninety percent of colon and rectal tumors develop from polyps, benign growths in the lining of the large intestine. Colorectal cancer is usually treated surgically, and a temporary or permanent colostomy is performed to attach a bag to collect bodily wastes. Chemotherapy or radiation is sometimes employed to shrink the tumor prior to surgery or afterward to prevent recurrence or prolong survival. Depending on the type of malignancy and its stage, survival rates range from 5 to 90 percent.

From the dietary view, colorectal cancer is caused primarily by long-term intake of overly yang foods, including meat, eggs, poultry, hard cheese, heavy fish and seafood, and other animal foods and by a lack of fiber from whole grains, fresh vegetables, beans and bean products, and other plant quality foods. The sigmoid colon and rectum are the most contracted part of the large intestine and especially affected by these foods. Too much baked, grilled, roasted, and other strongly cooked foods and too much salt and salted foods also contribute to an overly contracted condition. Though heavy animal foods are the main cause of colorectal malignancies, sugar, refined flour, light dairy products, alcohol, and other yin, expansive foods and beverages can cause the large intestine to become loose and sluggish. Tumors in the ascending colon are caused by proportionately more yin substances in combination with animal foods, while those in the transverse colon include yin to a lesser degree.

A sedentary lifestyle and irregular patterns of eating (especially eating late at night and before going to sleep) burden the intestines and contribute to digestive disorders. Drugs, medications, artificial electromagnetic radiation, and other environmental influences may also contribute to its development and accelerate its spread.

To help relieve colon cancer, discontinue all extreme foods and generally observe the dietary guidelines for Diet #2, for more yang conditions. All extreme foods are to be discontinued, especially all animal foods, including fish and seafood. In the event of cravings, a small volume of white-meat fish may be taken every 10 days for 2 or 3 months. After this time, it can be increased to once a week, but strictly avoid all tuna, salmon, and other dark fish and all shellfish. Also avoid all hard baked flour products, including high-quality whole-wheat sourdough bread, until the condition improves. A very small amount of sesame oil may be used in preparing sautéed vegetables for the first month and then gradually increased in amount and frequency.

Prepare brown rice as the main grain, combined or alternated day to day with millet or barley. Use a square of kombu the size of a postage stamp instead of salt in seasoning grains for sigmoid or rectal tumors. Sea salt may be used for other forms of colon cancer. Avoid buckwheat, soba noodles, and seitan altogether and, for 1 month, whole oats or oatmeal. Whole grain noodles or pasta may be used once or twice a week in small volume. Avoid raw salad for 1 month and then it may be used once in every 10 to 14 days.

One to 2 servings of soup are recommended daily, especially MISO SOUP cooked with wakame and onions, carrots, or other vegetables. A little shiitake mushroom may occasionally be added to miso soup or shoyu broth. Green leafy, round, and root vegetables are to be eaten daily, with a slight emphasis on leafy varieties for cancer in the ascending colon, round vegetables for that in the transverse colon, and round and root vegetables for the sigmoid colon or rectum. Special vegetable dishes can be prepared according to the dietary guidelines.

Follow the standard recommendations for beans and bean products, sea vegetables, and condiments. A little miso sautéed in sesame oil and a similar volume of chopped scallions may be used daily on grains. One teaspoon of sautéed whole dandelions is also helpful for this type of cancer. Among pickles, the rice bran kinds are the most suitable.

Minimize fruits until the condition improves, though a small volume of cooked apples or other temperate-climate fruit may be taken if cravings develop. Avoid raisins, all fruit juice, and cider. Avoid all sweets and desserts, including good-quality macrobiotic desserts, until the condition improves. Use sweet vegetables daily in cooking, SWEET VEGETABLE JAM, occasional AMASAKE, and if cravings arise, a little BARLEY MALT or BROWN RICE SYRUP. Avoid all nuts except chestnuts, and avoid nut butters. Unsalted blanched sunflower or pumpkin seeds may be consumed in small volume, up to 1 cup a week. Sea salt, miso, shoyu, and other seasoning is to be moderate. Avoid mirin, garlic, and all herbs and spices. BANCHA TWIG TEA should be the principal beverage. Strictly avoid all mineral or carbonated waters, soft drinks, iced beverages, and for 2 to 3 months grain coffee.

The following special dishes, drinks, or home remedies may be helpful for colon cancer:

I. Cook BROWN RICE PORRIDGE WITH GRATED DAIKON and UMEBOSHI. Eat 1 to 2 bowls of this porridge every day for 1 week to 10 days; and after that, 2 to 4 times a week for another 3 to 4 weeks.

2. Cook DRIED DAIKON, DAIKON LEAVES, ROASTED BROWN RICE, and SHIITAKE TEA. Drink 1 to 2 cups every day for 2 to

3 weeks; after that, reduce it to 3 to 4 times a week, and continue for another month.

3. PRESSED SALAD with daikon and daikon leaves and sea salt is beneficial for this condition. Wash the salad with water to remove excess salt before serving. Eat a small amount of this preparation with meals.

4. To help relieve bleeding, UME-KUZU is helpful. Drink 1 to 2 small cups every day for 3 days.

5. WATER-SAUTÉED DAIKON AND DAIKON LEAVES are also recommended. Season with a little miso or shoyu. Eat 1 small dish of this preparation every day.

6. If you have a tumor, prepare GRATED DAIKON AND POTATO JUICE. Drink one-third of a small cup of this preparation every day. You may add a little sea salt. But be careful not to take too much, as it can make you weak.

7. To relieve pain, a POTATO PLASTER may be helpful. Leave the plaster on for 3 to 4 hours; repeat every day for several days.

8. Make DAIKON AND DAIKON LEAVES QUICK PICKLES. Wash the salad with water to remove the excess salt before serving. Eat a small amount of this preparation with your meals.

9. If the descending colon or rectum is narrowed or blocked by a tumor, the channel may be opened by (1) 1–3 cups per day of liquid made by boiling dried shiitake, grated daikon, and a little grated ginger in water and cooking with a slight shoyu taste, (2) 2–3 cups of water in which dried tangerine or orange peel has been boiled, (3) MISO SOUP, 2–3 cups daily, cooked with sliced daikon or radish, garlic or ginger, and onion or scallion, or (4) cooked

agar-agar (kanten) seasoned with apple juice or barley malt and grated ginger twice a day.

Follow the standard way-of-life suggestions, especially remaining as hopeful and positive as possible. Depression, sadness, and melancholy commonly accompany this type of cancer, and singing a happy song every day will lift the spirits as well as facilitate energy flow and the discharge process. A daily BODY SCRUB is important; avoid wearing synthetic clothes, use cotton sheets and pillowcases, and avoid radiation from computers, television, and other sources, which tends to gather in the chest.

Kidney and Bladder Cancer. About one-third of malignancies in the urinary system occur in the kidney and two-thirds in the bladder, ureters, or urethra. Kidney and bladder cancer are more prevalent in men than women and tend to appear in middle or old age. About 30,000 new cases are diagnosed in the United States each year. Standard medical treatment involves surgical removal of the kidney along with adjacent lymph nodes and adrenal glands or partial or total removal of the bladder. Radiation is sometimes used internally or externally before surgery to destroy invasive tumors; chemotherapy is not used as a primary treatment, but occasionally it is employed to control pain after surgery. The survival rate for urinary cancers is about 50 to 75 percent.

Kidney cancer is caused by long-term consumption of dairy food and animal food high in saturated fats, along with sugar, chemicals, and artificial beverages. Cheese, eggs, and chicken are a frequent combination. Bladder cancer arises from overintake of dairy, sugar, fruits, juices, chemicals, stimulants, and foods that produce fat and mucus.

To relieve kidney or bladder cancer, follow the general dietary guidelines for Diet #3 for tumors arising as a result of both yin and yang dietary extremes. The kidneys control salt metabolism, and salt should be minimized for kidney or bladder cancer for several months, as it tends to solidify and harden the malignancy. Kombu may be used instead for seasoning. The use of miso and shoyu should also be light. Avoid all oily and greasy food, as well as refined flour products such as bread, cookies, and crackers. All cold foods, especially icy drinks, are to be eliminated. Though not the main cause, spices can accelerate cancer growth and should be discontinued. Avoid all animal food, including white-meat fish, unless cravings occur, in which case a small volume may be consumed once every 10–14 days. Avoid all hard baked flour products except for good-quality unyeasted sourdough bread, which may be taken 2–3 times a week. Avoid oil for the first month and then use sesame oil two or three times a week, brushed on the skillet, to sauté vegetables. Avoid raw salad and salad dressing for one month, and then eat once every 7–10 days.

Prepare brown rice as the main grain, combined or alternated day to day with millet or barley. Use a small square of kombu the size of a postage stamp instead of salt in cooking grain, though in some cases salt may be used. Avoid buckwheat and seitan for three months and, for 1 month, whole oats or oatmeal. Whole-grain noodles or pasta may be used a couple of times a week in small volume.

One to 2 servings of soup are recommended daily, especially MISO SOUP cooked with wakame and onions, carrots, or other vegetables. A small amount of shiitake mushroom may occasionally be added to miso soup or shoyu broth. Green leafy, round, and root vegetables are to be eaten daily, cooked in a variety of forms, mainly steamed, boiled, or, for the first month, water-sautéed. Special vegetable dishes can be prepared according to the dietary guidelines. Follow the standard recommendations for beans and bean products, but dried tofu is better for urinary cancers than fresh tofu. Sea vegetables are beneficial, especially a sheet of toasted nori, which may be taken daily and will strengthen the bladder. Follow the standard macrobiotic guidelines for pickles and condiments.

Minimize fruits until the condition improves, though a small volume of cooked apples or other temperate-climate fruit may be taken if cravings develop. Avoid raisins, all fruit juice, and cider. Avoid all sweets and desserts, including good-quality macrobiotic desserts, until the condition improves. Use sweet vegetables daily in cooking, SWEET VEGETABLE JAM, occasional AMASAKE, and if cravings arise, a little BARLEY MALT or BROWN RICE SYRUP. Avoid all nuts except chestnuts, and avoid nut butters. Unsalted lightly steamed or boiled sunflower or pumpkin seeds may be consumed in small volume, up to 1 cup a week. Limit rice cakes, popcorn, and other dry or baked snacks, as they may harden the tumor. Sea salt, miso, shoyu, and other seasoning is to be moderate. Avoid mirin, garlic, and all herbs and spices. BANCHA TWIG TEA should be the principal beverage. Strictly avoid all mineral or carbonated waters, soft drinks, iced beverages, and for two to three months grain coffee.

The following special dishes, drinks, or home remedies may be helpful for kidney cancer:

1. SWEET VEGETABLE DRINK, 1 small cup taken every day for 1 month and then every other day the second month.

2. CARROT-DAIKON DRINK is also beneficial. Take 1 small cup every day for 5 days, then every other day for 2 weeks, and then every 3 days for 1 month.

3. SHIITAKE-DAIKON TEA may be taken, 1 small cup once every three days for 1 month.

4. ADZUKI BEAN TEA can help restore smooth urination. Take 1–2 cups daily for up to several days.

5. RICE JUICE, the liquid that rises to the surface while cooking brown rice, may be used daily or regularly as a beverage.

6. BEET JUICE may be helpful in some cases. Take every day for 10 days, then every other day for 10 days.

7. In some cases, a plaster is beneficial. For pain on the kidney, a POTATO PLASTER or POTATO-CABBAGE PLASTER may be applied for 3 hours, preceded by a hot towel for 3–5 minutes. This may be repeated once or twice a day for several days.

8. LOTUS-POTATO PLASTER A plaster combining an equal volume of grated fresh lotus root and potato (mixed with a little white flour for consistency and 5 to 10 percent grated ginger) when applied to the back on the area of the kidneys for three to four hours is helpful for kidney cancer if used daily for 2 to 3 weeks. This should be preceded by a ginger compress for 3 to 5 minues.

9. A BODY SCRUB is recommended daily.

10. PALM HEALING on the kidney or bladder region is also helpful to control pain and discomfort.

For bladder cancer, one or more of the following may be helpful:

1. Cook DRIED DAIKON, DRIED DAIKON LEAVES, SHIITAKE, DRIED LOTUS ROOT, AND ROASTED BROWN RICE TEA. Have 1 cup every morning and evening for about 3 weeks. After that, continue about 3 times a week for another 3 to 4 weeks.

2. Cook HIJIKI WITH DRIED DAIKON AND SHIITAKE. A few drops of sesame oil can be added. Take ½ to ⅔ cup of this dish every day or every other day.

3. Cook MISO-SCALLION CONDIMENT. Have 1 teaspoon every day with the main grain at mealtime.

4. In case of bleeding, have 1 to 2 cups of UME-SHO KUZU or UME-SHO BANCHA every day for a few days.

5. In case of pain in the abdomen, make raw CABBAGE JUICE. Then simmer it slightly for about 3 minutes. Drink 1 to 2 cups daily for 3 to 4 days.

Follow the standard way-of-life suggestions. Especially avoid wool and synthetic fabrics such as nylon, which are irritating to the bladder. Artificial electromagnetic radiation is also depleting and can weaken the urinary system. Avoid or minimize television, computers, cell phones, and other electronic devices. The kidney and bladder are sensitive to cold. Keep these protected and warm, especially during the winter. A cotton band can be worn around the abdomen and back to prevent cold and chills.

Leukemia. Leukemia is a blood cancer that takes about 20,000 lives annually in the United States and accounts for nearly 30,000 new cases. Males are slightly more apt to get this disease than women. In leukemia, white blood cells are produced in abnormally large numbers. The acute forms grow quickly and affect children and young adults, while the chronic varieties grow slowly and occur in older age brackets. Among adults over 40, *acute myelocytic leukemia* (AML) is the most common form, while among children *acute lymphocytic* or *lymphoblastic leukemia* (ALL) occurs most frequently. *Chronic myelocytic* or *granulocytic leukemia* (CML) affects primarily young adults and the middle aged, while *chronic lymphocytic leukemia* (CLL) is found among the elderly. Chemotherapy is used to treat all types of leukemia, while surgery or radiation may also be employed if the lymph system is affected or the liver or spleen are enlarged. Bone-marrow transplants and blood transfusions are often performed to provide fresh red blood cells. The five-year survival rate for this disease is about one in three.

From the macrobiotic perspective, leukemia is primarily caused by extreme yin foods and beverages that weaken the blood and result in an imbalance of red and white blood cells. Milk, ice cream, and other dairy foods; sugar, honey, chocolate, and other concentrated sweeteners; soft drinks; excessive fruits and juices; frequent raw salads; tropical foods; spices; stimulants; alcohol; and drugs are included in this category. Chemicals used in growing or preserving foods may also be a main factor. In a small number of cases, leukemia is caused by strong yang factors, especially overuse of salt, too much baked flour, baked or roasted foods, and other contractive

items and cooking methods. In this type of leukemia, which accounts for only about 10 to 20 percent of all cases, animal food is usually not a primary factor. In the blood, too much salt and baked carbohydrates hinder red blood cell production. Strong yang environmental factors may also contribute to leukemia. For example, at the beach the strong, hot sun makes white blood cell counts go up and red blood cells go down as yin is attracted to the surface and yang is brought to the center.

For the more yin type of leukemia, observe the dietary guidelines for Diet #1, while for the more yang type follow Diet #2. In both cases, avoid all oily and fatty foods, including all animal foods, dairy products, and vegetable oils and dressings, as well as sugar and other sweets; refined and polished grains and flour products; tropical fruits and vegetables; coffee, tea, herbal drinks, mineral waters, and other stimulants; and spices. Tobacco, alcohol, and drugs are to be completely eliminated. All food is to be cooked and not eaten raw. Seasoning should be moderate, neither too salty nor too bland.

Prepare brown rice as the main grain, combined or alternated day to day with barley or millet. For more yin cases, either a pinch of sea salt or a square of kombu the size of a postage stamp may be used to season the grain during cooking. For more yang cases, frequently boil brown rice instead of pressure-cooking it, and use kombu for seasoning grains until the condition improves. For 1 month, avoid whole oats or oatmeal. Whole-grain noodles or pasta may be used a couple of times a week in small volume. Good-quality sourdough bread may be enjoyed two to three times a week, but all other hard baked flour products, including cookies, pie, cake, crackers, and pastries, are to be avoided. For both types, minimize buckwheat and seitan. The more yin type may use soba noodles occasionally.

One to 2 servings of soup are recommended daily, especially MISO SOUP cooked with wakame and onions, carrots or other vegetables. A small amount of shiitake mushroom may occasionally be added to miso soup or shoyu broth. MILLET AND SWEET VEGETABLE SOUP may be prepared often. Green leafy, round, and root vegetables are to be eaten daily in about equal volume for the more yin form of leukemia. Emphasize sweet vegetables for the more yang type, as well as steamed or boiled greens often. Special vegetable dishes can be prepared according to the dietary guidelines. Avoid the use of oil in cooking for 1 month, and then use a small volume of sesame oil to make fried rice, fried noodles, or sautéed vegetables several times a week. For more yin cases of leukemia, follow the standard recommendations for beans and bean products, sea vegetables, and pickles. However, for yang types of leukemia, a recommended dish is soybeans cooked with kombu, carrots, and onions with a light miso taste. Black soybeans may also be cooked with a small amount of chopped kombu and cooked for a long time to bring out their natural sweetness. Alternatively, a small volume of AMASAKE, BROWN RICE SYRUP, or BARLEY MALT may be added to beans for those with yang leukemia to give a light, sweet taste. A drop of oil may also be added to beans during cooking.

GOMASHIO may be used with a ratio of 1 part salt to 18 parts sesame seeds for two months and 1:16 thereafter.

Avoid animal food with the exception of white-meat fish, which may be eaten once a week. After 2 months, fish may be eaten twice a week if desired, especially by those with the more yin form of leukemia. Those with the more yang type of leukemia should avoid fish and seafood, though a small volume of white-meat fish may be taken once every 10–14 days if craved. The fish should be prepared steamed, boiled, or poached and garnished with grated daikon, lemon, or ginger. Minimize fruits until the condition improves, though a small volume of cooked apples or other temperate-climate fruit may be taken if cravings develop. Avoid raisins, all fruit juice, and cider. Avoid all sweets and desserts, including good-quality macrobiotic desserts, until the condition improves. Use sweet vegetables daily in cooking, sweet vegetable jam, occasional AMASAKE, and if cravings arise, a little BARLEY MALT or BROWN RICE SYRUP. Avoid all nuts except chestnuts, and avoid nut butters. Unsalted lightly steamed or boiled sunflower or pumpkin seeds may be consumed in small volume, up to 1 cup a week. Limit rice cakes, popcorn, and other dry or baked snacks, as they may harden the tumor. Sea salt, miso, shoyu, and other seasoning are to be moderate. Avoid mirin, garlic, and all herbs and spices. BANCHA TWIG TEA should be the principal beverage. Strictly avoid all mineral or carbonated waters, soft drinks, iced beverages, and for two to three months grain coffee.

The following special dishes, drinks, or home remedies may be helpful for leukemia:

1. Have MISO-ZOSUI made with brown rice or brown rice mixed with other grains every day, or 3 to 4 times a week. You can cook together burdock, daikon, carrot, cabbage, winter squash or pumpkin, onion, and leafy green vegetables, as well as a small amount of wakame, kombu, or nori.

2. Cook BROWN RICE WITH BEANS, using adzuki beans with a small piece of kombu. Have this with GOMASHIO or UMEBOSHI PLUM, chewing well. Take 1 to 2 bowls a day, for about 10 days.

3. NISHIME-STYLE ROOT VEGETABLES, with burdock, carrot, daikon, lotus, jinenjo (mountain potato), and kombu, is also good. Have 1 bowl every day or every other day, chewing well.

4. Make KOI-KOKU and have 1 bowl a day for 3 days. Ten days later, have 1 bowl of this every day for another 3 days. Repeat this sequence 3 times. If fish is not eaten, KINPIRA SOUP may be taken instead.

5. OHAGI, made with black sesame seed GOMASHIO, is good.

6. MASSAGE or PALM HEALING of the abdominal area may help improve digestion.

7. In case of frequent constipation or diarrhea, have light UME-KUZU or UME-SHO BANCHA every day or every other day for 2 weeks.

Follow the standard way-of-life suggestions. Deep breathing exercises and physical exercise, but not to the point of exhaustion, may be helpful. Keep the air in the home fresh and clean, adding green plants in each room and opening the windows from time to time. Avoid or limit television, computers, cellular phones, and other electronic or handheld devices that are weakening to the blood and circulatory system. Be bright and positive and sing a happy song every day.

Liver Cancer. Liver cancer kills about 15,000 Americans every year, affecting men and women about equally. Primary liver tumors often follow cirrhosis or hepatitis B or C. The organ is a frequent site for metastases from the breast, lung, and colon. Main types include *hepatomas,* tumors in the epithelial lining of both lobes; *cholangiocarcinomas,* which begin in the bile ducts and spread to the liver; *hemangiosarcomas,* mixed tumors of sarcoma cells and dilated blood vessels; *hepatoblastomas,* rare granular tumors in children; and *adenocarcinomas,* glandular tumors in the bile ducts. The survival rate for liver cancer is 1 percent, with most patients dying within six months of diagnosis. Most cases are inoperable, though surgery, chemotherapy, or radiation may be performed occasionally, especially in the early stages.

Liver cancer arises from predominantly extreme yang factors. The primary cause is animal protein and fat, especially eggs, salmon, tuna, shrimp, and other fatty meat, poultry, and seafood, in combination with cheese and other dairy products, sugar, sugary foods, stimulants, aromatic foods and beverages, alcohol, and chemically treated foods. Because the liver filters the blood of toxins, it is especially susceptible to irritation from drugs, medications, pesticides, plastics, and other chemicals in food, water, and the environment. Overeating also particularly stresses the liver and is often a primary factor in tumor development.

To relieve liver cancer, follow the general dietary guidelines for Diet #2 for disorders arising from excessive contractive factors. Avoid all animal food, including white-meat fish, unless cravings occur, in which case a small volume may be consumed once every 10–14 days. All flour products, including good-quality sour-dough bread, are to be avoided for several months. Avoid oil for the first month and then use sesame oil once or twice a week, brushed on the skillet, to sauté vegetables.

Prepare brown rice as the main grain, combined or alternated day to day with millet or barley. Generally use a square of kombu the size of a postage stamp instead of salt in cooking grain, though in some cases, such as when yin factors are present, salt may be used. Avoid buckwheat, soba noodles, and seitan altogether and, for 1 month, whole oats or oatmeal. Whole-grain noodles or pasta may be used a couple of times a week in small volume.

One to 2 servings of soup are recommended daily, especially MISO SOUP cooked with wakame and onions, carrots, or other vegetables. A small amount of shiitake mushroom may occasionally be added to miso soup or shoyu broth. Green leafy, round, and root vegetables are to be eaten daily, with a slight emphasis on green varieties such as broccoli, leafy green tops of carrots, turnips, daikon, and watercress. Special vegetable dishes can be prepared according to the dietary guidelines. Follow the standard recommendations for beans and bean products, sea vegetables, and pickles. GOMASHIO may be used with a ratio of 1 part salt to 18 to 20 parts sesame seeds.

Minimize fruits until the condition improves, though a small volume of cooked apples or other temperate-climate fruit may be taken if cravings develop. Avoid raisins, all fruit juice, and cider. Avoid all sweets and desserts, including good-quality macrobiotic desserts, until the condition improves. Use sweet vegetables daily in cooking, SWEET VEGETABLE JAM, occa-sional AMASAKE, and if cravings arise, a lit-tle BARLEY MALT or BROWN RICE SYRUP. Avoid all nuts except chestnuts and avoid nut butters. Unsalted lightly steamed or boiled sun-flower or pumpkin seeds may be consumed in small volume, up to 1 cup a week. Limit rice cakes, popcorn, and other dry or baked snacks, as they may harden the tumor. Sea salt, miso, shoyu, and other seasoning is to be moder-ate. Avoid mirin, garlic, and all herbs and spices. BANCHA TWIG TEA should be the principal beverage. Strictly avoid all mineral or carbon-ated waters, soft drinks, iced beverages, and for 2 to 3 months grain coffee.

The following special dishes, drinks, or home remedies may be helpful for liver cancer:

1. To help relieve liver tumors, prepare ROASTED BUCKWHEAT AND SCALLION TEA. Keep in a thermos and take 1 cup a day for 1 month.

2. A person with liver cancer frequently craves a sour taste. Sour foods create more up-ward energy, while liver tumors arise from the accumulation of more downward energy. A small amount of lemon juice may be taken fre-quently in tea or water. APPLE JUICE or apple cider may also be taken in small amounts and will provide a sour taste. If you develop jaun-dice, make 2 to 3 cups of SOUR GREEN APPLE SAUCE. This can be taken until the jaundice dis-appears. Be sure to use tart apples to make this.

3. A special dish, BROWN RICE AND BAR-LEY PORRIDGE WITH GRATED DAIKON, is recommended for liver cancer.

4. In some cases, a HATO MUGI–POTATO-CABBAGE PLASTER is recommended. Spread on cotton linen to a thickness of about 3 cm and apply directly over the liver. Keep on at least 4 hours. Repeat twice every day. If applied before bedtime, it may be kept on until morning.

5. Another helpful preparation is DRIED DAIKON, DRIED DAIKON LEAVES, BURDOCK, SHIITAKE, AND CABBAGE TEA. Drink every day 1 or 2 small cups. Continue for about 3 weeks. Thereafter, drink it 3 to 4 times per week, and continue for 3 or 4 weeks more.

6. Eat as little food as possible, and chew very well. The liver is particularly stressed by overeating. The more you chew, the better.

Follow the standard way-of-life suggestions. Avoid exposure to chemicals, plastics, synthetics, and other influences that are especially weakening to the liver and its functions. Avoid activities and exercise that produce exhaustion. Walking, breathing exercises, relaxation exercises, and other gentle activities are helpful.

Lung Cancer. Lung cancer causes more deaths in both men and women than any other malignancy, and its incidence is rising sharply. Middle-aged persons are at highest risk. *Squamous cell carcinoma,* arising in the central bronchi, is the most prevalent type in men and among smokers. *Adenocarcinoma,* the most common type in women and among nonsmokers, appears along the periphery of the lungs in the small bronchi and bronchioles. *Small cell lung cancer,* a very aggressive type, originates in the central bronchi, while *large cell carcinoma* manifests on the outer part of the lungs. Surgery is performed for most squamous cell tumors, adenocarcinomas, and large cell carcinomas, while small cell type is treated with a combination of chemotherapy and radia-

tion. The overall survival rate for lung cancer is 15 percent.

Lung cancer arises from a combination of dietary extremes. It appears in the upper body, showing that upward yin energy is involved, and yet the lungs are condensed organs, showing that strong inward-moving yang energy is also a factor. The primary cause is dairy food, especially cheese, which clogs the lungs and traps acids, wastes, and other toxins that are normally discharged by breathing. Eighty percent of lung cancer occurs in smokers, but generally only smokers who eat dairy food are at higher risk than nonsmokers. In addition to dairy, other animal foods are commonly involved, including meat, eggs, poultry, and seafood. From the yin category, sugar and other sweets, fruits and juices, spices and stimulants, and alcohol and other drugs are also usually consumed in excess. Relative to each other, squamous cell carcinoma and small cell lung cancer originating in the central part of the lungs are caused by proportionately more animal food and yang factors, while adenocarcinomas and large cell carcinomas, affecting the periphery, result from relatively more yin factors.

To help relieve lung cancer, observe the dietary guidelines for Diet #3, for conditions arising from a combination of factors. All extreme foods are to be discontinued, especially dairy foods and all animal foods, including fish and seafood. In the event of cravings, a small volume of white-meat fish may be taken every 10–14 days. Strictly avoid all tuna, salmon, and other dark fish and all shellfish. Avoid all hard baked flour products, including high-quality whole wheat sourdough bread, for 2–3 months or until the condition improves. No oil is to be consumed for 1 month, and then a very small amount of sesame oil may be used in preparing sautéed vegetables once or twice a week. Avoid raw salad for 1 month, and then eat it once every 10 to 14 days.

Prepare brown rice as the main grain, combined or alternated day to day with millet or barley. Use a square of kombu the size of a postage stamp instead of salt in seasoning grains for squamous cell carcinoma or small cell lung cancer. Sea salt may be used for adenocarcinomas and large cell carcinoma. Avoid buckwheat, soba noodles, and seitan altogether and, for 1 month, whole oats or oatmeal. Whole-grain noodles or pasta may be used once or twice a week in small volume.

One to 2 servings of soup are recommended daily, especially MISO SOUP cooked with wakame and onions, carrots or other vegetables. A little shiitake mushroom may occasionally be added to miso soup or shoyu broth. Green leafy, round, and root vegetables are to be eaten daily, with a slight emphasis on leafy varieties such as broccoli, carrot tops, turnip greens, daikon greens, and watercress. Lotus root is especially beneficial for all lung problems and will help ease breathing. It can be added to grains, soups, and other vegetable dishes. Special vegetable dishes can be prepared according to the dietary guidelines. Follow the standard recommendations for beans and bean products, sea vegetables, condiments, and pickles.

Minimize fruits until the condition improves, though a small volume of cooked apples or other temperate-climate fruit may be taken if cravings develop. Avoid raisins, all fruit juice, and cider. Avoid all sweets and desserts, including good-quality macrobiotic desserts, until the condition improves. Use sweet vegetables daily in cooking, SWEET VEGETABLE JAM, occasional AMASAKE, and if cravings arise, a little BARLEY MALT or BROWN RICE SYRUP. Avoid all nuts except chestnuts, and avoid nut butters. Unsalted blanched sunflower or pumpkin seeds may be consumed in small volume, up to 1 cup a week. Sea salt, miso, shoyu, and other seasoning is to be moderate. Avoid mirin, garlic, and all herbs and spices. BANCHA TWIG TEA should be the principal beverage. Strictly avoid all mineral or carbonated waters, soft drinks, iced beverages, and for 2 to 3 months grain coffee.

The following special dishes, drinks, or home remedies may be helpful for lung cancer:

1. Cook DRIED DAIKON, SHIITAKE, DRIED LOTUS ROOT, AND CARROT LEAF TEA. Drink 2 to 3 small cups of this preparation every day for 1 month. After that, drink it every other day for another 1 month.

2. Make GRATED DAIKON AND CARROT WITH SCALLIONS AND SHOYU, COOKED. Eat 1 small cup of this preparation every day for 10 days, and after that once every 3 days for 3 weeks.

3. To help relieve coughing, take LOTUS ROOT JUICE TEA. Drink ½ to ⅔ of a small cup of the juice. You may add a small amount of water and simmer it quickly. It is best to drink it from evening through night when you cough. It is helpful to drink it every day for 5 to 10 days. If your coughing has not then stopped, continue to drink the lotus juice.

4. Make BROWN RICE PORRIDGE WITH GRATED LOTUS ROOT. Eat 1 bowl of this preparation with UMEBOSHI (previously washed in water) every day for 10 days, and after that every other day or every 3 days for 1 month more. Note that you may add the remaining gratings that you squeezed from the remedy for lotus root juice mentioned above.

5. A small side dish of lotus seeds cooked with kombu or wakame seasoned with a moderate amount of shoyu or miso will help the lungs and may be eaten daily.

6. MASSAGE well the fingers, especially the thumbs and forefingers, 3 to 4 times every day. It is also helpful to rub both hands together until they are warm, 3 to 4 times daily.

7. In a few cases, a plaster may be beneficial. To loosen congestion in the lung, a LOTUS ROOT PLASTER can be applied and kept on a few hours. A MUSTARD PLASTER, placed over the front and then the back of the chest, can relieve severe coughing.

Follow the standard way-of-life suggestions, trying to keep as hopeful and positive as possible. Depression, sadness, and melancholy commonly accompany lung problems, and singing a happy song every day will lift the spirits as well as facilitate breathing, energy flow, and the discharge process. A daily BODY SCRUB is important. Avoid wearing synthetic clothes, use cotton sheets and pillowcases, and avoid radiation from computers, television, and other sources, which tends to gather in the chest. Avoid smoggy, dusty, and polluted air. Visit the seashore, countryside, or other natural environment as often as possible. Strictly avoid smoking or environments in which smoke is found.

Lymphoma and Hodgkin's Disease. Lymphatic system cancers take the lives of about 20,000 Americans annually, with nearly 50,000 new cases diagnosed. Lymphoma appears in men and women about equally. Hodgkin's disease primarily affects teens and young adults and adults over 50. It is accompanied by enlarged lymph nodes in the groin, armpit, or neck and may spread to the brain and adjacent lymph nodes. Non-Hodgkin's lymphomas appear in sites throughout the body, such as the digestive tract, and spread in a wide variety of ways. Radiation and chemotherapy are used to treat both types. The survival rate for Hodgkin's disease is up to 57 percent, while that for other lymphomas ranges from about 18 to 37 percent.

Lymphatic cancers primarily arise from overexpansion or inflammation of the lymph nodes and organs as a result of too much yin foods and beverages. Hodgkin's disease is the most expansive form of this disease, resulting from excessive intake of sugar, chocolate, and other sweets; milk, ice cream, and dairy; too much fruit and juice; excessive oily and greasy foods; alcohol; drugs; and chemicals. Non-Hodgkin's disease also usually involves extreme yin factors, but in less volume or frequency. There is also a more yang form of non-Hodgkin's lymphoma caused by taking too much salt, baked flour, and other contractive fare.

For the more yin type of Hodgkin's and non-Hodgkin's lymphomas, observe the dietary guidelines for Diet #1, while for the more yang type of non-Hodgkin's disease follow Diet #2. In both cases, avoid all dairy products; oily and fatty foods, including all animal foods and vegetable oils and dressings; sugar and other sweets; refined and polished grains and flour products; tropical fruits and vegetables; ice-cold foods and beverages; coffee, tea, herbal drinks, mineral waters, and other stimulants; and spices. Tobacco, alcohol, and drugs are to be completely eliminated. All food is to be cooked and not eaten raw. Seasoning should be moderate, neither too salty nor too bland.

Prepare brown rice as the main grain, combined or alternated day to day with barley or millet. For more yin lymphomas, either a pinch of sea salt or a square of kombu the size of a postage stamp may be used to season the grain during cooking. For the more yang form of lymphoma, frequently boil brown rice instead of pressure-cooking it, and use kombu for seasoning grains until the condition improves. For 1 month, avoid whole oats or oatmeal. Whole-grain noodles or pasta may be used a couple of times a week in small volume. Good-quality sourdough bread may be enjoyed two to three times a week, but all other hard, baked flour products, including cookies, pie, cake, crackers, and pastries, are to be avoided. For both types, minimize buckwheat and seitan. The more yin type may use soba noodles occasionally.

One to 2 servings of soup are recommended daily, especially MISO SOUP cooked with wakame and onions, carrots, or other vegetables. A small amount of shiitake mushroom may occasionally be added to miso soup or shoyu broth. Lotus root may be added to soup frequently. Green leafy, round, and root vegetables are to be eaten daily, with a slight emphasis on sweet vegetables. Steamed or boiled greens are to be eaten often. Special vegetable dishes can be prepared according to the dietary guidelines. Avoid the use of oil in cooking for 1 month, and then use a small volume of sesame oil to fry rice or noodles or sauté vegetables several times a week. For more yin cases of

lymphoma, follow the standard recommendations for beans and bean products, sea vegetables, and pickles. However, for the yang type of lymphoma, a recommended dish is soybeans cooked with kombu, carrots, and onions with a light miso taste. Black soybeans may also be cooked with a small amount of chopped kombu for a long time to bring out their natural sweetness. Alternatively, a small volume of AMASAKE, BROWN RICE SYRUP, or BARLEY MALT may be added to beans for those with yang lymphoma to give a light, sweet taste. A drop of oil may also be added to beans during cooking.

GOMASHIO may be used with a ratio of 1 part salt to 18 parts sesame seeds for 2 months and 1:16 thereafter.

Avoid animal food with the exception of white-meat fish, which may be eaten once a week. After 2 months, fish may be eaten twice a week if desired, especially by those with the more yin form of lymphoma. Those with the more yang type should avoid fish and seafood, though a small volume of white-meat fish may be taken once every 10–14 days if craved. The fish should be prepared steamed, boiled, or poached and garnished with grated daikon, lemon, or ginger. Minimize fruits until the condition improves, though a small volume of cooked apples or other temperate-climate fruit may be taken if cravings develop. Avoid raisins, all fruit juice, and cider. Avoid all sweets and desserts, including good-quality macrobiotic desserts, until the condition improves. Use sweet vegetables daily in cooking, SWEET VEGETABLE JAM, occasional AMASAKE, and if cravings arise, a little BARLEY MALT or BROWN RICE SYRUP. Avoid all nuts except chestnuts and avoid nut butters. Unsalted lightly steamed or boiled sunflower or pumpkin seeds may be consumed in small volume, up to 1 cup a week. Limit rice cakes, popcorn, and other dry or baked snacks, as they may harden the tumor. Sea salt, miso, shoyu, and other seasoning are to be moderate. Avoid mirin, garlic, and all herbs and spices. BANCHA TWIG TEA should be the principal beverage. Strictly avoid all mineral or carbonated waters, soft drinks, iced beverages, and for 2 to 3 months grain coffee.

The following special dishes, drinks, or home remedies may be helpful for lymphoma or Hodgkin's disease:

1. Make KINPIRA-STYLE BURDOCK, CARROT, AND KOMBU. Have a small dish of this every day or every other day for about a month. After that, take it occasionally.

2. Make DRIED DAIKON, DRIED DAIKON LEAVES, AND BURDOCK TEA and have ½ cup 1 to 2 times a day. Keep taking this for 3 weeks. After that, take it 2 to 3 times a week for 3 to 4 weeks.

3. SWEET VEGETABLE DRINK is also good. Take 1 cup a day for 3 to 4 weeks.

4. Make BROWN RICE, MILLET, BUCKWHEAT, AND VEGETABLE PORRIDGE, adding kombu and water. Have 1 bowl a day for 1 week, and then after that 3 times a week for 1 month.

5. Apply a KOMBU-CABBAGE PLASTER on swollen areas. Wrap them with cotton and keep the plaster on for about 4 hours. Do this twice a day; it is possible to keep this on overnight while you are sleeping. Continue this until the swelling disappears.

6. In the event of constipation, take 1 cup of UME-KUZU every day for 3 to 4 days; and then after that 2 to 3 times a week for about 1 month.

7. In case of excess sweating, take 1 cup of UME-KUZU, CABBBAGE TEA (cooled to room temperature), or DRIED DAIKON TEA.

8. Make a CABBAGE PLASTER. Directly apply it to the swollen spleen area for about 4 hours. Change it 2 to 3 times a day. Or apply it when you sleep, and keep it on overnight.

Follow the standard way-of-life suggestions. Deep breathing exercises and physical exercise, but not to the point of exhaustion, may be helpful. Minimize long baths and showers, which cause the body to lose minerals. Wear cotton next to the skin, and use all-cotton sheets and pillowcases. Keep the air in the home fresh and clean, adding green plants in each room and opening the windows from time to time. Avoid or limit television, computers, cellular phones, and other electronic or handheld devices that are weakening to the blood and circulatory system. Be bright and positive and sing a happy song every day.

Mouth and Upper Digestive Cancers. Cancers of the mouth, lips, gums, cheeks, larynx, pharynx, and esophagus account for about 25,000 deaths in the United States each year and 60,000 new cases. The prevalence is about twice as high in men as in women. The rates of esophageal and larynx cancers have soared in recent years. Surgery and radiation are standard treatments. Survival rates are: esophagus, 3 percent; pharynx, 21 percent; tongue, 32 percent; mouth, 45 percent; larynx, 63 percent, and lips, 84 percent.

Oral and upper digestive cancers are caused primarily by upward-rising yin energy that gathers and collects in the upper body. Primary causes are excessive intake of milk and dairy products, oily and greasy foods, sugar and other concentrated sweeteners, tropical fruits and vegetables, stimulants, spices, vitamin pills and protein supplements, alcohol, drugs, and medications. In Asia, the modern diet—high in white rice, sugar, poor-quality oil, chemical seasonings and flavorings, and betel for chewing, and, an assortment of spices—has contributed to one of the highest rates of mouth, throat, and esophageal cancers on the planet. However, cancer of the tongue, a small, compact organ, takes several forms. A tumor at the root of the tongue is caused by extreme yang factors, including eggs, baked flour and oil, fried foods, animal foods, and smoking. Cancer at the tip of the tongue is caused by extreme yin factors, including sugar, oil, deep fried foods, spices, and stimulants, while that in the middle of the tongue is caused by cheese, dairy fat, and more in-between factors. Throat cancer is also usually the result of dietary extremes, including sardines and cream cheese, smoked white fish cooked with spices, chicken and eggs, and other combinations of salt and fatty, oily, or greasy foods, as well as dairy, sugar, flour products, and too much fat and oil. Alcohol or tobacco use greatly enhances the risk of oral and upper digestive malignancies.

To relieve oral cancer and esophageal cancer, follow the general dietary guidelines for Diet #1 for tumors in the upper region, including the tip of the tongue, arising from predominantly extreme yin factors. Follow Diet #2 for cancer at the root of the tongue arising from extreme yang factors. Follow Diet #3 for tumors in the middle of the tongue or throat arising from a combination of extreme factors. In all cases, avoid all fatty and oily foods, including all ani-

mal foods, dairy products, and vegetable oils and dressings, as well as sugar and other sweets; refined and polished grains and flour products; tropical fruits and vegetables; coffee, tea, herbal drinks, mineral waters, and other stimulants; and spices. Tobacco, alcohol, and drugs are to be completely eliminated.

Prepare brown rice as the main grain, combined or alternated day to day with millet or barley. Generally use a square of kombu the size of a postage stamp instead of salt in cooking grain, though in some cases, such as when yin factors are present, salt may be used. Avoid buckwheat and seitan altogether and, for 1 month, whole oats or oatmeal. Whole-grain noodles or pasta may be used a couple times a week in small volume. Good-quality sourdough bread may be enjoyed two to three times a week, but all other hard baked flour products, including cookies, pie, cake, crackers, and pastries, are to be avoided.

One to 2 servings of soup are recommended daily, especially MISO SOUP cooked with wakame and onions, carrots, or other vegetables. A small amount of shiitake mushroom may occasionally be added to miso soup or shoyu broth. Green leafy, round, and root vegetables are to be eaten daily, with a slight emphasis on hard, leafy green varieties. Special vegetable dishes can be prepared according to the dietary guidelines. Follow the standard recommendations for beans and bean products, sea vegetables, and pickles. GOMASHIO may be used with a ratio of 1 part salt to 18 parts sesame seeds for two months and 1:16 thereafter.

Avoid animal food with the exception of white-meat fish, which may be eaten once a week. After 2 months, fish may be eaten twice a week, if desired. Minimize fruits until the condition improves, though a small volume of cooked apples or other temperate-climate fruit may be taken if cravings develop. Avoid raisins, all fruit juice, and cider. Avoid all sweets and desserts, including good-quality macrobiotic desserts, until the condition improves. Use sweet vegetables daily in cooking, SWEET VEGETABLE JAM, occasional AMASAKE, and if cravings arise, a little BARLEY MALT or BROWN RICE SYRUP. Avoid all nuts except chestnuts, and avoid nut butters. Unsalted lightly steamed or boiled squash or pumpkin seeds may be consumed in small volume, up to 1 cup a week. Limit rice cakes, popcorn, and other dry or baked snacks, as they may harden the tumor. Sea salt, miso, shoyu, and other seasoning is to be moderate. Avoid mirin, garlic, and all herbs and spices. BANCHA TWIG TEA should be the principal beverage. Strictly avoid all mineral or carbonated waters, soft drinks, iced beverages, and for 2 to 3 months grain coffee.

The following special dishes, drinks, or home remedies may be helpful for oral and upper digestive tumors:

1. SWEET VEGETABLE DRINK, 1 small cup taken every day for 1 month and then 2–3 times a week the second month.

2. CARROT-DAIKON DRINK, 1 small cup 2–3 times a week for 2–4 weeks and then once every 3 days for 1 month.

3. One teaspoon of SCALLION-MISO CONDIMENT may be taken frequently, but avoid a salty or strong taste.

4. To strengthen the blood and for general vitality, UME-SHO KUZU may be taken daily for a 1- to 2-week period and occasionally afterward.

5. For strength and vitality, KINPIRA SOUP may be eaten 2–3 times a week.

6. For the more yin malignancies, soba noodles or buckwheat paste is strengthening and may be taken 2–3 times a week. (The more yang types should avoid buckwheat.)

7. A half cup of fresh GRATED DAIKON with a few drops of shoyu may be taken 2 to 3 times a week and is good for melting fat deposits.

8. For throat cancer, make a HATO MUGI–POTATO-CABBAGE PLASTER. Spread this on a cotton linen and apply it directly to your throat for 3 to 4 hours twice a day; or sleep with it overnight. Do this for 2 to 3 weeks. This may also be helpful for thyroid cancer.

9. A CABBAGE PLASTER can be applied directly to the throat with the same conditions.

10. For throat cancer, take LOTUS-DAIKON-CABBAGE JUICE. Drink this twice a day for 10 days. Afterward, take once a day for another 10 days. Then have it every other day, or 3 to 4 times a week, for another 3 to 4 weeks.

11. In the event the person cannot eat or a tube has been inserted, the diet should be liquefied by cooking with more water and by mashing food in a hand food mill. GENUINE BROWN RICE CREAM is also helpful and may be eaten with MISO SOUP and other liquefied or mashed foods, including vegetables, beans, and sea vegetables.

12. MASSAGE the feet, from the toes up to the knees, for 10 minutes twice a day for 1 month.

13. A BODY SCRUB is recommended daily. PALM HEALING on the mouth or throat region is also helpful to control pain and discomfort.

Follow the standard way-of-life suggestions. Avoid synthetic clothing around the throat, neck, head, and chest, and use cotton as much as possible. Avoid or limit television, computers, cellular phones, and other electronic devices that are weakening to the blood and lymph and the upper body. Be bright and positive and sing a happy song every day.

Ovarian, Uterine, Cervical, and Other Female Cancers. Reproductive cancers are the most common form of cancer in American women after lung cancer and breast cancer. About 125,000 new cases develop and 25,000 women die every year. Ovarian cancer, which is hard to detect, accounts for a majority of fatalities and most patients live less than a year. Standard treatment is a hysterectomy and removal of the ovary and Fallopian tubes. Uterine and endometrial cancer are rising rapidly in incidence and are associated with the use of birth-control pills and hormone replacement therapy. Cervical cancer appears chiefly in women over 40 but increasingly affects younger women, especially those with cervical dysplasia or herpes type 2 virus. It can spread to the rectum, bladder, liver, lymph, and bones and is treated with a hysterectomy, radium implants, or chemotherapy. Vaginal cancer is rare, striking mostly older women, and tends to spread rapidly to the pelvic lymph nodes.

As a whole, cancer in the reproductive region is a result of extreme yang factors, as excess metabolic energy and toxins move downward and inward into the lower, deeper part of the female body. From a dietary perspective, ovarian cancer is caused primarily by long-term consumption of eggs and other animal foods high in protein and fat. Uterine tumors arise from beef, pork, and chicken. Hard cheese, as well as salty, baked, and roasted foods, make the muscles and tissues tight, also contributing to ovarian and uterine cancer. Cervical and vaginal cancers also result from the intake of fatty meats and animal protein, but proportionately more milk, ice cream, and other lighter dairy food is consumed, as well as excessive oil, fruits, juices, flour products, and other more expansive items. Sugar, chocolate, and other concentrated sweeteners; white flour in bread, cookies, crackers, and pastries; and foods and beverages that possess stimulant, aromatic, or fragrant qualities, including spices, coffee, soft drinks, herbal beverages, and alcohol, will help accelerate the spread of cancer in this region, though they are not main causes. Environmental and lifestyle factors also enhance the risk, especially the use of birth control pills, hormone replacement therapy, exposure to artificial electromagnetic radiation from computers and cell phones, synthetic fabrics, and other unnatural influences.

To relieve ovarian cancer, follow the dietary guidelines for Diet #2, for disorders caused by strong yang factors. To relieve uterine, endometrial, cervical, or vaginal tumors, observe Diet #3, for diseases arising from a combination of extreme yin and yang factors. In addition to discontinuing all of the foods and beverages noted above, all animal food, including fish and seafood, is to be avoided. However, in the event that animal food is craved, a small volume of white-meat fish may be taken once every 10–14 days. Strictly avoid tuna, salmon, and shellfish, which are often main causes of reproductive troubles. All hard baked flour products, including good-quality whole-grain sourdough bread, should also be avoided for several months. Women with ovarian cancer and other female tumors tend to like roasted, baked, or crunchy foods. These should be strictly avoided. Oil is also to be avoided completely for 1 month. Then sesame oil may be lightly brushed on the skillet once or twice a week to make sautéed vegetables or kinpira. Raw salad may be eaten by women with ovarian cancer once or twice a week, but those with other types of tumors should avoid raw salad for several months.

Prepare brown rice as the main grain, combined or alternated day to day with millet or barley. Use a square of kombu the size of a postage stamp instead of salt in seasoning grains though sea salt may be used for some cases with strong yin factors. Avoid buckwheat and soba noodles altogether for up to 6 months because they are too contracting, minimize seitan, and for 1 month avoid whole oats or oatmeal. Whole-grain noodles or pasta may be used once or twice a week in small volume.

One to 2 servings of soup are recommended daily, especially MISO SOUP cooked with wakame and onions, carrots, or other vegetables. A little shiitake mushroom may occasionally be added to miso soup or shoyu broth. Green leafy, round, and root vegetables are to be eaten daily in a variety of styles. Daikon and daikon greens are especially beneficial for reproductive tumors. Special vegetable dishes can be prepared according to the dietary guidelines. Follow the standard recommendations for beans and bean products, sea vegetables, pickles, and condiments. GOMASHIO is to be made with a ratio of 1 part sea salt to 18 to 20 parts sesame seeds.

Women with ovarian cancer may take a little fruit, including fresh fruit. But other types should minimize fruits until the condition improves. However, a small volume of cooked apples or other temperate-climate fruit may be taken if cravings develop. Avoid raisins, all fruit juice, and cider. Avoid all sweets and desserts, including good-quality macrobiotic desserts, until the condition improves. Use sweet vegetables daily in cooking, SWEET VEGETABLE JAM, occasional AMASAKE, and if cravings arise, a little BARLEY MALT or BROWN RICE SYRUP. Avoid all nuts except chestnuts, and avoid nut butters. Unsalted blanched sunflower or pumpkin seeds may be consumed in small volume, up to 1 cup a week. Sea salt, miso, shoyu, and other seasoning use is to be moderate. Avoid mirin, garlic, and all herbs and spices. BANCHA TWIG TEA should be the principal beverage. Strictly avoid all mineral or carbonated waters, soft drinks, iced beverages, and for two to three months grain coffee.

The following special dishes, drinks, or home remedies may be helpful for female reproductive cancers:

1. SWEET VEGETABLE DRINK, 1 to 1½ small cups taken every day for 1 month and then every other day for a second month.

2. CARROT-DAIKON DRINK, 1 small cup every day or every other day for 4–6 weeks and then once every 3 days for a second month.

3. Sea vegetable juice, 1–2 small cups daily of the liquid from arame or other sea vegetable boiled in water for 10 minutes. In the event of a hard tumor, a small volume of shiitake mushrooms may be taken every day cooked in soup or with vegetables. Prepare by cooking with daikon and seasoning with miso or shoyu.

4. For blocked Fallopian tubes or obstructions in other parts of the female reproductive area, ½–1cup of CARROT-DAIKON DRINK, cooked with nori and seasoned with miso or shoyu, may be taken daily for 5–7 days.

5. A half cup of fresh GRATED DAIKON with a few drops of shoyu may be taken 2 to 3 times a week and is good for all types of female tumors.

6. In the event of frequent vaginal discharges, a DAIKON HIP BATH will help discharge excessive fat and mucus. The hip bath can be taken every evening or every other evening for 5–10 days until the condition improves.

7. For ovarian cancer, make BROWN RICE PORRIDGE WITH GRATED DAIKON AND LEMON. Eat 1 small cup of this gruel every evening for about 2 weeks; after that, have it every other day or every 3 days for another 3 weeks.

8. Another special remedy for ovarian cancer is DRIED DAIKON, SHIITAKE, AND ONION TEA. Drink 1 small cup of this broth every morning and every evening for about 3 weeks. After that, take it 1 to 3 times a week for another 3 to 4 weeks.

9. For ovarian tumors, take KUMQUAT JAM. Eat 1 tablespoon of this jam every day for 3 to 4 weeks. You may also make KUMQUAT TEA by dissolving KUMQUAT JAM in BANCHA TWIG TEA or hot water.

10. You may make TANGERINE JAM and TANGERINE TEA following the above recipe.

11. A little lemon juice may be used from time to time for ovarian tumors to help cleanse the body of dairy. Grate ½ cup of daikon, add water, simmer, and add a little lemon juice. GRATED SOUR APPLE cooked with lemon is also good, as is MARINATED DAIKON AND CARROT.

12. A small amount of beets may also be used on occasion for ovarian conditions. Take ½ cup of raw BEET JUICE daily for 5 days, then every other day for 10 days, or cook the beets and eat them. Add a little lemon juice if the liver is stagnated.

13. When pain arises for ovarian cancer, take 1 to 2 small cups of SWEET VEGETABLE DRINK.

14. In some cases of ovarian cancer, a HATO MUGI–POTATO PLASTER is beneficial. Leave the plaster on for 4 hours or longer. Repeat twice a day, or leave the plaster on all night while sleeping, if possible. Continue every day for about 3 weeks.

15. For ovarian cancer, MASSAGE well the feet and all toes for about 15 minutes, 2 to 3 times every day. If the feet become so cold that you cannot sleep, you may use a HOT WATER BOTTLE, but do not soak your feet in hot water or do a ginger foot both.

16. For uterine tumors, take ROASTED BROWN RICE PORRIDGE WITH GRATED DAIKON AND SHOYU. Eat 1 to 2 small cups of the porridge every day for about 10 days, and after that every other day for 3 weeks. Then reduce it to twice a week and continue for another 1 month.

17. For uterine tumors, take DRIED DAIKON, DAIKON LEAVES, AND SHIITAKE TEA. Drink 1 to 3 small cups of this broth every day for 2 to 3 weeks; after that, 2 to 3 times a week for another 1 month.

18. For uterine cancer, take UME-SHISO BANCHA. Drink 1 small cup of this tea every day for 1 week; after that, every other day or every 3 days for another 2 weeks.

19. WATER-SAUTÉED DAIKON AND DAIKON LEAVES are especially good for uterine conditions. Eat 1 small dish of this preparation every day. Continue for 3 to 4 weeks.

20. For cervical cancer, make GRATED DAIKON AND CARROT WITH UMEBOSHI, SHISO, LEMON, and SHOYU. Eat 1 to 2 small cups of this preparation every day for 1 week, then every other day for 10 more days; after that, 2 to 3 times a week for another 1 month.

21. For cervical cancer, take DRIED DAIKON, DRIED DAIKON LEAVES, AND SHIITAKE TEA. Drink 1 to 2 small cups every day for 3 to 4 weeks; thereafter, 2 to 3 times a week for another 1 month.

22. For cervical tumors, take BROWN RICE PORRIDGE WITH GRATED DAIKON. Lightly season it with sea salt or miso. Eat 1 bowl of this every day for about 10 days; after that, 2 to 3 times a week for another 1 month.

23. For cervical conditions, make LOTUS SEED, SEAWEED, AND ONION TEA. This tea is nice to drink often.

24. CORN SOUP WITH LOTUS SEEDS is also helpful for cervical conditions. Take this soup 3 to 4 times a week for 4 to 5 weeks.

25. NABE-STYLE VEGETABLES WITH DIPPING SAUCE is also recommended to help relieve cervical tumors and may be taken often. But do not use udon noodles. Cook shiso leaves, Chinese cabbage, cabbage, and other leafy greens together. Tofu or yuba may also be added. Rather than ginger, use nori and chopped scallions for the dipping sauce. If you like, add a squeeze of yuzu (a type of lemon) or lemon juice to the dipping sauce.

26. For cervical cancer, MASSAGE the feet and toes well for 15 minutes. Repeat 2 to 3 times every day.

For all female reproductive tumors, follow the standard way-of-life suggestions, especially remaining as hopeful and positive as possible. Depression, sadness, and melancholy commonly accompany reproductive cancers, and singing a happy song every day will lift the spirits as well as facilitate energy flow and the discharge process. A daily BODY SCRUB is important. Avoid wearing synthetic clothes, use cotton sheets and pillowcases, and avoid radiation from computers, television, and other sources, which tends to gather in the reproductive area. Avoid artificial birth control methods, menopausal treatments, abortion, cesarean section, and other procedures and treatments as much as possible. Normal sexual activity, so long as it does not lead to exhaustion, may be observed, as well as breastfeeding. Avoid cold showers or washing the hair in cold water, as these may interfere with normal discharge. Use a wet towel or sponge to wash. Relaxation exercises, DO-IN or SHIATSU, light dancing, PALM HEALING, and other practices can help reduce physical and emotional discomfort, promote better energy flow, and enhance healing.

Pancreatic Cancer. Pancreatic cancer causes more than 27,000 deaths annually in the United States. Affecting primarily those over 60, it occurs in men about twice as often as in women. Over 90 percent of tumors are exocrine cell cancers, which involve cells that perform digestive functions, while the others are tumors of the islet cells, involved with sugar metabolism. Rarely diagnosed before it has spread, pancreatic cancer is considered incurable and there is no standard medical treatment. It may spread to the liver or small intestine.

The primary cause of pancreatic cancer is long-term consumption of poultry, eggs, meat, cheese, and shellfish such as shrimp, crabmeat, and lobster, as well as salty baked flour products that tighten the organ and interfere with digestive and hormonal functions. These include bread, chips, crackers, and cookies.

To relieve pancreatic cancer, follow the general dietary guidelines for Diet #2, for more yang disorders. Avoid all animal food, including white-meat fish, unless cravings occur, in which case a small volume may be consumed once every 10–14 days. All hard baked flour products, including good-quality sourdough bread, are to be avoided for several months. A small volume of sesame oil may be brushed on the skillet once or twice a week to sauté vegetables.

Prepare brown rice as the main grain, combined or alternated day to day with millet or barley. Use a square of kombu the size of a postage stamp instead of salt. Avoid buckwheat, soba noodles, and seitan altogether and, for 1 month, whole oats or oatmeal. Whole-grain noodles or pasta may be used a couple of times a week in small volume.

One to two servings of soup are recommended daily, especially MISO SOUP cooked with wakame and onions, carrots, or other vegetables. A small amount of shiitake mushroom may occasionally be added to miso soup or shoyu broth. MILLET AND SWEET VEGETABLE SOUP may also be taken daily or every other day. Green leafy, round, and root vegetables are to be eaten daily, with a slight emphasis on round varieties such as squash, pumpkin, onions, and cabbage. Emphasize lighter cooking, which preserves freshness and crispness. Special vegetable dishes can be prepared according to the dietary guidelines. ADZUKI BEAN, SQUASH, AND KOMBU DISH is particularly good for this condition. Slightly fewer beans may be taken than usual and a small amount of sea vegetables may be used in daily cooking, but minimize kombu. Follow the standard guidelines for pickles and condiments. GOMASHIO may be used with a ratio of 1 part salt to 18 to 20 parts sesame seeds.

Minimize fruits until the condition improves, though a small volume of cooked apples or other temperate-climate fruit may be taken if cravings develop. Avoid raisins, all fruit juice, and cider. Avoid all sweets and desserts, including good-quality macrobiotic desserts, until the condition improves. Use sweet vegetables daily in cooking, SWEET VEGETABLE JAM, occasional AMASAKE, and if cravings arise, a little BARLEY MALT or BROWN RICE SYRUP. Avoid all nuts except chestnuts, and avoid nut butters. Unsalted blanched sunflower or pumpkin seeds may be consumed in small volume, up to 1 cup a week. Limit rice cakes, popcorn, and other dry or baked snacks, as they may harden the tumor. Sea salt, miso, shoyu, and other seasoning is to be moderate. Avoid mirin, garlic, and all herbs and spices. BANCHA TWIG TEA should be the principal beverage. Strictly avoid all mineral or carbonated waters, soft drinks, iced beverages, and for 2 to 3 months grain coffee.

The following special dishes, drinks, or home remedies may be helpful for pancreatic cancer:

1. Take 1 small cup of SWEET VEGETABLE DRINK every morning and every evening for 3 to 4 weeks. After that, reduce it to once every other day, and continue for another 3 to 4 weeks.

2. If jaundice arises, add the same amount of FRESH APPLE JUICE to SWEET VEGETABLE DRINK, and simmer for about 2 minutes. Drink 2 to 3 small cups of this preparation every day for 3 to 5 days.

3. If the abdomen swells, prepare GRATED DAIKON AND CARROT WITH SHIITAKE TEA. Drink 2 small cups of this broth every day for 3 to 5 days.

4. Make DRIED DAIKON AND SHIITAKE TEA. Drink 2 small cups of this broth every day for 5 days.

5. Carrot juice, preferably heated, may be taken several times a week to relax the pancreas or relieve pain.

6. A compress may also be helpful in some cases. If the tumor can be felt on the pancreas or it has gotten harder, make a POTATO-CABBAGE–HATO MUGI PLASTER. Apply the plaster directly on the affected part. Tie with a cotton strip. Leave it on for 4 hours or overnight. Repeat every day for 1 week to 10 days.

7. MASSAGE well the feet and all toes for 10 to 15 minutes, 2 to 3 times every day.

8. Doing a FOOT BATH in moderately hot water for 3 to 5 minutes will promote better circulation.

9. It is also helpful to MASSAGE all over the whole body to eliminate stiffness, but be careful not to push near the pancreas.

10. For swelling or gas formation in the pancreatic region, apply a BUCKWHEAT PLASTER for 1–2 hours daily. Keep warm by placing a hot SALT PACK on top. Repeat daily for several days.

Follow the standard way-of-life suggestions, being careful to avoid artificial electromagnetic radiation, which is very weakening to the pancreatic area. Avoid activities and exercise that produce exhaustion. Walking, BREATHING EXERCISES, SHIATSU, PALM HEALING, and other gentle activities and exercises are helpful.

Prostate and Testicular Cancer. Prostate cancer, the most common type among men in the United States, causes nearly 40,000 deaths annually. Its incidence has skyrocketed, climbing about 80 percent in the last ten years and accounting for 200,000 new cases annually. African American men have the highest rates in the world, while it is rare in Africa, Asia, and most of the developing world. Eighty percent of cases are diagnosed in men over 65. Many cases of prostate cancer develop slowly, causing no symptoms and remaining inactive for years. However, others are very aggressive and spread to the bladder, rectum, and through the lymph travel to the bones, liver, lungs, and elsewhere. The standard treatment for prostate cancer is surgical removal of the prostate and adjacent lymph nodes. Radiation therapy is often combined with surgery, and injections of estrogen, a female hormone, can slow its growth. The overall survival rate is nearly 80 percent. Testicular cancer is the leading form of cancer in males between 15 and 35. The right testicle is affected more than the left, and the malignancy tends to spread to the lungs, liver, bones, and brain. Chemotherapy or removal of one or both testicles is the standard treatment.

From an energetic perspective, prostate cancer is classified as an extreme yang disorder. The prostate is situated in the lower part of the body and deep inside. The primary cause is high animal protein and fat, especially beef, pork, chicken, eggs, cheese, shrimp, crabmeat, scallops, and other fish and seafood. Too much hard baked food such as bread, cookies, crackers, and chips and too much salt and salty foods may also contribute to an overly contracted condition. Though not a direct cause, strong yin in the form of sugar, dairy, spices, stimulants, and alcohol should be avoided completely, as they can accelerate tumor growth. Testicular cancer may also involve heavy animal food, especially fish eggs, heavily salted meats, condensed dairy foods such as cheese, and high-fat, high-cholesterol shellfish or seafood, as well as oily, greasy foods, especially french fries. However, because the testes are more external than the prostate, extreme yin is often a major factor, especially animal fat, oil, and dairy, and some forms of testicular cancer are predominantly yin.

To relieve prostate cancer and the more yang form of testicular cancer, follow the general dietary guidelines for Diet #2. For testicular cancer arising from more yin factors, observe the guidelines for Diet #1 for conditions arising from overly expansive factors. Avoid all animal food, including white-meat fish, unless cravings occur, in which case a small volume may be consumed once every 10–14 days. All hard baked flour products, including good-quality sourdough bread, are to be avoided for several months, as well as all roasted, baked, or crunchy foods. Avoid oil for the first month and then use sesame oil once or twice a week, brushed on the skillet, to sauté vegetables.

Prepare brown rice as the main grain, combined or alternated day to day with millet or barley. Use a small square of kombu the size of a postage stamp instead of salt. Avoid buckwheat, soba noodles, and seitan altogether and, for 1 month, whole oats or oatmeal. Whole-grain noodles or pasta may be used a couple of times a week in small volume.

One to 2 servings of soup are recommended daily, especially MISO SOUP cooked with wakame and onions, carrots, or other vegetables. A little shiitake mushroom may occasionally be added to miso soup or shoyu broth. Green leafy, round, and root vegetables are to be eaten daily, with a slight emphasis on leafy varieties. Minimize burdock, which may be too contracting. Special vegetable dishes can be prepared according to the dietary guidelines. Follow the standard recommendations for beans and bean products, sea vegetables, and pickles. GOMASHIO may be used with a ratio of 1 part salt to 18 to 20 parts sesame seeds.

Minimize fruits until the condition improves, though a small volume of cooked apples or other temperate-climate fruit may be taken if cravings develop, and it may help reduce swelling. Tree fruits are preferable to ground fruits such as strawberries and watermelons. Avoid raisins, all fruit juice, and cider. Avoid all sweets and desserts, including good-quality macrobiotic desserts, until the condition improves. Use sweet vegetables daily in cooking, SWEET VEGETABLE JAM, occasional AMASAKE, and if cravings arise, a little BARLEY MALT or BROWN RICE SYRUP. Avoid all nuts except chestnuts, and avoid nut butters. Unsalted blanched sunflower or pumpkin seeds may be consumed in small volume, up to 1 cup a week. Limit rice cakes, popcorn, and other dry or baked snacks, as they may harden the tumor. Sea salt, miso, shoyu, and other seasoning is to be moderate. Avoid mirin, garlic, and all herbs and spices. BANCHA TWIG TEA should be the principal beverage. Strictly avoid all mineral or carbonated waters, soft drinks, iced beverages, and for two to three months grain coffee.

The following home remedies can help to reduce excess protein and fat, which are the cause of the cancer; to reduce cholesterol levels; and to assist recovery.

1. Take thin BROWN RICE LIQUID WITH DAIKON, UMEBOSHI, AND SHISO. Take 1 to 2 small cups of this gruel every day for about 2 weeks; after that, 3 to 4 times a week for another 1 month.

2. Take DRIED DAIKON, DAIKON LEAVES, AND SHIITAKE TEA. Drink 1 cup of this broth every evening for 3 weeks. After that, drink it occasionally.

3. MISO-ZOSUI with scallions may be taken frequently, 2 to 3 times a week.

4. Make TOMATO-MISO SAUCE WITH SCALLIONS AND CHINESE CABBAGE. Take 1 tablespoonful of this tomato sauce at dinnertime.

5. BANCHA TWIG TEA should be the principal beverage.

6. Eat light DAIKON LEAVES QUICK PICKLES (pickled briefly in sea salt). If they are salty, wash out the excess salt before eating.

7. BROWN RICE AND CORN PORRIDGE is also very healing for this condition.

8. If the lymph nodes are swollen, apply a KOMBU-CABBAGE PLASTER. Leave it on for 6 hours or more. Repeat once or twice every day. It may also be left on overnight while sleeping. Do this plaster every day for 2 to 3 weeks.

9. In the event of pain, take UME-SHO BANCHA, 1–2 cups. Kuzu may be substituted for bancha and will have a soothing effect.

10. For swelling of the abdominal region, apply a BUCKWHEAT PLASTER for 1 hour. Keep it warm by placing roasted hot sea salt wrapped in cotton towels on top. Repeat daily for several days.

11. For testicular cancer, a POTATO-CABBAGE PLASTER made from two-thirds taro potato or regular potato and one-third cabbage is helpful. Apply for 3–4 hours on the affected area, preceded by a GINGER COMPRESS for 3–5 minutes. Repeat daily for 2–3 weeks.

Follow the standard way-of-life suggestions, being careful to avoid artificial electromagnetic radiation, which is very weakening to the prostate area. Avoid activities and exercise that produce exhaustion. Walking, BREATHING EXERCISES, relaxation exercises, and other gentle activities are helpful. Avoid smoking, which can tighten the prostate. Normal sexual activity is not harmful, but avoid any artificial birth control methods, drugs, or medications to aid performance.

Skin Cancer and Melanoma. Skin cancer accounts for over 600,000 new cases in the United States each year and about 2,000 fatalities. Diagnosis is relatively easy, tumors spread slowly, and survival is much higher than in any other type of malignancy. However, malignant melanoma, a deadly form of this disease, is one of the fastest-rising cancers, accounting for about 35,000 new cases each year and 7,000 deaths. The most common form of skin cancer, *basal-cell carcinoma,* appears primarily on the face or back of the hands. *Kaposi's sarcoma,* another type of skin malignancy, often accompanies AIDS. Skin tumors are usually removed by surgery under local anesthesia, though radiation, chemotherapy, and immunotherapy may also be used. Melanoma commonly begins with a mole and spreads through the blood or lymph to the brain, lungs, liver, eye, intestines, reproductive organs, or other locations. Surgery is also standard treatment. Survival rates are 80–90 percent in early stages and about 14 percent among those with melanoma spread to distant lymph nodes.

Skin cancer is caused primarily by extreme yin factors that are discharged to the surface of the body. Primary causes are excessive intake of milk and dairy products, oily and greasy foods, sugar and other concentrated sweeteners, tropical fruits and vegetables, stimulants, spices, vitamin pills and protein supplements, alcohol, drugs, and medications. Several years ago, Kaposi's sarcoma was linked to herpes virus 8. However, from a macrobiotic perspective, this infectious agent arises primarily as a result of dietary imbalance that creates an acidic condition in the blood and body fluids. Various combinations of the foods noted above can contribute to this malignancy, especially in persons with AIDS whose immune function is weakened. The chief cause of melanoma is chicken, eggs, cheese, and other dairy food along with sugar and sweets, stimulants, spices, and baked flour products that accelerate its spread.

To relieve skin cancer, follow the general dietary guidelines for Diet #1, for disorders arising from predominantly extreme yin factors. Follow Diet #3 for malignant melanoma arising from a combination of extreme factors. In both cases, avoid all fatty and oily foods, including all animal foods, dairy products, and vegetable oils and dressings, as well as sugar and other sweets; refined and polished grains and flour products; tropical fruits and vegetables; coffee, tea, herbal drinks, mineral waters, and other stimulants; and spices. Tobacco, alcohol, and drugs are to be completely eliminated. All food is to be cooked and not eaten raw. Seasoning should be moderate, neither too salty nor too bland.

Prepare brown rice as the main grain, combined or alternated day to day with millet or barley. Either a pinch of sea salt or a square of kombu the size of a postage stamp may be used to season the grain during cooking. For 1 month, avoid whole oats or oatmeal. Whole-grain noodles or pasta may be used a couple of times a week in small volume. Good-quality sourdough bread may be enjoyed two to three times a week, but all other hard, baked flour products, including cookies, pie, cake, crackers, and pastries, are to be avoided.

One to two servings of soup are recommended daily, especially MISO SOUP cooked with wakame and onions, carrots, or other vegetables. A small amount of shiitake mushroom may occasionally be added to miso soup or shoyu broth. Green leafy, round, and root vegetables are to be eaten daily, with a slight emphasis on round vegetables such as cabbage, onions, pumpkin, and fall- and winter-season squashes. Special vegetable dishes can be prepared according to the dietary guidelines. Avoid the use of oil in cooking for 1–2 months, and then use a small volume of sesame oil to sauté vegetables several times a week. Follow the standard recommendations for beans and bean products, sea vegetables, and pickles. GO-MASHIO may be used with a ratio of 1 part salt to 18 parts sesame seeds for two months and 1:16 thereafter.

Avoid animal food with the exception of white-meat fish, which may be eaten once a week by those with skin cancer. After two months, fish may be eaten twice a week, if desired. Those with melanoma should avoid fish and seafood, though a small volume of white-meat fish may be taken once every 10–14 days if craved. The fish should be prepared steamed, boiled, or poached and garnished with grated daikon, lemon, or ginger. Minimize fruits until the condition improves, though a small volume of cooked apples or other temperate-climate fruit may be taken if cravings develop. Avoid raisins, all fruit juice, and cider. Avoid all sweets and desserts, including good-quality macrobiotic desserts, until the condition improves. Use sweet vegetables daily in cooking, SWEET VEGETABLE JAM, occasional AMASAKE, and if cravings arise, a little BARLEY MALT or BROWN RICE SYRUP. Avoid all nuts except chestnuts, and avoid nut butters. Unsalted lightly steamed or boiled squash or pumpkin seeds may be consumed in small volume, up to 1 cup a week. Limit rice cakes, popcorn, and other dry or baked snacks, as they may harden the tumor. Sea salt, miso, shoyu, and other seasoning is to be moderate. Avoid mirin, garlic, and all herbs and spices. BANCHA TWIG TEA should be the principal beverage. Strictly avoid all mineral or carbonated waters, soft drinks, iced beverages, and for 2 to 3 months grain coffee.

The following special dishes, drinks, or home remedies may be helpful for skin cancer or melanoma:

1. SWEET VEGETABLE DRINK, 1 to 2 small cups taken every day for 3 weeks, is helpful.

2. Cook DRIED DAIKON, SHIITAKE, AND KOMBU TEA. You may keep this tea in a thermos, and drink 1 to 2 cups a day for 3 weeks. After that, have it every other day, or about 3 times a week, for 3 more weeks.

3. Make BROWN RICE WITH MARINATED DRIED DAIKON. Have this once a day or every other day for about 3 weeks. After that, eat it 1 to 2 times a week for about 3 to 4 weeks.

4. KOMBU-LOTUS-SHIITAKE DRINK, 1 small cup daily for 3 weeks, then twice a week for 1 month. This is especially good for melanoma.

5. For strength and vitality, KINPIRA SOUP may be taken 2–3 times a week.

6. To strengthen the blood and for general vitality, UME-SHO KUZU may be taken daily for a 1–2 week period and occasionally afterward.

7. One teaspoon of MISO-SCALLION CONDIMENT may be used as a condiment.

8. A half cup of fresh GRATED DAIKON with a few drops of shoyu may be taken 2 to 3 times a week and is good for melting fat deposits.

9. A BODY SCRUB is recommended daily, and a rice bran (nuka) wash is also beneficial. Wood ash may also be used to wash the skin.

10. Fresh daikon is helpful to reduce itching, and sesame oil can be applied directly to the affected region where the skin has ruptured. Cover the area with cotton afterward for protection.

11. A kombu-grain compress, consisting of a 3-inch piece of kombu soaked and combined with ½ teaspoon of cooked rice or barley, may be put over the melanoma or other affected area. Cover with a cotton bandage and leave for several hours or overnight. Use daily for up to two weeks.

12. A DAIKON COMPRESS is also beneficial, applied on the affected area.

13. In the event of surgery, GENUINE BROWN RICE CREAM is recommended, 2–3 bowls a day, with a small volume of SCALLION-MISO CONDIMENT, GOMASHIO, TEKKA, or UMEBOSHI for several days, to promote healing. Thorough chewing is especially helpful at this time and may stimulate the removed portion of skin to regenerate itself over time.

Follow the standard way-of-life suggestions. Avoid wool or synthetic clothing, which is particularly irritating to the skin, as well as chemical deodorants, cosmetics, and other body care products. Among natural cosmetics, clay and rice bran (nuka) are the safest. Avoid direct exposure to the sun as much as possible, which may accelerate the spread of the malignancy. Avoid or limit television, computers, cellular phones, and other electronic devices, which are weakening to the blood, lymph, and skin. Be bright and positive and sing a happy song every day.

Stomach Cancer. Overall rates of stomach cancer have fallen in the United States over the last generation, but it is a leading cause of death in the Far East, Latin America, and Eastern Europe. It is more prevalent in men, blacks, and older people than in women, whites, and younger people. Surgical removal of the stomach is the standard treatment. However, because

it is often not diagnosed until later stages, many cases are inoperable. Chemotherapy or radiation may also be used, especially to prevent its spread to the blood or lymph system and other organs. The survival rate is about 20 percent.

From an energetic perspective, there are two types of stomach tumors: (1) those that arise in the upper part of the stomach, known as the *fundus* and the *body*, and (2) those that affect the lower region, known as the *pylorus*. The first type affects the more yin, expanded region of the stomach, where hydrochloric acid is released, and is caused primarily by long-term overconsumption of white rice, white flour, sugar, honey, chocolate, soft drinks, stimulants, spices, dairy, oily or greasy food, tropical foods, and chemicalized food, especially that prepared with MSG. The second type occurs in the more yang, contracted part of the stomach, where pepsin is released, and is caused primarily by cured and salted meats such as salami, bologna, and ham, as well as eggs, beef, pork, chicken, heavy cheese, hard baked flour products, and other more condensed foods. The more yin type is the leading malignancy in Japan and other Asian countries where white rice, sugar, milk, MSG, and other chemicals are regularly consumed. The more yang type declined in the United States when luncheon meats were replaced with hamburgers and other fast foods but is still widespread in Central and Eastern Europe, where cured meats are still popular.

To relieve stomach cancer, follow the general dietary guidelines for Diet #1 for tumors in the upper region, arising from predominantly extreme yin factors. Follow Diet #3 for tumors in the lower region, arising from a combination of extreme factors. In both cases, avoid all animal food, including white-meat fish, unless cravings occur, in which case a small volume may be consumed once every 10–14 days. Avoid all hard baked flour products except for good-quality unyeasted sourdough bread, which may be taken 2–3 times a week. Avoid oil for the first month and then use sesame oil two or three times a week, brushed on the skillet, to sauté vegetables. Avoid raw salad and salad dressing for several months.

Prepare brown rice as the main grain, combined or alternated day to day with millet or barley. Generally use a square of kombu the size of a postage stamp instead of salt in cooking grain, though in some cases, such as when yin factors are present, salt may be used. Avoid buckwheat and seitan altogether and, for 1 month, whole oats or oatmeal. Whole-grain noodles or pasta may be used a couple of times a week in small volume.

One to 2 servings of soup are recommended daily, especially MISO SOUP cooked with wakame and onions, carrots, or other vegetables. MILLET AND SWEET VEGETABLE SOUP may be enjoyed daily or often. A small amount of shiitake mushroom may occasionally be added to miso soup or shoyu broth. Green leafy, round, and root vegetables are to be eaten daily, with a slight emphasis on sweet round vegetables such as squash, cabbage, and onions. Special vegetable dishes can be prepared according to the dietary guidelines. Follow the standard recommendations for beans and bean products, sea vegetables, and pickles. GOMASHIO may be used with a ratio of 1 part salt to 18 parts sesame seeds for two months and 1:16 thereafter.

Minimize fruits until the condition improves, though a small volume of cooked apples or other temperate-climate fruit may be taken if cravings develop. Avoid raisins, all fruit juice, and cider. Avoid all sweets and desserts, including good-quality macrobiotic desserts, until the condition improves. Use sweet vegetables daily in cooking, SWEET VEGETABLE JAM, occasional AMASAKE, and if cravings arise, a little BARLEY MALT or BROWN RICE SYRUP. Avoid all nuts except chestnuts, and avoid nut butters. Unsalted lightly steamed or boiled sunflower or pumpkin seeds may be consumed in small volume, up to 1 cup a week. Limit rice cakes, popcorn, and other dry or baked snacks, as they may harden the tumor. Sea salt, miso, shoyu, and other seasoning is to be moderate. Avoid mirin, garlic, and all herbs and spices. BANCHA TWIG TEA should be the principal beverage. Strictly avoid all mineral or carbonated waters, soft drinks, iced beverages, and for two to three months grain coffee.

The following special dishes, drinks, or home remedies may be helpful for stomach cancer:

1. SWEET VEGETABLE DRINK, 1 small cup taken every day for one month and then 2–3 times a week the second month.

2. Cooked MILLET AND SWEET VEGETABLE PORRIDGE is also nice to eat daily or often.

3. Make GRATED DAIKON WITH CARROT AND SHOYU, COOKED. Eat 1 small cup of this preparation every day for 5 days, and after that 2 to 3 times a week for another month.

4. Eat 1 bowl of MISO-ZOSUI BROWN RICE AND MILLET every day for 10 days; after that, 3 to 4 times a week for another month.

5. Take BROWN RICE WITH WATER-SAUTÉED DAIKON AND DAIKON LEAVES.

6. In some cases, a POTATO-CABBAGE PLASTER may be beneficial. Put a hot towel on the affected area for about 3 minutes to promote better circulation, and then apply the potato and cabbage plaster directly on the skin. Tie it with a cotton strip and sleep with it so the plaster does not move. Leave the plaster on for 4 hours or for the whole night. Repeat every day for 2 weeks or more.

7. MASSAGE all the toes very well, especially the second and third toes, for about 15 minutes, 3 times every day.

8. If the stomach has been removed, GENUINE BROWN RICE CREAM is helpful. Take 2–3 bowls a day with a small volume of condiments such as SCALLION-MISO CONDIMENT, GOMASHIO, TEKKA or UMEBOSHI for several days. Then begin to introduce regular brown rice or other grains. Chewing will enhance healing. Sometimes the part of the stomach taken out will restore itself. If not, thorough chewing will aid digestion.

Follow the standard way-of-life suggestions, trying to be positive, happy, and outgoing. Doubt, anxiety, and skepticism are associated with stomach problems and will gradually be overcome with the new way of eating.

CAUTION

1. If someone has cancer or suspects that he may have cancer, he should promptly see a physician and have his condition diagnosed and evaluated. If he seeks a natural approach, he may then see a macrobiotic counselor for di-etary and lifestyle guidance. The choice of medical treatment should always be left up to the patient and his or her family. Even if medical treatment is not chosen, it is recommended that the person with cancer stay in touch with his physician and keep her or him informed of his progress following the macrobiotic approach.

2. Do not use a TARO PLASTER or GINGER COMPRESS on a cancerous condition without the guidance of an experienced macrobiotic teacher or counselor. In the past, taro has been used externally on certain tumors. However, its powerful effects may spread the cancer to surrounding organs, especially for malignancies deep inside the body. For tumors on the surface of the body, taro may be used in some cases. But a regular POTATO PLASTER or LEAFY GREENS PLASTER is much safer. Similarly, use a hot towel rather than a ginger compress for a few minutes prior to applying a cool compress. A ginger compress is often too stimulating and may cause the cancer to spread.

3. In some cases, the person with cancer will benefit from CHINESE MEDICINE, ACUPUNCTURE, or other traditional remedy, in addition to conventional medicine. Please consult with a qualified specialist if you feel this may be helpful.

MEDICAL EVIDENCE

MACROBIOTIC WOMEN PROCESS ESTROGEN MORE EFFICIENTLY

Macrobiotic and vegetarian women are at less risk for breast cancer. Researchers at New England Medical Center in Boston reported that macrobiotic and vegetarian women process estrogen more efficiently than women eating a modern diet and eliminate it more quickly from their bodies. The study involved 45 pre- and postmenopausal women, about half of whom were macrobiotic and vegetarian and half eating in a conventional way. The women took in about the same number of calories. But the macrobiotic and vegetarian women consumed only one-third as much animal protein and fat, yet excreted two to three times as much estrogen. "The difference in estrogen metabolism may explain the lower incidence of breast cancer in [macrobiotic] and vegetarian women," the study concluded.

Source: B. R. Goldin et al., "Effect of Diet on Excretion of Estrogens in Pre- and Postmenopausal Incidence of Breast Cancer in Vegetarian Women," *Cancer Research* 41:3771–73, 1981.

MACROBIOTIC WOMEN AT LOWER RISK FOR BREAST CANCER

In a case-control study of 104 women at high risk for breast cancer, researchers at the National Tumor Institute in Milan, Italy, reported that after four and a half months the women in the macrobiotic group showed improved hormonal and metabolic variables that are associated with developing breast cancer.

Source: F. Berrino et al., "Reducing Bioavailable Sex Hormones Through a Comprehensive Change in Diet: The Diet and Androgens (DIANA) Randomized Trial," *Cancer Epidemiology: Biomarkers & Prevention* 10:25–33, January 2001.

SEA VEGETABLES REDUCE LIKELIHOOD OF BREAST CANCER

Sea vegetables can reduce the risk of induced breast cancer in laboratory animals. In experiments at the Harvard School of Public Health, researchers reported that kombu resulted in de-layed onset of tumors, fewer tumors, slower spread, and longer life span. The study grew out of population studies showing that Japanese women had nine times less breast cancer than American women, and the scientists theorized that sea vegetables in their diet might be a protective factor. They concluded that it would be prudent for American women immediately to begin incorporating sea vegetables into their daily diets.

Source: J. Teas et al., "Dietary Seaweed [Laminaria] and Mammary Carcinogenesis in Rats," *Cancer Research* 44:2758–61, 1984.

DAIRY INTAKE LINKED TO LUNG CANCER

Dairy consumption increases the risk of lung cancer, according to Swedish researchers. In a case-control study of 308 men with the disease and 504 controls, higher milk consumption was linked with the disease in both smokers and nonsmokers. Lower intake of vegetables also raised the risk.

Source: R. Rylander et al., "Lung Cancer, Smoking and Diet Among Swedish Men," *Lung Cancer* 14 (Supplement 1):S75–83, 1996.

SUGAR ASSOCIATED WITH LUNG CANCER

Consumption of sugar-rich foods increases the risk of lung cancer by up to 55 percent, according to Latin American researchers. In a case-control study of 463 lung cancer patients and 465 controls, scientists found that foods high in sucrose, including rice pudding, marmalade, ice cream, custard, soft drinks, and coffee with sugar, substantially increased the risk.

Source: E. De Stefani et al., "Dietary Sugar and Lung Cancer: A Case-Control Study in Uruguay," *Nutrition and Cancer* 31(2):132–37, 1998.

RED MEAT CONSUMPTION LINKED TO LYMPHOMA

Red meat raises the risk of lymphoma. In a study of 35,156 women age 55–69, Iowa researchers reported that those who ate red meat 36 times or more a month developed lymphoma twice as much as women who ate meat 22 times or less.

Source: B. C. Chiu et al., "Diet and Risk of Non-Hodgkin Lymphoma in Older Women," *Journal of the American Medical Association* 275(17): 1315–21, 1996.

MISO SOUP REDUCES THE RISK OF CANCER

Miso protects against stomach cancer. In a study of 265,000 men and women over forty, Japan's National Cancer Center reported that those who ate miso soup daily were 33 percent less likely to contract stomach cancer and 10 percent less likely to develop cancer at other sites compared to those who never ate miso soup.

Source: T. Hirayama, "Relationship of Soybean Paste Soup Intake to Gastric Cancer Risk," *Nutrition and Cancer* 3:223–33, 1981.

COMPOUND IN SOY PROTECTS AGAINST CANCER

A diet high in soy products, especially miso soup, protects against cancer. German researchers at the Children's University Hospital in Heidelberg reported that genistein, the active ingredient in the soy foods, retarded the multiplication of cancer cells and choked off the small blood vessels that feed tumors. The scientists concluded that a soy-rich diet could help prevent and relieve solid tumors, including those of the brain, breast, and prostate.

Source: "Chemists Learn Why Vegetables Are Good for You," *New York Times*, April 13, 1993.

FERMENTED SOY FOODS LOWER CANCER RISK

In laboratory studies, researchers at the University of Alabama at Birmingham reported that miso, natto, shoyu, and other traditionally fermented soybean foods could reduce or offset the effects of induced breast cancer. "Organic compounds found in fermented soybean-based foods may exert a chemoprotective effect," the scientists concluded.

Source: J. E. Baggott et al., "Effect of Miso (Japanese Soybean Paste) and NaCl on DMBA-Induced Rat Mammary Tumors," *Nutrition and Cancer* 14:103–9, 1990.

MACROBIOTIC DIET LENGTHENS LIFE OF PANCREATIC PATIENTS

Survival rates among pancreatic cancer patients who followed a macrobiotic diet were significantly higher than usual patients. Tulane University researchers reported that the 1-year survival rate for the macrobiotic patients was 52 percent versus 9.7 percent for controls, while overall life expectancy was nearly three times longer on average among those who changed their diet. A case-control study of men with metastatic prostate cancer found that those who ate macrobiotically lived on average 177 months and enjoyed an improved quality of life compared to controls, who lived 91 months. "This exploratory analysis suggests that a strict macrobiotic diet is more likely to be effective in the long-term management of cancer than are diets that provide a variety of other foods," the study concluded.

Source: James P. Carter et al., "Hypothesis: Dietary Management May Improve Survival from Nutritionally Linked Cancers Based on Analysis of Representative Cases," *Journal of the American College of Nutrition* 12:209–26, 1993.

WHOLE GRAINS PROTECT AGAINST A VARIETY OF MALIGNANCIES

Consumption of whole grains lowers the risk of cancer, according to European scientists. In a review of case-control studies in Italy between 1983 and 1996 involving 15,000 people, researchers found that a high intake of whole-grain foods protected against cancers of the oral cavity, larynx, pharynx, esophagus, stomach, colon, rectum, liver, gallbladder, pancreas, breast, endometrium, ovary, prostate, bladder, kidney, and lymphatic system, as well as multiple myelomas. Reduced risk ranged from 10 to 80 percent depending on the type of malignancy. The researchers noted that the benefits were observed only with whole grains and their products, not refined grains. Refined bread, pasta, and rice, they stated, are associated with increased risk of stomach and colorectal cancer.

Source: L. Chatenoud et al., "Whole Grain Food Intake and Cancer Risk," *International Journal of Cancer* 77(1):24–28, 1998.

SAUERKRAUT HELPS PROTECT AGAINST BREAST CANCER

Polish women who move to the United States have substantially higher rates of breast cancer. In studies at the University of Illinois, researchers report that reduced consumption of sauerkraut may be a principal factor. Treating colonies of breast cancer cells with estrogen, the scientists found that sauerkraut or fermented Brussels sprouts not only slowed the growth of estrogen-fed cells but also blocked tumor promotion.

Source: "Fighting Cancer from the Cabbage Patch," *Science News,* September 23, 2000.

CANCER CASE HISTORIES

MACROBIOTICS HELPS OHIO AUTO WORKER WITH A BRAIN TUMOR

Brian Bonaventura, an auto worker in Columbus, Ohio, had been suffering flulike symptoms for several months and had suffered a seizure at work, when doctors discovered a benign tumor the size of a small orange in the right frontal lobe of his brain. He had surgery and cut back on fried foods at the urging of his doctor. However, several years later, as his marriage broke up, he started eating a high-fat, high-sugar diet again, and a new malignant tumor in his brain appeared. After another surgery, he started macrobiotics and his health greatly improved. His depression has lifted, he feels more stable than ever, and he has been cancer-free ever since.

Source: Ann Fawcett and the East West Foundation, *Cancer-Free: 30 Who Triumphed Over Cancer Naturally* (New York and Tokyo: Japan Publications, 1991).

PHYSICIST OVERCOMES INFLAMMATORY BREAST CANCER

Christine Akbar received a master's degree in high-energy physics and was working on her doctorate when she was diagnosed with inflammatory breast cancer. Her oncologist told her that she had only two to three months to live, even with medical treatment. She started chemotherapy, but the tumor remained. Her sister gave her a book on macrobiotics, and she realized that her cancer was the result of longtime consumption of dairy food, sugar, sweets, oils, flour products, and excess protein and fat. Following a consultation with Michio Kushi, Chris changed her diet and made four special home remedies: (1) grated daikon and carrot to help lose weight, (2) sweet vegetable drink to control sweet cravings, (3) ume-sho-kuzu for her chronic constipation, and (4) a hato mugi–cabbage plaster to soften and draw out excess fat and protein. After several months on the healing diet, she awoke on Good Friday with nearly uncontrollable diarrhea. To her amazement, she discovered that the soft mass of her tumor was suddenly gone. "Within two months under Michio Kushi's guidance, my cancer was gone," she exclaimed. "In the time that modern medicine predicted I would die, a macrobiotic diet had helped save my life." Chris went on to study and work at the Kushi Institute and has developed many scientific and medical research projects with the Kushis, including coordinating the National Institutes of Health study on macrobiotics and cancer.

Source: Christine R. Akbar, "Breast Cancer," in Gale Jack and Wendy Esko, editors, *Women's Health Guide* (Becket, Mass.: One Peaceful World Press, 1997), pp. 19–23.

METASTASIZED COLON CANCER YIELDS TO MACROBIOTICS

Osborn Woodford, a native of Macon, Georgia, enjoyed homemade food, but it was cooked in lard and seasoned with grease from bacon or fatback. During the next twenty years, he ate primarily fast food, highly processed foods, and excessive sugar. Diagnosed with colon cancer while in his early forties, Osborn was told by his doctors that he had six months to a year to live. During surgery, it was discovered that the cancer had metastasized to eleven lymph nodes. Searching for an alternative, Osborn started

macrobiotics and began eating whole grains, vegetables, beans, and sea vegetables every day. A little more than two years later, his oncologist could find no signs of recurrence or metastasis. Osborn went on to study at the Kushi Institute extension program and has been practicing and teaching macrobiotics for the last ten years in Cleveland.

Source: Ann Fawcett and the East West Foundation, *Cancer-Free: 30 Who Triumphed Over Cancer Naturally* (New York and Tokyo: Japan Publications, 1991).

EMMY AWARD WINNER HEALS HERSELF OF TERMINAL LEUKEMIA

Christina Pirello had become vegetarian at age fourteen. She stopped eating meat but ate lots of dairy foods, sugar, and refined foods. She had a difficult time healing cuts, and she bruised easily. She began hormone treatments to control her menstrual cycle. After her mother's death from colon cancer, Christina's fatigue worsened. Bruises began to appear throughout her body. She was finally diagnosed with leukemia and was told that she could live six months to a year with chemotherapy and a possible bone-marrow transplant, or three months without any treatment. Seeking an alternative, Christina started macrobiotics with the help of Bob Pirello. Her energy quickly returned, and within the next few months she began to discharge toxins that had accumulated in her body from past years. "Each blood test revealed an improvement in my white cell count. The doctors were amazed," she recalled. After thirteen months, her blood counts were normal, and the cancer was gone. For the last sixteen years, she has been cancer-free.

Christina went on to marry Bob Pirello and become a macrobiotic cooking teacher. Today she is the star of *Christina Cooks!* on national television, for which she won an Emmy Award, and she has written several best-selling books.

Source: Christina Pirello, "Macrobiotics: Getting Started," *MacroNews*, January/February 1990.

YOGA TEACHER WITH LIVER TUMOR NOW CANCER-FREE

Hilda Sorhagen had been suffering from poor digestion, fatigue, and nervousness for several years. Her husband had died, leaving her with a business to run and three demanding teenagers to raise. After the kids grew up, she turned the business over to a son and moved to a yoga ashram that followed a vegetarian diet high in dairy foods, spices, sweets, and fruit. When she experienced a tenderness in her liver area, nausea, diarrhea, constipation, and a skin color change to brownish-yellow, Hilda went for medical checkups, but tests failed to show anything. During a consultation, Michio Kushi evaluated her condition as cancerous. Her family physician subsequently confirmed that she had a tumor in the lower part of her liver. Hilda went to the Kushi Institute to study and take cooking classes. After about a year, her condition had greatly improved and the tumor went away. Hilda went on to teach cooking. "I have more energy now than my children," she reported. "This lifestyle has helped me to speed up my spiritual evolution and I have become a more loving person. I will continue to live a macrobiotic way of life because I love the food, and it saved my life." The 150-member ashram where Hilda lived subsequently adopted a semi-macrobiotic diet and experienced improved health at many levels.

Source: Michio Kushi and Alex Jack, *The Cancer Prevention Diet* (New York: St. Martin's Press, 1993), pp. 194–95.

NURSE OVERCOMES METASTATIC LUNG CANCER WITH MACROBIOTICS

Janet E. Vitt, R.N., had just turned forty-five when she was diagnosed with small cell adeno-carcinoma of the lung, Stage IV. The cancer had metastasized to her liver, pancreas, abdomen, and lymphatic system. As a registered nurse in the Cleveland area, she knew that her prognosis was very poor. She had surgery on the abdominal mass and had several chemotherapy treatments. But she lost one-third of her weight and further treatments were not recommended. Through her sister, she went to see Francois Roland, a macrobiotic counselor. "Observing my face and the palm of my hands, Francois asked questions related to diet. I will never forget the words he said to me: 'You could be healed.'" Meanwhile, her parents and family had come to assist in her final hours. Instead, they started cooking whole grains, organic vegetables, beans, sea vegetables, and preparing special home remedies for Janet. Looking back, she identified cheese as the main cause of her illness. "I was obsessed with cheese. Not a day passed when I didn't eat it. I loved cheese omelettes, I enjoyed cheese on hamburgers, and I added cheese to all my vegetables. On Tuesdays and Thursdays, after aerobics class, I would come home and eat cheese and crackers. I was a cheese-a-holic."

After ten months on the new way of eating,

the tumors were all gone. In addition, the migraine headaches she suffered from for over twenty years went away. Joint pain in her knees and ankles disappeared, and many other conditions cleared up. "My physicians were amazed at my recovery," she recalled. "At the hospital, the Tumor Board met to compare the new scans with my originals and couldn't believe they were taken of the same person."

Janet went on to complete studies at the Kushi Institute and become a macrobiotic cook and teacher. Cancer-free now for the last five years, she has helped countless other people adopt a natural way of life.

Source: Janet E. Vitt, R.N., "Healing Metastatic Cancer with Diet," *One Peaceful World Journal* 37:1–10, 1999.

FASHION DESIGNER RELIEVES INCURABLE LYMPHOMA WITH DIET

Judy MacKenney, a fashion designer and homemaker, was diagnosed with non-Hodgkin's lymphoma that would develop to Stage IV within a few weeks. The tumor was situated on the right side of her abdomen, the lymph nodes on the left side of her neck were swollen, and cancer cells were found in her bone marrow. Judy agreed to take oral chemotherapy, but the side effects were devastating. Her body swelled up and contorted, she developed ulcers, and her stomach burned with pain. While attending a support group for exceptional cancer patients inspired by Dr. Bernie Siegel, she came across *The Cancer Prevention Diet* and started macrobiotics. The sweet vegetable drink stabilized her blood sugar, and the ulcers went away. The ume-sho-kuzu strengthened her digestion and

restored her energy. Ginger compresses dissolved stagnation and stimulated blood circulation and energy flow. "After two weeks, I felt noticeable improvement. The pain in my joints and feet disappeared. My innards embraced the nourishing whole food and I started to discover energy I had not felt in years, and I was experiencing peaceful sleep at last," she recalled. Judy went on to recover completely. With her husband, Larry, she set up a macrobiotic bed-and-breakfast on the Gulf Coast of Florida. Both Judy and Larry graduated from the Kushi Institute teacher-training program and have managed the Way to Health program, sharing their knowledge and experience with many other cancer patients and their families. She has been cancer-free for the last nine years.

Source: Judy MacKenney, "Healing Lymphoma with Macrobiotics," *One Peaceful World Journal* 33:1–6, 1998.

BUSINESSWOMAN HEALS HERSELF OF MELANOMA

Marlene McKenna, a mother of four children, worked as a TV and radio commentator and investment broker in Providence, Rhode Island. After she complained of severe stomach pains, doctors discovered five tumors in her body. Several feet of her intestines were removed, and she was told she had six months to a year to live. Rejecting conventional therapy, Marlene started macrobiotics and bought a gas stove to replace her electric range. A devout Catholic, she prayed and read inspirational literature. "I promised God that if He walked me through this and helped me live, I would give Him life with life," she recalled. Within a year, she felt well enough to resume an active life and was nominated to run for state treasurer. She was also pregnant. Doctors confirmed that the cancer had disappeared, but warned her that she needed to have an abortion because of her previous illness and age (she was in her early forties). Marlene refused, realizing that going ahead with her pregnancy was part of her promise to give life with life. She lost the election but gave birth to a health baby boy. She has been cancer-free ever since and actively helping people around the country recover their health.

Source: *One Peaceful World Newsletter,* Autumn 1989.

JOURNALIST RECOVERS FROM METASTATIC OVARIAN CANCER

Mina Dobic was the program director for a large radio station in Belgrade, Yugoslavia, when tragedy struck. Following migraines, chronic tiredness, and pressure on her head, doctors diagnosed ovarian cancer that had already spread to the lymphatic system. After an operation, Mina declined further treatment because her prognosis was only two months to live, and started macrobiotics. She believed that her past way of eating—high in meat, dairy, and other animal foods, as well as oily, greasy foods—underlay her condition. Friends and associates raised funds to send Mina to the United States with her husband to have a consultation with Michio Kushi. Back in Yugoslavia, she supplemented her diet with daily body scrubs, self-massage, singing, meditation, and visualization. Lab tests indicated that she was getting better, and within five months the tumor disappeared. The Dobics, along with their two children, subsequently came to the United States,

worked and studied at the Kushi Institute, and settled in Los Angeles. Today, Mina is one of the leading macrobiotic cooks, teachers, and counselors on the West Coast and recently published her autobiography.

Source: Mina Dobic, *My Beautiful Life* (Forres, Scotland: Findhorn Press, 1999).

BUSINESSMAN WITH PANCREATIC CANCER SPREAD TO LIVER SURVIVES OVER TWENTY YEARS

Norman Arnold, a successful businessman in Columbia, South Carolina, was in his early fifties when he was diagnosed with pancreatic cancer that had spread to the liver. Doctors gave him three to nine months to live. While taking chemotherapy, he heard about macrobiotics and decided to take a dietary approach rather than continue drugs that left him depressed and feeling more pain than ever. On the new way of eating, he gradually began to recover his energy and a positive, optimistic view of life. "In time, I found that I had more energy and vitality than I had had for twenty years," he recalled. "My wife, who also had adhered strictly to the macrobiotic diet with me, had positive results both physically and psychologically." The Arnolds' children also benefited. Medical tests, including CAT scans, ultrasound, and blood tests, subsequently showed that the cancer was gone. For the last eighteen years, Norman has been cancer-free and testified before several congressional committees on the effectiveness of a dietary approach to cancer.

Source: Michio Kushi and Alex Jack, *The Cancer Prevention Diet* (New York: St. Martin's Press, 1993), pp. 217–18.

TABLE 18. CANCER*

1. More Yin Cause	2. More Yang Cause	3. Yin and Yang Combined
Breast (most cases)		Breast (some cases)
	Colon, rectum	Lung
Stomach (upper region)	Pancreas	Stomach (lower region)
Skin		Melanoma
Mouth		
Tongue (tip)	Tongue (root)	Tongue (middle)
Esophagus		Throat
		Kidney
		Bladder
Leukemia (most cases)	Leukemia (some cases)	Spleen
Hodgkin's disease	Bone (multiple myeloma)	
Lymphoma (most cases)	Lymphoma (some cases)	
Brain (outer region)	Brain (inner region)	
	Liver	
	Ovary	Uterus
	Cervix	Endometrium
Testicular (most cases)	Prostate	Testicular (some cases)

*These are general classifications. Within each category, there are tumors that may be further classified into more contractive or expansive types. The dietary approach will differ for each person according to his or her constitution, condition, age, sex, activity level, and personal needs, as well as the particular type of cancer.

FILM STAR WITH PROSTATE CANCER RECOVERS COMPLETELY

Dirk Benedict was a rising young film and TV actor when he got prostate cancer. Star of *Battleship Galactica, The A Team,* and several Broadway productions, Dirk retreated to his cabin in Montana to practice macrobiotics and cook for himself. He had grown up in the West and eaten a lot of fresh meat and other animal foods. His body responded to whole grains, vegetables, beans, and sea vegetables, and he completely recovered.

Source: Dirk Benedict, *Confessions of a Kamikaze Cowboy* (Garden City Park, N.Y.: Avery, 1991).

MEDICAL DOCTOR WITH METASTATIC PROSTATE CANCER RECALLED BY LIFE

Anthony Sattilaro, M.D., was president of the Methodist Hospital in Philadelphia when he came down with cancer in his mid-forties. As the malignancy spread from the prostate to the bones, skull, and throughout his body, he had aggressive treatment, including surgery, drugs, and hormone therapy. Finally his own oncology department told him his case was hopeless. One day Dr. Sattilaro uncharacteristically picked up two hitchhikers, who sensed that he was depressed. He told them that he was dying of cancer, and they suggested that he try macrobiotics. Dr. Sattilaro was skeptical, but he had nothing to lose. He arranged a consultation with Denny Waxman, the director of the East West Foundation in Philadelphia, changed his diet, and completely recovered. His hospital documented his recovery and the *Saturday Evening Post* and *Life* magazine wrote up his story. Dr. Sattilaro wrote his own best-selling book, *Recalled by Life,* detailing his recovery. Unfortunately, after seven years of good health, he went off the macrobiotic diet and started eating chicken, ice cream, and other foods he didn't usually consume. The cancer came back, and he passed away. However, he showed that even the most aggressive and incurable types of metastatic cancer could be relieved with diet, and he inspired thousands of people to begin a natural way of life.

Source: Anthony Sattilaro, M.D., with Tom Monte, *Recalled by Life* (Boston: Houghton-Mifflin, 1981).

UN DEPUTY SECRETARY GENERAL OVERCOMES TERMINAL STOMACH TUMOR WITH MACROBIOTICS

Katsuhide Kitatani, a senior administrator at the United Nations, was diagnosed with stomach cancer that had spread to the lymph system. Despite surgery and chemotherapy, doctors told him that he had only six to twelve months to live. One day at a reception, a woman who had lymph cancer related how all her hair

had quickly grown back after she started macrobiotics. "What kind of economics is that?" he asked. Kit, as he is known, went on to change his own way of eating, which was based on ice cream, spices, relishes, and other highly processed foods. After nine months practicing macrobiotics, the cancer went away completely. Kit went on to become deputy secretary-general of the United Nations and start 2050, a foundation that fosters social health programs in Southeast Asia and around the world. He has been cancer-free for the last sixteen years.

Source: Michio Kushi with Alex Jack, *One Peaceful World* (New York: St. Martin's Press, 1987).

HOUSEWIFE RELIEVES INCURABLE OVARIAN CANCER WITH DIET

Following prolonged menstrual bleeding, Elaine Nussbaum, a New Jersey housewife, was diagnosed with a uterine tumor. She had her ovaries and uterus removed, as well as radiation therapy, radium implants, hormone medication, and chemotherapy. After a compression fracture and the partial collapse of her vertebrae, she was put in a brace and wheelchair. Subsequent medical tests found that the cancer had spread to the spine and both lungs. Unable to ward off massive infections, she received several blood transfusions and massive doses of intravenous antibiotics. Realizing that her prognosis was hopeless, Elaine turned to macrobiotics and discontinued meat, dairy food, fruit, sugar, and gradually eliminated the thirty-eight pills she was taking daily. Within a few months, she was up and about from her sickbed, her chronic urinary disorder cleared up, and her hair grew back. "In six months I changed from a sick, depressed, pill-popping invalid to a happy, optimistic, and very grateful pain-free person," she recalled.

Elaine went on to get a degree in nutrition and teach macrobiotic cooking and work as a dietary counselor around the country. "I attribute the reversal of my cancer solely to macrobiotics. I hope that my story will be a source of hope and inspiration to others." She has been cancer-free for the last sixteen years and has written her autobiography.

Source: Elaine Nussbaum, *Recovery: From Cancer to Health through Macrobiotics* (Garden City Park, N.Y.: Avery Publishing Group, 1991).

⊚ DIGESTIVE PROBLEMS

Digestive ailments and disorders are one of the most common categories of health problems in modern society. These include appendicitis, colitis, diverticular disease, enteritis, gas and gas pains, hernia, hemorrhoids, and spastic or irritable colon. *See also "Lactose Intolerance" in "Allergies"; "Colon and Rectal Cancer" in "Cancer"; "Infectious Diseases," and "Stomach Problems."* Intestinal problems arise, for the most part, from improper eating, overeating, overwork, and a more sedentary lifestyle. Chaotic and irregular dietary habits, especially eating late at night, snacking between meals, and insufficient chewing, further enhance the burden on these organs.

SYMPTOMS

1. Intestinal pain
2. Cloudy or scattered thinking, lack of focus and concentration
3. Fatigue, physical or mental
4. Fever
5. Lung or breathing problems
6. Thumb problems or weakness
7. Depression, including sadness, melancholy, pessimistic view of life, and feeling disconnected from the whole
8. The intestines correspond with the lower lip. The top part of the lower lip corresponds to the small intestine, while the lower part of the lower lip corresponds to the large intestine. A swollen, puffy lower lip shows more yin tendencies, such as frequent diarrhea, constipation from weakening and loosening, and inflammation. An extremely contracted lower lip shows tight intestines and yang conditions, such as constipation from too much contractive food, a tendency to develop polyps, and hemorrhoids
9. The lower forehead also corresponds to the digestive and respiratory system, including the intestines. Wrinkles, discolorations, and other abnormalities here show developing problems in this region
10. The index finger and its root, down to the base of the palm, and the same region on the back of the hand correspond to the large intestine and its functions. The little finger and its root, on the back of the hand, corresponds with the small intestine and its function. Weakness, stiffness, rigidity, markings, or other abnormalities here show developing problems in the corresponding intestinal regions

CAUSES

From a large view, the environment and food govern life on our planet. Eating is the way species transform one into another. There is a complementary/antagonistic relation between the vegetable and animal kingdoms. Human beings, at the center of the spiral of natural growth and development, represent the culmination of billions of years of biological evolution. Whole cereal grains exemplify the apex of the plant world and serve as the principal food for human development. The stages of digestion include: (1) *cooking*, which prepares the food for easier digestion; (2) *chewing*, which stimulates the release of digestive juices in the mouth; (3) *digestion*, which coordinates the smooth breakdown of nutrients in the digestive tract through the alternate release of yin and yang acids by the stomach, liver, gallbladder, pancreas, and duodenum; (4) *absorption*, which assimilates metabolized food in the villi of the small intestine; and (5) *transmutation*, which transforms absorbed food into white blood cells, red blood cells, and ultimately body cells, tissues, organs, and consciousness. The following factors can interfere with this normal process:

1. Overeating, even of good-quality foods.

2. Overconsumption of foods that contribute to stagnation and tightness in the intestines, for example, an excess of flour products, including bread, cookies, muffins, crackers, chips, and cake.

3. Overconsumption of foods that loosen and weaken the intestines, for example, an excess of products made of simple sugars, including refined sugar, chocolate, and honey; and fruits, fruit juices, and soda.

4. Overconsumption of foods that tighten and harden the intestines, for example, meat, eggs, poultry, fish and seafood, and baked food.

5. Overconsumption of fat. An excess of animal foods high in fat, including meat, poultry, eggs, milk, cheese, and other dairy products, as well as vegetable-quality oils, can coat the intestines with fat and mucus and contribute to the formation of cysts, polyps, and tumors.

6. Underconsumption or overconsumption of salt: a deficiency of salt in the diet can loosen the intestines, while too much can harden them.

7. Excessive consumption of refined foods. These lead to digestive disorders due to lack of fiber, minerals, and vitamins.

8. Excessive intake of water and other fluids. This loosens the intestines and causes diarrhea and weakness. In the event that this condition becomes chronic, intestines that have been loosened completely can become constipated.

9. Midnight snacking or late-night eating. Frequent midnight snacking causes stagnation of the intestines.

10. Excessive intake of drugs or supplements. Proper doses and kinds of medications or supplements can temporarily help normalize digestive conditions, but taking them for too long can result in constipation, diarrhea, or more serious disorders.

11. Lack of exercise. In individuals with a sedentary lifestyle, digestion, absorption, and blood circulation do not function smoothly, and sluggish intestines commonly result.

12. Mental disorders. In people under extreme tension, neurosis, or stress, digestive problems often arise.

13. Disease. Various diseases, and the treatments for them, can lead to colonic disorders.

In this case, it is necessary to first recover from the original disease.

FORMS

Appendicitis. Modern science views the appendix, a small protuberance near the beginning of the large intestine, as a vestigial organ performing no useful function. It is surgically removed in case of appendicitis. From the macrobiotic view, the appendix, which is small, tight, and yang in structure, serves to balance energetically the rest of the large intestine, which is large, expanded, and yin. Taking out the appendix can lead to an overall decline in vitality and weakness in the lower body, including intestines, legs, and reproductive region. People who have had their appendix removed often have trouble walking or running for extended periods.

Appendicitis is caused primarily by consumption of too much meat, especially barbecued meats, eggs, poultry, seafood, and other strong yang foods. An attack often comes during a picnic or holiday meal following heavy animal food consumption and overeating. To relieve this condition, eat simply or fast for several days. Externally, a GINGER COMPRESS may be applied to the abdominal region for just a few minutes, followed by a TARO PLASTER, about ½ inch in thickness, and left on for about 2 hours. This combination will help cool down the inflammation and may be applied several times a day until relief is experienced. For pain, a BUCKWHEAT PLASTER may be applied to the site, also about ½ inch in thickness. A SALT PACK may be placed on top of this to help bring down the inflammation. If a high fever arises, apply a TOFU PLASTER to the forehead,

changing it every 90 minutes. The tofu plaster may also be placed near the appendix.

As long as the appendix is not ruptured, an operation is unnecessary. It should be sought only as a last resort. However, if there is danger of rupturing, if the appendix has ruptured, or if the above remedies are not working, immediate medical attention is required.

To prevent future attacks of appendicitis, observe Diet #2, adjusted for strong yang conditions.

Colitis. Inflammation of the large intestine, or colitis, usually involves persistent diarrhea, with discharge of copious mucus, pus, or blood in the bowels. Fatigue, fever, weight loss, pain, stiff joints, and other symptoms may accompany this condition. This condition is caused by long-term consumption of extreme foods in either the yin or yang category, or commonly both, creating an acidic blood and body condition. Excessive use of antibiotics and other drugs can also lead to colitis-like symptoms. To prevent or relieve colitis, follow the guidelines for Diet #3 for conditions caused by a combination of extreme yin and yang factors, as well as the recommendations below. As a special drink, UME-SHO KUZU with 1 teaspoon of grated daikon added at the end of cooking is very helpful. To relieve bleeding, add grated lotus root to this drink. Take either drink daily for about 10 days. BROWN RICE BALLS are also highly recommended for this condition. Chew up to 100 times per mouthful. A plain CABBAGE PLASTER may be applied to the affected region, but this is not usually needed and is optional.

Ulcerative colitis is a serious form of this disorder. It is characterized by tiny ulcers that form in the intestinal tract and are accompanied by loose, often bloody bowels, pain, and fever. Less serious cases may respond to dietary treatment and external applications such as described above for colitis. However, because this can be a life-threatening condition, serious cases of ulcerative colitis require prompt medical attention. In this case, a macrobiotic approach may be followed concurrently and over time may be beneficial.

Constipation. A healthy person has regular bowel movements, usually once a day. The stools are generally long, golden in color, floating, and pass without difficulty. In modern society, the majority of people experience eliminatory problems. Many of them suffer from constipation. This condition generally takes two forms. In the first, the bowel movements are hard, dense, and painful or difficult to pass. In the second, they go without a bowel movement for 3 or 4 days and, in some cases, 7 to 10 days or more. Constipation can accompany a wide range of intestinal disorders ranging from diverticulitis to hemorrhoids. In addition to dietary change, especially recommending more fiber, physicians treat constipation with laxatives, electrolyte solutions, or enemas.

The following symptoms may accompany constipation, and in some cases they can also cause it: fever, allergy, dermatitis, rash (especially on the face), diabetes or hypoglycemia, headache, fatigue, hearing difficulty, emphysema, irregular menstruation, insomnia, cancer or tumorous growth, or mental disorders, including irritation, stress, decline of thinking power and judgment, poor concentration, depression, loss of a positive outlook on life, and a tendency to depend on others.

Constipation shows up through diagnostic signs on the lips. The intestines correspond with the lower lip. The top part of the lower lip corresponds to the small intestine, while the lower part of the lower lip corresponds to the large intestine. A swollen, puffy lower lip shows constipation from weakening and loosening. An extremely contracted lower lip, sometimes to the point of a thin line, shows tight intestines and constipation from excessive yang intake.

There are two principal types of constipation. The more yin, or expansive, type results from lack of whole grains, beans and bean products, fresh vegetables (especially hard, leafy greens), sea vegetables, and other fiber-rich foods, proper minerals, and other strong, predominantly plant-quality foods or from overconsumption of refined flour, sugar and sweets, oil and greasy food, and other strong yin items. In this case, the intestines lack contractive power and are too weak to produce a bowel movement.

The other type of constipation results from excessive consumption of animal foods, baked foods, too much salt, and other strong yang intake. In this case, the intestines become clogged, hardened, or obstructed and the stools become small, compacted, and smelly.

For constipation caused by more yin factors, follow the guidelines for Diet #1. For constipation caused by more yang factors, follow the guidelines for Diet #2. Note the following: Eat whole grains, not refined grains, as the main dish of every meal. Reduce flour products to as little as possible. Noodles may be taken, but only a few times a week. Avoid simple sugars (refined sugar, honey, and chocolate). If you desire to eat animal food, it is best to choose fish or seafood, and then to consume it only a few times a week. Minimize fat consumption, including vegetable-quality oil. Do not take raw oil, such as in the form of salad dressings. Oil always should be cooked, for example, sautéed in the case of dressings, sauces, and dips. Sesame oil is most recommended. Avoid vegetables that originated in tropical regions, such as tomatoes, eggplants, and peppers. Avoid potatoes and yams, except taro potatoes and jinenjo (mountain potatoes), until you recover from constipation. Take hard leafy greens daily that are high in fiber (such as daikon greens and carrot tops) and take root vegetables (daikon, carrot, burdock, etc.) as whole as possible, without peeling them. The amount of salt (miso, shoyu, and sea salt) should be moderate. Cut down on water to a moderate level, but do not reduce it too much. Take a small amount of sea vegetables on a daily basis. Reduce the total volume of food, and chew more. Avoid late-night eating.

Home remedies may also be helpful to relieve constipation. In the case of constipation due to loose intestines, try one of the following:

I. Take a small cup of UME-SHO KUZU or UME-SHO BANCHA every morning for 10 days; after that, 2 to 3 times a week for another 3 to 4 weeks.

2. Eat 1 to 2 small rice-size bowls of stir-fried konnyaku every day for 5 days; and after that, 2 to 3 times a week for another 3 weeks. Konnyaku is a traditional Far Eastern potato that is high in fiber and cooks up gelatinous. It is available in Oriental or Japanese food stores.

3. Eat 1 small dish of SOYBEAN SPROUTS WITH LEEKS every day for 3 to 5 days.

4. Prepare BLACK SOYBEANS WITH KOMBU AND DRIED DAIKON. Eat a bowl of this dish once a day for 1 week.

5. COOKED BLACK SESAME SEEDS can also be effective.

6. Eat a small amount of KINPIRA-STYLE VEGETABLES every day. KINPIRA SOUP may also be taken several times a week.

7. Take SOBA WITH GRATED JINENJO occasionally to help with constipation.

8. For constipation due to an overly contracted condition, take more expansive items such as raw vegetables, lightly cooked vegetables, warm apple juice, fruit kanten, or other good quality yin to help stimulate elimination.

9. The following remedies are helpful to clean the bowels immediately: (a) Lightly simmer 3 to 4 tablespoons of SESAME OIL WITH SHOYU AND GRATED GINGER. Mix and drink slowly. (b) A BANCHA TEA AND SEA SALT ENEMA can also be effective.

10. For 7 to 10 days, SEMI-FASTING is effective; reduce the amount and number of meals and chew very well. However, avoid complete fasting for several days or more. Often an enormous appetite comes following resumption of eating, which cancels out the positive effect of the fast.

11. Various medications and supplements may be taken for a short time, if desired, but you should eliminate them as soon as possible, to avoid any harmful side effects and becoming dependent on them. CHINESE MEDICINE, ACUPUNCTURE, YOGA, and other traditional healing approaches may be used under the supervision of a professional practitioner. If you are suffering from other diseases, the treatments for them might be leading to constipation. In this case, discuss these treatments with your physician or health care professional.

Crohn's Disease. Crohn's disease is an intestinal disorder that involves chronic digestive problems, inflammation and weakness, and a variety of nonintestinal symptoms. Considered irreversible by modern medicine, it is characterized by sudden and severe attacks and may lead to disability or death. Crohn's disease usually affects the end of the small intestine or the colon but can occur anywhere along the intestinal tract. More frequent among women than men, it appears primarily in young adults age 20–40, though it may be found in infants and children. It is uncommon in those of Asian or African heritage. Depending on the severity, Crohn's disease is treated with anti-inflammatory drugs, a bland diet, and surgery, including partial or full removal of the colon.

From the macrobiotic view, the main cause of Crohn's disease is consumption of extreme yin foods and drinks, especially dairy food and sugar. These cause a slow deterioration of the intestinal wall, inflammation, and irritation. The intestines lose their elasticity, resulting in impaired digestion and absorption. To relieve this condition, it is important to discontinue these items and to eat a balanced standard diet, especially foods that will help restore natural contractive power such as whole grains, MISO SOUP regularly, sea vegetables, good-quality sea salt, shoyu, and other seasonings. Follow the guidelines for Diet #1, for conditions caused by extreme yin factors. High-quality condiments such as UMEBOSHI PLUMS, GOMASHIO, and TEKKA may also be strengthening. With this dietary approach, Crohn's disease can usually be controlled, and in some cases reversed.

Diarrhea. Normally, the bowel movement is large, long, light, soft, and floating. Small, compact, dark, hard stools are a sign of constipation (see earlier section), while loose or fragmentary bowels are a sign of diarrhea. Diarrhea or runny bowels takes two primary forms. The more yin type results from excessive consumption of extreme yin foods and beverages. Heavy, acute diarrhea of this type accompanied by a fever is frequently caused by taking sugar or ice cream. A mild, irregular bowel movement without a fever is usually produced by taking too much fruit, juice, or other liquid.

There is also a heavier, darker form of diarrhea caused by taking too much animal food, especially meat, poultry, fish, or seafood cooked in stews and combined with many other foods.

For the more yin type, take roasted rice, rice cakes, or dry toast. KUZU CREAM or UME-KUZU or UME-SHO KUZU will also help contract the intestines and prevent runny bowels. Other remedies include UMEBOSHI PLUMS or BLACK SOYBEAN TEA. If diarrhea arises from coldness, give BROWN RICE PORRIDGE with scallions and chives or GINGER TEA. For babies with runny bowels, give KUZU CREAM with BAKED KOMBO CONDIMENT or less strong UME-SHO BAN. Externally, a hot compress, such as a SALT PACK or GINGER COMPRESS, can be placed on the abdomen or intestines. For heavy diarrhea, a GINGER BATH is helpful.

For the more yang type, take GRATED DAIKON, KUZU CREAM, or ume concentrate made in the form of a tea. Externally, a TARO PLASTER or LEAFY GREENS PLASTER is helpful.

To prevent diarrhea in the future, the standard macrobiotic way of eating should be observed. Observe Diet #1 for a more yin condition or Diet #2 for a more yang condition. Whole grains, beans and bean products, vegetables from land and sea, and other staple foods are high in fiber and other nutrients that will normalize the intestinal function and result in healthy bowel movements.

Diverticular Disease. Diverticular disease, also known as *diverticulitis*, is characterized by the appearance of diverticula, or small pouches, in the walls of the large intestine. While they may develop anywhere in the colon, they are most frequent in the descending and sigmoid colons. In many cases, no symptoms are present, but in others severe cramping may be experienced, especially on the left side. Nausea, fever, and constipation and diarrhea may also occur. Diverticulitis may be both acute and chronic, involve inflammation or infection, and lead to abscesses, perforation of the bowel, and other serious complications. Diverticular disease is widespread in modern society, with an estimated half of all Americans over 50 eventually developing this disease. Modern medicine diagnoses diverticulitis with a barium enema or a sigmoidoscopy and treats serious cases with surgery. A diet low in fiber and high in refined foods is recognized to increase the risk.

From the macrobiotic view, this condition is primarily caused by extreme yin and yang foods, including meat, poultry, eggs, heavy cheese, too much fish and seafood, sugar, dairy, refined foods, tropical foods, spices, alcohol, and chemicalized foods. Too much baked food, especially hard baked flour products, and too much salt may be contributing factors. A centrally balanced way of eating may be observed, discontinuing extreme foods of all kinds and

moderating salt, condiments, and pickles until the condition improves. Follow the guidelines for Diet #3, for conditions caused by a combination of extreme yin and yang factors. For pain, a cool compress such as a POTATO PLASTER or LEAFY GREENS PLASTER may be applied over the affected area for up to 2 hours at a time, preceded by a hot towel for several minutes to stimulate blood circulation. Make a fresh compress and repeat the procedure, if necessary. Serious cases of diverticulosis may require medical attention.

Enteritis. Inflammation of the intestinal tract (enteritis) can arise from extremes of both yin and yang foods. It can be either acute or chronic and is typically accompanied by diarrhea, constipation, abdominal pain, fever, or other symptoms. Acute enteritis is accompanied by pain and sometimes diarrhea or fever. If this is the result of excessive yin foods and beverages, a hot application such as a GINGER COMPRESS or SALT PACK may be applied over the area. If this is the result of too many yang foods and drinks, a cool application such as a POTATO PLASTER or LEAFY GREENS PLASTER may be used. Of course, extreme foods of all kinds should be discontinued and a more centrally balanced way of eating adopted.

Chronic enteritis develops gradually and usually is caused by taking extremes from both categories. The primary symptom is irregular bowels and experiencing diarrhea on some occasions and constipation on others. The standard diet should be observed with special emphasis on miso, shoyu, natto, and other fermented foods. Follow the guidelines for Diet #3, for conditions caused by a combination of extreme yin and yang factors. UMEBOSHI PLUMS and pickles may also be taken frequently.

Gas and Gas Pains. Intestinal bloating, pain, and flatulence, as well as belching, commonly result from eating extreme foods, consuming improperly cooked foods, or observing chaotic and irregular dietary habits. Animal foods, dairy foods, refined carbohydrates, carbonated beverages, and other acid-forming foods can contribute to the buildup of bacteria that produce fermented gas in the intestines. Improperly prepared beans are a frequent cause of gas in modern society. However, properly prepared beans, especially those that are adequately soaked, seasoned, and thoroughly cooked, will not cause flatulence. On the contrary, macrobiotic-quality beans and bean products will enhance digestion, assimilation, and proper bowel elimination. People of African, Asian, and Native American ancestry often experience gas after eating dairy foods because they are lactose-intolerant *(see "Allergies")*. White bread sweetened with sugar and other sweetened flour products can also cause flatulence. To eliminate gas and gas pains, observe the standard way of eating, balancing for an overly yin or yang condition. Pay special attention to thorough chewing (ideally 50 times or more per mouthful), including beverages. Observe orderly dietary habits, including eating meals at regular times, avoiding overeating, no late night snacking, and minimizing snacking between meals. A kuzu drink, including UME-SHO KUZU or KUZU CREAM, may be beneficial in regulating digestion and preventing gas formation.

Hemorrhoids. Hemorrhoids are painful swellings or lumps in the veins near the anus. Tenderness or pain may be felt during bowel movements, frequent itching may be experienced, and bright red bleeding may occur. The yin form of hemorrhoids is caused by excessively expansive foods that cause the blood capillaries in the rectum to expand and rupture. The yang form is caused by excessively contractive foods that cause rectal tissues to contract and bleed. In both cases, the standard way of eating may be observed and extreme foods such as meat, poultry, eggs, sugar, and dairy should be discontinued. Those suffering from yin hemorrhoids should avoid fruit, juice, fresh salad, and excessive liquid until the condition improves, while for yang hemorrhoids avoid all animal foods, baked foods, and minimize salt and salt-based foods and condiments. Generally, follow Diet #3 for conditions arising from a combination of dietary extremes, taking plenty of green leafy vegetables steamed and boiled. For inflamed hemorrhoids, a CABBAGE PLASTER may be effective. As a special drink, take 1–2 cups of UME-KUZU-LOTUS TEA daily for 5 to 7 days. The lotus will help tighten the swollen area.

Hernia. A hernia develops when the wall of the intestines loosens, expands, and descends. While surgery is commonly performed, the intestines' normal contractive power can be restored only through proper diet and lifestyle. In most cases, a hernia can be relieved in four to six months by observing the guidelines for Diet #1, for more yin conditions and disorders, and discontinuing extreme foods, especially dairy, ice cream, fruit, juice, sugar, excessive beverages, and other yin foods. While the hernia is healing, even a few sections of an orange can loosen and expand the intestinal walls.

Tough, fibrous vegetables, such as leeks, kale, watercress, carrot tops, and daikon greens, should be eaten regularly to strengthen the intestines. Prepare a small side dish of HIJIKI sea vegetables daily or every other day for several weeks. Use only high-quality unrefined sea salt in cooking, along with unrefined vegetable oil. A CABBAGE PLASTER will sometimes help heal this condition. Avoid hot baths and showers because they cause the body to lose minerals and tissues to become loose. An athletic support may need to be worn. Light to moderate activity and physical exercise may be beneficial, but not strenuous or to exhaustion.

While excessive yin factors cause most hernias, extreme yang foods may sometimes enhance the condition, causing tightness and constipation that causes the intestinal tissue to descend and protrude through the anus. In this case, follow the guidelines for Diet #3 for conditions caused by both extreme yang and yin factors. If the intestinal tissue begins to come out through the anus, apply a hot, steaming towel over the region, apply a small amount of sesame oil, and push the protruding tissue back with a finger.

Irritable Bowel Syndrome. This condition, also known as spastic bowel or colon, involves chronic constipation or diarrhea, especially after meals, accompanied by intestinal cramps, bloating, or gas. Digestion frequently appears normal, but bowel movements are chaotic for weeks or months at a time. Considered to be the most common digestive disorder today, IBS is twice as frequent among women as men. The disorder may appear in children and often starts in early adulthood. It tends to arise during periods of stress and tension or following some major change in life. From the macrobiotic view, IBS may be caused by either extreme yin or yang factors, commonly both. Depending on the cause, follow Diet #1, #2, or #3. As a special drink, UME-SHO KUZU with 1 teaspoon of GRATED DAIKON added at the end of cooking is very helpful. To relieve bleeding, add grated lotus root to this drink. Take either drink daily for about 10 days. BROWN RICE BALLS are also highly recommended for this condition. Chew up to 100 times per mouthful. A plain CABBAGE PLASTER may be applied to the affected region, but this is not usually needed and is optional.

In traditional Oriental medicine, healthy intestines are associated with feelings of wholeness, security, and happiness. In combination with poor eating and a chaotic lifestyle, sudden changes in life, difficulties, and other challenges and stresses may contribute to this syndrome. In this case, moderate physical activity; DO-IN, SHIATSU, or other MASSAGE; and mental and spiritual exercises, such as MEDITATION, VISUALIZATION, and singing a happy song every day may be beneficial.

Motion Sickness. Motion sickness is marked by dizziness, sweating, nausea, and other symptoms of discomfort while traveling in a plane, car, bus, or train. It usually involves intestinal upset and may lead to vomiting. Conventional medicine treats this condition with antinausea pills, muscle relaxants in timed-release skin patches, and other medications. Simple, safe home remedies for motion sickness include GOMASHIO (taken alone or dissolved in BANCHA TWIG TEA), UMEBOSHI PLUMS (taken whole or dissolved in tea), and ginger (taken in powdered form in a tea or grated and squeezed out into juice and added to tea). As a compress, some people report that placing an umeboshi plum on the navel and securing it firmly during travel prevents motion sickness. DO-IN or MASSAGE may also be helpful. Press on Small Intestine 17, the point in the indentation at the back of the jawbone beneath the ear, for one minute while breathing deeply. Repeat several times on both sides. The ear governs overall balance and equilibrium. Pressing Heart Governor 6 in the center of the wrist, between the two bones of the forearm and about an inch from the beginning of the hand, will help soothe the nerves and prevent nausea. Apply firm pressure for about a minute, relax, and repeat several times on each arm.

SOLUTION

DIET

Observe the dietary guidelines noted above, with special emphasis on the following:

1. Eat whole grains, not refined grains or grain products, as the main dish of every meal. These are high in fiber and will help restore and maintain the health of the intestines. Reduce flour products to as little as possible. Noodles may be taken, but only a few times a week.

2. Avoid simple sugars (refined sugar, honey, and chocolate), which can destroy the intestinal flora and coat the villi of the intestines with mucus.

3. Avoid animal foods and dairy, which create stagnation in the intestines. If you desire to eat animal food, it is best to choose fish or seafood, and then to consume it only occasionally.

4. Minimize oil consumption, including vegetable-quality oil. Avoid raw oil, such as in the form of salad dressings.

5. Avoid vegetables that originated in tropical regions, such as tomatoes, eggplants, and peppers.

6. Take daily hard leafy greens that are high in fiber (such as daikon greens and carrot tops) and take root vegetables (daikon, carrot, burdock, etc.) as whole as possible.

7. Eat fermented foods frequently, including miso, shoyu, natto, and other soy products, as well as sauerkraut, umeboshi plums, and pickles. Fermented foods contain enzymes and bacteria that contribute to proper digestion and assimilation.

8. The amount of salt (miso, shoyu, and sea salt) should be moderate.

9. Cut down on water to a moderate level, but do not reduce it too much.

10. Follow the other standard dietary recommendations.

LIFESTYLE

Observe the standard way-of-life suggestions, focusing on the following:

1. Avoid exposing the abdominal region to cold air or consuming cold beverages, which have a paralyzing effect on the intestines. Keeping the abdominal region warm will help restore smooth digestive functions.

2. Intestinal problems are frequently accompanied by depression, sadness, and melancholy. It is important to keep a positive, optimistic, happy mood. Breathing exercises will help both lung function and the smooth operation of the intestines.

3. Avoid wearing wool or synthetic fibers next to the skin.

4. Avoid watching television or working at the computer for long stretches. Radiation weakens the intestinal area. X rays and other medical procedures should be limited whenever possible.

HOME REMEDIES

1. For most large intestine weaknesses, prepare the special LARGE INTESTINE DRINK.

2. For most small intestine problems, prepare the special SMALL INTESTINE DRINK.

3. For more yin intestinal conditions, take a cup of UME-SHO KUZU or UME-SHO BANCHA every morning for 10 days, and after that 2 to 3 times a week for another 3 to 4 weeks.

4. KINPIRA SOUP may also be taken 2–3 times a week for more yin digestive disorders.

5. A BODY SCRUB or GINGER BODY SCRUB every day or twice a day on the whole body, including the abdomen, will promote better circulation and activate physical and mental energies.

6. A HOT TOWEL COMPRESS can be used to relax the abdomen. Apply it hot to the area you wish to treat. Hold it in place until it cools, and then reheat the towel and apply again. Continue applying the hot towel for 5–10 minutes or until the area becomes red or warm. Note: hot towels or other hot applications should not be applied to areas of the body that are hot, swollen, or inflamed. Cool applications such as a TOFU PLASTER or LEAFY GREENS PLASTER are better for easing discomfort under these conditions.

7. A hot GINGER COMPRESS may be applied to the skin over the intestines several times a week to reduce stagnation and improve blood and energy flow. However, it should not be used in case of swelling or inflammation.

8. A SALT PACK may be used to warm and soothe any region where aches and pains are experienced. As with other hot applications, it should not be applied in cases of swelling, fever, or inflammation.

CAUTION

1. Intestinal disorders can lead to life-threatening or fatal complications. Please note the cautions described in the sections above on appendicitis, diverticulitis, and other conditions. Seek prompt medical attention when necessary.

2. For 7 to 10 days, it is effective to observe a semi-fast; reduce the amount and number of meals and chew very well. However, avoid complete fasting for several days or more; often following resumption of eating comes an enormous appetite that cancels out the positive effect of the fast.

3. Various medications and supplements may be taken for a short time, if desired, but you should eliminate them as soon as possible, to avoid any harmful side effects and becoming dependent on them.

4. CHINESE MEDICINE, ACUPUNCTURE, YOGA, and other traditional healing approaches may be used under the supervision of an experienced practitioner.

5. An ordinary enema or BANCHA TEA AND SEA SALT ENEMA may be used occasionally to help release obstructed bowels. However, avoid colonic enema therapies, colon cleansing, colonic irrigation, and other colonic remedies that typically involve several days' treatment and may put too much stress on the intestines.

MEDICAL EVIDENCE

TRADITIONAL JAPANESE DIET REDUCES RISK OF COLITIS

Japanese researchers reported that consumption of Western-style foods, especially bread, butter, margarine, cheese, and meats, was related to the onset of ulcerative colitis, while traditional Japanese foods, as well as vegetables and fruits, did not increase the risk.

Source: "A Case-Control Study of Ulcerative Colitis in Relation to Dietary and Other Factors in Japan," *Journal of Gastroenterology* 30 (Supplement 8): 9–12, 1995.

MEAT CONSUMPTION LINKED WITH INCREASED APPENDECTOMIES

British researchers reported that in a study of 11,000 appendectomies, those people who ate meat had a significantly higher risk of having this operation than vegetarians. "The results suggest that people who do not eat meat have a 50 percent lower risk of requiring an emergency appendectomy than those who do," the scientists concluded.

Source: P. Appleby et al., "Emergency Appendectomy and Meat Consumption in the U.K.," *Journal of Epidemiology and Community Health* 49(6): 594–606, 1995.

SOUTH AFRICAN DIET PROTECTS AGAINST HEMORRHOIDS

South African blacks have virtually no hemorrhoids compared to whites, who have high rates of this disorder. A researcher found that hemorrhoids were linked to a diet high in fat and low in fiber, the reverse of the traditional black South African way of eating.

Source: D. Burkitt, "Varicose Veins, Deep Vein Thrombosis and Hemorrhoids: Epidemiology and Suggested Aetiology," *British Medical Journal* 2:556, 1972.

MILK CONTAMINATION ASSOCIATED WITH CROHN'S DISEASE

Crohn's disease may be caused by a microorganism found in milk. According to a growing body of medical research, *Mycobacterium avium* subspecies *paratuberculosis*, or MAP, is epidemic in U.S. dairy herds and causes Johne's disease in cattle, a debilitating disorder similar to Crohn's disease. A study conducted by the National Animal Health Monitoring System found that 22 percent of American dairy herds have infected cows that secrete the mycobacterium in their milk. The microbe is not killed by ordinary pasteurization. Crohn's disease is found only in milk-drinking regions of the world, including Australia, southern Africa, Europe, North America, and New Zealand. It is rare in countries such as India, where the milk is drunk but boiled first. The spread of MAP constitutes "a public health disaster of tragic proportions," according to Dr. John Hermon-Taylor of St. George's Hospital Medical Center in London, an expert on the transmission of Crohn's.

Source: Thomas H. Maugh II, "Milk May Be the Carrier of Crohn's," *Los Angeles Times,* September 19, 2000.

DIGESTIVE ILLS ASSOCIATED WITH SWEETS, FATS, DAIRY

In a survey of the relation between diet and disease, a Canadian researcher found that people with Crohn's disease and ulcerative colitis experienced the strongest reactions to chocolate, dairy products, fats, and artificial sweeteners.

Source: G. Joachim, "The Relationship Between Habits of Food Consumption and Reported Reactions to Food in People with Inflammatory Bowel Disease," *Nutrition and Health* 13(2):69–83, 1999.

CASE HISTORIES

MACROBIOTIC DIET HELPS WOMAN RECOVER FROM CROHN'S DISEASE

Virginia Harper had suffered from intestinal disorders since she was fourteen. After eight years of agonizing, often paralyzing pain, discomfort, and disability, she was diagnosed with Crohn's disease and Takayasu arteritis, an autoimmune deficiency in which the blood vessels spontaneously create blockages. Doctors put her on prednisone, an anti-inflammatory drug, and recommended surgery, including a possible abortion when she became pregnant. From what they told her about the need for repeated surgeries, she was afraid that she wouldn't live to be thirty. Seeking an alternative, Virginia visited a macrobiotic counselor who told her, "You can turn this around." Virginia, who described herself as "a fast-food, junk-food, pre-prepared, vegetable-come-in-a-can baby boomer," started to eat whole, natural foods and experienced immediate relief. She gave birth to a beautiful daughter and has now been "symptom-free, drug-free, pain-free, doctor-free" for almost twenty years. She is a macrobiotic cook, counselor, and teacher in Nashville, Tennessee, helping many people, as is her daughter, who recently graduated from the Kushi Institute.

Source: Gale Jack and Wendy Esko, *Women's Health Guide* (Becket, Mass.: One Peaceful World Press, 1997), 7–10.

CHRONIC COLITIS DISAPPEARS AFTER DIETARY CHANGE

Andrew Weil, M.D., describes a woman with chronic ulcerative colitis for many years who took prednisone and other suppressive drugs. After starting macrobiotics, her colitis quickly disappeared.

Source: Andrew Weil, M.D., *Spontaneous Healing* (New York: Knopf, 1995).

TABLE 19. DIGESTIVE CONDITIONS AND DISORDERS

1. More Yin Cause	2. More Yang Cause	3. Yin and Yang Combined
Typical Symptoms		
Swelling	Constriction; some swelling	Swelling
Inflammation	Inflammation	Inflammation
Looseness of tissue	Hardening	
Enlargement of organs	Formation of pus and tumors	Production of pus and tumors
Spasmic pains		Lack of metabolic coordination
Slowness of metabolism	Fever	
Nausea, vomiting		
Belching, gas, flatulence		

1. More Yin Cause	2. More Yang Cause	3. Yin and Yang Combined
Diseases		
Some mouth and body odor	Some mouth and body odor	Some mouth and body odor
Toothache, tooth decay	Tooth erosion	Some toothache
Gingivitis, inflammation of the gums		Periodontal disease
Some abscess	Scurvy	Some abscess
Some TMJ		Some TMJ
Chronic constipation	Temporary constipation	
Chronic diarrhea	Temporary diarrhea	
Overweight	Underweight	Obesity
Stomachache, stomach cramps, stomach swelling		Enlarged spleen
Gastritis, gastroenteritis, heartburn		
Snoring		
Some drowsiness	Some drowsiness	Some drowsiness
Some insomnia	Some insomnia	Irregular sleeping
Oversleeping	Sleepwalking	
Motion sickness		Anorexia nervosa, bulimia
Allergies	Appendicitis	Hemorrhoids
Some irritable bowel syndrome	Some irritable bowel syndrome	Some irritable bowel syndrome
Lactose intolerance		
Crohn's disease		Colitis
Gastric ulcers	Duodenal ulcers	Enteritis
Hepatitis A	Hepatitis B	Hepatitis C
Cirrhosis	Jaundice	
Chronic pancreatitis	Acute pancreatitis	Diverticular disease
Diabetes	Hyperinsulinism	Hypoglycemia
Mumps		Gallstones
Upper stomach cancer	Colon cancer	Lower stomach cancer
Esophageal cancer	Rectal cancer	Spleen cancer
	Pancreatic cancer	
	Liver cancer	

◎ EAR AND HEARING PROBLEMS

Ear and hearing problems are on the rise in modern society. Nearly 30 million Americans suffer from some kind of hearing loss. Ear infections are common among infants, children, and teens, while clogged ossicles and auditory nerve damage are leading causes of hearing loss and deafness among adults and the elderly. As the principal organ processing sound and vibration, the ear and its functions govern overall balance and harmony of mind, body, and spirit. The auditory nerve connects with the muscles of the body, and through the vagus nerve, the inner ear connects with the heart, lungs, larynx, liver, stomach, kidneys, bladder, and intestines. The ear converts sound waves from an air medium to a fluid medium in the inner ear and then into electrical impulses that are sent to the brain.

In the embryo, the ear begins to develop in about the tenth week of pregnancy and is fully functional by four and a half months. The developing fetus is sensitive to the emotional tone of sounds, including the voices of the parents and other family members and the general vibration of the home or environment. Some congenital and childhood disorders have been linked with blockages or other abnormalities in the sonic bond between the pregnant mother and her child. Exposure to loud noise is the leading cause of hearing disability in the United States.

Sound plays a fundamental role in many of the world's creation myths, and early cultures used sound and music to heal. In Greek mythology, for example, Apollo was both the god of medicine and the god of music. He played a harp or lyre that could heal any illness. Orpheus, David (in the Bible), and other master musicians had the same ability.

A balanced way of eating will help prevent most hearing problems and often restore loss of hearing. Singing, playing music, and listening to harmonious sounds and rhythms will contribute to overall health and well-being as well as help recover from specific ailments and disorders.

SYMPTOMS

1. Buildup of wax in the ears
2. Ringing in the ears
3. Bleeding or discharge from the ears
4. Pain, irritation, or inflammation in the ears
5. Inability to hear certain sounds in both ears or one ear
6. Difficulty understanding conversation
7. Turning up the volume on the radio or TV
8. Dizziness, lack of coordination, loss of balance
9. Ringing or other abnormal sounds in the ears
10. Kidney problems

CAUSE

1. The buildup of fat and mucus in the ear, as a result of overconsumption of both extreme yin and yang foods and beverages, is the major cause of ear infections and hearing loss. These include meat, poultry, eggs, chicken, cheese and other dairy, and other animal foods, as well as refined grains, sugar and sugary foods, excessive

oil, fruit and juice, tropical foods, stimulants, spices, alcohol, and drugs.

2. In traditional Oriental medicine, the ear corresponds with the kidney, with which it shares a similar shape. Kidney problems as a rule lead to ear problems, while hearing difficulties in turn show underlying urinary system imbalance.

3. Cold foods, in particular, contract the kidneys and contribute to hearing difficulties. These include ice cream, yogurt, soft drinks, iced beverages, and other frozen foods.

4. Exposure to loud noises and other disharmonious sounds can cause damage to the ear or loss of hearing.

FORMS

Auditory Nerve Damage. The auditory nerve converts sound impulses into electrical impulses that are sent to the auditory centers of the brain. Resembling a fine hair, the auditory nerve can become coated with fat or mucus or become swollen and lose its ability to conduct sound. Long-term consumption of fat- and mucus-producing foods, especially animal foods, dairy food, hard baked flour products, sugar and sugar-treated foods, and too much fruit and juice, are the primary causes of auditory nerve damage. Discontinuing these foods and following the dietary guidelines for Diet #3 will help prevent or relieve this disorder.

Earache. Otitis media, an ear infection or inflammation, is the primary cause of earache. An infection of the middle ear, it commonly accompanies a cold, the flu, or other respiratory ailment. It is the most frequent cause of earache in infants and children, accounting for 30 million doctors' visits annually and $2 billion in antibiotic prescriptions. Otitis media can also affect adults and lead to hearing loss, perforated eardrum, meningitis, paralysis of the face, or other serious complication. In otitis media, the Eustachian tubes leading from the ear to the upper respiratory tract become swollen and inflamed, leading to fluid retention and a wide variety of symptoms. These include a sudden, sharp pain or dull, continuous pain in the ear, nasal congestion or discharge, fever, irritability, loss of appetite, and (in children) crying when lying down at night. Allergies to chemicals or environmental toxins, exposure to smoke and fumes, and lack of breastfeeding enhance the likelihood of getting earaches. Teeth and gum problems may also be accompanied by earaches.

The primary underlying cause of earache is dietary excess, especially extreme foods of both the yin and yang categories that create acidity in the blood, lymph, and fluids of the inner ear, creating susceptibility to viral or bacterial infections. Elimination of these foods, especially meat, poultry, eggs, and other strong animal foods, dairy food, sugar and sweets, refined grains and hard baked flour products, tropical foods, excessive fruit and juice, stimulants, spices, and alcohol and drugs, and adoption of a standard macrobiotic diet will help alleviate earaches and restore normal functioning. Whole grains as the central food, strong MISO SOUP daily, and regular consumption of sea vegetables will especially help this condition. Observe the guidelines for Diet #3.

Ménière's Disease. Ménière's disease, an inner ear disorder that afflicts about 2.5 million Americans, may be accompanied by a wide variety of symptoms, especially dizzy spells lasting from an hour or less to several days. All age groups may be affected, but middle adulthood is most common. In Menière's disease, too much fluid builds up in the inner ear, which governs balance, standing, lying down, and other body postures and movements. Hardening of the bones of the middle ear, infections, syphilis, leukemia, and other diseases can affect the fluids in the semicircular canals and bring on this condition. Excessive salt is also associated with the onset of Menière's disease. Conventional medicine uses diuretics, sedatives, antihistamines, and other medications to treat this disorder, but side effects are common. Surgery may also be performed, including removal of the labyrinth to stop severe vertigo.

Menière's disease can be prevented and alleviated by following a balanced way of eating and avoiding extreme foods, especially too much salt (which creates cravings for liquid) and too much fluid, including too much watery cooking. Observe the guidelines for Diet #2. The home remedies listed below, including DO-IN, may also be helpful.

Presbycusis. A progressive loss of hearing in the higher frequencies is known as *presbycusis*. It most commonly occurs among middle-aged men and affects their ability to understand women and children, who frequently speak in higher registers. In this disorder, the cilia, the thousands of tiny hairlike cells that line the cochlea of the ear, start to degenerate. This condition is caused primarily by taking too much milk, ice cream, yogurt, and other dairy food, as well as sugar, honey, fruit, fruit juice, raw salad, oil, mayonnaise and other oily, greasy foods, and other strong expansive items. In this case, yin foods and beverages repel yin high-frequency sounds. In other cases, strong yang foods, especially meat, eggs, poultry, and other animal foods, as well as too much hard baked flour products and salt, can cause the cilia to overly contract and lose their ability to conduct vibration. Discontinuing extreme foods and adopting a centrally balanced diet will help improve hearing in the higher registers. For a more yin condition, observe Diet #1, and for a more yang condition, observe Diet #2.

Ruptured Eardrum. A ruptured eardrum can be caused by an accident, injury, or infection. Blood and pus may ooze from the ear, accompanied by sudden pain, dizziness, ringing, and partial hearing loss. Surgery is performed to repair large tears, while antibiotics or a patch for the eardrum are used to treat less serious cases. While medical attention may be needed, especially in the case of an accident or injury, the eardrum will heal better if a balanced way of eating is observed. The ear should be protected from water or disturbances from nose blowing while healing. This can take about two months. During this time, a centrally balanced macrobiotic way should be observed, such as Diet #3.

Tinnitis. Ringing in the ears, or tinnitus, varies from mild discomfort to a severe condition that produces difficulty concentrating, loss of sleep, disability, and psychological stress, including suicide. In some cases, it can lead to hearing loss. An estimated 50 million American adults suffer from this condition, and 12 million each year receive medical treatment, including drugs, hearing aids, or surgery. Exposure to loud noise is the primary cause, and pilots, rock music performers and fans, construction workers, gun enthusiasts, and others who repeatedly are exposed to loud sounds are most affected. Reaction to aspirin or antibiotics can also cause this disorder, and tinnitus sometimes accompanies other conditions, including high blood pressure, allergies, anemia, underactive thyroid, TMJ, or infectious disease.

From the macrobiotic perspective, the major cause of tinnitus, apart from exposure to loud sounds that can cause permanent nerve damage to the cochlea, is the buildup of wax in the ear. Fatty and sticky foods, especially ice cream, yogurt, and other dairy products, as well as sugar, chocolate, honey, and other sugary foods; excessive fruit and fruit juice; tropical vegetables; and other predominantly yin, expansive substances are primary causes. Eliminating these foods, adopting a centrally balanced diet, and applying some of the remedies listed below will help reduce and in most cases eliminate ringing, whistling, buzzing, and other troublesome sounds. Observe the guidelines for Diet #1.

SOLUTION

DIET

Observe the dietary guidelines noted above, focusing on the following:

1. Eat whole grains as the main dish of every meal. Buckwheat is particularly strengthening for the ears (and its related organ, the kidneys), but avoid it if these organs are already too contracted. Black rice (such as wild rice) and other black or dark-colored grains are also nourishing for these organs.

2. Reduce flour products and refined grains as much as possible. Noodles may be taken several times a week, especially soba noodles (which contain buckwheat as well as whole wheat).

3. Avoid simple sugars (refined sugar, honey, and chocolate).

4. Avoid animal food, especially ice cream, yogurt, and other dairy products. Fish or seafood, preferably freshwater fish such as perch or trout, may be taken once or twice a week.

5. Beans are shaped like the ears and kidneys and are particularly strengthening. Select a variety of beans, particularly the smaller beans such as adzuki beans, lentils, chickpeas, and black soybeans. Bean products may also be eaten regularly, including tofu, tempeh, and natto.

6. Among vegetables, root vegetables and dried vegetables, including dried daikon and dried shiitake mushrooms, and winter vegetables such as kale particularly nourish the ears and their functions. Long-term pickles may also be strengthening if the condition is not already too contracted.

7. Sea vegetables are very nourishing, especially kombu.

8. The amount of salt (miso, shoyu, and sea salt) should be moderate.

9. As a rule, fruit and fruit juices should be limited or avoided, unless the condition is too yang and contracted.

10. Limit nuts and nut and seed butters until the condition improves. However, chestnuts and dark sesame seeds may be taken.

11. Among condiments, TEKKA and SHIO-KOMBU are strengthening.

12. Cut down on water to a moderate level, but do not reduce it too much. Besides BANCHA TWIG TEA, KOMBU TEA and MU TEA may be taken occasionally.

13. Reduce the total volume of food and chew more.

14. Avoid late-night eating.

LIFESTYLE

1. Avoid loud noises, including those caused by jackhammers, snowmobiles, tractors, shop tools, lawnmowers, vacuum cleaners, electric razors, automobile engines, gunshots, and rock concerts.

2. Avoid or limit the use of headphones, especially during jogging, cycling, or other physical activities, which can injure the delicate linings of the inner ear and lead to hearing loss.

3. Avoid inaudible, low-frequency sounds such as those of planes taking off and landing along an airport runway. Such powerful vibrations can stress inner organs and functions.

4. Proper chewing is essential to digestion. The ear's vestibular function influences the muscles involved in chewing.

5. Sing a happy song each day. This will contribute to balance at many levels, directly stimulating the ears, kidneys, lungs, large intestine, and other bodily organs and functions.

6. Take periodic "sound breaks" of 10 to 15 minutes during which you listen to music that energizes or relaxes you. Use sound and music to create a harmonious environment or produce desired physical or mental effects (see Table 20).

HOME REMEDIES

1. Many ear conditions are related to problems with the kidney. The following special drink will help normalize kidney functions and is beneficial for the ears and hearing problems. Prepare a mixture of 1 part adzuki beans, 1 part dried daikon, 1 part shiitake mushroom, and 1 part kombu. Add 5 times as much water, bring to a boil, and then simmer for about 25 minutes. Take 1 cup every day for 7–10 days. Don't eat the kombu.

2. A HOT TOWEL COMPRESS or a GINGER COMPRESS around the ears will help melt fat or mucus deposits in the ear.

3. A GINGER COMPRESS on the kidneys will have an energetic effect on the ears as well.

4. To help remove wax buildup, apply several drops of warm sesame oil with an eyedropper. Then rinse with warm BANCHA TWIG TEA with a pinch of sea salt added.

5. DO-IN, or self-massage, to the side of the head, including light banging with the fists to the sides of the head above the ears, is beneficial. Covering the ears with the palm of one hand and tapping hard with two fingers of the other hand, 50 to 100 times, is also helpful.

MEDICAL EVIDENCE

BALANCED DIET IMPROVES HEARING

Individuals who were given nutritional counseling and who observed a diet high in whole-grain cereals, vegetables, and fresh fruits and low in saturated fat, simple sugars, and table salt had improved hearing, in a study of more than 1,400 persons with inner ear symptoms conducted by the West Virginia University of Medicine. The diets encouraged vegetable consumption, replaced sugar-sweetened desserts and pastries with fruit, and avoided salty foods and adding salt to food at the table.

"The response to dietary management is dramatic in most patients," the researchers concluded. "With the otologic patient, dizziness clears promptly and the sensation of pressure in the ears and head is quickly relieved, along with associated headache. Hearing improves or stabilizes, evident in the pure tone audiogram and in the speech discrimination scores. Tinnitus often lessens in severity and sometimes even disappears. . . . General health also greatly improves, and elevated blood pressure often returns to normal. The patients have more energy and are free from headaches, their arthritic symptoms improve, and they often sleep better."

Source: J. T. Spencer, "Hyperlipoproteinemia, Hyperinsulinism, and Menière's Disease," *Southern Medical Journal* 74:1194–97, 1981.

EAR EXPERT WARNS AGAINST DAIRY CONSUMPTION

Albert Tomatis, M.D., the "Einstein of Sound," the world's foremost authority on the ear and its functioning, recommends a diet centered on whole grains and fresh foods. He warns against eating processed foods and acid-producing foods, especially yogurt and other dairy products, which he says can block the ear and its delicate structure and prevent normal hearing.

Source: Don Campbell, *The Mozart Effect* (New York: Avon Books, 1997), 39.

TABLE 20. HOW MUSIC IMPROVES HEALTH

1. Masks unpleasant sounds and feelings
2. Lifts mood and spirits
3. Slows down and equalizes brain waves
4. Stabilizes breathing and respiration
5. Regulates the heartbeat, pulse rate, and blood pressure
6. Reduces muscle tension and improves body movement and coordination
7. Raises or lowers body temperature
8. Increases endorphin levels and improves sense of well-being
9. Regulates stress-related hormones
10. Boosts the immune function
11. Changes the perception of time and space
12. Strengthens memory and learning
13. Boosts productivity and efficiency
14. Enhances romance and sexuality
15. Stimulates digestion
16. Increases stamina and endurance
17. Enhances receptivity to symbols and images
18. Promotes a sense of safety and well-being
19. Increases sensitivity to natural sounds and the environment
20. Contributes to awareness, compassion, and spiritual insight
Source: Don Campbell and Alex Jack, *The Mozart Effect*, 1997

TABLE 21. EAR AND HEARING CONDITIONS AND DISORDERS

I. More Yin Cause	2. More Yang Cause	3. Yin and Yang Combined
Typical Symptoms		
Dulled sense of hearing	Sharp sense of hearing	
Soft, quiet behavior	Loud, noisy behavior	Combination of both
Attraction to loud or formless sounds and music	Attraction to quiet or orderly sounds and music	Attraction to irregular or chaotic sounds and music
Diseases		
		Earache
Loose eardrum		
Cochlea problems	Ménière's disease	Clogged auditory ossicles
Tinnitis	Presbycusis (most cases)	Auditory nerve damage
Transmission and peripheral deafness		Central deafness
		Auditory hallucinations

◉ ENDOCRINE DISORDERS

The endocrine system consists of specialized glands that release hormones that influence the functioning of the organs and aid in the digestion of food. These include the pituitary gland, thyroid and parathyroid glands, adrenal glands, and specialized cells in the pancreas, duodenum, kidneys, and gonads. Conventional medicine treats endocrine disorders with a wide variety of medications, surgery, radiation, and other invasive treatments. They are viewed largely as biochemical imbalances that can be corrected with drugs rather than as dietary and energetic imbalances that can be corrected with proper nutrition and other lifestyle changes. The macrobiotic approach to endocrine disorders emphasizes an integrated approach in which the daily way of eating and mental and physical activities play a central role. *See also "Diabetes" and "Hypoglycemia" in "Pancreatic Problems," and "High Blood Pressure" and "Low Blood Pressure" in "Heart Disease and Circulatory Problems."*

SYMPTOMS

The following symptoms may accompany endocrine disorders:

1. Rapid weight loss or gain
2. Increased or decreased metabolism, including heart rate, blood pressure, nervous sensitivity, perspiration, sensitivity to temperature and pressure
3. Muscle weakness
4. Tingling, numbness, or tremors
5. Rapid growth or cessation of growth

6. Tenderness in the glands of the neck
7. Bulging eyes
8. Thickened skin
9. Abnormal blood pressure
10. Fluctuations in blood sugar levels
11. Abnormal sexual development, appetite, or change in orientation
12. Abnormal sexual characteristics including hair quality, muscle development, skin texture and thickness, and voice quality

CAUSES

1. Overall, the endocrine glands are small, dense, and compact—yang. They therefore are easily damaged by overintake of meat, poultry, eggs, cheese, and other animal foods, as well as too much salt, hard baked flour, and other strong yang items. The endocrine glands also attract extreme yin in the form of metabolic energy from consumption of sugar, chocolate, honey, and other refined sweeteners; polished grains; fruits and juices; tropical foods; spices; stimulants; alcohol; and especially drugs and medications.

2. The more yang hormones of the endocrine system are related to the functioning of the sympathetic nerves, while the more yin hormones are related to the parasympathetic nerves.

3. In general, there are two major types of endocrine disorders: (1) *hyposecretion*, in which not enough of a particular hormone is secreted, and (2) *hypersecretion*, in which too much of a hormone is secreted.

4. Hyposecretion of a yin hormone produces an overly yang condition, while hyposecretion of a yang hormone produces an overly yin condition.

5. Hypersecretion of a yin hormone produces an overly yin condition, while hypersecretion of a yang hormone produces an overly yang condition.

FORMS

Adrenal Disorders. The adrenal glands are located near the top of each kidney. The *medulla*, or inner part, secretes adrenaline, which affects blood pressure, heart rate, sweating, and other activities. The *cortex*, or outer part, secretes androgens, corticosteroids, and other hormones associated with development of male features, controls blood pressure, and regulates levels of salt and potassium in the body. The principal adrenal disorder is *Addison's disease*, characterized by a degeneration of the cortex region, resulting in fatigue, low blood pressure, reduced basal metabolism, muscular weakness, abnormal skin color, and other symptoms. Addison's results from underactive adrenal glands and the insufficient production of corticosteroids. Conventional medicine treats this potentially life-threatening disease with prednisone or other steroids, administered orally or intravenously for the rest of the person's life. From a macrobiotic perspective, Addison's disease is primarily yin, resulting from excessive consumption of sugar, chocolate, honey, and other refined sweeteners; refined or polished grains; excessive fruits and juice; tropical vegetables; spices; stimulants; alcohol; drugs; and other overly expansive foods and beverages. However, long-time overconsumption of beef, pork, chicken, eggs, and other animal foods, as well as too much salt and salty foods, can also cause the adrenals to become overworked and lose their contractive power, resulting in a hormonal insufficiency. Extreme foods of all kinds should be avoided and a more centrally balanced way of eating adopted. Generally, observe Diet #3.

Hypersecretion of androgens in the cortex can lead to *virilization* or the development of exaggerated male features in either men or women, sexual precocity, or the failure of the sex organs to develop. In later life, this condition can result in a tendency to reverse sexual orientation. Overproduction of corticosteroids can lead to *Cushing's syndrome*, a disease marked by excessive fat deposits throughout the trunk and top of the back, a large, round face, muscle weakness, a tendency to bruising, high blood pressure, weakened bones, and increased susceptibility to infection, kidney stones, and diabetes. Cushing's syndrome is associated with pituitary malfunctions, a benign tumor in the adrenals, or lung tumors. Surgery or radiation of the pituitary or adrenal glands is commonly prescribed. From an energetic perspective, these conditions are extremely yang, resulting from taking too much meat, poultry, eggs, fish and seafood, cheese and hard dairy, and other animal foods, as well as too much salt and hard baked flour products. A standard way of eating, slightly oriented in a lighter, yin direction, will help offset overactive adrenals and restore balance. Observe Diet #2.

To help activate the adrenals, SHIATSU may be performed on the bladder meridian running along either side of the spine.

Pituitary Disorders. The pituitary gland is the body's master endocrine gland and to a large extent regulates the thyroid, parathyroid, adrenals, pancreatic alpha and beta cells, go-

nads, and duodenal mucosa. Located at the base of the brain, the pituitary secretes several hormones, including (1) *human growth hormone*, which regulates growth, (2) *thyrotropic hormone*, which regulates the thyroid gland, (3) *gonadotropic hormones*, which regulate the sex organs, (4) *lactogenic hormone* or *prolactin*, which initiates the secretion of milk by the mammary glands, (5) *adrenocorticotropic hormone*, which regulates the adrenal cortex, (6) *vasopressin* (also known as *pitressin* or *ADH*), which causes the blood vessels to contract and inhibits urination, and (7) *oxygocin*, which causes the uterus to contract.

From a macrobiotic perspective, the first five hormones listed above are classified as yin. They are released by the anterior or front lobe of the pituitary gland. The last two hormones are classified as yang. They are released by the posterior or back lobe.

Hyposecretion of a yin hormone such as human growth hormone results in *dwarfism* in early childhood or in pituitary *cachexia* if it begins at a later age. Both conditions are overly contracted, or yang. Hyposecretion of vasopressin (ADH) creates *diabetes insipidis*, an excessive loss of body fluids due to a large increase in the frequency of urination. This is a more expansive or yin condition.

Hypersecretion of human growth hormone in early childhood creates *giantism* or *acromegaly* if it begins at a later age. These are extremely yin conditions. Hypersecretion of ADH results in difficulty urinating, a more yang, contractive condition.

Over- or undersecretion of the other pituitary hormones results in a similar pattern of imbalances.

To prevent or relieve pituitary problems, observe the guidelines for Diet #1 or Diet #2, adjusting slightly for a more yin or yang condition. SHIATSU performed along the Governing Vessel meridian on the back will be beneficial for pituitary conditions, especially on GV 20, GV 15, GV 16, and GV 12 (see a standard meridian chart or acupuncture text).

Thyroid Disorders. The thyroid is a small gland in the neck just below the Adam's apple that influences many basic metabolic processes. Hyposecretion of thyroxin, the principal hormone released by the thyroid, can lead to (1) *simple goiter*, an enlargement of the thyroid gland that results primarily from a lack of iodine in the diet, and (2) *myxedema* or *Gull's disease* in adults and *cretinism* in children. These conditions are commonly characterized by a bulge in the neck and mental retardation, low body temperature, slow heartbeat, thickened skin, and abnormal metabolism. Modern diets low in iodine and other trace minerals found in whole grains, vegetables from land and sea, and other fresh foods are the primary cause of simple goiter. Since iodine was added to table salt, this disorder has virtually disappeared in the United States. Synthetic oral hormones, including those made from animals, are commonly prescribed for hypothyroidism. To relieve hypothyroidism, follow the guidelines for Diet #2, for more yang conditions. A touch of sea vegetables may be used for this condition, but too many minerals can aggravate an overly yang condition. As an external treatment, a compress made from 50 percent regular potato and 50 percent cabbage (with a little flour and water) can be applied to the affected area. Leave

on for several hours and apply daily for several weeks or until the condition improves.

Hypersecretion of thyroxin can result in (1) *exophthalmic goiter* or *Graves' disease* or (2) *toxic goiter*. The former involves a swollen throat, rapid heartbeat, muscular weakness, shortness of breath, nervous malfunctions, irritability, tremors, prolonged staring, protruding eyeballs, and increased metabolism. Toxic goiter is caused by a tumor in the thyroid and the symptoms are similar to Graves' disease except for the absence of protruding eyeballs. Hyperthyroidism is commonly treated with drugs, surgery, or radioactive iodine. Radioactive iodine, however, commonly destroys the thyroid, and is a cause of hypothyroidism (see above). Hyperthyroidism is caused primarily by excessive intake of overly yin foods and beverages that expand, loosen, and weaken the thyroid, resulting in an oversecretion of thyroxin. These include sugar, dairy, oil, fruits (including both citrus and tropical fruits), hot spices, and alcohol, as well as chicken and eggs. A diet centered on whole grains and vegetables will help relieve Graves' disease and toxic goiter. Follow the guidelines for Diet #1. Use of seasoning, sea vegetables, and other mineral-rich foods should be light to moderate until the condition improves.

Prepare the special THYROID DRINK.

In addition, there are four parathyroid glands that are situated near the thyroid gland that regulate levels of calcium in the blood that are instrumental in the development of bones and teeth. Hyposecretion of parathormone, the principal hormone, can lead to *tetany* accompanied by cramps and muscle spasms. Hypersecretion of parathormone results in the release of calcium from the bones into the blood.

Known as *osteitis fibrosa*, this condition can produce structural changes in the bones, skeletal deformities, and a buildup of calcium in the kidneys. Tetany is classified as an extreme yin disorder, while osteitis fibrosa is very yang. A balanced macrobiotic way of eating should be followed to alleviate parathyroid conditions, adjusting in a slightly more yang way for tetany and a more yin way for osteitis fibrosa.

To help treat thyroid problems, SHIATSU can be performed on the major points along the lung meridian.

SOLUTION

DIET

Follow the dietary guidelines noted above, paying special attention to the following:

1. In the event not enough of a particular yin hormone is secreted, eat a slightly more yin diet.

2. If an excess of a yang hormone is secreted, eat a slightly more yin diet.

3. If not enough of a yang hormone is secreted, eat a slightly more yang diet.

4. If an excess of a yin hormone is secreted, eat a slightly more yang diet.

LIFESTYLE

1. The endocrine glands are highly charged by electromagnetic energy from the environment. Their functioning can be improved by stimulating the meridians through SHIATSU, MOXIBUSTION, or ACUPUNCTURE.

2. Avoid synthetic clothing, especially next to the skin, confined environments, and exposure to artificial electromagnetic radiation. These im-pede the natural exchange of energy between the body and the natural environment. They also produce extremely weakening vibrational effects that can contribute to hormone imbalances.

3. Exposure to nuclear radiation can cause thyroid disorders, including cancer.

HOME REMEDIES

See the remedies noted above.

CAUTION

1. A physician should be consulted for any life-threatening condition or one that does not clear up using the dietary approach recommended above.

2. As the condition improves with diet and lifestyle adjustments, drugs and medications for endocrine disorders usually can be reduced or discontinued. Please consult your doctor or health professional for advice.

3. Human growth hormone "harvested" from the pituitary glands of cadavers is associated with the human form of mad cow disease.

MEDICAL EVIDENCE

ATOMIC BOMB TESTS CAUSED THOUSANDS OF THYROID MALIGNANCIES

Nuclear weapons tests in the 1950s and early 1960s released fallout that exposed millions of people, especially children, to large amounts of radioactive iodine that caused thyroid problems in future years, including an estimated 50,000 cases of thyroid cancer. According to the National Cancer Institute, the release of radiation was much larger than previous estimates at the time and at least 10 times larger than those caused by the Soviet nuclear accident in Chernobyl in 1986. Vast regions of the United States, including the West, Midwest, and Northeast, were affected.

Source: Matthew Wald, "U.S. Atomic Tests in '50s Exposed Millions to Risk," *New York Times,* July 29, 1997.

TABLE 22. ENDOCRINE DISORDERS

1. More Yin Cause	2. More Yang Cause	3. Yin and Yang Combined
Typical Symptoms		
Oversecretion of yin hormones	Undersecretion of yin hormones	Irregular and unbalanced secretion of yin and yang hormones
Undersecretion of yang hormones	Oversecretion of yang hormones	
Expansion in growth	Constriction in growth	Imbalanced growth
General fatigue	General irritability	General frustration
Diseases		
Graves' disease	Simple goiter	Imbalanced and complex symptoms combined
Toxic goiter		
Acromegaly	Myxedema (Gull's disease)	Irregular growth
Giantism	Dwarfism	
Pituitary basophilism	Pituitary cachexia	
Diabetes mellitus	Diabetes insipidus	Hypoglycemia
Tetany	Hyperinsulinism	
Addison's disease	Osteitis fibrosa	
Cushing's syndrome	Adrenogenital syndrome	
Undersecretion of the testes	Sexual precocity	Irregular menstruation
Hypogonadism	Virilism	
Underactive sexual libido	Overactive sexual libido	Frequent change of sexual and physical vitalities
Some menstrual disorders, irregularity	Some menstrual disorders, irregularity	Menopausal irregularities

TABLE 23. MAJOR HORMONES

Hormone	Energy	Produced by	Function
Adrenaline (epinephrine)	Yang	Adrenal glands	Controls fight-or-flight response and influences circulation, the muscles, and sugar metabolism
Aldosterone	Yang	Adrenal glands	Regulates salt and water balance and excretes potassium
Antidiuretic hormone	Yang	Pituitary gland	Controls water retention in the kidneys and blood pressure
Corticosteroid	Yin	Adrenal glands	Anti-inflammatory effects, maintains blood sugar, blood pressure, muscle strength
Corticotropin	Yin	Pituitary gland	Regulates adrenal cortex production and secretion of hormones
Erythopoietin	Yang	Kidneys	Stimulates red blood cell production
Estrogen	Yin	Ovaries	Regulates female sex characteristics and reproduction
Glucagon	Yin	Pancreas	Elevates blood sugar levels
Growth hormone	Yin	Pituitary gland	Regulates growth and development and protein production
Insulin	Yang	Pancreas	Lowers blood sugar levels; influences glucose, protein, and fat metabolism in the body
Luteinizing hormone and follicle-stimulating hormone	Yin	Pituitary gland	Governs reproductive functions, including sperm and egg growth, menstrual cycle, female and male sexual characteristics

Hormone	Energy	Produced by	Function
Oxytocin	Yang	Pituitary gland	Contracts uterine and milk ducts in breast muscles
Parathyroid hormone	Yang	Parathyroid glands	Regulates bone formation and elimination of calcium and phosphorus
Progesterone	Yang	Ovaries	Affects mammary glands and milk secretion and the uterine lining for implantation of fertilized egg
Prolactin	Yin	Pituitary gland	Initiates and maintains milk production in the breast
Renin and angiotensin	Yang	Kidneys	Helps regulate blood pressure
Testosterone	Yang	Testes, adrenal glands, ovaries	Gives strong, aggressive energy and male sex characteristics
Thyroid hormone	Yin	Thyroid gland	Influences growth, development, and maturation
Thyroid-stimulating hormone	Yin	Pituitary gland	Stimulates thyroid gland to produce and secrete hormones

◎ EYE AND VISION PROBLEMS

Eye and vision problems range from styes and other simple ailments to cataracts, glaucoma, macular degeneration, and other serious disorders that may lead to blindness. In modern society, eye problems are treated as a separate branch of medicine, ophthalmology, and widely considered an accompaniment of aging. From a macrobiotic view, dietary imbalance is the underlying cause of most eye problems, and the need for eyeglasses, bifocals, drugs, and surgery can be reduced, controlled, or sometimes avoided altogether.

SYMPTOMS

The following symptoms may accompany eye problems:

1. Eyestrain
2. Blurred vision
3. Bloodshot eyes
4. Itchiness
5. Flashing-light sensations, floating objects in the field of vision
6. Loss of focus
7. Inability to distinguish colors, especially red and green in dim light
8. Difficulty seeing in dim light or twilight
9. Pain

CAUSES

1. In traditional Oriental medicine, the eyes correspond with the liver, whose meridian passes through the eye. Imbalances in the liver, whose many functions include detoxification of the blood, often translate into eye troubles. Avoidance of foods and beverages that stress the liver (and to a lesser extent the spleen, which governs the lymphatic system and the left side of the body, including the left eye) and observance of a centrally balanced way of eating are important to healthy vision.

2. Excessive yang foods, including meat, eggs, chicken, fish, seafood, salted cheese, and other animal products, as well as hard baked flour products and too much salt, can contract the eyeball, the lens, the pupils, the optic nerve, and other parts of the eye, contributing to a wide variety of symptoms and disorders.

3. Excessive yin foods, including refined grains, milk and light dairy products, sugar and sweets, excessive fruit and juice, tropical foods, stimulants, spices, alcohol, drugs, and other expansive foods, can expand the eye and its structures and weaken its functions.

FORMS

Cataracts. A cataract is a milky film that may develop over the eye, blocking light. It typically develops in the crystalline lens or capsule of the eye and may eventually lead to blindness. This condition is generally treated with surgery, but cataracts tend to reappear unless the diet is corrected. The main type of cataract is caused by long-term consumption of expansive yin foods, especially dairy products, too much fruit and juice (especially citrus), sugar and refined sweets, alcohol, and drugs. Another type of cataract forms when the gelatinous lens becomes encased in fat and cholesterol, from too much meat, eggs, cheese, butter, and other animal foods. In many cases, these types of cataract form together. To prevent or relieve cataracts, avoid extreme foods and generally observe the guidelines for Diet #3, for conditions arising from a combination of yin and yang factors.

As an external remedy for cataracts, apply a hot towel, rinsed in ginger water and squeezed out, over the closed eyes for several minutes five or six times a day. Also rub fresh grated ginger on the front of the face around the outside of the eyes to stimulate circulation. The ginger towel may also be placed on the back of the neck and on the big toe. The liver meridian runs through both of these places, and cataracts are related to underlying liver imbalances.

One or two drops of sesame oil strained through a piece of sanitized cotton may be applied to the eyes daily before sleep to accelerate the discharge of yin in the case of cataracts caused by too much expansive food. In many cases, cataracts can be relieved in three to four months with this approach without the need for surgery.

The special home remedies described below for liver conditions are also recommended.

Conjunctivitis. Conjunctivitis refers to an inflammation of the transparent membrane that lines the eyeball and eyelid. It is associated with bacterial or viral infection, allergic reactions to pollen, smoke, or other irritants, or a congenital type that appears in newborns. Symptoms may include burning, itchy eyes; the discharge of heavy, sticky mucus; excessive tears; and redness. Overall, this condition is more yin, resulting from excessive milk and dairy food, too much fruit and juice, raw foods, too much oil and fat, tropical foods, stimulants, alcohol, and other excessive yin foods. However, animal fat and pro-

tein will contribute to underlying acidity and should also be avoided. With a balanced macrobiotic way of eating, conjunctivitis will generally clear up in a few days. Follow the guidelines for Diet #1. A BANCHA TEA COMPRESS may be applied to the eyes for temporary relief.

Detached Retina. Normally light focuses on the retina of the eye, creating an image that is relayed to the brain by the optic nerve. The retina, a sensitive membrane containing many nerve endings, is attached to the rear wall of the eyeball. When it starts to separate or detach, light no longer focuses on the retina and blindness may result. Medically, this condition is treated with surgery. However, the retina tends to detach again in several years, as the underlying cause is not addressed. From the macrobiotic view, the primary cause of detached retina is overconsumption of more yin, expansive foods and beverages, including too much fluid, oil, fruit and juice, sugar and sugar-treated foods, raw vegetables, alcohol, and watery cooking. Discontinue these items, follow a centrally balanced macrobiotic way of eating, and be especially careful to use roasted dark sesame oil in cooking, instead of corn oil or other usual vegetable oils, until the condition improves. Observe the guidelines for Diet #1.

Glaucoma. Glaucoma occurs when the fluid in the eyeball builds up and starts to exert pressure on the eye as a whole, threatening to damage the retina and the optic nerve. The result may be blindness. Modern medicine treats this condition by draining the eye of excess liquid, but the buildup of fluid usually recurs several weeks or months later. Diabetes is a major risk factor in the onset of glaucoma. The basic cause of this disorder is long-term consumption of too many yin foods and beverages, especially milk and dairy products, fruit and juice, soft drinks, sugar and sweets, stimulants, alcohol, and other expansive items. Too much liquid intake and watery cooking may also be contributing factors. To relieve or control the progression of glaucoma, observe a centrally balanced macrobiotic way of eating. Follow the guidelines for Diet #1.

Macular Degeneration. Macular degeneration affects 13 million Americans and is the leading cause of vision loss in the country. Symptoms include dim, blurred, or distorted vision during reading, loss of central vision, and blank spots in the field of sight. Produced by scarring of the macula, a tiny spot in the center of the retina, macular degeneration begins with loss of focus and concentration. In the dry form, small yellow deposits form beneath the macula from the thinning of nerve tissue. In the wet form, abnormal blood vessels arise beneath the macula, leaking blood and fluid onto the retina, causing blurring and blank spots to appear. Medically, macular degeneration is considered irreversible. Magnifying glasses and large-print reading material are widely used to offset the dry type, while laser surgery is used for the wet type.

From the macrobiotic view, macular degeneration is primarily a more yin disorder, resulting in loss of yang, central vision. Excess fat and mucus build up beneath the macula, resulting in scarring and loss of focus. However, relative to each other, the dry type is slightly more yang, resulting from strong animal foods, baked flour, and salt, in combination with extreme yin such as sugar and sweets, dairy food, spices, tropical vegetables, excessive oil, fruit, juice, alcohol,

drugs, and other expansive items. The wet type involves predominantly the extreme expansive items and less yang factors. Both types can be controlled and to some extent improved through a macrobiotic way of eating. Follow the guidelines for Diet #1 for macular degeneration caused by excessive yin factors or Diet #3 for that arising from a combination of strong yin and yang factors.

Retinitis Pigmentosis. Retinitis pigmentosis is a hereditary disorder that involves the progressive deterioration of the retina, leading to eventual blindness. Symptoms usually begin in early childhood with gradual loss of peripheral vision. It is considered irreversible by modern medicine, and people with this disease are commonly counseled not to have children. From the macrobiotic perspective, congenital weakness, especially the influence of the mother's way of eating in pregnancy, may lead to the onset of this disorder. However, dietary practices from infancy and childhood forward largely control the rate and extent of vision loss. Extreme foods will accelerate the progression of retinitis pigmentosis, especially chicken and eggs, while a balanced diet centered around whole grains and vegetables will maintain vision at optimal levels, though glasses or corrective lens may still need to be worn. Observe Diet #3 for this condition, avoiding extremes of all kinds.

Stye. A stye is an inflammation along the edge of the eyelid. It may be in the corner or in the middle of the eyelid and usually reddens and forms a pimple that may ooze pus. Styes are caused by extreme foods, especially oily and fatty foods of either animal or vegetable origin, but also too much liquid, sugar and sweet foods, tropical foods, spices, alcohol, and drugs. Avoid these items, adopt a macrobiotic way of eating, and apply a BANCHA TEA COMPRESS over the eyes to help relieve pain and promote healing. Most styes will clear up naturally in a few days to a week. Follow Diet #3, avoiding extremes of both kinds.

SOLUTION

DIET

Follow the above suggestions, paying special attention to the following:

1. Eat whole grains as the center of each meal, including brown rice regularly. Grains that particularly nourish the liver, and hence the eyes, include whole wheat berries, whole barley, and whole rye. These may be cooked together in small amounts with brown rice or occasionally prepared as a small dish.

2. Avoid all animal products with the occasional exception of white-meat fish until the condition improves. Chicken and eggs are particularly bad for the eyes because a chicken has poor vision, especially at night, and these energetic qualities are absorbed when eating these foods.

3. Avoid refined grains, simple sugars (refined sugar, honey, and chocolate), soft drinks, excessive oil, fruits, juices, tropical foods, stimulants, spices, alcohol, drugs, and other strong yin foods and beverages that can weaken eyes and contribute to vision problems.

4. Avoid chemically grown and treated foods that burden the liver and enhance eye problems.

5. Take daily hard leafy greens, orange and yellow vegetables, and other foods that are high in carotenoids, including kale, mustard greens, parsley, broccoli, pumpkins, green peas, Brussels sprouts, and others.

6. Avoid any food artificially enhanced with beta-carotene, including genetically engineered rice, as well as vitamin supplements, herbs, and other symptomatic remedies.

7. The amount of salt (miso, shoyu, and sea salt) should be moderate.

8. Use a moderate amount of water in cooking and drinking, neither too little nor too much.

9. Take a small amount of sea vegetables on a daily basis.

10. Reduce the total volume of food and chew more.

11. Avoid late-night eating, which overburdens the liver and hence the liver meridian and eyes.

LIFESTYLE

Follow the standard way of life suggestions and note the following:

1. Eye exercises will help strengthen the eyes. One simple exercise consists of closing the eyes, covering them with the palms, and moving the eyeballs up and down, then left and right, and then rotating them in a clockwise direction and then a counterclockwise direction. Each motion can be repeated about thirty times before moving on to the next step in the exercise.

2. Light massage on the sides of the head and back of the neck will help release tension and improve eye functioning.

3. MOXIBUSTION on points related to the eye may be useful.

HOME REMEDIES

1. Sesame oil is helpful for the eyes. Heat a small amount and pour through a piece of sanitized cotton. This strained oil may be stored in a small jar. Apply one or two drops directly to the eyes with an eye dropper once a day until the condition improves. The oil serves to repel water and discharge excess fluid retention in the eye.

2. RAW RICE has traditionally been used to treat eye problems, including inflammations, bloodshot eyes, glaucoma, and cataracts. Eat daily for 4–5 days. The rice's gathering, downward energy will help clear up these conditions.

3. FRIED MISO is good for more yin, expanded eye conditions such as nearsightedness, glaucoma, and detached retina. Take 1 teaspoon of this condiment with rice or vegetables.

4. SESAME SEED TEA can improve troubled eyesight. Drink 2 to 3 cups daily, unstrained.

5. A BANCHA TEA COMPRESS is beneficial for many eye diseases, including styes and eye tiredness. Apply over the eyes 3 times a day for 10 to 15 minutes.

6. The following drink is beneficial for the liver and hence for most eye conditions. Combine 1 part dried shiitake mushrooms, 1 part soy or mung bean sprouts, 1 part daikon greens, and 1 part buckwheat groats. Add 4 to 5 times as much water and boil 25 to 30 minutes to make a tea. Drink 1 to 2 cups for about 3 weeks and then every other day for 3 more weeks.

CAUTION

Many vision problems will respond to the approach recommended in this section. However, if symptoms persist or serious complications result, a physician or ophthalmologist should be consulted promptly. Proper diet, external applications, and simple vision exercises can accompany medical treatment, if required.

MEDICAL EVIDENCE

PLANT FOODS PROTECT AGAINST CATARACTS

Vegetables and fruits protect against cataracts, according to a research study at Brigham and Women's Hospital in Boston. Researchers reported that 1,380 people age 40 to 79 who ate vitamin-rich vegetables, fruits, and other nutritious foods had 37 percent less risk of developing cataracts.

Source: M. C. Leske et al., "The Lens Opacities Case-Control Study: Risk Factors for Cataract," *Archives of Ophthalmology* 109(2):244–51, 1991.

VEGETABLES LOWER RISK OF MACULAR DEGENERATION

Green leafy vegetables such as kale, collards, turnip greens, and mustard greens can help protect against macular degeneration. In a study involving nearly 900 patients, Harvard Medical School researchers reported that people who had the highest intake of carotenoids, especially from dark green leafy vegetables, had a 43 percent lower risk of developing this vision disorder.

Source: W. S. Christen, "Dietary Carotenoids, Vitamins A, C, and E, and Macular Degeneration," *Journal of the American Medical Association* 273(23):1835, 1995.

CASE HISTORY

MACROBIOTICS AIDS MINISTER SUFFERING FROM GLAUCOMA AND BLINDNESS

In the early 1960s, when he was living in Cambridge, Michio Kushi met a minister in his seventies suffering from glaucoma. The man was legally blind and one night dreamed he recovered his sight. The next day, a woman in his neighborhood told him about macrobiotics and recommended that he see Mr. Kushi. Michio met with him and his wife, and they both started macrobiotics. In his case, excessive liquid was the main cause of his condition, and Michio told him to strictly control the amount of water in cooking as well as beverage intake. After several months, he came for another consultation. He was very thin and dry, and Michio recommended that he increase the amount of soup in his diet and add more green vegetables. Two weeks later the man returned without his wife and exclaimed that his sight was returning. He came regularly after that and soon could get about without a white cane. His sight came back, and he was extremely happy.

TABLE 24. EYE AND VISION CONDITIONS AND DISORDERS

I. More Yin Cause	2. More Yang Cause	3. Yin and Yang Combined
Typical Symptoms		
Eyestrain (some cases)	Eyestrain (some cases)	
Pupil dilation	Pupil constriction	
Bloodshot eyes		
Excessive blinking	Excessive staring	Fixed or unblinking stare
Diseases		
Myopia (nearsightedness)	Farsightedness	
Eyes going outward	Crossed eyes	
Color blindness (some)	Color blindness (some)	Night blindness
Stye		
Astigmatism (some cases)	Astigmatism (some cases)	
Conjunctivitis		
Detached retina		
Glaucoma		Cataract
Macular degeneration (wet type)	Macular degeneration (dry type)	
		Retinitis pigmentosis
Blindness (some cases)	Blindness (some cases)	Blindness (some cases)
		Visual hallucinations

◎ FOOT AND LEG PROBLEMS

Foot and leg problems include aches, pain, and cramps, as well as athlete's foot, corns, and edema. On the one hand, people today are more overweight and sedentary than in the past and walk, climb, and use their feet less often. On the other hand, professional sports, specialized occupations, and increased leisure time have resulted in a new branch of medicine, known as sports medicine, and athletic footwear has become an international phenomenon. An assortment of steroids, painkillers, and other drugs is used to boost speed, endurance, and performance. A natural approach, focusing on diet and lifestyle, ultimately offers a more rewarding approach to healthy feet and legs, contributing to flexibility, physical lightness and mobility, and adaptability at all levels. *See "Tarsal Tunnel Syndrome" in "Repetitive Stress Injuries"; "Bunion" in "Bone and Joint Disorders"; "Vein Disorders" in "Heart Disease and Circulatory Problems"; and "Cramps and Spasms" in "Muscle Problems."*

SYMPTOMS

The following symptoms may accompany feet and leg problems:

1. Aches, pains, or cramping
2. Toes curving inward or outward
3. Bow legs
4. Knock knees
5. High or low arches
6. Discolorations on the feet
7. Calluses
8. Shaking legs

CAUSE

1. The legs and feet mirror the entire physical, mental, and spiritual constitution and condition, and disorders in the feet tend to correspond with the middle organs.

2. The different parts of the legs and feet correspond to different organs as a result of parallel development in the embryo. The ankles correspond to the sex organs, the shins and calves to the intestines, and the knees to the liver and spleen. Problems in these areas show corresponding problems in the respective organs and their functions.

3. Higher arches indicate tightly contracted muscles, allowing for active functioning of the feet, and are essential for athletes, dancers, and other physically active professionals. They result from the intake of more yang foods, including animal foods, salt, and baked food, while lower arches show a tendency for more yin items such as fruits, juices, and liquids.

4. Lack of flexibility in the legs and feet results primarily from hardening of the arteries, muscles, and joints as a result of too much food high in saturated fat and cholesterol.

5. Feet that point outward while walking show that the base of the spine is too contracted from consumption of animal-quality foods, while feet that point inward show that the spine is more open from consumption of more vegetable-quality foods.

FORMS

Ankle Problems. Sprained ankles, swollen ankles (edema), bruised ankles, and other ankle problems indicate problems in the sexual, reproductive, and excretory functions. In the fetal position during pregnancy, the ankles of the developing baby grew alongside the genitals. Hence, weakness or stagnation in the ankles commonly mirrors similar problems in the reproductive organs. The liver, kidney, and bladder meridians also pass through the ankle region, so that these organs and their functions may also be affected. The Achilles tendon at the back of the ankle should ordinarily be tight. If the tendon is too hard or tight, it shows an overly yang condition from too much animal food, salt, or baked food. If it is too loose and soft, it shows an overly yin condition from too much sugar, dairy, fruit, tropical foods, stimulants, alcohol, and other expansive foods.

For a sprained ankle, apply a TOFU PLASTER to help relieve inflammation and pain. This will help to neutralize the heat and bring down the swelling. Change every two or three hours or when it becomes hot; use until the condition improves. Tofu is more effective than ice. If tofu is not available, a LEAFY GREENS PLASTER or DAIKON PLASTER can be used. For immediate relief while the compress is being made, put large, leafy green leaves such as collard leaves or others that grow upward directly on the bruised ankle (CABBAGE LEAF COMPRESS). The leaves will absorb the initial heat and reduce swelling. Eat simply until the condition heals. In addition to a balance of whole grains, beans, and vegetables, take strong MISO SOUP for several days, slightly more sea vegetables than usual to help restore elasticity to the ankle, and UMESHO BANCHA for strength and vitality.

Athlete's Foot. A scaly rash between the toes that is itchy, may produce blisters, and become infected is known as athlete's foot. It affects both sexes but is more common in males, and is associated with a fungal infection that also causes jock itch. Antifungal powder, proper hygiene, and drugs are commonly used to treat this condition. From the macrobiotic view, *athlete's food* is the underlying cause of *athlete's foot*. Too much animal protein, fat, and dairy products, as well as white flour and refined grains, sugar and sweets, fruit, juice, soft drinks, tropical foods (especially nightshades), stimulants, alcohol, and drugs (especially prior antibiotic use) create an overacidic blood condition that is susceptible to parasitic infections. Follow Diet #1 for conditions arising from primarily strong yin factors. Observing a balanced way of eating, discontinuing the above foods and beverages, and wearing all-natural cotton socks and porous shoes (made of leather or fabric) instead of water-resistant synthetics will help prevent and relieve this condition. Some of the home remedies listed below may also help to relieve pain and accelerate the healing process.

Corns and Calluses. Corns typically arise on the toes and balls of the feet. *Hard corns* are composed of small areas of thickened, dead skin on the top or outside of the toe or sole of the foot. *Soft corns* are red, sensitive areas of skin about a half inch in size that develop on the side of a toe and have a smooth, thin skin. A *callus* is an area of hardened, dead skin up to an inch in diameter on the soles of the feet (or hands). In some cases, corns and calluses develop from pressure or friction, such as tight shoes or repeated motions, in most cases they represent an abnormal discharge of fat and mucus to the surface of the body as a result of dietary excess. For example, a callus on the sole of the foot at the end of the kidney meridian arises from an overconsumption of flour products, fats and oils, and sugar and sweets. The kidneys are stagnated and excess is being transported and released by the kidney meridian at this point.

An assortment of over-the-counter medications, including Epsom salts for foot baths, hydrocortisone cream, and rubbing oils, is used to treat these conditions. A pumice can help gently scrape dead skin off a callus, but unless the way of eating is changed, it will usually come back. A balanced macrobiotic way of eating will usually prevent new calluses from forming and gradually cause old ones to disappear.

The most common site is in the center of the ball of the foot at the beginning point of the kidney meridian. This shows that calluses are the discharge of excess, impurities, and toxins that are not being eliminated through normal urinary channels. Hard baked flour products, saturated fats and cholesterol, and excessive vegetable-quality oil are a primary cause of calluses. Even calluses that have hardened and thickened over many years will gradually disappear when these items are discontinued and a balanced way of eating, centered on whole grains and vegetables, is adopted. Soaking the feet in hot ginger water for 10 to 15 minutes can help soften calluses and ease stiffness, pain, or tightness in the feet and toes.

Hard calluses around the heel indicate overconsumption of bread and other hard baked flour products that are stagnating the intestines. These will usually go away in several days if flour products are strictly avoided.

Knee Problems. Knee problems can arise from many sources, including injury, ligament or cartilage damage, athletic overexertion (runner's knee, biker's knee, jumper's knee), rheumatoid arthritis, bursitis, osteoarthritis, and bone or joint infection. In traditional Oriental medicine and philosophy, the knees are related to the liver and spleen on account of their parallel development in embryo. Also the liver and gallbladder meridians run up the inside and outside of the legs, and the kidney and bladder meridians run up the inside and back of the legs. Among its many functions, the liver helps filter the blood and eliminate toxins from the body, while the spleen regulates the lymphatic system and the gallbladder stores bile from the liver to help digest fat and oil. The kidneys and bladder overall regulate reproductive functions and sleeping. Dietary extremes tend to gather in these organs and their corresponding meridians, weakening the knees and making them more susceptible to injury, infection, or disease. Fatty and oily foods such as hamburger, french fries, mayonnaise, salad dressings, and others are particularly stagnating, while too much sugar, sweets, fruits, juices, tropical beverages, stimulants, and other expansive foods, including too many beverages, will cause the spleen and lymphatic system to become overactive and weaken the knees. Clasping the knees during the night will help relieve insomnia.

If knee pain arises while walking or running, it is generally from a more yang cause, while if it arises while climbing stairs, it is primarily yin in origin. Follow the standard way of eating to help recover from knee problems, adjusting slightly for more yin or yang factors. Observe Diet #1, #2, or #3 depending on the cause. Some of the special dishes and home remedies suggested in the liver section may be helpful. A HOT TOWEL COMPRESS or a GINGER COMPRESS may help ease aches and pains in the knees. However, if swelling or inflammation is present, use a cool application instead such as a TOFU PLASTER or LEAFY GREENS PLASTER to help absorb the heat and fever.

In children, *knock knees* occurs when a child's legs curve abnormally in, resulting in a gap between the feet when the knees are in contact. This is an overly yang condition that can be corrected by eating the standard macrobiotic diet with a slight emphasis on yin factors. If a child that has started to walk returns to crawling on its knees, excessive salt is usually responsible. Temporarily discontinuing salt and making the diet slightly more yin will allow normal development to continue, at which point a little good-quality sea salt can be introduced. Follow the guidelines for Diet #2 for more yang conditions and the recommendations below.

SOLUTION

DIET

Follow the standard macrobiotic diet, adjusting slightly for a more yin or yang cause and following the dietary guidelines for the organs and functions corresponding with leg and foot problems.

LIFESTYLE

Follow the standard way-of-life suggestions, including the following:

I. Get up early and go to bed early. Lead an active life, both physically and mentally.

2. It is advisable to walk daily, about a half hour or more. Avoid strenuous exercise and activities, including running, jogging, fast dancing, and active sports, until the condition improves.

3. SHIATSU, DO-IN, YOGA, martial arts, folk dancing and other traditional dancing, and other practices can help open the energy channels and improve energy flow in the legs and feet.

HOME REMEDIES

I. A BODY SCRUB every day or twice a day with a towel dipped in hot water or hot ginger water, including the arm, hands, and each finger, will promote better circulation and activate physical and mental energies.

2. A HOT TOWEL COMPRESS can be used to relax specific areas of the legs, feet, or toes for the relief of aches, pains, and stiffness. Apply it hot to the area you wish to treat. Hold it in place until it cools, and then reheat the towel and apply again. Continue applying the hot towel for 5–10 minutes or until the area becomes red or warm. Note: Hot towels or other hot applications should not be applied to joints or other parts of the body that are hot, swollen, or inflamed. Cool applications such as a TOFU PLASTER or LEAFY GREENS PLASTER are better for easing discomfort under these conditions.

3. A hot GINGER COMPRESS may be applied to the corresponding region of the legs, knees, feet, ankles, or toes several times a week to reduce stagnation and improve blood and energy flow. For example, pains and aches in the second and third toes are associated with the stomach meridian. A compress on the abdomen will help reduce stagnation in the stomach as well as the meridian as a whole. A ginger compress may be applied on the leg or foot itself. However, it should not be used on areas that are hot, swollen, or inflamed.

4. Apply a raw TOFU PLASTER to draw out a fever or help ease swelling or inflammation in the legs, knees, feet, ankles, or toes.

5. A LEAFY GREENS PLASTER can also be used to lower fevers or ease swelling and inflammation in the legs or feet. Apply directly to the affected area. Change every several hours or leave on until the greens become warm.

6. A TOFU AND LEAFY GREENS PLASTER combines the effectiveness of raw tofu and leafy greens and will help bring down a fever or ease swelling and inflammation. Apply as above.

7. A SALT PACK may be used to warm and soothe any region where aches and pains are experienced. As with other hot applications, it should not be applied in cases of swelling, fever, or inflammation.

◉ GALLBLADDER PROBLEMS

The gallbladder, a small, muscular organ near the liver, secretes bile, the greenish-yellow, viscid digestive fluid produced by the liver. Bile helps to emulsify, or digest, fats and certain vitamins and flows from the gallbladder to the upper intestine a few inches below the stomach. Bile contains bile salts, electrolytes, bile pigments such as bilirubin, cholesterol, and other substances. The most common gallbladder problem is gallstones. However, blockages along the gallbladder meridian, which is one of the longest in the body and runs from the face and top of the head, down the inside of the torso and side of the legs and feet, is a frequent source of pain in modern society.

SYMPTOMS

The following symptoms may accompany gallbladder troubles:

1. Tightness, swelling, pain, or soreness in the gallbladder or abdominal area, especially after a meal or in the middle of the night.

2. Acute pain in the upper right part of the abdomen, extending often to the upper back; indigestion; fever and shivering, severe nausea and vomiting, and jaundice.

3. Swelling, pain, or other abnormalities on the fourth toe, where the gallbladder meridian runs.

4. Hardness, stiffness, or swelling along the gallbladder meridian, which has several branches running from the face and head through the neck, shoulders and chest, down the trunk to the gallbladder and hip, outside the leg, crossing above the ankle bone, and running to the fourth toe.

5. One or more vertical lines in the center of the forehead between the eyebrows or puffiness in this region. Deep lines tend to be caused by contraction and show too much animal food consumption, salt, or baked food. Lines with puffiness tend to be caused by expansive, yin items such as sugar, alcohol, and too much fat and oil.

6. Impatience, upset, anger, rage, aggression, and violent thoughts, emotions, or actions

7. Inability to stay in one place and tendency to move about constantly

8. Headaches on either or both sides of the head, above or behind the ears.

CAUSE

1. Overeating, even of good-quality foods, particularly affects the gallbladder.

2. Overconsumption of foods that contribute to stagnation and tightness of the gallbladder or gallbladder meridian, especially an excess of hard baked flour products, including bread, cookies, muffins, crackers, chips, and cake.

3. Overconsumption of foods that loosen and weaken the gallbladder, for example, an excess of products made of simple sugars, including refined sugar, chocolate, and honey; fruits, fruit juices, and soda; and vegetable-quality oils, dressings, sauces, and spreads.

4. Overconsumption of foods high in fat and cholesterol that cause the gallbladder to become hard and swollen, including meat, poultry, eggs, milk, cheese, and other dairy products.

5. Over- or underconsumption of salt. A deficiency of salt in the diet can weaken the gallbladder, while too much salt can harden it.

6. Midnight snacking or late-night eating. Frequent snacking burdens the gallbladder at night and does not allow it to rest.

7. Excessive intake of drugs or supplements. Proper doses and kinds of medications or supplements can temporarily help alleviate certain conditions, but taking them for too long can particularly burden the gallbladder.

8. Lack of exercise. In individuals with a sedentary lifestyle, digestion, absorption, and blood circulation do not function smoothly, and gallbladder function may be affected.

9. Tension and stress. Too much conflict or stress in the home or workplace can place additional stress on the gallbladder and contribute to mental and emotional problems, especially irritability, anger, and upset.

10. Various diseases, and the treatments for them, may contribute to gallbladder problems. In this case, it is necessary to first recover from the original disease.

FORMS

Gallstones may obstruct the flow of bile from the gallbladder, causing pain (biliary colic) or gallbladder inflammation (cholecystitis). Stones may also migrate from the gallbladder to the bile duct, where they can cause jaundice by blocking normal flow of bile to the intestine. The flow can also be blocked by tumors and other less common causes. In size, gallstones range from minuscule, the size of a grain of sand, to as large as a marble or Ping-Pong ball. They can be soft or hard, smooth or rough, single or multiple. About 10 percent of Americans will develop gallstones at some time in their life. Many cases are mild, but gallstones can cause obstruction and blockages when they become lodged in one of the ducts, leading to inflammation, infection, and damage to the gallbladder, liver, pancreas or small intestine. Women are about four times more likely to have gallstones than men, and those over 40 are more likely to develop gallstones than younger people. In less serious cases, modern medicine treats this condition with bile salt tablets that may help dissolve stones caused by excessive cholesterol buildup. In serious cases, the gallbladder is removed surgically.

Gallstones commonly result from eating too much animal food, saturated oils, and other foods that cause the liver to produce excessive cholesterol. In the gallbladder, bile acids are not able to break down the cholesterol, and it begins to solidify and form crystals and stones. Oily, greasy, sticky foods, as well as sugar, white flour, and other mucus-producing foods, may also lead to the development of gallstones independent of cholesterol formation. Soft drinks and other sugary beverages are often contributing factors, as cold fluids accelerate contraction and the buildup of crystals, leading to the formation of stones.

To prevent the formation of gallstones, stop eating foods that contribute to the formation of cholesterol, mucus, and fat and accelerate the dissolution and discharge of existing stones. Eat in a slightly more yang way, consuming burdock and different varieties of fall squash and pumpkins often. Follow the dietary guidelines for Diet #3 arising from a combination of dietary extremes. A hot GINGER COMPRESS is very helpful in melting stones to a size that allows them to pass through the bile duct. This can be extremely painful. In this case, drink several cups of hot BANCHA TWIG TEA. This will expand the duct and should allow the stone to quickly pass through.

SOLUTION

DIET

For gallbladder disorders, follow the standard macrobiotic diet, paying special attention to the following:

1. Eat whole grains, not refined grains, as the main dish of every meal. Grains that especially nourish the gallbladder are whole barley, whole wheat, and hato mugi (prepared alone or cooked together with other grains). Natural, un-yeasted sourdough bread, udon noodles, seitan, and other whole-wheat products may also be taken from time to time, especially after the condition improves, but avoid hard baked products.

2. Eat organically grown food as much as possible, as pesticides, chemical fertilizers, and other additives irritate the gallbladder.

3. Avoid simple sugars (refined sugar, honey, and chocolate).

4. Avoid animal food as much as possible. Eat only white-meat fish, if craved, in small volume, once every 10 to 14 days, and serve with grated daikon.

5. Minimize fat consumption, and also reduce vegetable-quality oil. Avoid raw oil, such as in salad dressings, sauces, and dips.

6. Leafy greens, especially dandelions, chives, and scallions, in the spring help to release stagnation in the body caused by previous consumption of more contracted foods during the winter.

7. Avoid vegetables that originated in tropical regions, such as tomatoes, eggplants, and peppers.

8. The amount of salt (miso, shoyu, and sea salt) should be moderate.

9. Cut down on water to a moderate level, but do not reduce it too much.

10. Take a small amount of sea vegetables on a daily basis.

11. Natural fermentation is a product of earth's rising or expansive energy. Naturally processed miso made from barley and soybeans is especially good for the gallbladder, as are UMEBOSHI PLUMS, sauerkraut, and pickled vegetables, especially light or quick pickles. Be careful of the salt in pickled foods.

12. A sour flavor naturally nourishes the gallbladder and its functions. It counteracts the effects of rich, greasy food, functioning as a solvent and breaking down fats and protein. Examples: lemon, lime, pickles, sauerkraut, sour apple, sour plum, vinegar, leek, apple, blackberry, mango, raspberry, sourdough bread, tangerine, and tomato (which can be used medicinally for very contracted conditions).

13. Barley malt also releases tightness in the gallbladder, but use sparingly.

14. Reduce the total volume of food, and chew more, ideally 50 to 200 times per mouthful.

15. Avoid late-night eating.

LIFESTYLE

1. Get up early and go to bed early. Lead an active life, both physically and mentally.

2. It is advisable to exercise moderately.

3. Eat two to three meals a day, at regular times.

4. Avoid unnatural environments, such as those with high electromagnetic radiation. Avoid excessive use of air conditioners or heaters and exposure to stagnated air.

5. Keep your personal things clean and in order.

6. Avoid relationships that cause you stress.

7. Spend time in nature as often as possible.

HOME REMEDIES

1. For gallbladder problems caused by excessive yin food consumption, UMEBOSHI PLUM may be taken for several days, or UME-SHO KUZU may be taken, 1 cup a day, for several days.

2. For gallbladder problems caused by excessive yang food consumption, apple cider or BARLEY MALT may be added to KUZU TEA and taken 1 cup a day for several days. Other remedies for this condition include pouring hot BANCHA TWIG TEA over shiso leaves, eating the leaves, and drinking the tea; taking a little rice vinegar or ume vinegar; eating a small side dish of baked or stewed apples; or adding fresh scallions as a garnish to MISO SOUP or vegetable side dishes.

3. To release old fats and oils in the gallbladder, take CARROT-DAIKON DRINK 3 times a week for several weeks.

4. To help eliminate excess protein, especially animal-quality protein that has gathered in the gallbladder, LEAFY GREENS JUICE is helpful.

5. DO-IN can stimulate the gallbladder: rub the fourth toe of each foot. Also rotate the fourth toe about 50 times in each direction.

6. If experiencing pain, first apply a hot GINGER COMPRESS over the gallbladder or gallbladder region, followed by a TARO PLASTER. In some cases, a person with this condition will also experience abdominal swelling due to the retention of fluid. In this case, after applying the ginger compress, apply a BUCKWHEAT PLASTER to the swollen region.

CAUTION

1. Many gallbladder problems result from overeating. For several days, it is effective to eat small quantities of food or observe a semi-fast. Reduce the amount and number of meals and chew very well, up to 200 times per mouthful. After FASTING or SEMI-FASTING, eat only brown rice soup with leafy green vegetables for a brief period. If miso is added to the soup, use only a small amount. After several days, widen the diet to include the standard dietary guidelines, but avoid all animal foods until the condition has improved.

2. Avoid or limit unnecessary medications, supplements, vitamins, and others as much as possible, as these put an added burden on the gallbladder.

MEDICAL EVIDENCE

VEGETARIAN WOMEN HAVE FEWER GALLSTONES

British researchers reported that vegetarian women have 50 percent fewer gallstones than women eating the standard modern diet. In a study of over 700 women, age 40 to 69, Oxford University scientists found that nonvegetarians had nearly twice the risk of developing gallstones as a result of eating more fat and less fiber.

Source: F. Pixley et al., "Effect of Vegetarianism on Development of Gall Stones in Women," *British Medical Journal* 291:11–12, 1985.

HORMONE THERAPY INCREASES RISK OF GALLSTONES

Synthetic hormone therapy for menopause increases the risk of developing gallbladder disease, as well as blood clots and uterine cancer.

Source: Susan Love, M.D., "Sometimes Mother Nature Knows Best," *New York Times,* March 20, 1997.

◎ HEADACHES

Headaches range from mild, infrequent pain in the front, back, or sides of the head to chronic, severe migraines deep inside the head. They may accompany underlying conditions and disorders such as anemia, brain tumors, chronic fatigue syndrome, eyestrain, fibromyalgia, food allergies, menopause, premenstrual syndrome,

sinusitis, stroke, or TMJ. Headaches are generally classified into four main types: (1) *tension headaches*, characterized by a dull, steady pain that feels like a tight band around the head; (2) *sinus headaches*, accompanied by pain in the forehead, eyes, and nasal region; (3) *cluster headaches*, which cause severe, sharp pain around one eye, occur with nasal congestion and a flushed face, and tend to recur every few hours or days, especially several hours after going to sleep; and (4) *migraines*, which are intense, debilitating headaches deep inside the head or on one side of the head, usually accompanied by pinpoints of light, strange odors, or unusual sounds. Modern medicine treats tension headaches with aspirin, acetaminophen, or ibuprofen. Antibiotics and decongestants are used to treat sinus headache. A variety of stronger drugs and medications, including corticosteroids, calcium channel blockers or beta blockers, and antidepressants, are used to relieve migraines. Biofeedback, meditation, visualization, and other alternative methods may also be recommended. In most cases, headaches arise from underlying dietary imbalance, especially food or beverages consumed shortly before the onset of symptoms. A balanced macrobiotic way of eating will help eliminate headaches and prevent their recurrence.

SYMPTOMS

The following symptoms result from headaches and can also cause them:

1. Constipation
2. Indigestion
3. Irregular menses

4. Fatigue
5. Pain in the neck, back or shoulders; stiffness
6. Low blood sugar (hypoglycemia)
7. Overweight
8. Irregular heartbeat
9. Coldness
10. Disorders of the liver
11. Disorders of the endocrine system
12. Disorders of the lymphatic system
13. Emphysema
14. Allergies
15. Congestion and disease of the eyes, such as glaucoma
16. High blood pressure
17. Hearing difficulty or otitis interna
18. Dizziness
19. Mental or emotional problems such as irritation, depression, excitability, short temper, anger, complaining, discontentment, forgetfulness, self-abandonment, obstinacy, and unsociability

CAUSES

1. Headaches are caused primarily by eating extreme foods or beverages. Stress or tension may enhance the pain but rarely gives rise to a headache. In the modern macrobiotic community, it is common for adults and children to go through the entire year without a single headache. They may still face many pressures and challenges in their daily life, but they no longer experience headaches or feel the need to take aspirin or other medications.

2. From an energetic view, headaches can be distinguished into four types, those arising in the front, back, side, or deep inside the head.

These are classified according to their location as relatively more contracted or expanded. Simple, safe home remedies are then recommended based on an understanding of yin and yang.

3. Headaches in the front of the head are caused by excessive consumption of strong yin foods or beverages, including sugar, chocolate, honey, and other sweeteners; fruits and fruit juice; beer, wine, and other alcohol; aspirin, birth control pills, and other drugs and medications. The pain is usually throbbing or sharp, stabbing, or explosive. Heat or warm weather makes it worse. Some types of tension headaches and most sinus and cluster headaches fall into this category.

4. Headaches in the back of the head are caused by excessive consumption of strong yang foods, including too much meat, poultry, eggs, salty cheese, grilled fish and seafood, as well as salt and salty foods, and too much hard baked flour products such as bread, cookies, crackers, and rice cakes. The pain is generally dull, squeezing or viselike, and nonthrobbing. It tends to worsen in cold surroundings. Some tension headaches fall into this category.

5. Headaches in the side of the head are often caused by the intake of oily and greasy foods or other foods that affect the smooth functioning of the liver and gallbladder and their meridians, which extend to the head. The pain may be dull or sharp. Some tension headaches fall into this category. Those on the left side of the head also commonly involve excessive intake of simple sugars; fruit and fruit juice; soft drinks; and spices and stimulants. Those on the right side of the head may also result from excessive consumption of animal food, including meat, poultry, eggs, cheese, and other dairy products; salty foods; baked flour products; and stimulants.

6. Headaches deep inside the head are caused by the overconsumption of animal food high in protein and fat, especially salted meat, eggs, caviar, and salted fish. They are usually accompanied by strong pressure and pain in the brain. These correspond with migraines.

7. Sharp headaches, besides the above cause, often result from excessive intake of hot spices (for example, cayenne pepper and mustard) or stimulants (for example, alcohol, coffee, mint tea, and peppermint tea).

8. Dull headaches, besides the above mentioned causes, may result from excessive intake of water or oil; overeating as a whole; and excessive consumption of foods that do not digest easily.

9. In addition, excess intake of cold foods and beverages, ice cream, raw oil, and alcohol also cause headaches.

10. Overeating and excessive drinking may also cause headaches.

11. Excessive intake of medications or supplements is also an occasional cause.

SOLUTION

DIET

1. Take whole cereal grains (for example, brown rice, barley, wheat, millet including *awa* or *hie,* and corn) at every meal. If you have an ache on the back of the head or deep inside the head, do not take buckwheat. It is better to avoid baked flour products such as bread.

2. Avoid fried rice and fried noodles when you have an ache on the sides of the head, but it is all right to take them about once a week if you have another type of headache.

3. MISO SOUP or clear shoyu broth may be taken every day, but the taste must be light.

4. Eat a variety of vegetables, but avoid potatoes, tomatoes, avocados, and others that originated in tropical regions. Also avoid yams of any kind, except jinenjo (mountain potatoes).

5. Avoid raw salad.

6. Avoid cooking with a lot of oil.

7. Follow the standard guidelines for beans and sea vegetables.

8. It is better to avoid animal food, even fish and seafood. But if desired, once a week prepare white-meat fish that is low in fat.

9. Avoid fruit if possible. If cravings arise, cooked fruits or dried fruits are preferred. If you have fresh fruit, sprinkle it with a pinch of sea salt.

10. Avoid nuts because they are high in fat. Sesame seeds and pumpkin seeds may be taken, but avoid sunflower seeds, as they are more oily.

11. For beverages, follow the standard dietary recommendations, and completely avoid stimulants (such as coffee, alcohol, mint tea, and peppermint tea).

12. The amount of salt must be moderate.

13. Avoid midnight snacks.

14. It is important to chew well. Try to chew each mouthful at least 50 times.

LIFESTYLE

Follow the standard way-of-life suggestions.

HOME REMEDIES

1. For frontal headaches, take a small cup of SHOYO-BAN TEA, UME-SHO BANCHA, or UME-SHO KUZU. A small handful of

GOMASHIO or a teaspoon of TEKKA is also helpful. These are very contractive and will counteract the expansive energy that is producing the pain and ache. Externally, a TOFU PLASTER, LEAFY GREENS PLASTER, or other cold compress placed on the front of the head will provide relief. A towel drenched in cold water or ice can be used but is not as effective. Also, you can rub APPLE JUICE, daikon juice, sesame oil, or SESAME OIL WITH GINGER on the painful area. To bring the energy down from the head to the lower part of the body, soak the feet in salted water, preferably cold. Massaging the second and third toes on each foot will stimulate the stomach meridian and facilitate the discharge of excessive yin through these pathways. If you have an ache on one side of the head, massage the toe of same side. The way to massage is to do so strongly, pulling the toes a little.

2. For rear headaches, take a small cup of APPLE JUICE, orange juice, or AME KUZU TEA or take a small volume of ume concentrate. A towel drenched in hot water and squeezed out can be applied to the back of the head or neck to provide relief. Soaking the feet in hot water is helpful, as is massaging the ball of the foot where the kidney meridian ends. Massage the fifth toe.

3. For side headaches, grate 2 tablespoons of fresh daikon, add a cup of hot water, simmer, and add a little shoyu. AME KUZU TEA, or kuzu made with barley malt, is also relaxing and will help relieve the pain. A little grated ginger may be added to this tea. MISO SOUP with scallions or onions is also recommended. Externally, alternate compresses on the side of the head with towels drenched in hot water and squeezed out and then another towel with cold water. Soaking the feet in lukewarm water is

helpful, as is massaging the fourth toe. This will help to bring the energy down from the head to the feet and stimulate discharge through the gallbladder and bladder meridians.

4. For deep, inside headaches, take cooked apples, heated APPLE JUICE, or hot water mixed with 1 teaspoon of rice vinegar or 1 teaspoon of barley malt or rice honey. UMEBOSHI PLUMS are also helpful to neutralize extremes. Massage the big toe on each foot, including both the outside and inside regions, where the ends of the liver and spleen meridians are located. This will help stimulate these organs, release pressure and blockages, and reduce pain.

5. Every morning and every evening, twice a day, do a BODY SCRUB to promote better circulation.

6. When constipation accompanies the headache, take a cup of UME-SHO KUZU or UME-SHO BANCHA every day for about 5 days; after that, every other day for another 10 days to 2 weeks.

7. A GINGER COMPRESS over the kidneys and on the abdomen (over the intestines), for 15 minutes on each area, will provide relief and get energy circulating. Continue this every day for a few days, or twice a week for 1 month. If you have a stiff neck, shoulders, or back, reduce your meals to once a day for about 5 days. Do a GINGER COMPRESS on your neck, shoulders, or back once a day during that time.

8. SHIATSU, ACUPUNCTURE, and other practices can help you recover from headaches.

9. It is helpful to practice SEMI-FASTING or FASTING, but it must be limited to 1 week to 10 days. Take water or tea at that time. At this time, you may take BROWN RICE PORRIDGE, a thick rice gruel. It is also helpful to take a cup of SWEET VEGETABLE DRINK every morning and every evening.

CAUTION

1. Certain medications or supplements can cause headaches. In this case, it is necessary to recover from the original disease and reduce the medications and supplements at the same time. Please consult a physician about reducing or withdrawing from any prescription medicine.

2. Analgesics can help temporarily but will probably not result in a complete recovery or will drive the imbalance deeper into the body, where it will resurface later.

3. Prepare food moderately. It should not be extremely salty or extremely sweet. Try instead to season your food mildly.

4. When those who have taken coffee or alcohol for a long time quit, a headache sometimes occurs for 3 to 5 days. This withdrawal headache occurs when the cells of the brain, which have become expanded from the coffee or alcohol, begin contracting. In this case, ½ to 1 cup of SWEET VEGETABLE DRINK, APPLE JUICE, or apple cider can help to relieve the headache. But this type of headache should clear up in 2 to 3 days without these drinks.

5. Headaches may also be caused by brain tumors or other serious disease. Consult a physician for any persistent headache that does not clear up with the approach recommended above.

MEDICAL RESEARCH

MIGRAINES LINKED TO SPECIFIC FOODS

Specific foods can trigger migraine attacks in susceptible individuals, according to a Spanish medical study. These include chocolate, cheese, citrus fruits, bananas, nuts, cured meats, dairy products, hot dogs, pizza, food additives (including MSG), stimulants, soft drinks, and alcohol.

Source: R. Leira and R. Rodriguez, "Diet and Migraine," *Revue Neurol* 24(129):534–38, 1996.

CASE HISTORY

MEDICAL DOCTOR RELIEVES HER MIGRAINES WITH MACROBIOTICS

Dr. Helen V. Farrell, a former medical consultant for the Department of National Health and Welfare in Canada, used macrobiotics to recover from chronic migraines. She had suffered from severe, debilitating headaches since she was 11 years old, experiencing scintillating scotomas, dysplasia, transient parasthesias, and vomiting. The headaches diminished as she grew older, and they disappeared when she discontinued dairy food altogether. However, they recurred and she turned to macrobiotic home remedies for a solution. "By the time I got home twenty minutes later," she reported after one attack, "I could barely see, and the pounding migraine pain was just starting. I headed straight for the pantry and the umeboshi plum paste. I had been reading about the condiment and its contractiveness, so I thought I would experiment and see if it worked or not. After about 2 teaspoons and within 2 minutes, the visual symptoms disappeared completely. I couldn't believe it!" she exclaimed. Dr. Farrell continued eating a little more umeboshi and within two hours she "got up, feeling completely normal with no headache, nausea, or tingling." She went on to incorporate macrobiotics into her own medical practice and found it especially effective for PMS and other women's health problems.

Source: H. V. Farrell, M.D., "PMS Is Not PMS," in Michio Kushi, ed., *Doctors Look at Macrobiotics* (Tokyo and New York: Japan Publications, 1988), pp. 177–91.

◎ HEART DISEASE AND CIRCULATORY PROBLEMS

Cardiovascular disease is the leading cause of death in the world today. Approximately 50 percent of all people in the United States, Europe, Japan, and other industrialized societies will die of a heart attack, stroke, hypertension-related illness, peripheral artery disease, or other circulatory disorder. Heart disease is also increasing rapidly in the developing world and is projected to surpass infectious disease as the leading cause of death and disability in the next twenty years. Today, Americans spend one-seventh of all their food money on hamburgers, fried chicken, beef tacos, and other fast food. Next to home cooking, it is the second most important source of nutrition. In the United States the average person lives within three miles of a McDonald's restaurant.

In traditional societies, heart attacks, strokes, and even blood pressure rising with age are virtually unknown. Heart disease was the first major degenerative disease linked by medical and scientific research to the modern way of life, especially the modern way of eating. The Framingham Heart Study and pioneering studies on the macrobiotic community in Boston by researchers at Harvard Medical School helped establish diet as a main risk factor in the development of high blood pressure, heart attacks, and strokes. Modern medical science has subsequently discovered that many heart conditions, including advanced coronary disease, are not only preventable but also reversible, especially with the help of a balanced diet, moderate activity and exercise, and a healthy lifestyle.

SYMPTOMS AND SIGNS

Signs of developing heart and circulatory problems often manifest long before symptoms appear. In the traditional medicine and philosophy of the Far East and other regions, the following are often evaluated:

I. A reddish color to the face shows an overworked heart and circulatory system from the expansion of blood capillaries beneath the skin toward the surface. Except in cold weather or when blushing, when the face naturally turns red, a red color often indicates elevated blood pressure. A swollen, puffy face, accompanied by this color, shows that the heart muscle itself is expanded and weakened from too many yin foods and beverages. From chronic redness, the facial color may turn to purple, which shows a dangerous overworking of the heart muscle and developing low blood pressure. A pale color to the face may indicate the heart is becoming tight from too much animal food and salt and a yang form of low blood pressure is developing.

2. The nose develops in unison with the heart in embryo, and abnormalities on the nose show underlying heart problems. A swollen nose, for example, shows that the heart is swollen and laboring to provide oxygen to cells and tissues. This condition is caused by excessive intake of strong yin, including sugar, sweets, and beverages; too much fruit and juices; and alcohol or drugs. In some cases, this is a sign of developing congestive heart failure. A hardened tip on the nose shows a buildup of saturated fat and cholesterol in the coronary arteries and the buildup of fat around the heart and other inner organs from the intake of excessive meat, poultry, cheese, and dairy, as well as margarine, dressings, and other oily, greasy foods. Unless the way of eating is changed, hardening at the end of the nose may lead to a heart attack or stroke. A purple color to the nose, accompanied by a hardened tip, is a traditional warning sign of an imminent heart attack or stroke. A cleft in the nose shows the presence of a heart murmur.

3. The hands also show the condition of the heart. The left hand corresponds with the left chamber, the right hand with the right chamber. In the left hand, with palm facing up, blood circulation mirrors an imaginary line extending from the tip of the little finger tracing an arc down to the base of the palm and up to the top of the thumb. In the right hand, blood flow follows a line from the thumb down to the base of the palm and up to the end of the little finger. Any symptom or discoloration along these lines correlates with circulatory changes in the respective chambers. The center of the palms indicate the condition of the main heart valves between the atria and ventricles. Swelling, discolorations, or other abnormal signs here, or feeling pain when pressed, shows looseness, leaking, or weakness in the tricuspid or mitral valves.

4. The heart and condition of the arteries can be evaluated by the handshake or grip. A weak, limp grip shows a deficiency in the heart and circulatory system, while a crushing one shows high blood pressure and overactive pumping action of the heart. Reddish or hot hands also show an overburdened heart and a tendency toward high blood pressure. Moist or wet hands show an overworked heart as a result of consuming too many fluids, sweets, and other strong expansive foods.

5. Hold the palms of the hands together and press. If the hands are not able to bend perpendicular to the extended arms at a 90-degree angle, hardening of the arteries is present.

6. The heart meridian runs along the lower inside of each arm to the inside of the little finger. Tension, tightness, hardening, stiffness, flabbiness, or loosening along this region shows corresponding heart and circulatory problems. A heart attack is often accompanied by pain running along this channel of electromagnetic energy along the left arm. CPR practitioners are sometimes taught to employ the traditional Oriental first aid technique of biting the nail of the little finger to stimulate the heart in the event of a coronary, stroke, or sudden cardiac arrest. Massaging the inside of the little finger and the meridian along the arm is also very effective.

7. Excitability, excessive talking, hysteria, and similar emotions show developing heart problems. Stuttering, stammering, lisping, and other speech difficulties also often show underlying cardiovascular problems. Stuttering indicates a heart murmur, overactive heartbeat, or other irregularity caused by too much dairy or other fatty food. Electrical impulse disturbances and a tired, overworked heart produce stammering. Rapid speaking signifies a tendency toward high blood pressure, especially from spices, sugar, and oily food.

8. A narrow, rigid view of life, prejudice and discrimination, and other mental and psychological imbalances often accompany hardening of the arteries and other heart problems. As these are relieved, the person's view of life usually becomes more broad and flexible and more tolerant of others and the dynamics of change.

9. Laughter is proverbially one of the best medicines, but excessive laughter, giggling, and joking show a swollen, overactive heart. Excessive intake of fruit and juices, as well as sugar and sweets, raw foods, tropical foods, stimulants, and alcohol, as well as other extreme foods, contribute to this condition.

10. Heart problems are most pronounced between about 10 A.M. and 2 P.M., when the circulatory system is most active, according to the Far Eastern theory of the five transformations. Similarly, in the yearly calendar, the summer corresponds with the heart, and chest pains, cramps, hyperactivity, and other symptoms are usually heightened during this season. Medical studies have corroborated this traditional wisdom, finding that the peak period for heart attacks is 1:30 P.M. and during the month of July.

11. There are other simple, safe diagnostic techniques that can be used to evaluate the condition of the heart and circulatory system. These include pulse diagnosis, iridology, and voice diagnosis. These are easily learned but take time and practice to master.

UNDERLYING CONDITIONS

The conditions underlying most forms of contemporary heart disease include the following:

High blood pressure. High blood pressure, also known as *hypertension*, is generally caused by consumption of a combination of meat and sugar, eggs and poultry, dairy foods, and other extreme foods from both the extreme yang and extreme yin categories. Excessive salt and too much hard baked flour products are also frequently involved. The arteries become constricted and narrowed, while the heart becomes swollen, enlarged, and expanded. With proper eating and lifestyle, normal blood pressure can usually be reestablished in 3 to 4 months.

The most common type of high blood pressure is *systolic hypertension*. It occurs frequently in those over 50 and is characterized by hardening of the larger arteries and arteriosclerosis in the smaller arteries and vessels. Systolic pressure (the pressure of the heart when beating) commonly rises to 160–200 or more, while the diastolic pressure (the pressure of the heart at rest) falls to 50–60 or lower. Though often benign, systolic hypertension can progress to coronary heart disease or congestive heart failure. To prevent or relieve this condition, avoid or reduce meat, dairy, poultry, eggs, and other animal products (with the exception of occasional white-meat fish, if desired), hard baked flour products, and refined salt. Sugar, spices, stimulants, alcohol, and other strong expansive foods commonly contribute to high blood pressure and should also be limited. A standard macrobiotic diet can be observed, with slightly lighter cooking and seasoning. Follow the dietary guidelines for Diet #2. Special dishes include a small side dish of dried DAIKON WITH KOMBU; boiled salad, steamed leafy greens, and a small volume of grated daikon with shoyu (3 times a week for 3 weeks) to help eliminate hardened fats and toxins from the body. A BODY SCRUB once or twice daily is advisable, as is light to moderate exercise, but strong, vigorous exercise should be avoided.

Diastolic hypertension occurs when both systolic and diastolic pressures are elevated to abnormally high levels, typically 200/125 or more. The burden that this increase places on the pumping action of the heart can lead to left heart failure, congestive heart failure, stroke, or weakened kidneys. While chronic consumption of animal food is typically involved, overconsumption of sugar, sweets, milk and other light dairy, oily and greasy foods, juices and fruits, tropical foods, alcohol, spices, and other more expansive foods are typical. Overall, there is a tendency toward ingesting sugar, liquid, juicy, and raw foods. Follow the guidelines for Diet #1. In addition to the standard macrobiotic diet, special dishes for this type of high blood pressure include STEAMED LEAFY GREENS daily, DRIED DAIKON WITH KOMBU, and NISHIME-STYLE VEGETABLES several times a week. A daily BODY SCRUB is advisable, but long, hot showers or baths are not recommended, as they result in mineral loss and further weakness.

Low blood pressure. Low blood pressure, or *hypotension*, commonly takes two forms. The first is the culmination of high blood pressure. Overburdened by hardened arteries and swollen left chambers, the heart gives out and blood pressure drops from abnormally high levels to precipitously low ones. This yin, more expansive form of low blood pressure is caused by lack of good-quality salt and minerals, whole grains, and fresh vegetables and other plant-quality foods, along with excessive intake of

sugar, sweets, fruit, juices, soda, and other extreme expansive foods. A slightly stronger standard diet should be followed to offset this condition, including sea vegetables, especially kombu, emphasized in daily cooking. Follow the guidelines for Diet #1 for this type of low blood pressure.

The second form of low blood pressure arises from an extreme yang or an overly contracted condition. The heart becomes too tight from long-term consumption of too much meat and other animal foods, salt, baked food, flour products, and heavy, long-cooked food and, corresponding lack of light or more centrally balanced foods. This condition may be relieved by the standard diet with slightly lighter cooking and seasoning, with an emphasis on STEAMED LEAFY GREENS and other green and white leafy vegetables. Observe the guidelines for Diet #2.

High cholesterol. High cholesterol, a waxy, fatlike component in the blood, is a major risk factor for developing heart disease. Americans typically have cholesterol levels of 200 to 300 mg/dL. In the body, the liver naturally produces cholesterol, especially HDL, the "good" cholesterol, associated with maintaining cell walls, serving as a precursor to bile acids, vitamin D, and some hormones, and contributing to other beneficial effects. However, foods high in saturated fat and in dietary cholesterol, including meat, poultry and eggs, dairy food, and fatty fish and seafood, as well as selected saturated vegetable oils such as palm oil and coconut oil, raise levels of serum cholesterol and contribute to cardiovascular disease. The foods in the standard macrobiotic way of eating contain virtually no saturated fat or dietary cholesterol. Whole grains, beans and bean products, and fresh vegetables all contribute to the maintenance of high HDL levels and protect against the effects of LDL, the "bad" cholesterol. Harvard researchers reported that after two years of dietary practice, cholesterol levels in the macrobiotic community in Boston on average fell to 126 mg/dL, a level where heart disease is virtually nonexistent. To lower cholesterol, observe Diet #2, for overly yang conditions. For conditions arising from a combination of extreme yin and yang, follow Diet #3.

Atherosclerosis. Atherosclerosis, the buildup of plaque in and around the arteries, is the underlying cause of coronary heart disease, many strokes, peripheral artery disease, and other cardiovascular conditions. Once thought to be an inevitable accompaniment of the aging process and one that manifested in middle age or old age, cardiologists agree that in society today atherosclerosis is a slow, cumulative process directly connected to the modern diet, centered around foods high in saturated fat and dietary cholesterol. It begins with tiny injuries to the endothelial lining of the arteries in infancy, advances through fatty streaks in childhood, and results in raised lesions and fibrous plaque in the aorta and coronary arteries by the late teens and early adulthood. By the thirties and forties, calcification commonly sets in, with plaque forming in the heart and major blood vessels, extending from the brain to the pelvis. Atherosclerosis can be prevented, and even reversed, through a return to a more balanced way of eating, especially one high in whole grains and vegetables and low in animal-quality foods and fatty, oily foods of plant origin. Observe the guidelines for Diet #3, for conditions arising from a combination of dietary extremes. The home remedies below detail several special dishes to open and restore elasticity to hardened blood vessels

FORMS

Heart and other cardiovascular disease take many forms, including the following:

Aneurysm. An aneurysm results when an artery weakens and its wall bulges into the surrounding tissue. This balloonlike bulge may enlarge and rupture, leading to hemorrhaging and death. The lower part of the aorta is the most frequent site for an aneurysm. A *dissecting aneurysm* occurs when the sac erupts into the artery itself, impeding blood flow and blocking connecting vessels. Atherosclerosis underlies this condition. Heavy fat intake along with strong yin in the form of sugar, alcohol, or other expansive foods can cause a *regular aneurysm*, while proportionately strong yin, including chocolate, sweets, spices, stimulants, drugs, and chemicals, produces a dissecting aneurysm. To prevent or relieve an aneurysm, follow the guidelines for Diet #3, for conditions arising from dietary extremes.

Angina. Angina pectoris is a form of advanced coronary heart disease accompanied by chronic chest pains that reaches a threshold at certain levels of activity, shortness of breath, pounding of the heart, light perspiration, and feelings of apprehension. When not enough oxygen is available to perform daily activities, an angina attack occurs. Such pain commonly occurs after eating a large meal and may lead to a heart attack. Modern medicine prescribes nitroglycerin, isosorbide, and beta blockers to lower the strain on the heart. Angina can be relieved using the guidelines for coronary heart disease below and observing Diet #2.

Cardiomyopathy. Cardiomyopathy involves the dangerous overexpansion of one of the ventricles or the heart cavity as a whole. It leads to shortness of breath, chest pain, irregular heartbeat, development of thrombi and emboli, and ultimately death. This degenerative condition is considered irreversible and is the leading cause of heart transplants. Almost unknown until recently, it is now appearing frequently, especially in young people. *Congestive cardiomyopathy* produces swelling and stretching of the entire heart as fibrous tissue replaces normal muscle cells; the ventricles weaken, and congestive heart failure results. *Hypertrophic cardiomyopathy* involves the progressive enlargement of the ventricular muscle itself, most commonly the left, but sometimes the right. Teenagers and young adults are more likely to have this type. Combinations of extreme yin and yang foods, especially meat, oily and greasy food, and salty foods, combined with sugar, chocolate, sweets, stimulants, and alcohol, may cause these conditions. Hypertrophic cardiomyopathy is more yin than the congestive type. Pizza, french fries, candy bars, and other highly processed fast foods should especially be avoided. The progressive degeneration of the heart and its muscles can be arrested, controlled, and in some cases reversed by observing a centrally balanced way of eating. Observe Diet #3, for conditions

arising from a combination of dietary extremes. Focus on whole grains as the center of each meal. MISO SOUP should be taken daily, along with hard green leafy vegetables and other articles in the standard macrobiotic diet, including moderate use of salt in cooking. A small volume of sesame or other good-quality vegetable oil may be used occasionally for SAUTÉED VEGETABLES, but refined oil and raw oil should be avoided. Consumption of bread and other baked flour products, fruits, and juices should be avoided or minimized for several months. The special dishes listed under heart failure below may also be taken in case of extreme fatigue, weakness, or loss of vitality.

Congenital Defects. Congenital heart disease produces defects or abnormalities in the heart at birth. It includes *ventricular septal defect*, or incomplete fusion in the tissues that divide the lower chambers of the heart; *atrial septal defect*, incomplete fusion in the upper chambers; *patent ductus arteriosus*, irregularities in the tissues connecting the aorta and pulmonary artery; *coarctation of the aorta*, a severe narrowing of the major blood vessel leading away from the heart; *valve stenosis* and *atresia*, or abnormal narrowing or closing of the valves; and *endocardial fibroelastosis*, or thickening of the inner lining of the heart. Congenital defects occur primarily because of dietary imbalances and nutritional deficiencies in the mother's way of eating during pregnancy, especially lack of complex carbohydrates, fiber, and minerals that produce a strong contractive effect, flexibility, and elasticity to the heart and blood vessels. The consumption of extreme yin foods and beverages, including sugar, too much fruit and juice, soft drinks, drugs, medications, alcohol, and other more expansive items are frequently involved.

As noted above, the hand corresponds to the heart. A baby's hand grasp is normally strong and tight, correlating with the strength and contractive power of the heart. If the mother has been taking too many yin foods during pregnancy, her baby's grasp will be weak. Surgery is necessary for immediate life-threatening cases. However, many congenital defects can be corrected through proper diet in infancy and childhood. Parents are sometimes told that their child will need elective surgery to correct serious heart problems in later childhood. Often these are unnecessary if the diet and way of life are corrected in time, though medical supervision is still strongly advised to monitor the child's development. The standard macrobiotic way of eating will help control, improve, or restore normal heart functions and overall balance. Follow the guidelines for Diet #1. Whole cereal grains as the foundation of the child's diet are essential, along with other good-quality contractive foods, including hard, fibrous leafy greens, sea vegetables, and mineral-rich condiments and seasonings. Expansive foods such as fruits, juices, raw foods, fats and oils, fluids, and others should be limited for a time until the condition improves. Breastfeeding mothers with babies with heart defects may take KOI-KOKU, KINPIRA SOUP, MOCHI, or AMASAKE to strengthening nursing and offset weakness.

Coronary Disease and Heart Attack. The buildup of atherosclerotic plaque in the coronary arteries can obstruct blood flow and oxygen supply to the heart. Generally the obstruction that causes a *myocardial infarction*, or heart attack, is partial, only about 50 to 70 percent. A heart attack may also arise when a *thrombus*, or blood clot, forms over the plaque, closing off the flow of blood. The long-term intake of strong yang animal foods, including meat, eggs, poultry, dairy food, and fatty fish and seafood, are principal causes, while sugar, chocolate, and other refined sweets, excessive fruit and fruit juices, tropical foods, stimulants, alcohol, spices, and drugs are enhancing factors. Coronary heart disease is commonly treated with bypass surgery, in which a vein from the leg or arm is attached to the aorta to bypass the obstruction. But plaque or blood clots return within 6 months in about 20 to 30 percent of cases. To help prevent or relieve a heart attack, follow the dietary guidelines for Diet #2. Special dishes to help relieve the development of coronary disease include MISO SOUP daily, STEAMED LEAFY GREENS daily, DRIED DAIKON WITH KOMBU often, and a small volume of grated daikon with shoyu eaten occasionally (for a 3-week period) to help discharge accumulations of fat and cholesterol.

Heart Failure. Heart failure is a general term referring to any weakening of the left or right ventricle that impedes pumping. It may result from high blood pressure, atherosclerosis, heart attack, stroke, or other cardiovascular disorder. When fluid accumulates in the pumping chamber, it is known *as congestive heart failure. Left heart failure,* the most common type, affects the left ventricle and arises from high blood pressure or hardening of the arteries. Blood congests the lungs, breathing shortens, and panting and gasping may result. *Right heart failure* (a more yin form) usually arises from lung diseases and complications, valve problems, or congestion in peripheral blood vessels. Right ventricle weakness causes the blood to back up in the veins, the leaking of fluid into surrounding tissues and cells, and progressive swelling of the abdomen and lower extremities. Depending on its severity, heart failure may be mild, serious, or potentially life threatening. Because it may arise from many conditions, there is no single diet for heart failure, though a more centrally balanced macrobiotic way of eating may be safely followed in most cases. Special dishes to strengthen the heart include KOI-KOKU, KINPIRA SOUP, FRIED BROWN RICE, RAN-SHO taken for no more than 3 days, or EGG OIL taken in small volume for a few days.

Rheumatic, Pulmonary, and Infectious Heart Disease. Infectious forms of heart disease were prevalent in America and other modern societies in the first half of the twentieth century. Though now eclipsed by coronary heart disease and stroke, infectious heart disease is widespread in the developing world. *Rheumatic fever,* a childhood affliction associated with a streptococcal throat infection, can result in mitral stenosis and other valve deformities, leading to possible heart failure. Another form is *rheumatic carditis,* which develops when the endocardium covering the heart values becomes inflamed. In this case, the heart valves may also become deformed, leading to disability or death. Penicillin and other antibiotics are used to treat these disorders, but new drug-resistant strains of microorganisms may be immune to this form of treatment.

Rheumatic heart problems generally arise from the intake of extreme foods in both the yin and yang categories, especially eggs and foods containing eggs in which the streptococcal microbes thrive. The overconsumption of other animal foods, sugar, chocolate, tropical foods, soft drinks (especially cold beverages), and other imbalanced foods also contribute to susceptibility to infection. Rheumatic fever may be relieved with a balanced macrobiotic diet, including MISO SOUP with brown rice or barley cooked in it. Follow the guidelines for Diet #3. All animal food, including fish and seafood, as well as salads and raw food and fruits and juices should be discontinued until the condition improves. Rheumatic carditis requires medical attention in acute cases. Less serious cases can also be improved with diet, as well as the application of a CARP PLASTER externally to bring down the high fever.

Pulmonary heart disease, known as *chronic cor pulmonale,* may result from several lung problems and usually leads to pulmonary hypertension, a dangerous elevation of blood pressure and susceptibility to clots, emboli, or heart failure. This disorder is predominantly caused by excessive yin intake, especially ice cream, milk, butter, cheese, yogurt, and other dairy foods, as well as icy beverages, sugar, chocolate, sweets, tropical foods, fruits, juices, and other cold, expansive substances. Follow a slightly more yang way of eating as described in Diet #1. Special dishes include NISHIME-STYLE VEGETABLES such as carrots, carrot tops, lotus root, and kombu cooked together; a small, regular volume of KINPIRA-STYLE BURDOCK or lotus root; regular MISO SOUP; a small volume of kombu condiment; and UME-SHO KUZU twice a day for 3 days. A MUSTARD PLASTER may be applied to the front of the chest once a day for several days to bring down the fever. Light breathing exercises may also be helpful.

Other infectious heart conditions include *pericarditis*, where the outer protective layer of the heart becomes inflamed or infected; *myocarditis,* in which the muscle of the heart is infected; and *infectious endocarditis*, in which the surface lining of the heart loosens. Extremes of yin and yang create infectious conditions such as these, especially dairy food in combination with fatty, oily food, soft drinks, alcohol, and other overly expansive items. Besides discontinuing these items, all baked flour products need to be avoided to prevent the production of mucus. Observe Diet #3. Helpful side dishes include steamed DAIKON AND DAIKON LEAVES with a slight shoyu or miso taste; dried daikon cooked with carrots and kombu with moderate seasoning; and UME-SHO KUZU once or twice a day for 3 days. Applying a LEAFY GREENS COMPRESS to the chest may cool down the fever and ease breathing. Acute cases of infectious endocarditis are life-threatening and immediate medical treatment is advised.

Stroke. Impeded blood flow to the brain can produce a stroke or *cerebral vascular disease.* Strokes range from mild to severe or fatal and often result in speech loss, motor function loss, or paralysis. The principal type of stroke is a *cerebral thrombosis*, which is similar to a heart attack. Atherosclerotic plaque builds up in the arteries leading to the head, narrowing, hardening, and finally cutting off the supply of oxygen to the brain. The next most common type is a *cerebral hemorrhage*, which results when an artery ruptures and blood discharges into the tissue or surface of the brain. This more yin type of stroke is especially common among black people in the South or others eating a diet high in pork or other animal fat, oily and greasy foods, herbs and spices, and sugar. Overall, compared to coronary heart disease, strokes are slightly more yin. Excessive yin in the form of sugar, chocolate, sweets, milk, ice cream, tropical foods, fruits and juices, soft drinks, alcohol, and drugs or medications are commonly consumed, along with strong animal-quality food. For the more yin type of stroke, follow the guidelines for Diet #1 and for the type arising from a combination of dietary extremes observe Diet #3. Emphasize slightly more yang factors, especially sea vegetables, unrefined vegetable oil in small volume, NISHIME-STYLE VEGETABLES cooked often (including daikon, carrots, and kombu cooked together), and GENUINE BROWN RICE CREAM with umeboshi plum. Condiments such as TEKKA, UMEBOSHI PLUMS, and SHIO-KOMBU are also helpful. To bring down the high fever that often accompanies stroke, apply a TOFU PLASTER repeatedly to the head over the region affected. Proper rest and avoidance of strenuous activity and even exercise temporarily are advised. A foot massage is helpful for a stroke, especially the first toe. This will help bring the energy down, promote circulation, and increase body warmth.

Thrombosis and Embolism. A *thrombus*, or blood clot, may obstruct a blood vessel, impeding blood flow and causing other complications. When a clot breaks off and becomes lodged in another, usually smaller vessel, it is called an *embolus*. This is a serious, potentially life-threatening condition. Excruciating pain, cold, numbness, and localized paralysis may result from thrombi or emboli. Anticoagulant drugs or surgery is the standard medical treatment. Both conditions are associated with the atherosclerotic process and result from longtime consumption of extreme yang and yin foods, usually in combination. Excessive intake of poor-quality salt is often a factor. Follow the guidelines for Diet #3 to help relieve this condition. In addition, 1 tablespoon of GRATED DAIKON WITH SHOYU may be taken daily for several days. A small side dish of daikon, daikon greens, and kombu cooked together with a light shoyu or miso taste is also helpful. A HOT TOWEL COMPRESS and a COLD TOWEL COMPRESS may be applied alternately on the area affected.

Valve Disorders. The four valves of the heart may become infected, inflamed, or fail to perform properly. In this case, the blood may back up or leak, leading to heart murmurs and congestive heart failure. Major forms of value diseases include *aortic regurgitation*, in which the left ventricle ejects up to half the blood during the diastolic, or filling, phase of the pumping cycle; *aortic stenosis*, in which the left ventricle labors to pump blood through a narrowed aortic value; *mitral regurgitation*, in which blood leaks back from the left ventricle to the left atrium; and *mitral stenosis*, in which the blood coming in the left ventricle is impeded by a narrowed valve. Valve disorders usually develop in pregnancy or infancy from lack of proper complex carbohydrates and minerals in the diet and corresponding overintake of excessive yin. This includes sugar, chocolate, and other sweets, fruit, juices, tropical foods, chemicalized and artificial foods, and drugs and medications that cause lack of contracting power, resulting in looseness of the valves or narrowing from scar tissue or calcified deposits

arising from fever or infection. Congenital valve problems may be controlled to some extent, if not entirely reversed, with a standard way of eating, emphasizing a slightly more yang diet. Follow the guidelines for Diet #1. SAUTÉED VEGETABLES, especially cabbages, onions, and carrots, may be taken frequently. A small dish of HIJIKI or ARAME cooked with a little oil and shoyu taste may also be helpful. MISO SOUP should be taken regularly and will help restore balance to the affected areas.

Vein Disorders. Blood vessels that carry returning blood to the heart and lungs are called veins. They are thinner, more flexible, and transport blood under less pressure than arteries, which carry blood away from the heart. Still, veins are liable to inflammation, swelling, or obstruction by a blood clot or embolus. *Varicose veins*, in which the surface veins of the legs swell, affect a majority of adult women in modern society and about 25 percent of men. Though primarily cosmetic, they may contribute to fatigue, tiredness, and an overall feeling of heaviness. In traditional societies, where the modern diet has not been widely adopted, varicosity in both sexes is virtually nonexistent. Varicose veins are not caused by pressure on the legs or feet, prolonged standing, or other external factors. This condition arises from the intake of extreme yin and yang foods and beverages, especially heavy meat, poultry, dairy, and eggs, in combination with oil, flour, sugar, sweets, and other more expansive items. The blood becomes stuck from stagnating yang energy and excess yin makes the veins expand. Varicose veins can be relieved by following Diet #3, including regular consumption of MISO SOUP, a small side dish of ADZUKI BEANS regularly, frequent consumption of nishime-style root vegetables such as daikon, carrots, and lotus root, cooked together with kombu; and SAUTÉED VEGETABLES or FRIED BROWN RICE two to three times a week. As a special drink, combine 3 parts dried shredded daikon and 1 part shiitake mushroom, and add 5 times as much water. Cook for about 25 minutes and take 1–2 cups every day for 2 weeks.

Externally, a HOT TOWEL COMPRESS may be applied over the affected area for 5 minutes, followed by a COLD TOWEL COMPRESS. Repeat a second time, alternating hot and cold towels. Do this twice a day for several days until the condition improves. This will also help with *spider veins.*

Another vein problem is *phlebitis,* which occurs when a blood clot lodges in a vein and obstructs the blood flow to the heart. Most commonly, phlebitis develops in the legs and is treated primarily with anticoagulant drugs. If a part of the clot breaks off inside a vein, it can travel to the lungs. In the United States every year, 50,000 people die from a pulmonary embolism arising from this condition. Improper diet is the underlying cause of phlebitis, including potatoes, tomatoes, and other tropical foods (consumed in a temperate climate), refined salt, and meat, poultry, eggs, and other animal foods. Observing centrally balanced Diet #3 will help relieve this disorder, including MISO SOUP regularly, dried daikon cooked with carrots, lotus root, and kombu, and hard green leafy vegetables steamed or water-sautéed. Alternating HOT TOWEL COMPRESS and COLD TOWEL COMPRESS as noted above may also be useful.

SOLUTION

DIET

Besides the dietary advice for specific heart conditions listed above, the following guidelines may be observed to strengthen the heart and prevent the development of cardiovascular disease:

1. Center the diet on whole grains and consume whole grains primarily in whole form. This gives the strongest, most balanced energy, contributes to proper development of the heart and circulatory system, and creates strong sperm, eggs, and genetic material to be passed on to future generations.

2. Among whole grains, whole corn especially nourishes the heart and its physical and psychological functions. Good-quality corn (open-pollinated or heirloom variety, organically grown as much as possible, and non-genetically-engineered) may be taken frequently throughout the year in the form of fresh corn on the cob, dried corn, *masa* (whole corn dough) used to make tortillas, *arepas,* and other corn dishes, and popcorn (without poor-quality salt or oil). A minor portion may be consumed in the form of corn products such as grits, cornmeal, and corn flour.

3. The heart is nourished by foods with a slightly bitter taste. Watercress, mustard greens, dandelion greens, turnip greens, and burdock stimulate the heart and circulatory system. GOMASHIO (roasted sesame salt) and lightly roasted sesame seeds are helpful to restore flexibility to hardened arteries and vessels. Note that digitalis, a drug often prescribed for heart patients, has a bitter taste.

4. Round vegetables, especially those with a heart shape, are beneficial. These include autumn and winter squashes, onions, rutabagas, turnips, and radishes.

5. Use unrefined vegetable-quality oils in cooking to prepare sautéed vegetables, stir-fries, tempura, and other dishes. Organic corn oil may be used as a major supplemental oil to sesame oil, though it is very difficult to find at the present time. Good-quality plant oils will contribute to the elasticity of the heart and blood vessels, but too much oil of any kind may be detrimental.

6. Beans and bean products, especially soy products such as tofu, tempeh, and natto, lower cholesterol in the blood and are associated with increased cardiovascular health in many scientific and medical studies.

7. Eat sea vegetables regularly in small volume. Not only do these supply good-quality minerals, but edible seaweeds also contribute to maintaining the natural flexibility of the arteries, veins, and other blood vessels. Hardened, narrowed arteries can be reversed with a diet that includes these dynamic foods from the sea.

8. Reduce animal-quality foods and avoid or minimize dairy food. These particularly affect the heart and blood vessels, beginning in infancy, even among vegetarians eating just low-fat milk, ice cream, yogurt, and cheese.

9. Avoid simple sugars (refined sugar, honey, and chocolate), which can expand the heart and weaken the blood vessels.

10. If you are living in a temperate climate, minimize vegetables that originated in tropical regions, such as potato, tomato, and eggplant.

11. The amount of salt (miso, shoyu, and sea salt) should be moderate, neither too much nor too little. Modern table salt, consisting of 99.99 percent sodium, is associated in many studies with high blood pressure. Harvard scientists reported that blood pressure did not rise with increased consumption of sea salt (lower in sodium and higher in trace minerals) among individuals following a macrobiotic diet.

12. A small amount of beer, sake, or other alcoholic beverages may be taken infrequently, if desired. These are not essential for the health of the heart or circulatory system, or good health in general, but contribute to enjoyment, relaxation, and sociability. Moderate consumption of wine and other alcoholic drinks is often recommended to help prevent heart disease, because medical studies show that the French, who customarily drink wine with each meal, have lower rates of heart disease than nondrinkers. Wine, in this case, serves to keep the blood vessels open and less susceptible to clotting caused by heavy animal food consumption. Wine, however, may contribute to the development of stroke or other afflictions.

13. Eat less total volume of food, and chew more. Avoid late-night snacks.

LIFESTYLE

1. The heart is situated near the heart chakra, the energy center that governs the emotions. Emotional stability and balance are integral to the proper functioning of the heart and circulatory system. Emotional shock, trauma, or heavy stress can trigger a coronary spasm that can cause the arteries to compress, resulting in damage and, in extreme cases, even sudden cardiac death. Hardening of the arteries or other degenerative condition need not be present for this to occur. Cultivating gentleness, tranquility, intuitive comprehension, spiritual oneness, and a merry, humorous expression will strengthen the heart.

2. Maintain a balance between physical and mental activity. Get proper rest and a good night's sleep.

3. Moderate exercise is beneficial to the heart, especially walking about a half hour every day. Avoid isometric exercises, in which static, tension-producing movements are emphasized. These can raise blood pressure, produce irregular heartbeat, and diminish pumping capacity. Heart attacks often occur during snow shoveling or other isometric activity. *Aerobic* activities in which the body moves comprehensively, including dancing, yoga, martial arts, gardening, and cleaning, are preferred.

4. Listening to peaceful, harmonious music or playing an instrument can stimulate the heart and cardiovascular system. Gregorian chants, shakuhachi music, and Mozart are especially beneficial. Singing a happy song each day will also nourish the heart and lungs and raise your spirits.

5. Reading aloud or reciting poetry every day will strengthen the heart, expand the lungs, and promote better circulation. All types of literature are recommended, including scripture, myths, epics, short stories, and novels. Plays from Elizabethan England, written in iambic pentameter, almost perfectly mirror the natural cadence of the heartbeat. Because of their form as well as their content, the dramatic works of Marlowe and Shakespeare find universal resonance around the world, even in traditional cultures with no knowledge of English.

6. Keep green plants in your home. These will supply oxygen and contribute to better respiratory and circulatory functions.

7. Simplify your life, embrace all joys and sorrows, and regard everyone as your brother and sister on the infinite journey of life.

HOME REMEDIES

1. To strengthen the heart or for most heart problems, prepare the special HEART DRINK. To stimulate the heartbeat and blood circulation, especially in the event of a heart attack or stroke, prepare RAN-SHO. Drink slowly. Use only once a day and for no more than 3 days. Do not use for easing overly yang conditions, such as atherosclerosis or high blood pressure.

2. In other cases when the heart is seriously weakened, EGG OIL may be taken to strengthen the heart and circulatory functions. Take in small quantities for 2 to 3 days.

3. To help discharge accumulations of saturated fat and cholesterol from the body, take a cup of CARROT-DAIKON DRINK once a day for 5 days; after that, 2 to 3 times a week for another 1 month.

4. SHIITAKE TEA can relax an overly tense, stressful condition and dissolve animal fats that have accumulated in the body. Drink ½ cup at a time, 2 to 3 times a week.

5. For congestive heart failure and other weakened conditions, KINPIRA SOUP may be taken 2 to 3 times a week for strength and vitality.

6. SHIATSU, DO-IN, PALM HEALING, BREATHING EXERCISES, STRETCHING EXERCISES, ACUPUNCTURE, YOGA, or MEDITATION may be used at the same time to strengthen heart and circulatory functions.

7. Simplify your living conditions and human relations as a whole.

CAUTION

1. In the event of surgery, drug therapy, hormonal therapy, or other medical intervention, the macrobiotic dietary guidelines may need further modification to balance the effects of the treatment as well as the underlying heart condition.

2. If you have some illness or are on prescription medicine, you may wish to seek the advice of specialists, including your doctor, in addition to trying to practice the above recommendations.

MEDICAL EVIDENCE

MACROBIOTIC DIET PROTECTS AGAINST ELEVATED CHOLESTEROL AND HIGH BLOOD PRESSURE

In a pioneering study, researchers at Harvard Medical School reported that people living in the Boston area who ate a macrobiotic diet of whole grains, beans, fresh vegetables, sea vegetables, and fermented soy products had significantly lower levels of cholesterol and triglycerides and lower blood pressure than people eating the standard American diet of meat, sugar, dairy foods, and highly processed, chemicalized foods.

The macrobiotic group had average serum cholesterol levels of 126 mg/dL versus 184 for subjects enrolled in the Framingham Heart Study. Cholesterol and fat levels rose significantly when dairy foods and eggs were added to the macrobiotic diet. "The low plasma lipid levels in the vegetarians," the researchers concluded, "resemble those reported for populations in nonindustrialized societies," where heart disease, cancer, and other degenerative illnesses are uncommon.

Source: F. M. Sacks et al., "Plasma Lipids and Lipoproteins in Vegetarians and Controls," *New England Journal of Medicine* 292:1148–51, 1975.

ANIMAL FOOD CONSUMPTION RAISES BLOOD PRESSURE

In another pioneering dietary study on the Boston macrobiotic community, scientists reported the first direct evidence that animal food raised blood pressure. In a study of 21 people eating primarily whole grains and vegetables, Harvard Medical School researchers found that the addition of 250 grams of beef per day for four weeks to their diet raised cholesterol levels 19 percent. Systolic blood pressure also rose significantly. Cholesterol and blood pressure values returned to previous levels after the beef was discontinued.

Source: F. M. Sacks et al., "Effects of Ingestion of Meat on Plasma Cholesterol of Vegetarians," *Journal of the American Medical Association* 246:640–44, 1981.

MACROBIOTIC PRACTITIONERS HAVE HEALTHIER HEARTS THAN TRAINED ATHLETES

Dr. William Castelli, director of the Framingham Heart Study, the nation's oldest and largest cardiovascular research project, and a participant in research on macrobiotic diet at Harvard Medical School, noted that vegetarians and those eating a macrobiotic diet have healthier hearts and circulatory systems than conditioned athletes: "What a person eats every day is a very important aspect of how his or her health will be in every day as well as later life. Supporting this view is the fact that macrobiotic people studied had a ratio [of HDL to total cholesterol] of 2.5 and Boston marathon runners were at 3.4, ratios at which rarely, if ever, is coronary heart disease seen. Studies and observations such as these are a clear indicator that people need to take a critical look at their diet with the intention of making changes now."

Source: William P. Castelli, "Summary of Lessons from the Framingham Heart Study," Framingham, Mass., September 1983.

Patients suffering from angina pectoris, a form of coronary heart disease, experienced significantly improved blood pressure values and lowered coronary risk factors after ten weeks on a macrobiotic diet, according to researchers at Columbia-Presbyterian Hospital in New York City. Cholesterol levels declined from an average 300 to 220 mg/dL, levels of blood pressure also dropped, patients could walk about 20 percent farther in stress tests, and three patients with severe angina showed no symptoms at the end of the study. The participants, mostly businessmen and their wives, learned how to cook and ate together at the Natural Gourmet Cookery School under the direction of macrobiotic and natural foods cook Annemarie Colbin. In this study, funded and monitored by the New York Cardiac Center, the lead researcher reported that there was "tremendous enthusiasm and adherence" to the new way of eating.

Source: Michio Kushi and Alex Jack, *Diet for a Strong Heart* (New York: St. Martin's Press, 1985), p. 131.

MISO SOUP PROTECTS AGAINST HEART DISEASE

Miso soup, a daily staple in the macrobiotic way of eating, can help prevent heart disease. In a 13-year study involving about 265,000 men and women over 40, Japan's National Cancer Center reported that people who never ate miso soup daily had a 43 percent higher death rate from coronary heart disease than those who consumed miso soup daily. Those who abstained from miso also had 29 percent more fatal strokes, three and a half times more deaths resulting from high blood pressure, and higher mortality from all other causes.

Source: T. Hirayama, "Relationship of Soybean Paste Soup Intake to Gastric Cancer Risk," *Nutrition and Cancer* 3:223–33, 1981.

TEENAGERS AND YOUNG ADULTS AT RISK FOR HEART ATTACK

Many American teenagers and young adults have clogged arteries and are at risk for heart attack. In a study conducted by the American Heart Association journal *Circulation*, researchers examined the coronary arteries of 760 males who had died as a result of accident, homicide, or suicide. Two percent of those between the ages of 15 and 19 and 20 percent of those 30 to 34 years of age had advanced plaque in their arteries. Girls from 15 to 19 did not have plaque, but 8 percent of young women in their early thirties did have signs of advanced heart disease.

Source: "Clogged Arteries Found in Many U.S. Teenagers," Reuters, July 25, 2000.

HIGH HOMOCYSTEINE LEVELS LINKED TO CARDIOVASCULAR DISEASE

High levels of homocysteine, a substance in blood, may be an important factor in the development of cardiovascular disease and other ills. High levels of homocysteine result from eating a diet high in animal protein. Animal protein is rich in methionine, an amino acid that is the source of the principal compound found in homocysteine. Researchers for the Physicians' Health Study found that those with a level of 15 micromoles or higher had a heart attack rate three times higher than those with lower levels in the course of five years. Dr. William Castelli, former director of the Framingham Heart Study, said that levels above 9 micromoles are elevated and place people at risk for heart attack or stroke. Homocysteine can damage the walls of arteries and lead to blockages, causing cholesterol buildup and obstruction of vessels. In addition to meat and dairy consumption, homocysteine levels are increased by diets low in B vitamins, smoking, consumption of unfiltered coffee, low thyroid levels, estrogen deficiency, organ transplants, and chronic kidney failure. In addition to heart attack, stroke, and blood clots in the veins, high homocysteine levels are associated with dementia in Alzheimer's disease, recurrent miscarriage, birth defects, premature delivery, very low birth weight, osteoporosis, and presbyopia or aging eyes.

Source: Jane E. Brody, "Health Sleuths Assess Homocysteine as Culprit," *New York Times*, June 13, 2000.

CASE HISTORIES

AIRCRAFT ENGINEER RECOVERS FROM HEART ATTACK WITH MACROBIOTIC DIET

Jack Saunders, an aircraft engineer and designer at the General Electric plant in Lynn, Massachusetts, was diagnosed in a routine company medical examination as having suffered from a "silent heart attack." Though he did not experience symptoms, permanent damage to the heart can result or be followed by more serious attacks in the future. Saunders began macrobiotics, and his cardiovascular condition quickly improved. EKG tests and other heart evalua-

tions showed no sign of further problems. "On my previous diet, I was not able to deal as well with people or to reconcile various differences between people. Macrobiotics has not only changed my physical health," he reported, "it has changed my entire life."

Source: Jack Saunders, "Case History," in Michio Kushi, *Cancer and Heart Disease* (Tokyo: Japan Publications, 1982).

EX-MARINE REDUCES BLOOD PRESSURE FOLLOWING DIETARY CHANGE

After twenty-six years in the Marine Corps, Fletcher Sojourner retired and found work as a hospital administrator. At an employee clinic, doctors told him his blood pressure was an elevated 145/114 and put him on medication. Meanwhile, his wife started macrobiotics, and he also began to change his diet. Within three months, he lost forty-five pounds and his weight stabilized at 170 pounds. After six weeks, he stopped taking all drugs, and doctors found that his blood pressure dropped to an ideal 122/72. "My energy level has increased immeasurably," he reported. "My stamina is phenomenal. Friends are very inquisitive. They see me running at lunch hour and wonder why they can't do the same thing. But they can't give up their meat or martinis."

Source: Michio Kushi and Alex Jack, *Diet for a Strong Heart* (New York: St. Martin's Press, 1985), p. 319.

WAITRESS ELIMINATES VARICOSE VEINS ON MACROBIOTIC REGIMEN

Patricia Goodwin had a tendency toward rheumatoid arthritis and suffered from a variety of aches and pains. She also had varicose veins that were tender, swollen, and throbbing.

Sometimes the pain was so sharp she could hardly walk. After beginning a new job as a waitress in a macrobiotic restaurant in Boston, Patricia noticed that her arthritic condition began to improve. The varicose veins quickly disappeared. When she became pregnant a few years later, she feared that the varicosity might return, but she had a smooth, trouble-free delivery. She has been healthy and energetic ever since.

Source: Patricia M. Goodwin, "Case History," in *Macrobiotic Case Histories*, No. 5 (Boston: East West Foundation), 1978.

MACROBIOTICS HELPS BABY WITH CONGENITAL HEART DEFECT AVOID SURGERY

Jessica Brown was born with atrial septal defect, a congenital heart condition characterized by a small hole between the upper chambers of her heart. Doctors told her parents that she would have to have open-heart surgery before she was five to close the hole. Meanwhile, Debby Brown, her mother, started macrobiotics and met with Michio Kushi for a consultation. "Michio told us to especially avoid fruits," she recalled. "He said that in two years, the murmur

TABLE 25. HEART AND CIRCULATORY CONDITIONS AND DISEASES

1. More Yin Cause	2. More Yang Cause	3. Yin and Yang Combined
Cushing's syndrome	Systolic hypertension	Diastolic hypertension
	Eclampsia	Renal hypertension
Low blood pressure (some)	Low blood pressure (some)	
	Coronary heart disease	Arteriosclerosis
Fibrillation	Heart attack (myocardial infarction)	Atherosclerosis
	Angina pectoris	Prinzmetal angina
Stroke (cerebral hemorrhage and some cerebral thrombosis)		Stroke (some cerebral thrombosis)
Heart failure (some)	Heart failure (some)	Heart failure (some)
Tachycardia	Bradycardia	Irregular heartbeat
Pulmonary heart disease		Rheumatic heart disease
Valve disorders		Infectious heart disease
		Arteriosclerosis obliterans
Raynaud's phenomenon	Buerger's disease	Acute thrombosis or embolism
		Aneurysm
		Varicose veins
		Phlebitis
Congenital heart defects		Cardiomyopathy

resulting from the congenital defect would be gone. He said there was nothing to worry about so long as we all ate well." When their little girl was four, the Browns took her back to the physician who made the original diagnosis. He could find no signs of any heart problems and pronounced her in perfect health. The hole had closed up naturally without the need of potentially life-threatening surgery. As an afterword to this heartwarming story, Jessica's grandmother, Virginia, a nurse, was diagnosed with malignant melanoma, Stage IV. As a result of Jessica's improvement, Virginia went on a macrobiotic diet and completely recovered from what her doctors told her was a terminal condition.

Source: Michio Kushi with Alex Jack, *Diet for a Strong Heart* (New York: St. Martin's Press, 1985), pp. 330–31.

◎ INFECTIOUS DISEASE

Infectious diseases, such as tuberculosis, malaria, and cholera, which killed millions of people in recent centuries, were believed to have been largely eradicated with the spread of penicillin, streptomycin, and other miracle drugs in the mid-20th century. However, in recent years, new multiple-drug-resistant strains of many bacterial and viral diseases have emerged. Infectious diseases have now reached epidemic proportions in many affluent countries and are still widespread in the developing world. Also following the anthrax attacks on the United States, public health officials are concerned that this extremely lethal bacterial disease, as well as smallpox and other viral infections, may be released by bioterrorists in the future. *See also*

"AIDS," "Pneumonia" in "Lung Problems," and "Mad Cow Disease."

SYMPTOMS

Modern medicine diagnoses infection by blood tests that show the presence of antibodies to the virus or bacteria in the body. But many people do not symptomatize for long periods, and many others are simply carriers, spreading disease organisms to others without knowing it. The tendency toward infectious disease is shown by the following:

1. Fatigue, lack of energy and vitality
2. Colds, infection, light fever
3. Skin rashes or allergies, a milky skin texture, or skin that easily ruptures
4. Intestinal disorders, including gas formation, constipation, and frequent diarrhea
5. Nausea, especially after eating or drinking
6. Irregular appetite, including extreme appetite, frequent change of food preferences, or no or little appetite
7. Night perspiration, including light fever and shivering
8. Liver inflammation or infection
9. Swelling of lymph glands, especially in the groin, armpit, neck, and chest area
10. Red or purple face
11. Slow body movement and weak coordination
12. Dulled mental focus and concentration

CAUSE

1. Bacteria, viruses, and other microorganisms are an integral part of life on our planet.

They are instrumental in creating fertile soil and in helping to digest foods in the human intestines. Every person has trillions of microorganisms (about 4 pounds on average) living on his or her body, including the digestive system, the skin, hair, glands, and other areas. These are predominantly benign, living in symbiosis, and performing many beneficial functions. A healthy person enjoys natural resistance to disease, including the ability to harmonize or neutralize undesirable viruses and bacteria by producing antibodies. However, if we become out of balance with nature, especially through improper eating, potentially harmful microbes may gather and overwhelm our natural capacity to resist disease. Our blood, lymph, and other immune functions may become too weak to protect us from infection.

2. Most epidemics in human history are associated with the spread of infectious diseases from animals to human beings. Hence, smallpox spread from cowpox, pneumonia is linked to avian or swine flu, and AIDS is believed to have evolved from a monkey-borne virus. Because animal food putrefies before it is cooked, eating animal food, especially contaminated or improperly cooked animal food, lies at the root of many epidemics. Recent outbreaks of deadly *E. coli* bacteria are linked to hamburger; consumption of contaminated beef or milk underlies the human form of mad cow disease; and salmonella typically follows eating tainted eggs or egg salad. The rise of drug-resistant microorganisms is directly connected with the spread of antibiotics. These may kill 99.99 percent of the harmful microbes, but they allow the remaining 0.01 percent to evolve into supermicrobes resistant to the drug. The increased use of chemical

pesticides and fertilizers, and genetically altered foods has also contributed to the spread of infectious disorders.

3. Monocropping and other modern agricultural practices that upset the delicate balance of microorganisms in the soil are a major factor in the emergence of new, more virulent strains of microorganisms. In the absence of the usual checks and balances that have developed for thousands and often millions of years, these new strains of microbes have evolved, causing chaos and disorder throughout the ecosystem. Easily transported by jet airplanes or cargo ships to far-distant regions, they enter radically new environments where they may have no natural predators, producing what environmentalists call *bioinvasion*. The appearance of West Nile virus in North America from its homeland in the Middle East is a recent example.

4. The environmental crisis is also a major factor in the spread of infectious disease. In South America, herbicides introduced into the pampas altered the ecology, leading to the creation of a new mouse that was the carrier of a deadly virus that produced Argentine hemorrhagic fever, a new disease. The worldwide decline of songbirds and frogs, to take another example, is leading to the catastrophic increase in mosquitoes, fleas, and other insects that spread viral and bacterial diseases. Global warming, the thinning of the protective ozone layer around the earth, and other environmental changes are believed to be major factors in the decline of biodiversity.

5. In many cases of infection, microbes multiply within the body, especially in the blood, body fluids, the interior of the intestines, and the reproductive organs. However, another mechanism by which infection may develop is through the transformation of normal human body cells into bacteria, viruses, and fragments of DNA. This process, known as *biological degeneration* or *reverse evolution,* is now being investigated by modern medicine for the first time. In other words, in some case of infectious diseases, the harmful microbes are not introduced from outside but are self-caused, the end result of the body's own cells and tissues decomposing into more primitive forms of life, usually as a result of long-term dietary imbalance and a chaotic lifestyle. The process may take place in less developed cells, including blood cells (especially white blood cells) and reproductive follicles.

6. The combination of these dietary, environmental, and way of life factors is the principal cause of infectious disease. Conditions that influence the spread of infectious disease include the following:

a. Infectious diseases arise and spread more often in warmer climates than in colder ones. Tropical and semitropical areas are more affected than northern areas and colder areas. However, recently global warming has raised temperatures around the world and caused infectious diseases to gradually spread to more northern latitudes, for example, the West Nile virus in New York City.

b. Bacteria, viruses, and other microorganisms are more active in the late spring, summer, and early autumn in temperate regions and less active in the late autumn, winter, and early spring.

c. Bacteria and viruses are more active in a humid environment than a dry one and in the rainy season than the dry season.

d. Bacteria and viruses are more likely to spread in large urban populations than in small towns and cities or in rural areas.

e. Poor sanitation, pollution of the water and air, poverty and hunger, social unrest and war, natural disasters, refugee camps and congested population centers, and other adverse social and environmental conditions foster the spread of undesirable microorganisms and epidemic disease.

f. Individuals consuming the following foods or combinations of foods are especially susceptible to infection: foods high in animal protein and fat, including meat, poultry, eggs, fatty fish, and dairy food; foods high in simple sugar such as refined white sugar, chocolate, honey, ice cream, and soft drinks; and frequent consumption of fruit and fruit juice, especially of a tropical and semitropical variety. Those who consume acidic foods, including the above items; white flour and baked goods, including bread, cookies, crackers, doughnuts, bagels, and similar foods; tomatoes, potatoes, and other members of the nightshade family; and oily, greasy food, including fried and deep-fried foods, are also liable to infection. Raw salad, raw oil, and other raw foods should also be avoided.

g. Communities that depend upon transportation of food from a different climatic zone, especially a hotter and more humid region, are more liable to infection.

h. Drug abuse and promiscuous sexual activity are often involved in the spread of infectious disease.

i. In temperate regions, men are more frequently infected than women because they are more easily weakened by simple sugar, fruit, alcohol, and other more yin, acid-producing foods and by drugs. However, in tropical regions, men and women are affected about equally.

j. Bacteria tend to be more yang than viruses because they are denser, have a nucleus, and produce stronger effects.

The possible means of transmitting infectious microorganisms are generally as follows:

1. Breathing contaminated air, drinking contaminated water, or eating contaminated food, as in the case of inhaling airborne microbes associated with tuberculosis, ingesting waterborne microbes that spread cholera, or eating meat that harbors the deadly *E. coli* bacteria.

2. Shaking hands, touching, hugging, and other forms of nonintimate physical contact will usually not transmit infectious diseases. Generally, kissing, while it exchanges bodily fluids, does not transmit microbes, because the yang, alkaline quality of saliva serves to offset the yin, acid condition of the microbes. But an open wound, ulcerated rupture, allergic rash, cancerous tumor, or other inflamed condition may allow transmission to occur at these locations.

3. Blood transfusions, including not only blood donated by people who have used drugs, alcohol, or unsafe sexual practices, but also by those who have eaten an extreme or chaotic diet that has weakened the quality of their blood.

4. Nine thousand Americans die from food poisoning every year. Disease may also be spread from contaminated or stagnant water, especially in rural areas, in hot climates, or in areas of high humidity. Cooking food rather than eating it raw, cooking food at high temperatures in some cases rather than at low temperatures, and adding salt or mineral-rich food in cooking such as sea vegetables (rather than as a condiment at the table) all help to prevent transmission. Drinking or cooking with chlorinated or other chemically treated water, however, may kill beneficial microbes in our body as well as potentially harmful ones, enhancing the likelihood of disease.

5. Sexual intercourse, as in the case of many sexually transmitted diseases and AIDS, including vaginal, oral, and anal sex.

6. The use of needles for intravenous drug use.

7. Iatrogenic or doctor-caused disease is one of the leading causes of death in modern society. Modern hospitals and clinics are a breeding zone for harmful viruses and bacteria. One in 20 patients in the United States acquires an infection in the hospital, including 1 in 7 intensive-care patients. One-third of all pneumonia in America is contracted in the hospital, and one-third of these cases are fatal. The use of invasive medical procedures or unsterilized medical instruments, including surgical implements, dental treatment, abortion, chemotherapy, and acupuncture needles, may spread disease directly or weaken the patient and make him or her more susceptible to infection. Organ transplants, especially xenotransplants—the transfer of organs between humans and other species—are one of the most dangerous procedures and carry a high risk of infection.

8. Embryonic transmission through the mother's umbilical cord or fluids in the uterus during pregnancy, as a direct result of her chaotic and unhealthy eating, drug or alcohol abuse, overmedication, or other factors enhancing susceptibility to disease.

9. Transmission by insects, such as mosquitoes that carry the organisms associated with malaria, yellow fever, and other diseases. Mosquitoes are commonly attracted to the blood of people eating sugar, fruit, and other sweet-tasting foods and beverages.

10. Modern technology, including air-conditioning, airplane and cruise ship ventilation, and supermarket food misters, have been associated with transmitting Legionnaire's disease, pneumonia, flu, and other infectious conditions.

FORMS

Anthrax. Following the terrorist attacks on the United States on September 11, 2001, anthrax was released through the mails and five persons died. Anthrax was traditionally known as "wool gatherer's disease" because it primarily infected people who worked with ruminants, wool, or animal hides. As a bioweapon, anthrax is highly refined and processed into a powder that releases tiny spores that penetrate deeply into the lungs, where they become activated on contact with fluid. Extremely stable, the anthrax spores remain resistant to sunlight, heat, and many disinfectants and can survive in a dormant state for decades and possibly centuries.

Cutaneous anthrax, the most common type,

occurs following skin contact with contaminated meat, wool, hides, or leather from infected animals. The incubation period is from 1 to 12 days. The skin infection begins as a small papule and progresses to a vesicle in 1–2 days, followed by a black necrotic ulcer. The lesion is usually painless, but patients may also have fever, malaise, headache, and regional swelling in the lymph glands. *Inhalation anthrax* produces symptoms similar initially to the flu or common cold, but then breathing problems, hemorrhage, edema, and shock may develop, followed by death. Research suggests that from 4,000 to 5,000 spores need to be present to cause an infection, but authorities suspect that far fewer may be involved in some of the fatal terrorist cases in the United States. The incubation period ranges from 1 to 7 days and up to 60 days. Cutaneous anthrax is less dangerous than the inhalation variety, though fewer spores are required to induce illness. The third form, *gastrointestinal anthrax,* usually follows the consumption of raw or undercooked contaminated meat and has an incubation period of 1–7 days.

Anthrax does not spread from person to person. Early treatment of cutaneous anthrax with antibiotics is extremely effective, with a success rate of 99 percent. Without antibiotics, the mortality rate is about 20 percent. The death rate for inhaled anthrax is about 75 percent, even following antibiotic treatment. While Cipro, the principal antibiotic used to prevent infection, is often effective, it may produce severe side effects, result in antibiotic resistance, and lead to weakness and susceptibility to other infections and disorders in the future. Some postal workers exposed to anthrax stopped taking antibiotics because of their debilitating effects. Similarly, the anthrax vaccine is linked to severe reactions, especially among U.S. military personnel during the first Persian Gulf War. Some medical authorities are warning against using it. The Centers for Disease Control and Prevention has discouraged use of both antibiotics and the vaccine unless directly exposed and warned that the risks and benefits must be carefully weighed.

Following the anthrax attacks, some people in the macrobiotic and natural foods communities in New York, Washington, Florida, and other areas started taking UMEBOSHI PLUMS, miso, sea vegetables, and other healing foods as a preventive measure to help reduce the risk of infection. These foods are traditionally taken in the Far East to strengthen the blood, lymph, and other body fluids and to increase natural immunity to disease, especially bacterial and viral infection.

As noted above, extreme foods should be strictly avoided and a standard macrobiotic way of eating be observed. All raw foods, including fresh salad, should temporarily be discontinued. Observe Diet #1 for more yin conditions and disorders or, if substantial animal food is being consumed, observe Diet #3 to balance both extremes.

The principal home remedy to prevent anthrax infection is UME-SHO BANCHA, a tea made with umeboshi plum, shoyu, and bancha twig tea. Take 1 small cup daily for up to 3 weeks, then every other day, or occasionally as needed for several weeks, and then stop or taper off.

MISO SOUP, made from fermented soybean paste, will also help alkalinize the blood, strengthen the liver and spleen, and ward off infection. Organic barley, brown rice, or hatcho (all-soybean) miso that has aged a minimum of 2 years has the strongest effect.

Sea vegetables also have strong, detoxifying properties and may be used in small volume daily in soup, as a condiment, or as a small side dish. During a crisis, slightly more volume and frequency may be taken.

Anthrax particularly affects the lymphatic system. To strengthen the spleen and other lymphatic organs, often prepare millet, sweet rice, winter squash (such as butternut, buttercup, acorn, and others), cabbage, onions, and other sweet vegetables. See MILLET AND SWEET VEGETABLE PORRIDGE and MILLET AND SWEET VEGETABLE SOUP. These will particularly nourish the lymphatic vessels and organs and help reduce susceptibility to infection.

In the event of actual infection by anthrax or the appearance of symptoms from another terrorist-related microbial disease, please seek prompt medical attention. At the same time, the above dietary recommendations and home remedies may be continued to strengthen immunity and minimize any side effects of treatment.

Influenza. While most cases of influenza or the flu are mild, every several decades an especially virulent form appears, such as the pandemic of 1918 in which an estimated 20 million people around the world died. Flu, colds, and other viral infections commonly appear in the autumn, spring, or after other major change in season, weather, or temperature. In the autumn, the body begins to discharge the excess yin (from sugar, sweets, fruits, liquid, raw foods, oil, etc.) accumulated during the summer, while in the spring the body commonly discharges excess yang (from salt, meat, chicken, fish, and other animal food, and hard baked flour products). Symptoms include aching muscles, sore throat, headache, sneezing, runny nose, cough, high fever, and possible vomiting or diarrhea and usually last for several days to a week or more. Annual shots or vaccines are widely used to combat influenza, but these lead to overall weakening of the body and susceptibility to future infection. Severe influenza can lead to pneumonia.

Follow the guidelines for Diet #3, for conditions caused by a combination of extreme yin and yang factors, as well as the recommendations below. To help neutralize the common viruses associated with these conditions, UMEBOSHI PLUMS or preparations with ume may be taken, especially UME-SHO BANCHA as well as KUZU TEA or KUZU CREAM.

Lyme Disease. Lyme disease first appeared in Lyme, Connecticut, in 1975. Since then it has spread to 46 of the 48 states in the continental United States and is the most prevalent insect-borne disease in the country today. Spread by ticks, Lyme disease is a classic example of an emerging new epidemic that resulted from ecological disruption. As urban development replaced forests in New England, weedy grasses and shrubs multiplied, providing protection to rodents. As bears, wolves, and other large animals disappeared, deer proliferated. Originally the ticks were confined to the small rodent population, but deer became their intermediate hosts, spreading the Lyme organisms to the human habitats where they foraged for food. Because it is usually accompanied by flulike, arthritic symptoms or knee pain, Lyme disease

is often misdiagnosed. Its distinctive mark is a circular, bull's-eye rash, which may grow to 8 inches in diameter and last several weeks. On the other hand, about 75 percent of people who think they have been bitten by a Lyme tick prove not to be infected. Lyme disease is treated with antibiotics, but many advanced cases are considered incurable.

The main cause of Lyme disease is excessive intake of chicken, eggs, and chocolate. Other extreme foods also contribute to this condition, especially baked flour products, cheese and dairy food, citrus and tropical fruits, and sugar, honey, maple syrup, and other concentrated sweeteners. However, poultry items and chocolate, in the form of candy, ice cream, brownies, and other sweets and desserts, are the principal factors. People eating these foods are more susceptible to getting infected. These foods create sweet and fatty blood that attracts ticks and in which the Lyme organism can thrive and spread. Of course, all these items must be discontinued, including vinegar, spices, stimulants, and other items that may enhance the condition.

Following the standard macrobiotic diet will help prevent and relieve this condition. Observe the guidelines for Diet #3 for conditions caused by extreme yin and yang factors, as well as the following suggestions. In order to bring the blood, lymph, and bodily fluids back into balance, it is important to eat MISO SOUP daily or regularly, as well as sea vegetables, UMEBOSHI PLUM (as a condiment or seasoning), and other strengthening foods. Avoid oil for the first 3 weeks, then use a small amount of sesame oil brushed on the skillet for SAUTÉED VEGETABLES 2–3 times a week. Later a little more oil, including different types of vegetable oil, may be used as the condition improves. Also avoid raw foods, especially raw salad, until the condition improves. Take KINPIRA SOUP several times a week. MISO-ZOSUI is also very good and may be taken frequently. NISHIME-STYLE VEGETABLES are also recommended. Take SWEET VEGETABLE DRINK, 1 small cup every day for 1 month, then every other day for another month, and then occasionally. Two or three pieces of SHIO-KOMBU may be taken at every meal each day to strengthen the blood.

Lyme disease is frequently accompanied by pain and swelling in the joints, especially the knees, similar to rheumatoid arthritis. A GINGER COMPRESS or HOT TOWEL COMPRESS on the joints is good in this case. UME-SHO KUZU may be taken twice a week to strengthen the blood and circulation. The compress and drink will help loosen fat from chicken and eggs that has accumulated in the joints.

Malaria. Malaria may arise following exposure to a mosquito that carries the parasite that causes infection. Worldwide an estimated 3 million people die every year from this potentially deadly disease. New drug-resistant strains of malaria have recently developed, especially in Southeast Asia, and standard treatments are often no longer effective. With the advent of global warming, malaria is gradually spreading north and is expected to reach temperate latitudes in North America and other regions in the early decades of the 21st century. The parasites commonly infect the liver, multiplying rapidly and causing severe fevers with hot and cold chills. Anemia, kidney failure, rupture of

the spleen, seizures, or coma may follow. Cerebral malaria can leave survivors mentally impaired.

Follow the guidelines for Diet #1, for conditions caused by extreme yin factors, as well as the following suggestions. Mugwort is traditionally used to treat malaria, especially when prepared in MOCHI. Select young, soft mugwort leaves, wash them, and boil for 2–3 minutes (discarding the water). Then add the leaves when pounding the mochi. Mugwort mochi then can be pan-fried (without oil), steamed, or boiled and taken regularly. UMEBOSHI PLUMS are also very good to help prevent or relieve this condition.

Tuberculosis. Tuberculosis or TB is one of the deadliest scourges in human history. Prior to the development of penicillin in the mid-20th century, TB was the leading cause of death in modern society. Since then it has been replaced by heart disease and cancer. Today it is still one of the leading causes of mortality around the world. Every year an estimated 3 million people die. New drug-resistant strains have appeared in the United States, Russia, and other advanced countries, and it has returned as a major public health problem, especially in hospitals, prisons, and schools, where hundreds of people may be infected by one carrier. One in every three people around the world today carries the TB bacillus. While only a small percentage will get sick, many of them are at risk of infection in the future, especially if food quality continues to decline, the environmental crisis accelerates, and other imbalanced social and lifestyle conditions continue.

Tuberculosis may arise in the bones and joints, kidneys, bladder, intestines, lymph glands, or in any part of the body. However, the most common form of TB appears in the lungs. In the primary stage, which is noninfectious, the lymph nodes in the central part of the lung, around the entrance to the bronchi, become enlarged and calcified. The second stage involves the formation of cavities in the lungs. These cavities, or *tubercules*, continue to calcify and grow in size, causing the inner lung tissue to decompose. This stage of disease creates active infection. The TB bacilli thrive in the highly acidic environment of the lung cavities and may be transmitted through breathing.

Sun baths are often recommended for TB patients. TB bacilli are easily killed by sunlight, since they are very yin and weak. But as the disease progresses, the tiny blood vessels within the lungs may weaken and rupture, causing blood to be coughed up by exposure to sunlight which stimulates blood production. It is better for someone with this condition to remain inside or go out with a hat or sunscreen.

Tuberculosis is caused by long-term consumption of a modern diet, including extremes of meat and sugar, eggs and dairy, tropical foods and beverages, and other items that create a strong acid condition in the blood. This acidic condition, in turn, produces a buffer reaction that draws on the body's reserve of minerals. The body's stored minerals consist of about 40 percent calcium, which is the element most involved in this process. In the case of minor acidosis, the body's natural buffer mechanisms maintain the necessary alkaline condition in the blood, and the effects are minimal. However, when the consumption of excess exceeds the bloodstream's capacity to neutralize it, deposits of fatty acid and mucus begin to accumulate in the lungs, kidneys, lymph nodes, and other areas. In an effort to offset these increased acidic deposits, buffer reactions begin to occur around the site of the localization. Calcification is the end result. Dairy food is usually a primary cause of tuberculosis, especially milk, cream, butter, ice cream, yogurt, and other light forms of dairy.

To prevent or treat tuberculosis, it is necessary to stop the consumption of dairy, sugar, fruit, meat, soft drinks, eggs, fish, refined grains, and other foods that create an acidic condition in the blood. Follow the guidelines for Diet #1, for conditions caused by predominantly extreme yin factors. Emphasize well-cooked whole grains and vegetables as the primary food and be careful to control liquid consumption. Drink when thirsty, but do not overconsume beverages and fluids. MISO SOUP and condiments made with miso are especially good to help prevent infection. FRIED MISO is especially helpful; 1 teaspoon of this may be taken with rice and vegetables. CARBONIZED UME-BOSHI plum is good for intestinal TB. Externally, a TARO PLASTER is beneficial for some cases of tuberculosis to help reduce inflammation and draw out toxins and other stagnant matter. Apply repeatedly until the condition eases.

Other Infectious Diseases. There is an array of other infectious diseases. These include infections caused by rickettsiae, tiny microorganisms that live inside the linings of small blood vessels and are spread by ticks, mites, fleas, and lice. *Typhus,* once a worldwide epidemic spread by lice, and *Rocky Mountain spotted fever*, a tick-borne disorder spread by rabbits, squirrels, deer, and other animals, are examples.

Bacterial disease spread by tiny, single-cell organisms include *cholera, diphtheria, typhoid, staph infections, strep infections, pneumonia, meningitis*, and *leprosy*. A newly recognized staph infection is *toxic shock syndrome*, a disorder that affects primarily young women using superabsorbent tampons. This is a potentially fatal disease that produces a high fever, severe headache, vomiting, diarrhea, and a body-wide rash followed by severe shock within 48 hours and damage to major organs. Other new bacterial diseases include *Legionnaire's disease*, spread by air-conditioning ducts and super-market misters, and *necrotizing fasciitis*, a strep infection that causes large areas of flesh to be consumed. Though largely quiescent in recent centuries, the *plague*, or black death, has surfaced in the desert southwest of the United States and assorted countries in recent years. It has two main forms: *bubonic*, which results in swollen lymph nodes (buboes) and inflames the liver and spleen, and *pneumonic*, which affects the lungs.

Most bacterial diseases respond to prompt antibiotic treatment, but new strains are forming that are resistant to drugs. Vancomycin, the last antibiotic capable of treating many staph infections, recently yielded to drug resistance for the first time. A case turned up in Japan that could not be treated with this powerful drug, then several in the United States, and soon vancomycin-resistant bacteria appeared around the world.

Other viral diseases include *rabies*, which is transmitted by the bites or saliva of infected animals and affects the brain and spinal cord; *hantavirus* infection, which is spread by rodents and damages the lungs and kidneys; *yellow fever*, a once major epidemic disease spread by infected mosquitoes; *Ebola*, a deadly hemorrhaghic fever that recently appeared in Central Africa and may be associated with consuming contaminated monkey meat; *West Nile virus*, a potentially fatal disorder spread by mosquitoes; SARS (Severe Acute Respiratory Syndrome), a respiratory illness with pneumonia-like symptoms that may prove lethal.

Dysentery, an infectious condition associated with exposure to contaminated water and the bane of travelers, commonly arises following exposure to amoebas, worms, or bacteria. There is also a non-infectious type caused by a chemical toxin.

In general, the dietary and lifestyle approach recommended in this section may be followed for these and other infectious diseases. However, the precise foods or combinations of foods that give rise to each disorder will vary slightly, and the recommendations may need to be adjusted in a slightly more yin or yang direction. Typically, infectious diseases arise from a more yin cause and the person's condition is more yin. In this case, observe Diet #1. In some cases, especially where strong animal food is still being consumed, the disease arises from a combination of dietary extremes and Diet #3 should be followed.

SOLUTION

DIET

Dietary extremes, especially the consumption of strong acid-producing foods and beverages, are the primary cause of viral and bacterial infections. Observe the dietary recommendations noted above for each condition and the more extended special diets.

LIFESTYLE

1. Live each day happily without worry, especially anxiety over exposure to microbes in your immediate environment.

2. Walk outdoors every day for a half hour or longer.

3. Keep green plants in the home to produce oxygen and freshen the air.

4. Wear 100 percent cotton clothing next to the skin, and use cotton sheets and pillowcases to allow better exchange of natural electromagnetic energy with the environment.

5. Avoid microwave or electric cooking and use gas, wood, or some other form of natural energy or fire. Microwaved food in particular may increase microbial activity and should strictly be avoided.

6. Avoid or limit watching television, using computers, or exposure to other artificial electromagnetic fields, especially until the condition improves.

7. A few minutes each day, meditate, pray, or visualize healthy, positive feelings and images. Do not visualize negative images such as the destruction of harmful microbes; rather, visualize the blood, lymph, and other factors becoming stronger and peacefully, gently, and naturally eliminating virulent microorganisms and toxins from the body through the lungs, skin, urine, and bowel movement.

8. Practice safe sex.

9. Strictly avoid all drug use, minimize X rays, and avoid invasive medical procedures as much as possible.

10. Maintain a clean, orderly environment. Use food-based or other natural body-care products and nontoxic home cleaning products. Scientific studies have found that many common household cleansers containing strong chemicals only spread the germs more widely through the home.

11. Sing a happy song each day.

HOME REMEDIES

1. For energy and vitality, KOI-KOKU may be taken, 1 bowl for no more than 3 days in a row.

2. Instead of koi-koku or as an alternative, KINPIRA SOUP may be taken 2–3 times a week to strengthen the blood.

3. For anemia that accompanies an infectious condition, small dried fish *(iriko)* may be eaten, sautéed in a little water or oil with shoyu at the end of cooking, 2 small pieces a day.

4. For some cases, a compress, poultice, or other external application may be needed to help neutralize the infection or gradually help draw out excess mucus and fat from the body. Miso is particularly effective in helping to neutralize viruses and bacteria and prevent infection from spreading. Besides MISO SOUP eaten regularly, it may be used externally as a MISO PLASTER.

5. A BODY SCRUB is helpful to promote better circulation of blood, lymph, and other body fluids, as well as to activate physical and mental energies.

6. When traveling to a new environment, including most international travel, take a large supply of UMEBOSHI PLUMS, enough for one or two every day, along with BANCHA TWIG TEA (in the form of twigs or tea bags), to neutralize harmful viruses or bacteria that may be encountered in contaminated food or water.

CAUTION

1. Persons who have received or who are currently undergoing medical treatment may need to make further dietary modifications. Please consult your medical doctor, nutritionist, or other health care professional.

2. The bacteria, virus, and other microorganisms in stored blood can usually be eliminated by heat treatment, but this treatment may not have been applied in some cases. The safest measure of blood transfusion is to collect blood from a member of the immediate family, relative, or close friend who has the same blood type and whose blood has been tested for safety prior to the transfusion.

3. If the condition worsens, other lack of improvement is experienced, or a serious, potentially life-threatening condition develops, such as toxic shock syndrome, prompt medical attention is necessary.

4. Life-threatening infectious diseases such as cholera, diphtheria, rabies, and others may need to be reported to public health authorities, even if a macrobiotic or alternative approach is taken.

MEDICAL EVIDENCE

NATURAL ANTIBIOTICS GO BACK THOUSANDS OF YEARS

"More than four thousand years ago the Chinese routinely treated skin wounds and infections with a paste made from moldy soybeans," explains Jeffrey A. Fisher, M.D, an expert on epidemic diseases. "Almost identical remedies are described in the Hebrew Talmud. . . . The ancient practices all had as a common denominator the use of fermented grains, with molds, yeast and fungi as the fermenting agents.

"Until the 1960s, when scientists at pharmaceutical companies began developing synthetic versions of antibiotics, the naturally produced ones were derived from similar sources: molds, sewage or soil. As the bacteria or fungi producing these early antibiotics have been around for millions of years, it is likely that the pastes, packs or liquids used by these early healers contained antibiotics."

Source: Jeffrey A. Fisher, M.D., *The Plague Makers: How We Are Creating Catastrophic New Epidemics—And What We Must Do to Avert Them,* New York: Simon & Schuster, 1994.

INFECTIOUS DISEASE TRACED TO ANIMAL INFECTIONS

Most infectious diseases have been transferred to human beings from domesticated animals. "Measles, for example, is probably related to rinderpest and/or canine distemper; smallpox is certainly connected closely with cowpox and with a cluster of other animal infections; influenza is shared by humans and hogs," explains historian William H. McNeill. Today 26 diseases are shared by humans and poultry, 42 with pigs, 46 with sheep and goats, and 50 with cattle.

Source: William H. McNeill, *Plagues and Peoples* (Garden City, N.Y.: Anchor Press/Doubleday, 1976), p. 51.

VACCINATIONS PROMOTE SURVIVAL OF THE FITTEST MICROBES

"The present efforts to control infectious diseases generally do not involve assessment of evolutionary stability," explains Paul Ewald, a biologist, in *Evolution of Infectious Diseases.* "Rather, researches focus on vulnerable aspects of a pathogen, such as biochemical components that can be used in a vaccine.... If the individuals in a pathogen species always wore the same uniform, identifying and destroying them would be as easy as it was with smallpox. But most parasites practice guerrilla warfare ... vaccines generated against sexually reproducing parasites like malaria or mutation-prone viruses like HIV and influenza can be expected to provide partial and unstable solutions. Vaccination has already nullified easy adversaries. We are now left with the more wily ones, which probably will evade our vaccination efforts by changing their coats."

Instead of public vaccination campaigns to eradicate germs, Ewald proposes that we "use our knowledge about them to make them evolve into less dangerous organisms." Not only are many vaccines unsafe and infective, they ultimately produce microorganisms with increased virulence.

Source: Paul Ewald, *Evolution of Infectious Diseases*, Oxford University Press, 1994 pp. 207–215.

HAZARDS OF ANTIBIOTICS

The use of antibiotics to treat bacterial diseases is counterproductive, according to public health research Marc Lappé. "For four decades now, we have thrown hundreds of tons of antibiotics against our Hollywood imagination of microscopic enemies. In the process we have sown seeds for a whole new array of actual germs and disease.... We favor simple technological fixes for complex disease entities, while our medical complex fosters a near-sighted one-germ, one-chemical mentality. Together,

these positions contribute to a world view that encourages the proliferation of new chemotherapeutic agents, and in turn, the proliferation of new disease entities.... The answer clearly does not consist of throwing more troops into a losing battle."

Source: Marc Lappé, *When Antibiotics Fail: Restoring the Ecology of the Body* North Atlantic Books, 1995 p. 190–192.

NUTRITIONAL DEFICIENCIES CAUSE GERMS TO MUTATE

Nutritional deficiencies in their hosts can cause viruses to mutate and become lethal. In the first study on the effect of nutrients on viral growth and development, scientists at the University of North Carolina reported that a human virus introduced into mice mutated from being harmless to damaging their hearts after selenium, a nutrient found naturally in whole grains and vegetables, was limited. Dr. Melina A. Beck, the lead researcher, said that nutritional deficiencies may cause viruses and bacteria to become more virulent and be involved in the spread of influenza, hepatitis, meningitis, and other epidemics. The viruses used in the study were associated with sore throats, colds, aches and inflammation, as well as polio and some types of heart disease, meningitis, and diabetes. "Perhaps virus evolution does depend on what we eat or what we do not eat," an editorial in the journal concluded.

Source: M. A. Beck et al., "Rapid Genomic Evolution of a Non-Virulent Coxsackievirus B3 in Selenium-Deficient Mice Results in Selection of Identical Virulent Isolates," *Natural Medicine* 1(5):433–36, 1995.

INFECTIOUS DISEASES MAY BE INTERNALLY GENERATED

Early in the 20th century, an infectious disease expert reported that in laboratory experiments, pneumococci, the microbes that cause pneumonia, could be transformed into streptococci, the microbes that cause strep infections. E. C. Rosenow of the Memorial Institute for Infectious Diseases in Chicago concluded that nutritional and environmental factors may cause bacteria and viruses to transmute into potentially harmful species within the body without outside stimulation or intervention.

Source: E. C. Rosenow, "Transmutations Within the Streptococcus-Pneumococcus Group," *Journal of Infectious Diseases,* vol. 14, 1914.

AIDS MAY BE SELF-CAUSED

In his book on modern epidemics, Dr. Robert Gallo, the co-discoverer of HIV, mentions the theory that AIDS and other new viral diseases may be self-caused. "Some scientists have speculated that in a weird case of reverse evolution, viruses are descended from more complex parasites, adapting by shedding their ingredients to the barest form capable of survival."

Source: Robert Gallo, *Virus Hunting: AIDS, Cancer, and the Human Retrovirus,* Basic Books, 1991, p. 52.

DEADLY *E. COLI* INFECTION LINKED TO HAMBURGERS

Nearly half the cattle at feed lots in the United States carry the deadly bacteria *E. coli* O157:H7 in the summer, according to a new U.S. Department of Agriculture study. This is 10 times more than previously estimated. Each year about 60 people die from eating infected hamburgers and another 73,000 become sick. In the winter the presence of *E. coli* drops to 1 percent, but then shoots up in the warmer months. At the present time, testing is required only on ground beef and not on other cattle products.

Source: "*E. coli* Levels in Cattle Higher Than Thought," *Boston Globe,* March 1, 2000.

ANTIBIOTICS FOR ANTHRAX ASSOCIATED WITH STRONG ADVERSE EFFECTS

Medical researchers expressed concern that antibiotics used to prevent or treat anthrax may have serious consequences. Following the anthrax attacks after September 11, 2001, the *Boston Globe* reported that scientists were concerned "that the drugs will cause severe side effects and possibly create a mutant strain that resists treatment." Cipro causes severe side effects such as diarrhea, nausea, tendinitis, ruptured tendons, joint pain, nerve damage, and allergic reactions that can become life threatening in 2–7 percent of people who take the drug. "It made me so dizzy that I just couldn't take it," Patricia Soloman, a Washington postal employee, stated. "Since we use this drug as a last resort in many patients, we run the risk of creating super bugs that are resistant to all drugs," Stuart Levy, an antibiotic specialist at Tufts University, further noted.

Meanwhile, the FDA, consumer groups, and the *New England Journal of Medicine* demanded that Bayer, the manufacturer of Cipro, withdraw from sale Baytrill, its sister antibiotic, used in breeding poultry. Health authorities warned that people who eat chicken could develop resistance to Cipro and other antibiotics. In chickens, Baytrill destroys campylobacter, the bacteria that are the most common cause of food-borne illness and which are linked to 2 million cases of food poisoning in the United States every year. Experts expressed concern that the widespread use of Cipro by the public following bioterrorist attacks would increase the number of serious cases of food-borne illness and increase the risk of drug resistance spreading to other microbes. After Baytrill was approved for use in breeding chickens in 1995, drug-resistant germs in the human gut soared from 1 percent to 17 percent.

Sources: Tasha Robertson, "As Use Becomes Widespread, Mutant Strains Feared," *Boston Globe,* October 31, 2001; Philip J. Hilts, "Drug for Poultry Stirs Resistance Concerns," *New York Times,* October 30, 2001.

ANTHRAX VACCINATIONS CAUSE WIDESPREAD REACTIONS

Prior to the September 11 attacks, a congressional panel investigating the Pentagon's campaign to vaccinate American troops against anthrax called for the vaccination to be halted. The House Committee on Government Reform warned that the program was based on incomplete, obsolete science and that those in the military should not be required to have shots until more reliable data were obtained about the inoculation's effectiveness and adverse side effects.

A follow-up study by the General Accounting Office found that 86 percent of those who had received the shots experienced some type of adverse reaction. A previous anthrax vaccine administered to U.S. soldiers in the Persian Gulf in the early 1990s is a suspected cause of Gulf War syndrome, whose symptoms include chronic pain, skin rashes, nausea, memory loss, and concentration problems.

Meryl Nass, M.D., an expert on anthrax vaccines, reported that "10–35% of vaccine recipients develop illnesses resembling chronic fatigue syndrome, fibromyalgia, multiple chemical sensitivity, autoimmune illnesses, and/or neuropathies. . . . You will never find me lining up for my dose," she vowed. After the anthrax attacks, the U.S. government offered to inoculate postal employees, but many refused. "Those vaccinations can cause all kind of harm," William M. Smith, president of the New York Metro Area Postal Workers Union, asserted. "Until I see the Supreme Court and the Congress taking those vaccinations, I don't want them to be giving it to us."

Sources: "FAQs About Anthrax," Centers for Disease Control and Prevention, November 15, 2001; Meryl Nass, M.D., "The Anthrax Vaccine Saga: How Not to Develop a Vaccine Program," www.anthrax vaccine.org, September 10, 2001 (see also updates, October 21, October 26, and November 1, 2001); Meryl Nass, M.D., "Response to Those Seeking Anthrax Vaccine Information and/or Vaccination," www.anthraxvaccine.org, September 20, 2001; "Unon Head Objects to Anthrax Vaccine Program," *New York Times,* December 25, 2001.

CASE HISTORY

TUBERCULOSIS OVERCOME WITH MACROBIOTIC DIET

Yukikazu Sakurazawa, a young man suffering from tuberculosis, came upon a small book, *The Curative Method by Diet.* Sakurazawa lived in Kyoto, the old capital of Japan, in the early part of the twentieth century and had already lost his mother and brothers to this dread affliction. Sagen Ishizuka, M.D., the author of the book, explained that TB and most other infectious diseases could be relieved by diet. He recomended avoiding meat and other animal foods, sugar, refined grains, and other highly processed foods and eating brown rice and other whole cereal grains, miso soup, cooked vegetables, sea vegetables, and other traditional foods. Given only a short time to live by his doctors, Sakurazawa had nothing to lose and,

though skeptical, began to cook and eat according to these guidelines. Soon his case of advanced tuberculosis cleared up, and he resolved to devote himself to this method. Adopting the pen name George Ohsawa, he went on to become the founder of modern macrobiotics in Japan and traveled around the world tirelessly over the next fifty years, spreading these traditional teachings.

Source: Michio Kushi with Alex Jack, *The Book of Macrobiotics* (Tokyo and New York: Japan Publications, revised edition 1986), pp. 25–26

TABLE 26. INFECTIOUS DISEASES AND EPIDEMICS

Disease	Region	Transmission	Dietary Factor	Social Factor
Viral Epidemics (more yin)				
AIDS	USA, Caribbean, 1980s; Africa, global, 1990s–	Sexual contact, needles, transfusion	Sugar, tropical foods, oil, dairy, fat	Ecological imbalance, antibiotic and drug use
Argentine hemorrhagic fever	Argentina, 1958–	Rodents	Beef, sugar, chemicals	Modern farming, pesticides
Dengue	Cuba, 1981; Asia, Africa, Australia	Mosquitoes, monkey/human	Sugar, fruit, dairy	Urbanization, open water
Ebola hemorrhagic fever	Zaire, Sudan, 1976–	Possibly monkeys	Sugar, dairy, oil, fat, contaminated meat	Ecological imbalance
Hantavirus	Asia, U.S., 1993–	Rodents	Meat, sugar	Monoculture
Hepatitis A, B, C, D, E	Tropics, U.S., global, 1990s–	Poor hygiene, food, or water (A, E); contaminated blood, needles, sex (B, D); transfusions, needles (C)	Meat, sugar, tropical foods, shellfish	Travel, contaminated food, unsanitary conditions, medication
Herpes	U.S., global, 1980s–	Sexual contact	Meat, sugar, dairy, fat	Sexual revolution, cultural values

Disease	Region	Transmission	Dietary Factor	Social Factor
Human T-cell leukemia	Caribbean 1979–, Japan, 1983–, global	Humans	Sugar, fruit, dairy, oil, fat	Medical technology, transfusions
Influenza	Global, 1918; various strains, 1968, 1977	Fowl, swine	Meat, sugar, dairy, oil, fat	Pork and poultry production
Lassa fever	West Africa, 1969–	Rodents	Sugar, dairy	Mining
Marburg disease	Germany, 1967; Africa, 1975	Monkeys	Sugar, dairy, fruit, oil, fat	Polio vaccine, hospitals
Polio	U.S., 20th century; global, sporadic	Waterborne, contaminated feces	Sugar, dairy, fruit, oil, fat	Poor hygiene, hot weather, reaction to vaccination
SARS (Severe Acute Respiratory Syndrome)	Asia, Europe, North America, 2003	Humans	Possibly sugar, fat, dairy, and other acid-producing foods	Jet travel
West Nile virus	Israel, 1990s; U.S., 2000	Mosquitoes, birds	Sugar, dairy, oil, fat, fruit	Chemical farming, travel
Yellow fever	South America and North America, 17th century; East Africa, 1980s–	Monkeys, mosquitoes	Fruit, sugar, chocolate, dairy	Plantation farming, medical technology

Bacterial Epidemics (more yang)

Disease	Region	Transmission	Dietary Factor	Social Factor
Cholera	Europe, Asia, 18th century; tropics, 1980s–	Waterborne	Sugar, dairy, eggs, white flour, fruit, spices	Antibiotic resistance, chemicalization
Diphtheria	Global, 19th century; Russia, 1990s–	Airborne	Meat, sugar, potatoes, white flour, fruit, oil, dairy	Urbanization, overcrowding, poverty, hunger
E. coli infections	U.S., Mexico, SE Asia, 1980s–	Food-, air-, and waterborne	Hamburger, chicken, sugar, dairy, chemicals	Chemical farming, soil depletion, fast food
Legionnaire's disease	U.S., 1976–	Air- and waterborne	Meat, sugar, dairy, oil, fat	Air-conditioning ducts, travel

Disease	Region	Transmission	Dietary Factor	Social Factor
Leprosy (Hansen's disease)	Global, sporadic, from ancient times	Living in prolonged contact with patient	Fungi, sugar, dairy, raw and undercooked food	Unsanitary conditions, poverty
Lyme disease	U.S., Europe, Australia, 1980s–	Deer tick	Sugar, chocolate, fruit, fat	Urbanization, pesticides
Necrotizing fasciitis (flesh-eating disease)	Australia, 1960s; U.K., U.S., 1994–	Air-, hospital-borne strep infection	Sugar, chocolate, diary, fruit, oil, fat	Resistance to antibiotics, medicalization
Plague (bubonic and pneumonic)	Eurasia, 14th century; India, U.S. Southwest, 1990s–	Rats, fleas	Sugar, dairy, fruit, fat, tropical foods	World food trade, transportation, poor hygiene
Pneumonia	Global, since ancient times	Airborne	Meat, eggs, poultry, sweets, dairy, oil, spice	Extreme weather, resistance to antibiotics
Salmonella	Iran, 1963–73; global 1980s–	Food-, airborne	Meat, sugar, dairy, oil, fat	Contaminated meat, poultry
Shigella dysentery	Japan, 1955; tropics, 1980s–	Water-, air-, foodborne	Sugar, milk, tropical foods	Resistance to antibiotics
Staph infections	Global, 1980s–	Airborne	Sugar, fruit	Antibiotics
Toxic shock syndrome	U.S., 1978–	Superabsorbent tampons, surgery	Meat, sugar, dairy, oil, fast foods, chemicals	Chemicalization, medication
Tuberculosis	Global, 19th century; Russia, U.S., 1980s–	Air-, hospital-borne	Fruit, sugar, milk, fat, oil, white flour	Antibiotic resistance, AIDS
Typhoid fever	Global, 19th century; sporadic today	Water-, foodborne, contamined feces and urine	Oil, fat, dairy, white flour, potatoes, tropical foods	Poor sanitation, poverty, overcrowding
Other Epidemics (yin, yang, or combination of both)				
Candidiasis	U.S., 1980s–	Fungal or yeast infection in the mouth or vagina	Sugar, chocolate, white flour, fruit, juice, diet colas	Fast foods, chemicals, pesticides, drugs, medication

Disease	Region	Transmission	Dietary Factor	Social Factor
Gulf War syndrome	U.S., 1990s–	Unknown	Military rations, fast food, irregular eating	Possible exposure to nerve gas, vaccination, depleted uranium, chemicals
Mad cow disease (variant Creutzfeldt-Jakob disease)	U.K., Europe, 1990s–	Prions or infectious proteins in beef, milk, or dairy products; contact with bone meal, drugs, medicines, and extracts made with cow parts	Rendered beef or dairy, possible chemical or pesticide contamination	New food technology, chemical farming and food processing, medical procedures and contamination
Malaria	Europe, Asia, Africa, from ancient times; global, today	Plasmodium parasite transmitted by mosquitoes	Fruit, sugar, sweets, milk, oil, spices	Monocropping, poverty, hunger, pesticides, drug resistance
Rocky Mountain spotted fever	Continental U.S.	Ticks infected with *Rickettsia rickettsii* transmitted by rabbits, squirrels, deer, bears, dogs, and humans	Meat, sugar, dairy, oil, chemicals, and fast foods	Urbanization, chemical farming, pesticides
Typhus	Global, 19th century	Fleas carrying *Rickettsia typhi* carried by rats, mice, and other rodents	Meat, sugar, white flour, oil, fruit, potatoes, tropical foods	Urbanization, poverty, slums, hunger, poor sanitation

◎ KIDNEY AND BLADDER PROBLEMS

Urinary system problems are common in modern society. These include kidney and bladder infections, kidney and bladder stones, uremia, and incontinence. Located in the upper part of the abdominal cavity near the spinal column, the kidneys filter impurities from the blood and discharge excess wastes from the body in a fluid known as urine. In filtering the blood, the kidneys regulate its volume and chemical makeup. They maintain the fluid-electrolyte and acid-base balances, e.g., the salt-water balance in the body, as well as produce hormones (such as erythropoietin, which stimulates red blood cell production) and enzymes (such as renin, which regulates blood pressure and kidney function).

The kidneys also convert vitamin D to a more active form.

The other major components of the urinary system are the ureters, long, narrow tubes that convey the urine from each kidney to the bladder by muscular action. The bladder is a Y-shaped organ situated in the pelvis, which serves as a reservoir for urine. It can hold about 1 pint. The urethra is the canal through which the urine is discharged in the body and is about five times as long in men as in women. The urethra is divided into a prostatic portion and penile portion in men and is largely separate from the reproductive system in women.

In traditional Oriental medicine, the kidneys and bladder are most highly charged during the night and broadly govern sleep, reproductive functions, and overall vitality and regeneration. *See also "Kidney and Bladder Cancer" in "Cancer."* Through a balanced way of eating, most urinary system problems can be prevented or relieved.

SYMPTOMS

1. Snoring
2. Groaning
3. Bed-wetting
4. Urinary problems
5. Lower back pain
6. Swelling of the legs
7. Getting up too early or too late
8. Getting up to urinate in the night
9. Sleeping problems such as tossing and turning
10. Insomnia
11. Nightmares
12. Nausea
13. Vomiting
14. Lethargy
15. Drowsiness
16. Mental and psychological symptoms and disorders, for example, fear, timidity, shyness, hesitation, indecision, lack of clarity, paranoia, schizophrenia
17. Decline of mental and physical vitality
18. Reproductive system problems

SIGNS

Traditional Oriental diagnosis offers further insight into developing kidney and bladder problems:

1. Darkness or blackness on the skin under the eyes shows kidney stagnation and toxic blood as a result of tight kidneys. This may result from too much animal food, salt, chips, baked food, or other strong contractive substances.

2. Bags under the eyes show kidney problems. The first type is watery and swollen and shows that too much fluid is accumulating, the kidneys are swollen, and urination is frequent. Foods that cause this type include beverages of all kinds, fruits, and juices. The second type is fatty and indicates fat and mucus accumulation in the kidney tissues. Small pimples or dark spots on this type of fatty eyebag show that kidney stones are forming. Foods that cause this fatty type of eye bags include dairy foods, meat, poultry, refined flour, sugar, and oil.

3. The ears are kidney-shaped and also correspond with these organs. A red coloration around the outer edge of the ear shows the kidneys are swollen from too much sugar, dairy, fruit, and

juices. Too much animal protein can lead to moles or warts on the ear. The left kidney is reflected in the left ear, the right kidney in the right ear. Fatty deposits in the ureter correspond with wax buildup in the ears.

4. Wet or damp hands and feet result from too much fluid consumption and show overburdened kidneys and bladder.

5. Pain or hardness at the beginning of the kidney meridian at the bottom of the foot shows developing kidney problems. Calluses on this spot indicate an accumulation of excess mucus, protein, and fat in the kidney and its related meridian from dairy, animal fats, oils, sugar, and flour products.

6. The upper part of the forehead shows the condition of the bladder. Lines or ridges in this area show swelling or accumulation of fluid in that organ.

7. Poor posture shows kidney troubles. Leaning forward while sitting, standing, or walking shows tight kidneys, while leaning backward, leaning against things, slouching, or the inability to sit up very long on the floor show expanded, overly yin kidneys.

CAUSES

1. Most of the excess that the body takes in in the form of extreme foods and beverages, as well as chemicals, toxins, and undesirable microorganisms, are processed by the kidneys and eliminated through the bladder in the form of urine. The kidneys can easily become overworked from overeating and overdrinking or having to filter too many impurities from the blood.

2. Overconsumption of meat, poultry, eggs, fish and seafood, bread and other hard baked flour products, and other contractive foods can tighten and harden the kidneys and cause them to become encased in fat or mucus, restricting blood flow and urination.

3. Overconsumption of refined grains, tropical foods, excessive fruit and juice, sugar and sweets, too much liquid, alcohol, coffee and other stimulants, drugs, and other more expansive substances can loosen and cause the kidneys to swell, leading to excessive water retention or elimination and incomplete filtration of the blood.

4. Cold and frozen foods are particularly contracting to the kidneys and bladder. These include soft drinks, mineral waters, beer, and iced drinks of all kinds.

5. High-protein foods, especially those of animal quality, create excessive urea, a solid waste that is processed by the kidneys.

6. Kidney stone formation is associated with a high level of calcium oxalate in the urine. Foods high in oxalate include spinach, rhubarb, cocoa, pepper, nuts, and black tea.

7. Excessive intake of salt or water, or in some cases a deficiency of salt or water, can lead to urinary system problems.

8. Too many sweets, especially sugar, chocolate, and other refined sweets but also good-quality natural sweeteners, can overburden the pancreas, which regulates blood sugar levels in the body, and weaken the kidneys and bladder.

FORMS

Abnormal Urination. Normally the urine is amber or yellow in color, forms a mildly acidic reaction, and has a slight odor and a salty taste.

Unhealthy urine may have high levels of albumin, sugar, blood, pus, acetone, fat, chyle, cellular material, bacteria, and other impurities. Overconsumption of too much salt, animal food, or other yang fare will turn the urine dark, while too much fluid intake, sugar, and other expansive substances will turn the urine lighter in color or colorless. Normal urination is about three to four times a day. Urinating more frequently can arise from either too much yang or too much yin food and beverage consumption. Too much liquid intake or consumption of sugar and other expansive foods that contain large amounts of liquid can produce excessive fluid in the body and lead to frequent urination. Too much salt, baked food, or other yang substances can cause the bladder to shrink in size and cause frequent urination.

Producing too little urine, or *oliguria*, may result from excessive sweating following intense physical activity or hot weather. Edema, loss of blood, diarrhea, or kidney disease are other possible factors. Difficulty or pain urinating, or *dysuria*, is usually caused by cystitis or urethritis. Burning pain in this case is usually the result of excessive yang factors in the diet, including meat, eggs, baked flour, or salt. In men, trouble urinating may also be associated with prostate problems. *Anuria,* or complete failure to produce urine, usually arises from a sudden drop in blood pressure or uremia *(see "Kidney Disease," below).* It may arise from strong yin factors or a combination of strong yin and yang factors.

For urination problems arising from yin factors, observe Diet #1; for those stemming from yang factors, observe Diet #2; and for combined factors, follow Diet #3. The home remedies below may be helpful.

Kidney or Bladder Infections. Urinary tract infections are commonly accompanied by pain, high fever, the constant desire to urinate even when the bladder is empty, bloody or cloudy urine, and severe nausea or vomiting. A burning sensation when urinating and urine with a powerful bad odor tend to accompany bladder infections. Women have many more bladder infections (cystitis) than men. These tend to be mild but are likely to recur and can lead to more serious kidney infections. In men, bladder infections tend to arise from prostate problems and may indicate a more serious disorder.

Associated with *E. coli* or other common bacteria, kidney infections may lead to serious complications, including chronic kidney disease, blood poisoning, or loss of the fetus (in the case of pregnant women). Conventional medicine treats urinary infections with antibiotics and a large volume of fluids to help flush out the bacteria. From the macrobiotic view, the bacteria associated with these infections are normally harmless. They become harmful only as a result of an acidic condition in the blood, lymph, body fluids, and digestive and urinary tract as a result of overconsumption of extreme foods and beverages. Overall, susceptibility to infections such as this is more yin, as a result of the intake of excessive dairy food, sugar, chocolate, soft drinks, fruits, juices, alcohol, and other expansive substances. However, too much animal food will also create overacidity and lead to microbial imbalance.

The macrobiotic approach to urinary tract infections is to observe the standard diet, with strong, regular consumption of MISO SOUP, sea vegetables, and proper seasonings (including shoyu and sea salt) to help alkalinize the blood and bodily systems. Then the infection will clear up naturally without the need for drugs or medications. Follow the guidelines for Diet #1.

Kidney or Bladder Stones. Overconsumption of extreme foods from the yin and yang category can lead over time to the formation of stones in the kidney or bladder. Excessive mucus and fatty acid can build up in and around these organs, leading to the formation of crystals, stones, cysts, and eventually tumors. These hardened deposits, which may vary in size from that of a grain of sand to a marble or a golf ball, commonly obstruct the fine network of cells in the interior of the kidneys, ureters, or the bladder, leading to water accumulation in the legs, swelling, and weakness. Many foods in the modern way of eating can create stones in the urinary tract. One of the most frequent combinations is high-fat, high-protein foods, including animal foods of all kinds, combined with cold, frozen, or chilled foods, including ice cream, sherbet, yogurt, frozen juices, soft drinks, ice water, and other foods and beverages that lower the body temperature, contract the kidneys, and harden developing deposits and crystals.

Kidney stones are usually accompanied by excruciating pains radiating from the side of the affected kidney moving down toward the groin, nausea and vomiting, excessive sweating, and blood in the urine. They are more common in younger and middle-aged adults than in the elderly, and women are more likely to have stones than men. Since most stones will naturally pass through the urine of their own accord, physicians commonly prescribe plenty of water and pain medication. Surgery is performed if an infection persists, total blockage of the ureter prevents urination, or any other serious complication develops. Other modern medical treatments include laser beams, sound therapy, or high-energy shock waves to break up the kidney stones into smaller pieces.

Such methods may relieve pain and eliminate obstructions. However, they do not address the underlying cause of the problem and, in many cases, kidney stones will form again in the future unless the diet is changed. Observe the centrally balanced guidelines for Diet #3 to help prevent the formation of stones in the kidneys or bladder. To relieve existing stones, a GINGER COMPRESS should be applied over the kidneys continuously, especially during a kidney stone attack or strong pain. Plenty of hot fluids may be taken, especially hot BANCHA TWIG TEA, to help ease the obstruction and flush out the stone.

Kidney Disease. Kidney disease refers to the loss of kidney function, a potentially fatal degenerative condition. Symptoms may include swollen hands and feet, the constant desire to urinate, shortness of breath, rising blood pressure, constant thirst, unpleasant taste in the mouth, and unpleasant odor of the breath. Kidney disease may result from diabetes, atherosclerosis, high blood pressure, or other chronic condition that interferes with the proper flow of blood to this organ. Congenital disorders, exposure to toxins or chemicals, drug abuse, active sports, and other factors can also lead to kidney degeneration or failure. One of the most common symptoms is *uremia*, or an excessive amount of urea and other nitrogenous wastes in the blood. The kidneys normally excrete urea in the urine. But through long-term consumption of dietary excess, kidney function is impaired and these wastes spill over into the blood, producing nausea, vomiting, lethargy, drowsiness, and eventual kidney failure. Conventional treatments for kidney disease include drugs to help slow the deterioration, kidney dialysis in which the blood is artificially filtered by mechanical devices, and kidney transplant.

A balanced macrobiotic way of eating can prevent and slow down the progression of kidney disease and, in some cases, relieve it. Observe the guidelines for Diet #3.

Nephritis. Nephritis is an inflammation of the kidneys. Generally arising from an infection or an irregular immune reaction, it can occur in the glomeruli (the initial part of the kidneys' filtration system), the tubules and tissues surrounding them, or the blood vessels in the kidneys. Symptoms may include the sudden appearance of blood, protein, or clumps of red blood cells in the urine; fluid retention with tissue swelling; low urine volume; and dark or abnormally colored urine. While no treatment is available in most cases, some nephritis lends itself to antibiotic therapy. A diet low in protein and salt is recommended. High blood pressure is commonly controlled with drugs. Nephritis often leads to progressive kidney failure and the need for dialysis. From the macrobiotic perspective, nephritis is caused by long-term consumption of dietary extremes from both the yin and yang category. To help relieve this condition, observe Diet #3. Daikon is recommended to help discharge excess protein, fat, and mucus that have gathered in the kidney and impaired

its functioning. Take GRATED DAIKON cooked in water. Also daikon may be cooked by preparing ½ cup daikon, adding twice as much water, and boiling for a short time. A special drink for this condition consists of 1 part shiitake, soaked and chopped, 2 parts soaked adzuki beans, 1 part shredded dried daikon, and 3 to 4 parts water. This will relax and normalize the kidneys. Also soaking the feet in hot salt water for 5 to 7 minutes is helpful. A GINGER COMPRESS on the kidney will also help dissolve stagnation and improve blood and energy flow.

Tight Kidneys. Tight kidneys and bladder can result in frequent urination (see above), discomfort, and pain. They may also lead to more serious urinary conditions, including renal hypertension. Excessive protein and fat, particularly from animal sources, are a principal cause of tightness and hardness in the kidneys. Too much salt, or poor-quality salt such as refined table salt or unrefined gray sea salt, can also create an overly contracted condition. Baked flour products, including too much bread, crackers, cookies, and chips, also contribute to this condition. To relieve tight kidneys, follow the guidelines for Diet #2, using only light to moderate salt and seasonings. Beans can be prepared with a sweet taste, especially ADZUKI BEANS with a little rice syrup, lima beans with barley malt, or black soybeans with amasake. These become very sweet when cooked together and will relax the kidneys and bladder.

Daikon is also good for an overly contracted kidney condition. Take GRATED DAIKON cooked in water. Daikon may also be cooked by preparing ½ cup daikon, adding twice as much water, and boiling for a short time. A special drink to relax the kidneys is given in the home remedies section below. Also soaking the feet in hot salt water for 5 to 7 minutes is helpful. A GINGER COMPRESS on the kidney will also help dissolve stagnation and improve blood and energy flow.

SOLUTION

DIET

Follow the standard macrobiotic way of eating with emphasis on the following:

1. Eat whole grains, not refined grains, as the main dish of every meal. Buckwheat is particularly strengthening for the kidneys and bladder, but avoid if these organs are already too contracted. Black rice (such as wild rice) and other black or dark-colored grains are also nourishing for the urinary system.

2. Reduce hard baked flour products as much as possible. However, noodles may be taken several times a week, especially soba noodles (which contain buckwheat as well as whole wheat).

3. Avoid simple sugars (refined sugar, honey, and chocolate).

4. Avoid animal food with the exception of fish or seafood (preferably freshwater fish such as perch or trout) once or twice a week.

5. Beans are shaped like the kidneys and are particularly strengthening for the urinary system. Select among a variety of beans, particularly the smaller beans such as adzuki beans, lentils, chickpeas, and black soybeans. Bean products may also be eaten regularly, especially dried tofu.

6. Among vegetables, root vegetables and dried vegetables, including dried daikon and dried shiitake mushrooms, and winter vegetables such as kale particularly nourish the kidney function. Long-term pickles may also strengthen the urinary system, if not already too contracted.

7. Sea vegetables are very nourishing for the kidneys and bladder, especially kombu, unless the condition is too contracted.

8. The amount of salt (miso, shoyu, and sea salt) should be moderate.

9. As a rule, fruit and fruit juices should be limited or avoided, except in the case of overly contracted kidneys and bladder, in which case a small volume may be taken. Dried fruit, dark or black fruits such as blackberries, and watermelon are very relaxing for the kidneys and bladder.

10. Limit nuts and nut and seed butters until the condition improves. However, chestnuts and dark sesame seeds may be taken.

11. Among condiments, TEKKA, SHIO-KOMBU, shio nori, and dried fish condiment are strengthening.

12. Cut down on water to a moderate level, but do not reduce it too much. Besides BANCHA TWIG TEA, teas that nourish the kidney include KOMBU TEA and MU TEA.

13. Reduce the total volume of food, and chew more.

14. Avoid late-night eating, which puts stress on the urinary function.

15. Generally, for the kidneys and bladder use less liquid in cooking, use more oil and seasoning, and emphasize slightly longer cooking, including stewing, simmering, long-time pressing, marinating, and multiple food preparation techniques such as frying and then baking, blanching and then marinating, pickling and then sautéing.

16. Strengthening foods include FRIED RICE BALLS, MILLET CROQUETTES, rice pressure cooked with another grain, overnight oats, adzuki croquettes, baked beans, BLACK SOYBEANS WITH CHESTNUTS, and bean or grain stews.

LIFESTYLE

Follow the standard way-of-life suggestions, emphasizing the following:

1. Get up early and go to bed early. Lead an active life, both physically and mentally.

2. It is advisable to exercise moderately but not to exhaustion.

3. Avoid exposure to artificial electromagnetic radiation as much as possible, for example, from computers, television, cell phones, and other electronic devices.

4. Avoid wearing wool and synthetic clothing, especially nylon, which is irritating to the bladder. Wear cotton underwear and use cotton sheets and pillowcases.

5. The kidneys govern the body's overall vitality, including reproductive functions, and should always be protected and kept warm, especially during the winter or when it is cold.

6. Avoid long baths or showers, which can deplete the body of minerals.

7. Keep a positive mind and spirit.

8. Keep your personal things clean and in order.

9. Avoid relationships that cause you stress.

10. Spend time in nature as often as possible.

HOME REMEDIES

1. For most kidney conditions, prepare the special KIDNEY DRINK.

2. ADZUKI BEAN TEA is beneficial for the kidneys and bladder. Take 1 or 2 cups cooked with a little sea salt or a piece of kombu to help restore smooth urination and other functions.

3. CARROT-DAIKON DRINK will help eliminate fat and oil that have accumulated in the kidney or induce urination. Take 1 small cup every day for 5 days and then every second or third day for several weeks.

4. SHIITAKE-DAIKON TEA is also good to help eliminate the accumulation of fat. Take 1 small cup once every third day for 1 month.

5. For strength and vitality, especially for weakened conditions, KINPIRA SOUP may be taken 2 to 3 times a week.

6. RICE JUICE, the liquid that rises to the surface after cooking brown rice, may be taken frequently to harmonize the kidney, bladder, and their functions.

7. DAIKON NORI GINGER TEA can help stimulate the bladder and open the urinary passages.

8. For yang disorders, BLACK SOYBEAN TEA may be taken 3 times a day for several days.

9. For yin disorders, UME-SHO KUZU may be taken once every 3 days for several weeks.

10. A BODY SCRUB every day or twice a day, including over the kidney region, will promote better circulation and activate physical and mental energies.

11. A hot GINGER COMPRESS may be applied over the kidneys in the case of kidney stones. Repeat as necessary to help dissolve the obstruction and allow the stone to pass.

TABLE 27. KIDNEY AND BLADDER CONDITIONS AND DISORDERS

1. More Yin Cause	2. More Yang Cause	3. Yin and Yang Combined
Typical Symptoms		
Swelling	Swelling, especially joints	Swelling
Water intoxication	Water retention	
Sweating	Sweating	Sweating
Colorless urine	Dark urine	
Expansion of urinary systems	Constriction of urinary passages	Constriction or expansion of urinary tract
General fatigue		
Some frequent urination	Some frequent urination	
	Urination difficulty	Accumulation of mucus and fat in organs
Some pain and inflammation		Some pain and inflammation
Diseases		
Chronic oversleeping (most cases)	Chronic getting up early	Irregular rising
Insomnia: trouble sleeping before 2 A.M.	Insomnia: trouble sleeping after 2 a.m.	Irregular sleeping pattern
Fragmented dreams	Vivid or disturbing dreams	Nightmares
Cystitis	Oliguria	Uremia
Enuresis (bed-wetting) (most cases)	Dysuria	
Pyelitis		Nephritis
Moveable kidney		
Some retention	Some retention	Edema
Some anuria	Some stricture	Some anuria
		Kidney stone
Incontinence		Bladder cancer
		Kidney cancer

CAUTION

1. Kidney disorders commonly lead to high blood pressure and heart problems, so the heart and circulatory system may also need to be strengthened.

2. A macrobiotic way of eating may benefit a person undergoing kidney dialysis or taking strong medications for deteriorating kidney and bladder functions. Please consult your physician about gradually reducing such treatment or medication as improvement is experienced as a result of dietary or lifestyle changes.

MEDICAL EVIDENCE

PLANT FOODS PROTECT AGAINST URINARY IMBALANCES

British researchers report that increased intake of foods high in fiber and complex carbohydrate such as whole grains and reduced intake of animal protein, sugar, and refined carbohydrates reduced the excretion of calcium, oxalate, and uric acid in the urine.

Source: P. N. Rao et al., "Dietary Management of Urinary Risk Factors in Renal Stone Formers," *British Journal of Urology* 54:578–83, 1982.

◎ LIVER PROBLEMS

The liver performs many operations in the body, actively coordinating various digestive, circulatory, and excretory functions. It filters toxins from the blood, makes and transports bile, controls blood sugar levels, converts carbohydrates, fat, and protein into one another, and manufactures hormones and enzymes, creating proteins, especially those needed for the blood to clot. The liver is such an important organ that the *Yellow Emperor's Classic*, the ancient authority on Oriental medicine and philosophy, compares it to the general of the army, second in importance only to the heart. While it is impossible to live without a liver, even if up to 80 percent of the organ has been removed, it will regenerate and continue to function.

In addition to hepatitis, jaundice, cirrhosis, and liver cancer *(see "Cancer")*, the major liver disorders, a variety of strong emotions and abnormal behaviors are associated with this organ. A healthy liver contributes to a calm, patient character and disposition, courage and endurance, a clear vision or goal to be achieved and an adventurous spirit. A balanced diet, centered on whole grains and vegetable-quality food, will lead to the development of these qualities, as well as help recover from past liver troubles.

SYMPTOMS

The following symptoms may accompany liver troubles:

1. Tightness, swelling, pain, or soreness in the liver or liver area. To diagnose yourself, place your fingers under the rib cage on the right side. If you can't insert your fingers here without encountering hardness or if you feel pain or tension, the liver is swollen. If the liver is healthy, you should be able to insert all four fingers without any pain or discomfort

2. Tightness in the abdominal center on the left side of the body

3. Swelling, pain, or other abnormalities on

the big toe, especially on the inside part of the toe along the liver meridian

4. Hardness, stiffness, or swelling along the liver meridian, which runs up the inside back of the legs, etc.

5. One or more vertical lines in the center of the forehead between the eyebrows or puffiness in this region. Deep lines tend to be caused by contraction and show too much consumption of animal food, salt, or baked food. Lines with puffiness tend to be caused by yin, expansive items such as sugar, alcohol, and too much fat and oil.

6. Eye problems are associated with the liver, since the liver meridian passes through the eyes. They may become inflamed, swollen, or lose focus.

7. Impatience, upset, anger, rage, aggression, and violent thoughts, emotions, or actions.

8. Inability to stay in one place and tendency to move about constantly.

CAUSE

I. In structure and activity, the liver is compact, active, and centrally located, making it one of the most yang organs of the body. Thus it is especially affected by eating too many yang animal foods, including beef, chicken, eggs, pork, dairy, fish, and seafood, as well as salt and baked foods. It also attracts its opposite, strong yin, in the form of sugar, alcohol, and oily, greasy foods of both animal and vegetable origin. All of these items are extremely weakening to the liver. For example, excess sugar in the body is stored by the liver in the form of glycogen. If we consume large amounts of simple carbohydrates, such as white flour, white sugar, fruit, dairy, and honey, they will quickly exceed the liver's storage capacity. This will not only overtax the liver, but also allow the carbohydrates to get into the bloodstream, weakening the body as a whole and reducing natural immunity to disease. Chemicals, pesticides, genetically modified organisms, and other potentially hazardous material also particularly affect the liver, because of its role in filtering the blood of toxins.

2. In traditional Far Eastern medicine, the word for anger is *kan-shaku*, or "liver pain." A hard, swollen liver creates irritability, frustration, and impatience that can easily manifest as anger, rage, aggression, and violence. Typically, heavy animal food tightens and hardens the liver, while sugar, alcohol, drugs, or other strong yin are like the match that sets off the explosion. Hence, much hyperactivity and violence arise from eating candy bars, soft drinks, and other sugary foods, as well as beer and whiskey, and drugs of all kinds. A great deal of disruptive and antisocial behavior in the home, school, workplace, and community and among nations stems from underlying liver imbalances. Specific causes include the following:

a. Overeating, even of good-quality foods.

b. Overconsumption of foods that contribute to stagnation and tightness of the liver, for example, an excess of flour products, including bread, cookies, muffins, crackers, chips, and cake.

c. Overconsumption of foods that loosen and weaken the liver, for example, an excess of products made of simple sugars, including refined sugar, chocolate, and honey; fruits, fruit juices, and soda;

vegetable-quality oils, dressings, sauces, and spreads.

d. Overconsumption of foods high in fat and cholesterol, including meat, poultry, eggs, milk, cheese, and other dairy products, which cause the liver to become hard and swollen.

e. Over- or underconsumption of salt. A deficiency of salt in the diet can weaken the liver, while too much salt can harden the liver.

f. Midnight snacking or late-night eating, which burdens the liver at night and does not allow it to rest.

g. Excessive intake of drugs or supplements. Proper doses and kinds of medications or supplements can temporarily help alleviate certain conditions, but taking them for too long can particularly burden the liver.

h. Lack of exercise. In individuals with a sedentary lifestyle, digestion, absorption, and blood circulation do not function smoothly, and liver function may be affected.

i. Tension and stress. Too much conflict or stress in the home or workplace can place additional stress on the liver and contribute to mental and emotional problems, especially irritability, anger, and upset.

j. Disease: various diseases, and the treatments for them, may contribute to liver problems. In this case, it is necessary to first recover from the original disease.

FORMS

Cirrhosis. Cirrhosis of the liver is the destruction of normal liver tissue that leaves non-functioning scar tissue surrounding areas of functioning liver tissue. The most common cause of cirrhosis is alcohol abuse. Among people age 45 to 65, cirrhosis is the third most common cause of death, after heart disease and cancer. In many parts of Asia and Africa, chronic hepatitis is a major cause of cirrhosis. Some people may have no symptoms; others are weak, have a poor appetite, feel sick, and lose weight. Other possible symptoms include jaundice, cough or vomiting of large amounts of blood, muscle wasting, redness of the palms, a curling up of the fingers, small spiderlike veins in the skin, breast enlargement in men, salivary gland enlargement in the cheeks, hair loss, shrinking of the testes, and abnormal nerve function.

In *primary biliary cirrhosis*, a latticework of scar tissue develops throughout the liver, beginning with the bile ducts, blocking the flow of bile out of the liver and causing the bile to spill into the bloodstream. About 50 percent of cases have an enlarged liver, and 25 percent have an enlarged spleen. About 15 percent have small yellow deposits in the skin or eyelids. This condition is treated medically with supplements of calcium and vitamins A, D, and K, which are not properly absorbed where there is insufficient bile. While nutritional supplementation is moving in the right direction, a comprehensive dietary approach such as that offered below offers more lasting relief. As a degenerative disorder, cirrhosis may involve structural and functional changes to the liver, and advanced cases may be difficult to reverse. However, improvement will generally be experienced on a macrobiotic diet. Observe the standard guidelines for Diet #1 for conditions caused primarily by extreme yin dietary factors.

Hepatitis. Hepatitis is an inflammation of the liver. The most common cause is a virus, particularly one of five hepatitis viruses named A, B, C, D, and E. However, hepatitis can also be caused by infectious mononucleosis, yellow fever, or cytomegalovirus infection. Major non-viral causes are alcohol and drugs. Hepatitis can be acute (lasting less than 6 months) or chronic.

Hepatitis A spreads primarily from the bowel movements of one person to the mouth of another, usually from poor hygiene. Water- and food-borne epidemics are common in developing countries. Eating contaminated raw shellfish can spread hepatitis A. *Hepatitis B* is commonly spread through contaminated blood or blood products, especially among injecting drug users who share needles, as well as between sexual partners, both heterosexual and homosexual. A pregnant woman can transmit the virus to her baby at birth. Hepatitis B can be carried by healthy people who are chronic carriers. *Hepatitis C* is linked to 80 percent of the hepatitis cases that arise from blood transfusions. It usually comes from shared needles, and sexual transmission is rare. Hepatitis C often leads to chronic hepatitis and some cases of cirrhosis and liver cancer. It is also associated with alcoholic liver disease. *Hepatitis D* occurs only as a co-infection with B and makes it more severe. *Hepatitis E* causes occasional epidemics similar to those caused by A, mostly in developing countries.

The symptoms of acute viral hepatitis usually appear suddenly. They include poor appetite, a feeling of being ill, nausea, vomiting, often a fever, distaste for smoking (especially among smokers), dark urine, and worsening jaundice. Jaundice usually peaks in 1–2 weeks and fades after 2–4 weeks. It can range from minor to serious and even fatal. Usually hepatitis B is more serious than hepatitis A. Hepatitis C is unpredictable. Acute hepatitis usually lasts 4 to 8 weeks, even without treatment. Hepatitis A rarely, if ever, becomes chronic. Hepatitis B becomes chronic in 5–10 percent of cases. Hepatitis C becomes chronic in 75 percent of cases, though is often mild and without symptoms; 20 percent of those with this form develop cirrhosis. Modern medicine uses vaccines to treat hepatitis A and B, but there are none for hepatitis C, D, or E.

Chronic hepatitis, though much less common, can last for years. Though usually mild, it can lead to cirrhosis and liver failure. About one-third of cases develop after a bout of acute viral hepatitis.

Overall, hepatitis arises from consumption of extreme foods, including sugar, chocolate, and other sweets; soft drinks and other carbonated drinks; milk, yogurt, ice cream, and other light dairy foods; refined grains and pasta; tropical foods, excessive fruit and juice, spices and herbs, too much fat and oil, and other predominantly expansive items. Relative to each other, hepatitis A is slightly more yin, caused primarily by sugar, sweets, milk, and ice cream; hepatitis B is more yang, commonly also involving the intake of animal food and greasy and fatty food; and hepatitis C arises from yin and yang combined, including too much oily, greasy food, foods high in fat and protein, alcohol, stimulants, and sugar and chocolate. Lifestyle and environmental influences as well as dietary practices may contribute to the onset of hepatitis. These include electrical and microwave cooking, exposure to other artificial electromagnetic fields, and vaccines, X rays, and other medical procedures and operations.

To recover from hepatitis, observe the standard guidelines for Diet #1 for hepatitis A and E; Diet #2 for hepatitis B and D; and Diet #3 for hepatitis C. All foods are to be cooked. Avoid all raw foods, especially raw salad. No hard baked flour products are to be taken for 1 month, though noodles may be taken once a week if well cooked and served in soup. Oil should be avoided for 1 month, after which a small volume may be used 2 to 3 times a week. No animal food is recommended, not even fish and seafood. Avoid ginger, garlic, spices, and stimulants that can cause the virus to spread. Avoid fruits and juice for the first month. Then a small amount of cooked fruit, stewed with a pinch of sea salt, may be taken. Avoid nuts. Avoid vinegar for two months, even brown rice and umeboshi vinegar. Then a small amount may be taken 2–3 times a week. Overall, a moderate salt taste should be used in cooking.

As special drinks or dishes, SWEET VEGE-TABLE DRINK is helpful, 1 small cup daily, adding burdock and dried shiitake mushroom in cooking. UME-KUZU is also helpful taken daily or every other day for several days to strengthen the blood. KINPIRA SOUP may be taken twice a week, including leafy green vegetables cooked in the soup. The special drink for liver conditions in the home remedies section below is helpful for all types of hepatitis.

If jaundice accompanies the condition, take one of the following: (1) sour apple juice, 2 cups daily for 5 days; (2) stewed sour apple, once a day for 5 days; (3) sour apple grated with a little water to make applesauce, adding a pinch of sea salt at the end of cooking, 1 cup daily for 5 days.

If the liver is infected and swollen, apply a CABBAGE PLASTER over the affected region. The plaster may also be applied on all of the toes, especially the first toe. First apply a hot towel on the region for 3 minutes to improve circulation. Leave the cabbage plaster on for 3–4 hours every day. If the liver is too active, apply the compress only on the feet. A cabbage plaster may also be applied on the throat and the eyes in some cases. Apply for just a couple of hours daily. The liver meridian runs through these areas and the plaster will help calm down the liver energy.

Jaundice. Bile is secreted by the liver and normally flows either to the gallbladder or the duodenum where it aids in the emulsifying, or breakdown, of fats and oils. When the bile ducts become blocked or obstructed, bile gets into the bloodstream and its yellowish color may produce a yellowish facial and skin discoloration. The urine may also turn a dark color from the discharge of excessive bile pigments. Heavy animal foods, dairy food, sugar, oily and greasy foods of both animal and vegetable origin, and other foods that create fat and mucus in the body are the main causes of blockage in the bile ducts. In addition to discontinuing these foods and eating a standard diet, avoid all fish and seafood until the condition improves. Follow the standard guidelines for Diet #2, for conditions caused by more yang factors. Hard, green leafy vegetables should be taken regularly, especially daikon greens, to help dissolve fat and mucus in the bile ducts. Mugwort tea is helpful for jaundice. The liver drink in the home remedies section below is helpful.

A sour taste is also recommended for this

condition. Take one of the following: (1) sour apple juice, 2 cups daily for 5 days; (2) stewed sour apple, once a day for 5 days; (3) sour apple grated with a little water to make applesauce, adding a pinch of sea salt at the end of cooking, 1 cup daily for 5 days.

Externally, a GINGER COMPRESS may be applied over the liver and gallbladder regions to help melt the obstructions. These can be applied daily until the skin color returns to normal.

SOLUTION

DIET

For liver disorders, follow the standard guidelines noted above, paying special attention to the following:

1. Eat whole grains, not refined grains, as the main dish of every meal. Grains that especially nourish the liver are whole barley, whole wheat, and hato mugi (prepared alone or cooked together with other grains). Natural, unyeasted sourdough bread, udon noodles, seitan, and other whole-wheat products may also be taken from time to time, but avoid hard baked products until the condition improves.

2. Eat organically grown food as much as possible, as pesticides, chemical fertilizers, and other additives irritate the liver.

3. Avoid simple sugars (refined sugar, honey, and chocolate) that in excess are converted into fatty acid and stored in the liver.

4. Avoid animal food as much as possible that can overburden and stagnate the liver. Eat only white-meat fish, if craved, in small volume, once every 10 to 14 days, and serve with grated daikon.

5. Minimize fat consumption, including reducing vegetable-quality oil. Avoid raw oil, such as in salad dressings, sauces, and dips.

6. Leafy greens, especially dandelions, chives, and scallions in the spring, help to release stagnation in the body caused by consumption of yang foods during the autumn and winter and are especially soothing to the liver.

7. Avoid vegetables that originated in tropical regions, such as tomatoes, eggplants, and peppers.

8. The amount of salt (miso, shoyu, and sea salt) should be moderate.

9. Cut down on water to a moderate level, but do not reduce it too much.

10. Take a small amount of sea vegetables on a daily basis.

11. Natural fermentation is a product of earth's rising or expansive energy. Naturally processed miso made from barley and soybeans is especially good for the liver, as are UMEBOSHI PLUMS, sauerkraut, and pickled vegetables, especially light or quick pickles. Be careful of the salt in pickled foods.

12. A sour flavor naturally nourishes the liver and its functions. It counteracts the effects of rich, greasy food, functioning as a solvent and breaking down fats and protein. Examples: lemon, lime, pickles, sauerkraut, sour apple, sour plum, vinegar, leek, apple, blackberry, raspberry, sourdough bread, tangerine, and tomato (which can be used medicinally for very contracted conditions). However, if the liver is infected, swollen, or inflamed, a sour taste should be avoided, including brown rice vinegar and umeboshi vinegar, for up to several months or until the condition improves.

13. BARLEY MALT also releases tightness in

the liver, but use sparingly. Avoid raisins and raisin bread, which are not good for the liver.

14. Reduce the total volume of food, and chew more, ideally 50 to 200 times per mouthful.

15. Avoid late-night eating.

LIFESTYLE

Observe the standard way-of-life suggestions, emphasizing the following:

1. Irritability, upset, and anger accompany many liver problems. Try to develop patience and be as calm and peaceful as possible.

2. Keep physically active, walking outdoors a half hour each day and doing light to moderate exercise. Stretching exercises, including yoga and tai chi, are very helpful.

3. A healthy liver contributes to vision, idealism, and values. Focusing more on aesthetic, mental, cultural, and spiritual pursuits and less on material achievements will gradually strengthen and stabilize the liver and its functions.

4. Use only cotton garments next to the skin and avoid leather, metal, and other materials on or near the liver.

5. The eyes correspond to the liver. Keeping the eyes in good health will benefit the liver. Avoid eyestrain, particularly from too much television or computer use. Eye exercises, birdwatching, stargazing, and other activities that naturally stimulate the eyes may be helpful.

HOME REMEDIES

1. For most liver conditions, the following special drink will be helpful. Prepare it with 1 part dried shiitake, 1 part sprouts (such as soy or mung bean sprouts), 1 part daikon greens, and 1 part buckwheat groats. Add 4 to 5 times as much water and boil 25 to 30 minutes to make a tea. Drink 1 to 2 cups for about 3 weeks and then every other day for 3 more weeks. In the case of jaundice, use sour apple juice instead. Drink 1 cup a day for 3 to 4 days.

2. Avoid dried daikon for most liver conditions, as this will make them worse. Fresh daikon is helpful.

3. Dried shiitake is beneficial for the liver, especially for a more yang, contracted condition. A maximum of 3 medium shiitakes may be taken daily.

4. For liver problems caused by excessive yin food consumption, 1 UMEBOSHI PLUM may be taken for several days, or UME-SHO KUZU may be taken 1 cup a day for several days.

5. For liver problems caused by excessive yang food consumption, apple cider or barley malt may be added to KUZU DRINK and taken 1 cup a day for several days. Other remedies for this condition include pouring hot BANCHA TWIG TEA over shiso leaves, eating the leaves, and drinking the tea; taking a little rice vinegar or ume vinegar; eating a small side dish of baked or stewed apples; or adding fresh scallions as a garnish to MISO SOUP or vegetable side dishes.

6. To release old fats and oils in the liver, take CARROT-DAIKON DRINK 3 times a week for several weeks.

7. GRATED DAIKON WITH SHOYU is beneficial to help release fats and oil.

8. Lemon is beneficial for the liver. Cook lemon in water after slicing. A little sweet taste, such as from barley malt, may be added. Sour green apple, cooked with 3 to 4 drops of lemon, is also helpful for the liver.

9. To help eliminate excess protein, especially animal-quality protein, that has gathered in the liver, LEAFY GREENS JUICE is helpful.

10. DO-IN self-massage can stimulate the liver; rub the two large toes of each foot together. Also rotate the large toes about 50 times in each direction.

11. Since the eyes and liver correspond, exercises to stimulate the eyes may be helpful. Rub the palms until they are hot and cover the eyes. Leaving the eyes open, move them up and down and then right to left approximately 30 times.

12. If experiencing pain, first apply a HOT TOWEL COMPRESS over the liver region for a few minutes, followed by a POTATO PLASTER or LEAFY GREENS PLASTER for about 2 hours. In some cases, a person with this condition will also experience abdominal swelling due to the retention of liquid. In this case, after applying a hot towel, apply a BUCKWHEAT PLASTER to the swollen region.

CAUTION

1. Many liver problems result from overeating. It is effective to eat small quantities of food or observe a semi-fast for several days. Reduce the amount and number of meals and chew very well, up to 200 times per mouthful. After FASTING or SEMI-FASTING, eat only brown rice soup with leafy green vegetables for a brief period. If miso is added to the soup, use only a small amount. After several days, widen the diet to include the standard dietary guidelines, but avoid all animal foods until the condition has improved.

2. Avoid or limit unnecessary medications, supplements, vitamins, and others as much as possible, as these put an added burden on the liver.

MEDICAL EVIDENCE

DAIRY LINKED WITH HEPATITIS B

In a study of the effects of hepatitis B virus and animal food intake on the development of liver cancer, Stanford University researchers reported that reducing the amount of dairy protein in the diet significantly reduced hepatitis B infection in laboratory experiments.

Source: J. F. Hu, "Repression of Hepatitis B Virus (HBV) Transgene and HBV-Induced Liver Injury by Low Protein Diet," *Oncogene* 15(23):2795–801, 1997.

CASE HISTORY

MACROBIOTICS HELPS TRAVELER OVERCOME HEPATITIS A

While traveling in India, Yuko Horio began to eat a lot of tropical fruits, hot tea with milk and sugar, and sugar cane juice served with ice. She had practiced macrobiotics in her native Japan, but not strictly, and the hot temperature and humidity of the tropics made these foods seem very appealing. After several days, she felt extremely tired, lost her appetite, and had diarrhea. The sugar cane juice satisfied her cravings for liquid. Back home, her symptoms persisted for a month. In early autumn, jaundice set in and she was diagnosed with acute hepatitis A. Her doctor recommended immediate hospitalization and steroid treatment and warned that if her condition worsened to fulminant hepatitis, she could die within a week. A nurse told her she had never before seen such dangerously abnormal liver function levels. Meanwhile, a macrobiotic friend inspired her to use food as medicine. At home she observed a strict healing diet, consisting of brown rice, gomashio, miso soup, cooked konnyaku (dried gourd), and other simple dishes and chewed her food more than 100 times per mouthful. Gradually, improvement came and the 34-year-old woman was able to return to work in a few weeks. Within another month, her liver tests were almost normal, and she has been healthy ever since.

Source: Gale Jack and Wendy Esko, editors, *Women's Health Guide* (Becket, Mass.: One Peaceful World Press, 1997), pp. 11–13.

◎ LUNG PROBLEMS

Problems with the lungs, the main organs of the respiratory system, range from simple coughs and congestion to asthma, bronchitis, and other moderate illnesses to pneumonia, pleurisy, and other serious disorders. Besides the lungs, the respiratory system includes the nasal passages and sinuses, the larynx and vocal cords, trachea or windpipe, bronchi and bronchioli, alveoli or air sacs, and the thoracic or pleural cavity. Respiratory problems affect millions of people, and nasal and sinus congestion are among the most common ailments in modern society. About 70 percent of the waste excreted from the body is discharged in the form of carbon dioxide and other gases through the lungs. A healthy diet and lifestyle will eliminate the buildup of mucus in the lungs and sinuses (the main cause of respiratory problems) and contribute to proper breathing and the improved health of these organs. *See also "Lung Cancer" in "Cancer," and "Tuberculosis" in "Infectious Diseases."*

SYMPTOMS

The following symptoms may accompany lung problems:

1. Coughing
2. Shortness of breath, labored breathing, chest pain
3. Respiratory infections
4. Soreness or tightness in the chest
5. Sallow, pale, or slightly puffy appearance on the cheeks
6. Rounding and tensing of the shoulders
7. Drooping posture

The cheeks correspond with the lungs in traditional Oriental diagnosis. Evaluating these and other signs may show developing lung problems.

1. Pimples on the cheeks show accumulation of fatty acid and mucus from dairy and sugar.

2. White cheeks show too much dairy accumulating in the lungs.

3. Red cheeks show overactive blood capillaries in the lungs from excessive fruit, juice, spices, sugar, and stimulants.

4. Drawn, overly tight cheeks result from too much salt, fish, poultry, dry or baked foods.

5. Vertical lines on the cheeks indicate restricted blood flow, contracted alveoli, and tightened chest muscles.

6. Brown blotches on the cheeks show acidosis from excessive sugar intake.

7. Beauty marks on the cheeks indicate past fever in the lungs, while moles show excessive protein and sugar intake.

8. Constipation and other intestinal difficulties correspond with overactive lungs.

9. Discolorations, blemishes, hardness, looseness, or other abnormalities along the lung meridian may show developing lung problems. The lung meridian runs from the stomach through the large intestine, lungs, throat, shoulder, and down the inner arm to the seam between the thumb and first finger and to the outer corner of the thumbnail.

10. Weakness or tension in the thumb commonly shows lung problems.

CAUSES

1. The primary cause of most respiratory disorders is long-term dietary imbalance. Pollution, smoking, and exposure to other chemicals and toxins in the environment are often contributory factors, but diet governs underlying susceptibility to these influences.

2. The lungs are located in the upper body, showing the influence of earth's expansive force. At the same time, they are extremely contracted in their structure, showing the influence of heaven's force. The lungs, as a result, attract both types of energy, and excessive intake of extreme foods from either category can harm the lungs. These include meat, eggs, poultry, dairy products, refined flour, sugar, fats and oils, excessive fruits and juices, excessive baked foods, alcohol, stimulants, chemicals, and drugs.

3. Overconsumption of acid foods, mucus-forming foods, and fatty foods can lead to the accumulation of excess in the lungs. Mucus can coat the bronchi, air sacs, and capillaries in the lungs, become firmly lodged, and remain a long time. Dairy foods especially, but also hard baked flour products and refined grains, can produce mucus in the lungs.

4. If the lungs are burdened with fat and mucus, especially from dairy food, heavy carbon compounds and other particulates from tobacco may become trapped in the lungs, further irritating these organs and leading to the development of tumors.

FORMS

Asthma. This chronic lung disease is accompanied by tightening of the chest during breathing, constant coughing, copious mucus, and congestion. Typically, sufferers experience asthma attacks triggered by exposure to pollen, grass, dust, mold, cigarette smoke, animal hair, or other environmental stimuli, as well as certain medications and foods high in sulfites. These may be mild or severe and be of short duration or persist for a day or more. A recurrence is common, often lasting much longer, days or weeks. An estimated 15 million Americans suffer from asthma, especially children, for whom it is the leading cause of school absences. Physicians usually treat asthma with bronchodilators, drugs designed to keep the airways open. These come in the form of inhalers or are taken orally and may have serious side effects, including high blood pressure.

While environmental or chemical triggers can bring on an attack, the main cause of asthma is overconsumption of strong yin foods and beverages, especially mucus-producing foods such as dairy food, refined flour products, and sugar and sugary foods and beverages. The excessive intake of these items can cause obstruction in the respiratory passages as a result of spasm of the muscles in the bronchial tubes or the oversecretion of mucus.

To relieve asthma, the standard way of eating should be observed, following the guidelines in Diet #1 for more yin conditions. Be careful to limit the amount of fluids consumed or used in cooking as well as cutting back sharply on the intake of fruit, juice, fresh salads, and other expansive items. Of course, extreme foods of all kinds should be discontinued. With proper diet, asthma can usually be relieved within several weeks.

To prevent or relieve an asthma attack, apply a hot GINGER COMPRESS repeatedly to the chest region. A small amount of GOMASHIO or UMEBOSHI PLUMS may be taken. These will cause the alveoli to contract, offering immediate relief. Asthma occurs more frequently in wet, humid climates, so a drier environment may be helpful while recovering. Using a dehumidifier to reduce moisture in the air; exposure to a bright, sunny environment, and access to fresh air (including putting green plants in every room) are also beneficial.

Bronchitis. Bronchitis is an inflammation of the bronchial passages. It is accompanied by strong, constant coughing; the discharge of yellow, white, or green mucus; fever and chills; soreness or tightness in the chest; and pain during deep breathing. The acute form of the disease comes and goes rapidly, usually a matter of days, and is associated with a viral or bacterial infection. The chronic form of bronchitis is more serious, affecting primarily obese people and heavy smok-

ers. Like emphysema, it can be life-threatening and usually requires medical attention.

The chief cause of bronchitis is the intake of excessive foods and beverages in the strong yin category, including cold drinks, fruit, ice cream, and sugar. To relieve this condition, discontinue these foods, as well as extreme yang foods, which can also have an acidic effect. Start the standard macrobiotic way of eating, focusing on slightly more yang adjustments, such as stronger seasoning, longer cooking, proportionately more root vegetables, sea vegetables, and stronger condiments. Observe Diet #1 for strong yin conditions.

The fever that accompanies bronchitis is generally mild and serves to help burn off these items. However, if the fever becomes too high, a TOFU PLASTER or LEAFY GREENS PLASTER may be applied to the forehead. Meanwhile, a hot GINGER COMPRESS or MUSTARD PLASTER can be applied regularly to the chest to help loosen mucus and improve breathing.

Coughing. Coughing accompanies many conditions and disorders. It may be mild or severe, acute or chronic. Medically, coughing is often suppressed with medication or drugs. However, from the macrobiotic view, coughing is simply an abnormal discharge mechanism by which the body attempts to eliminate mucus, toxins, or other excessive metabolic energy that cannot be processed through normal eliminatory channels. Coughs can be classified as more yin or more yang. The more yin type of cough is generally milder, located more superficially in the chest, longer-lasting (often chronic), and is wet, commonly resulting in copious mucus being discharged from the lungs and bronchi. A yang cough is strong (explosive, barking, hacking), located deeper in the chest, less long-lasting (often acute), and dry. Extreme yin foods, especially milk, ice cream, and other dairy food, as well as sugar and sweets, soft drinks, spices, and stimulants, are frequent causes of yin, wet coughs. Hard baked flour products, too much animal food, and too much salt or salty foods can cause a yang, dry cough.

While mild coughs can usually be allowed to run their course, coughs that become uncomfortable or painful can be controlled through special dishes and drinks. To relieve a more yin cough, prepare any of the following: LOTUS ROOT TEA, MU TEA, or brown rice and lotus tea (made by roasting a handful of brown rice, adding a handful of chopped lotus root, and adding a small volume of shiso leaves; add 3 cups of water and boil down to 1 cup).

To relieve a more yang, dry cough, prepare any of the following: SHIITAKE TEA, rice tea with citrus rind (made by roasting a handful of rice and adding chopped lemon or orange rind; add 3 to 4 cups of water and boil down to 1 cup), BLACK SOYBEAN TEA, or ame-daikon tea (made by combining rice syrup with grated daikon in equal amounts, pouring hot BANCHA TWIG TEA over the mixture, and taking 1–2 tablespoons every day).

Cystic Fibrosis. Cystic fibrosis results when the walls of the bronchi become covered with mucus, leading to deep wheezing and coughing. The alveoli can fill with phlegm, making breathing more difficult and choking off the blood supply. The main cause of cystic fibrosis is frequent consumption of dairy food, sugar, fruit, and saturated fats. In addition to following the standard macrobiotic diet, mucus buildup can be relieved with a LOTUS PLASTER or MUSTARD PLASTER. Follow the standard dietary guidelines for Diet #3 for conditions arising from both extreme yin and yang factors.

Emphysema. Emphysema is a degenerative ailment in which the lungs lose their elasticity, leading to chronic coughing, shortness of breath, and sometimes wheezing. Men between 50 and 70, especially heavy smokers, are most affected, but it is increasingly frequent in women. Emphysema is considered irreversible and is the leading cause of death from lung ailments in the United States. From the macrobiotic perspective, the underlying cause of this disorder is primarily consumption of excessive yin foods and beverages, especially milk and other dairy foods, sugar and sweets, soft drinks, too much fruit and juice, frozen foods, chemicalized foods, stimulants, spices, and other more expansive items. These cause the alveoli, or air sacs, to dilate and fuse or burst. Bursting reduces the surface area in which oxygen and carbon dioxide are exchanged, causing breathing to become more rapid and burdensome. The end result is breathlessness, increased pressure on the heart, disability, and eventual death. A balanced standard macrobiotic diet can help control, slow, and often stop the progression of this disease. But once the alveoli have begun to fuse, it is difficult to reverse the process completely or increase the surface area of the lung tissue. Hence, strong yang factors, especially meat, poultry, and other animal foods, as well as smoking (which has a contracting effect), can aggravate the condition. Observe the standard guidelines for Diet #3 for conditions arising from a combination of dietary extremes.

Pleurisy. Pleurisy, an inflammation of the pleura, the membrane surrounding the lungs and rib cage, is generally accompanied by severe sharp chest pain, a high fever, and pooling of liquid in between the chest membranes. It is generally a complication of pneumonia, tuberculosis, congestive heart failure, or other disease that affects the lungs and its protective membrane. Pleurisy patients usually remain bedridden for 1 to 3 months until their condition improves. Antibiotics, anti-inflammatory drugs, aspirin or other analgesics, or cough syrup with codeine are commonly prescribed to treat pleurisy or its symptoms.

From the macrobiotic perspective, pleurisy is caused primarily by the overconsumption of liquid, especially cold or iced soft drinks, frozen fruit juices, and carbonated or mineral waters. Watery foods, sugary foods, and other foods and beverages that increase fluids in the body or dissolve rapidly into water are contributing factors. Through a balanced diet, pleurisy can be relieved in 1 or 2 weeks in many cases. Follow the dietary guidelines for Diet #1 for strong yin conditions.

Pneumonia. Pneumonia is an inflammation of the lungs that is associated with exposure to various viral, bacterial, fungal, or chemical agents. *Viral pneumonia,* the milder form, is usually accompanied by chest pains, coughing, muscle aches, sore throat, enlarged lymph nodes in the neck, and low fever and chills. *Bacterial pneumonia* is more serious, involving sharp chest pains, labored breathing, severe fatigue, high fever, and coughing up thick mucus and blood. Until the advent of antibiotics, bacterial pneumonia was often fatal. Today the emergence of drug-resistant strains of pneumonia have made treatment increasingly difficult, and mortality rates are on the rise. From the macrobiotic view, pneumonia is caused by the repeated consumption of meat, eggs, and other strong animal foods. It is more prevalent in the spring and summer. While the underlying cause is yang, symptoms are activated by strong yin, including dairy, sugar, excessive fruit and fruit juice, cold drinks, and other expansive foods and beverages. In addition to discontinuing all these foods and observing the dietary guidelines for Diet #3, arising from a combination of strong yin and yang factors, a cold application may be placed over the lungs to bring down the high fever. In the Far East, a CARP PLASTER was traditionally used. The carp is a very yin fish and proved to be very effective to bring down the temperature. If carp is not available, a TOFU PLASTER, LEAFY GREENS PLASTER, or POTATO PLASTER may be applied, and even ice or cold ground beef may be beneficial.

SOLUTION

DIET

Observe the standard macrobiotic diet, paying special attention to the following:

1. Eat whole grains as the principal food at every meal. Brown rice is especially beneficial for the lungs. It may be prepared in a variety of ways, including pressure-cooked, boiled, fried, and made into rice balls. Rye is also beneficial and may be taken in small volume, especially cooked together with rice.

2. Hard baked flour products should be

avoided or minimized until the condition improves, as they can create mucus and stagnation in the lungs. However, if cravings arise, a small volume of unyeasted sourdough bread may be taken. If the condition is not too contracted, seitan or wheat gluten may be taken in moderate amounts.

3. Avoid foods from both extremes, including meat, eggs, poultry, and dairy, as well as refined grains and grain products; sugar, chocolate, and other refined sweets; nuts and nut and seed butters (with the exception of chestnuts); tropical foods; excessive fruit and juice; alcohol; stimulants; spices; and drugs.

4. Black soybeans are especially good for the lungs. As the condition permits, deep-fried tofu or tempeh, as well as miso and natto, may be eaten.

5. Among vegetables, the small, more compact leafy greens, including watercress, arugula, mustard greens, and parsley, are recommended. Overall, root vegetables nourish the lungs, including burdock, carrot, daikon, red radish, and jinenjo. Broccoli, cauliflower, and Brussels sprouts are also very beneficial to the lungs.

6. The lotus plant, including roots and seeds, is especially beneficial to the lungs.

7. Among sea vegetables, HIJIKI is especially good for the lungs.

8. Generally, fish and seafood should be avoided until the condition improves, especially for more contracted conditions. In the event that fish is craved, a small volume of white-meat fish may be eaten once every 7 to 10 days. Small, compact ocean fish such as smelt are best for the lungs.

9. A pungent taste is strengthening to the lungs. Good-quality soy sauce, ginger, mustard, rice vinegar, or horseradish may be used as seasonings.

10. TEKKA, GOMASHIO, roasted sea vegetable powder, and sesame seeds may be taken as condiments.

11. Sweets and sweeteners should be avoided as much as possible. However, if cravings arise, a small volume of grain-based sweetener, especially BROWN RICE SYRUP, may be taken.

12. In addition to BANCHA TWIG TEA, roasted brown rice tea may be taken and is harmonizing for the lungs.

13. Among cooking styles, stronger cooking nourishes the lungs, except in the case of overly contracted conditions. These styles include baking, broiling, kinpira, long sautéing, nishime-style dishes, and slightly more oil, salt, and seasoning. A little more pressure, less liquid, and longer cooking time may also be used.

LIFESTYLE

1. Get up early and breathe in the fresh, early morning air.

2. Avoid synthetic fibers, wool and silk, and other fabrics that may impede breathing and energy exchange. Wear cotton next to the skin and use cotton sheets and pillowcases.

3. Avoid industrial fumes and gases, smoggy and dusty air, and other polluted environments. Walk in the woods, along the seashore, or in the fields where the air is clean.

4. Avoid home furnishings that may include asbestos fibers, including aprons, potholders, cooking fabrics, and some floor tiles and building and construction materials. Use natural materials as much as possible.

5. Place green plants in every room to provide a fresh supply of oxygen in the home.

6. Do a BODY SCRUB every day to promote better circulation, energy flow, and breathing.

7. Artificial electromagnetic radiation is especially weakening to the lungs and respiratory system. Avoid excessive exposure to television, computers, cell phones, and handheld electrical appliances as much as possible.

8. Avoid wearing metallic jewelry, especially on the fingers and hands, as it can transmit an electromagnetic charge along the lung meridian.

9. Strictly avoid smoking or secondhand smoke, which can irritate the lungs.

10. Lung conditions correlate to the proper functioning of the intestines. Regular bowel movements can contribute to improved breathing and lung activity. Proper chewing will help restore normal elimination and help the lungs at the same time. Chew very well, up to 100 times or more per mouthful.

11. Sadness, depression, and melancholy commonly accompany lung problems. Strive to be positive, optimistic, hopeful, and happy.

12. Breathing exercises are helpful, but not to exhaustion.

13. Sing a happy song each day and listen to music that lifts your spirits.

HOME REMEDIES

1. For most lung conditions, prepare the special LUNG DRINK.

2. A LOTUS ROOT PLASTER can help relieve congestion in the lungs, the throat, or the bronchi. First apply a GINGER COMPRESS for a few minutes, then the lotus root plaster for several hours. Depending on the condition, it may be used daily for 7 to 10 days to help dislodge and discharge heavy mucus.

3. A MUSTARD PLASTER can be applied on the chest, as well as the back of the chest, to help reduce severe coughing. This is good for bronchitis and asthma. Apply 3 to 4 times a day as needed.

4. A TOFU PLASTER, LEAFY GREENS PLASTER, or other cold compress can be applied on the chest to reduce inflammation or fever in the case of a more yang, contracted condition.

5. LOTUS ROOT JUICE TEA is helpful to dissolve and eliminate excess mucus in the lungs, throat, or sinuses. Drink ½ cup of liquid squeezed from grated fresh lotus root and cooked like a tea with ½ cup of water. Take once or twice a day for several days, as needed. This is very helpful for wet conditions where mucus, phlegm, and fluids are involved, but not for dry, contracted conditions.

6. Lotus seeds may be cooked with kombu or wakame and seasoned with a little miso or shoyu. Take 1 cup daily for several days.

7. CARROT-DAIKON DRINK may help eliminate fats and oils that have accumulated in the lungs. Take one small cup every day or every other day for 2 to 4 weeks, then 2 to 3 times a week for the next 2 to 4 weeks. Fresh lotus root may be substituted for daikon.

8. SWEET VEGETABLE DRINK will nourish the lungs and their functions. Take 1 small cup daily for 1 month, then every other day for the second month.

9. GRATED DAIKON WITH SHOYU may be taken 2 to 3 times a week.

10. To relax the lungs in case of a dry cough or more yang condition, take a small cup of black bean juice once or twice a day. This is the liquid in which black beans are cooked.

TABLE 28. RESPIRATORY CONDITIONS AND DISORDERS

1. More Yin Cause	2. More Yang Cause	3. Yin and Yang Combined
Typical Symptoms		
Dilation	Constriction	Expansion or constriction
Breathing difficulty	Breathing difficulty	Breathing difficulty
Inflammation, swelling	Inflammation	Inflammation
Infectious conditions	Shortness of breath	
Some coughing	Some coughing	Some coughing
Sneezing, hiccuping		Guttural voice
Yawning, snoring		
Sighing, crying, sobbing		
Stuttering		
Diseases		
Sinusitis		Mucus and fat accumulation
Asthma		
Bronchitis		Pneumonia
Croup		Emphysema
Diphtheria		
Some emphysema		Some emphysema
Hay fever		
Pleurisy		Cystic fibrosis
Tonsilitis		
Tuberculosis		
Whooping cough		
Some cyanosis	Some cyanosis	
Collapsed lung		Consolidation
		Lung cancer
		Throat cancer

11. A BROWN RICE–GINGER COM-PRESS is helpful for relieving tightness in the lungs and muscle pains. Prepare by roasting rice in a pan and add a few slices of raw ginger-root. Wrap the rice and ginger mixture in cheesecloth or other cotton and apply it on the chest.

12. For pneumonia, a CARP PLASTER may be placed over the lungs to neutralize the fever.

CAUTION

1. If blood is coughed up from the lungs, there may be internal bleeding, and immediate medical attention is required.

2. Chest X rays, mammograms, MRIs, CAT scans, and other high-tech diagnostic tools may be advisable in some cases but can produce weakening effects. Avoid or limit as much as possible.

MEDICAL EVIDENCE

FAT INTAKE LINKED TO ASTHMA

Asthma is related to high fat consumption, according to a Swedish study. "Men with asthma have a significantly higher intake of fat than men without asthma," the researchers found.

Source: K. Strom et al., "Asthma but Not Smoking-Related Airflow Limitation Is Associated with a High Fat Diet in Men," *Monaldi Archives of Chest Diseases* 51(1):16–21, 1996.

WHOLE GRAINS AND VITAMIN E-RICH FOODS PROTECT AGAINST ASTHMA

A diet high in foods containing vitamin E may protect against asthma, according to the American Lung Association. In a study of 77,866 women, Harvard scientists reported that eating foods high in this nutrient, especially whole grains and vegetables, reduced the risk of asthma.

Source: R. J. Troisi et al., "A Prospective Study of Diet and Adult-Onset Asthma," *American Journal of Respiratory and Critical Care Medicine* 151(5):1401–8, 1995.

VITAMIN A MAY HELP REVERSE EMPHYSEMA

In laboratory studies, nutritional researchers have been able to reverse emphysema and regenerate alveoli, the small air sacs that are damaged by this chronic lung disease. Adult rats given retinoic acid, a derivative of vitamin A (found in many common vegetables and fruits), repaired damaged air sacs. "For the first time, we have been able to induce the formation of alveoli," Dr. Donald Massaro, a Georgetown University School of Medicine researcher, explained.

Source: Warren E. Leary, "Animal Studies Show How Vitamin Treatment May Reverse the Effects of Emphysema," *New York Times,* May 28, 1998.

◎ MAD COW DISEASE (VARIANT CREUTZFELDT-JAKOB DISEASE)

Mad cow disease, one of the major epidemics in recent times, appeared in herds of British cattle in the late 1980s and is believed to have spread to the human population through consumption of contaminated beef or dairy products or contact with bone meal, tallow, or other products made from cows. The official name for the disease is *bovine spongiform encephelopathy*

(BSE), and the human form is known as *variant Creutzfeldt-Jakob Disease* (vCJD). The disease affects the brain and central nervous system, and all cases to date have been fatal. Nearly 1 million cattle and about 125 people have died, though medical experts say that the average incubation period of 10 years or more may result in thousands, hundreds of thousands, and even millions of human deaths in the future. There is no medical treatment or cure. The disease is believed to be spread by prions, infectious "rogue" proteins in the body that are impervious to boiling, pasteurization, or radiation. It affects predominantly younger persons, age 15 to 40, including vegetarians who have not eaten meat in over a decade but who have eaten dairy food.

SYMPTOMS

1. Loss of coordination
2. Nervous dysfunction
3. Spongy holes in the brain

CAUSES

1. Mad cow disease emerged following the introduction of *rendering*, a new food recycling technology in which British cows were fed ground-up animal parts, including the carcasses and inedible parts of sheep and other cows, road kill, and euthanized pets from animal shelters. Scrapie, a brain disease that afflicts sheep, evidently passed to the cattle and evolved into BSE, which in turn passed to humans.

2. An alternative theory is that BSE originated from the spread of organophosphate pesticides that the British government required farmers to use on their cattle to kill warble fly, a

parasite. The chemical used in the treatment is similar to thalidomide, a drug that resulted in many deformed babies a generation ago.

3. Several people who have died of vCJD worked in garden supply stores and were exposed to bone meal, a soil additive made from cattle ingredients that is commonly used in gardening.

4. Since prions contain no DNA, it is not known how they reproduce and spread in the body. Lack of DNA, however, is very yin. It is not natural for cows, which normally are vegetarian and eat grass, to consume animal food, especially other cows. When yang animals such as cows take in yang foods (other cows), it changes into yin. The cows fed rendered meat become weaker, degenerate, and begin to lose the DNA in the yang center of their cells. Extreme yin manifests as prions, and yin energy rises and expands, appearing as holes in the brain. The intestines, pancreas, and reproductive organs may also be affected. Overall, this is the same process by which the modern diet is leading to infertility, allergies, and immune function disorders. Sugar, alcohol, drugs, and chemicals, especially in combination with animal foods, are causing the DNA in sperm and eggs to lose its vitality.

SOLUTION

DIET

Observe the dietary guidelines for Diet #3, especially noting the following:

1. Avoid all animal-quality foods, especially beef, dairy food, organ meats, gelatin, and other food made from cows. Also avoid all factory-raised chicken, pork, lamb, and fish (especially

salmon, trout, and other varieties) that may be produced through rendered food, including contaminated cattle parts. In the United States, rendered food may no longer contain cattle or sheep parts, but it may legally include cow's blood and gelatin. Hamburger may include cow brains, so especially avoid.

2. Avoid hunting or eating deer, elk, squirrel, mink, and other wild game that may be contaminated from ingesting infected cow parts in the wild, fast-food leftovers foraged in national parks, or "downer" cows and road kill.

3. Though they are not main causes of transmission, avoid sugar, refined grains, tropical foods, spices, stimulants, and chemicalized foods that may weaken natural immunity and contribute to greater susceptibility to infection.

4. Avoid raw salad, fruit, and juice as much as possible, and other raw foods until the condition improves.

5. To strengthen DNA, eat organically grown brown rice and other cooked whole grains. Other seeds will also be helpful to restore DNA, especially sesame seeds and pumpkin seeds. These may be prepared in various ways.

LIFESTYLE

Observe the standard way-of-life suggestions as well as the following:

1. Avoid contact with household or garden items that may include contaminated cattle parts made from bones, hides, and muscles, including bone meal, tallow, candles, floor wax, moisteners, face cream, shampoos, cosmetics, potting soil, lipstick, contact lenses, soap, cooking oil, capsules, tablets, and leather products.

2. Avoid medical products that may include contaminated cattle parts, including growth hormones, gelatin capsules, sutures, contact lenses, allantoin, amino acids, cholesterol, elastin, cortisone, fatty acids, keratin, nucleic acid, polysorbates, stearic acid, and heparin.

3. Avoid using cattle manure for gardening or farming or handling foods and produce that have been grown using it.

4. Since vCJD may be transmitted by contaminated blood, the American Red Cross has recently prohibited people who lived in or visited Britain for three months or more between 1980 and 1996 from donating blood. Avoid transfusions of blood and blood products unless you have an uncontaminated source from a friend or relative.

5. In the United States, transmissible encephalopathies similar to BSE have spread into the wild animal population, especially mink, elk, deer, squirrels, and sheep. Known as chronic wasting disease, it has reached epidemic proportions among deer in Colorado, other western states, and the Midwest.

HOME REMEDIES

1. Take UMEBOSHI PLUMS, once a day or frequently, to strengthen the blood.

2. To restore energy and vitality, UME-SHO KUZU may be taken several times a week for 3 or 4 weeks or until the condition improves.

3. To further strengthen the blood and give energy, KINPIRA SOUP may be taken several times a week.

4. BAKED KOMBU CONDIMENT may also be helpful for this condition. Bake some kombu in a dry skillet until it is black and crush it into powder. Then mix it with baked dried shiitake and roasted black sesame seeds and crush in a suribachi. Take 1 teaspoon daily for 10 days, then every other day for 10 days, and then occasionally as desired for 4 to 6 weeks.

CAUTION

Sporadic Creutzfeldt-Jakob disease strikes about 1 in every 1 million people in modern society and is unrelated to the new variant form of the disease. It primarily affects older people, especially men and until recently men of Mediterranean or Jewish background. Recently, however, its incidence appears to be increasing and its symptoms are similar to Alzheimer's disease. There is growing concern that many Alzheimer's cases in the U.S. may, in fact, be part of an invisible epidemic of CJD or vCJD. The macrobiotic dietary approach for sporadic CJD is similar to that outlined above for vCJD. Though contaminated cow products may not be the underlying cause, some kind of abnormal animal food consumption (such as eating the brains or inner organs of infected squirrels or other animals not usually consumed) may be involved.

MEDICAL EVIDENCE

U.S. AT RISK FOR MAD COW EPIDEMIC

From Britain, vCJD has spread to a half dozen European countries. While only one case has been confirmed in the United States (in a girl who lived in Britain), it may only be a matter of time until the epidemic spreads. "Will BSE come to America?" Richard Rhodes, a Pulitzer Prize–winning science writer asks. "The answer seems to be: it's already here, in native form, a low-level infection that industrial

cannibalism could amplify to epidemic scale. We still feed meat-and-bone meal to cattle. And an estimated 77 million Americans eat beef every day." No population anywhere in the world that eats meats is entirely free of risk, he concludes.

Source: Richard Rhodes, *Deadly Feasts: Tracking the Secrets of a Terrifying New Plague* (New York: Simon & Schuster, 1997), p. 229.

CASE HISTORY

VEGETARIANS AT RISK FOR MAD COW DISEASE

Several vegetarians have died from the human form of mad cow disease. Clare Tomkins, 24, died in 1998, two years after symptoms first appeared. A strict vegetarian, she had not eaten meat for a dozen years, but she did take cheese and drink milk. She worked in the pet section of a garden supply store near her residence in Tonbridge, Kent, and had contact with bone meal, cow manure, and other cattle products commonly used in gardening.

Source: "Vegetarian Woman Dies from 'Mad Cow' Disease," PA News, April 22, 1998.

⊚ MENTAL AND EMOTIONAL PROBLEMS

An estimated 10 percent of people today suffer from mental illness, including depression, schizophrenia, bipolar disorder, paranoia, and other clinical disorders. Many others suffer from anxiety, chronic anger, abuse and neglect, insecurity, and phobias. Around the world, mental and emotional problems are among the most rapidly rising disorders. Modern society treats mental problems as though they were independent from physical problems and refers major mental and emotional disturbances to psychiatrists, social workers, and other mental health experts. Until recently, extreme manifestations of mental illness were treated primarily with drugs, surgery (including lobotomy), electroshock, or incarceration in a mental hospital. Dietary and lifestyle factors, including nutrition and biochemical imbalances, are now under active investigation by the scientific and medical profession, as well as related psychological, sociological, and correctional disciplines.

From the macrobiotic view, physical imbalance and mental and emotional imbalance cannot be separated. Physical sicknesses are frequently the immediate causes of mental and emotional disorders, and thoughts and feelings directly affect the physical condition. Many psychological approaches to health and happiness are unaware of the cause of unhappiness. Drugs, medicines, and psychotherapy all fail to get to the root of the problem because they ignore day-to-day food, as well as consciousness and other lifestyle factors. Thousands of people today live their whole lives in mental hospitals because they and their doctors don't know the cause of their psychological problems or how to deal with them. Food's vibrational energy creates immediate emotional change. Chicken, for example, causes people to focus on minute details (like a hen pecking) and ask endless questions. Sugar leads to dispersion of energy, forgetfulness, and memory loss. Alcohol, especially in combination with meat or other strong animal food, often leads to boasting and exaggerated emotions, delusional thinking, and wild, crazy be-

havior. A balanced way of eating centered on whole grains and vegetables can help prevent, relieve, or control many mental and emotional problems.

For depression and mood swings, see "Hypoglycemia" in "Pancreatic Problems."

SYMPTOMS

The following symptoms may accompany mental or emotional problems:

Physical Symptoms
1. Flushed face
2. Irregular pulse
3. Allergy, dermatitis, or freckles
4. Constipation or diarrhea
5. Catatonia, shooting pain, numbness
6. Headache
7. Tendency toward enteritis and hepatitis
8. Candidiasis
9. Tendency toward cancer
10. Viral disease, including hepatitis, HIV, etc.
11. Rheumatism
12. Frigidity
13. Infertility and miscarriage
14. Dizziness such as with anemia
15. Shaking in the whole body
16. Reduced vitality
17. Acidic conditions and buffer reactions
18. Osteoporosis
19. Irregular eating

Mental and Social Symptoms
1. Forgetfulness
2. Memory loss
3. Cloudy or unfocused thinking
4. Talking too much or not at all

5. Fatigue

6. Stress

7. Sensitivity

8. Overexcitability

9. Loss of direction, reduced ambition

10. Loss of discipline

11. Decreased creativity

12. Anxiety, doubt, insecurity

13. Anger, irritability

14. Sadness or depression

15. Apprehensions, fears, and phobias

16. Overcaution or recklessness

17. Euphoria or excitement

18. Mood swings

19. Inability to cope with daily life

20. Inappropriate speech or behavior

21. Bizarre or unstable actions

22. Delusions, hallucinations

23. Suicidal or violent thoughts

24. Dependence on artificial social support systems

25. Divorce or separation

26. Violence and criminal behavior

27. Opportunistic and shallow relationships

28. Arguing, complaining

29. Collapse of family

CAUSES

1. If we do not live in harmony with our environment, imbalance arises, leading eventually to sickness and disease. The first stage is general fatigue, both physical and mental, which manifests as tiredness, complaining, a gradual loss of clear thinking and behavior, and frequent changes of mind. The next stage is physical aches and pains and feelings of sadness, gradual loss of self-confidence, forgetful-ness, vague memory, stubbornness, and a focus on small or insignificant matters. The following stage is a weakening in blood quality. As red and white blood cells and blood plasma weaken, acidosis, high and low blood pressure, anemia, and other conditions, including skin diseases, appear. These may be accompanied by nervousness, hypersensitivity, fear and irritability, depression, timidity, and general loss of direction in life.

2. If the blood quality continues to weaken without correcting the diet or lifestyle, anger, impatience, frustration, overexcitement, suspicion and skepticism, withdrawal, conceptual and delusional beliefs and thinking, and other chronic emotional imbalances will arise.

3. The next stage, organic disease, gives rise to structural changes, malfunctions, and degeneration of inner organs and glands. Physically, this manifests as heart disease, cancer, multiple sclerosis, and other degenerative disorders. Mentally, this manifests as chronic stubbornness, prejudice, narrow-mindedness, a rigid view of life, and a general inability to cope with daily life. An underlying inferiority or superiority complex may develop as egocentric thinking prevails.

4. Various nervous disorders may arise in the next stage as the degenerative tendency continues. Physically, this manifests as loss of coordination, partial or complete paralysis, and other musculoskeletal conditions. Mentally, a negative view of life prevails, frequently manifesting as loss of self-discipline, chaotic behavior and thinking, schizophrenia or paranoia, and suicidal or destructive tendencies.

5. Finally, in the last stage, arrogance emerges, including selfishness, egocentricity, vanity, self-

pride, exclusivity, and self-justification. People commonly feel that the whole world is against them and that their sicknesses and difficulties are totally unconnected to their diet, lifestyle, and behavior. They may make active attempts to control or force others or completely give up and withdraw into an inner world of fantasy and illusion.

6. The brain corresponds in structure and function to the intestines. Both organs are long, compacted tubes with many coils and convolutions. Where the intestines process physical food, the brain processes mental food in the form of waves and vibrations. Problems in the intestines are commonly mirrored in ordinary consciousness. For example, constipation gives rise to frustrated thinking and inability to carry things through to completion. Diarrhea may precede or be accompanied by too much talking, nonstop talking, or other verbal discharges.

7. The chakras, or energy centers, also contribute to consciousness and mental and psychological processes. The crown chakra, at the top of the head, governs universal consciousness. The chakra in the midbrain (sometimes called the third eye) coordinates overall intuition and mental processing. The chakra in the region of the throat governs speech and expression. The heart chakra governs overall destiny, including emotional development and love. The solar plexus chakra, branching off to the liver, spleen, kidneys, and middle organs, governs intellect, courage, sympathy, patience, and other qualities. The hara or intestinal chakra governs overall social development. The chakra in the reproductive region governs regeneration at all levels, including emotional and spiritual.

8. Sugar and other extreme yin foods are among the major causes of mental and emotional problems. Clear judgment is affected by sugar, chocolate, honey, and other refined sweeteners. Microorganisms live in the intestines that are responsible for synthesizing the group of B vitamins that are transported to the brain and in the form of glutamic acid stimulate the nerves and higher consciousness centers. Simple sugars interfere with this process, expanding the brain cells and tissues, resulting in loss of focus, concentration, and clear thinking. From childhood, blood sugar levels commonly grow out of balance, leading to depression and sadness.

9. Strong contractive foods also create emotional problems, especially attachment, possessiveness, and guilt. Life is not always smooth, and almost everyone experiences some great hardship, difficulty, or unhappiness. Some people are able to let go of these negative experiences and live happily, while others are attached and cannot release old memories and are constantly reliving events that happened in the past. This comes principally from consuming too much bread and baked food, which then harden and contract the brain, nerves, and chakras, preventing memories from being released. Meat, eggs, poultry, fish and seafood, and other animal food, as well as too much salt, will also hold the emotions inside and prevent their release.

10. Excessive talking and wild, hyperactive behavior are commonly caused by garlic. Raw onions and scallions, too much ginger, and other herbs and spices can also result in hyperactivity.

11. In the Far East, the ideogram for "anger" means "liver disease." Short temper, anger, irritability, and aggressive behavior commonly result from an overactive or stagnant liver or gallbladder condition as these organs discharge excessive metabolic energy in a wild, chaotic way. Conversely, a healthy liver and gallbladder are associated with calm, patience, perseverance, and other stable qualities. Animal foods in particular can give rise to anger and irritability, especially meat, poultry, eggs, cheese, and too much fish or seafood. Too much salt or salty food, hard baked food (including bread and chips), and other strong yang foods and processing methods or cooking methods can also tighten and overburden the liver. Meanwhile, sugar and other refined sweeteners, fatty and oily foods, too much fruit and juice, refined grains, milk and light dairy, spices, stimulants, and other strong yin foods can contribute to liver stagnation or cause yang energy gathering in the liver or gallbladder to be discharged rapidly and chaotically, something like a volcanic eruption.

12. Anxiety, doubt, skepticism, and jealousy are associated with imbalances in the spleen, pancreas, and stomach. Healthy conditions of these organs correspond with sympathy, wisdom, compassion, and understanding. Depending on the underlying imbalance, mental and psychological symptoms may range from simple worry and general uneasiness to moderate anxiety and skepticism and even to deep feelings of inadequacy and lowered self-esteem or total suspicion of others. Animal foods in particular can give rise to anxiety and doubt, especially eggs, poultry, meat, salty cheese, and too much shellfish or fish. Overintake of salt or salty food, hard baked food (including bread and chips), and other strong yang foods and processing methods or cooking methods can also tighten and

overburden the pancreas, spleen, and stomach. Meanwhile, sugar and other refined sweeteners, fatty and oily foods, too much fruit and juice, refined grains, milk and light dairy, spices, stimulants, and other strong yin foods can contribute to overacidity in the stomach and digestive system, contribute to an imbalance in blood sugar levels, and overburden these central organs.

13. Timidity, fear, lack of self-esteem, hopelessness, and paranoia are related to imbalances in the kidney and bladder functions. In traditional Oriental medicine, healthy conditions in these organs contribute to confidence, courage, inspiration, and trust. Animal foods in particular can give rise to a fearful mind, especially eggs, poultry, meat, dairy foods of all kinds, and too much shellfish or fish, as the kidneys become overburdened with excessive protein. Animal foods also carry the vibration of the animals that were killed. Conditions in modern slaughterhouses are often overcrowded and the assembly-line process of slaughtering is often accompanied by fear and terror. Such conditions can result in the excessive release of adrenaline and other hormones and chemicals in the animal that, in turn, are absorbed by those who eat them. Overintake of salt or salty food, hard baked food (including bread and chips), and other extreme yang foods and processing or cooking methods can also tighten and overburden the kidneys and bladder. Paranoia and paranoid tendencies in which the persons distrust everyone around them and see a vast conspiracy directed against them almost always involve too much animal food, animal extracts, salt, or some other strong, contractive substance. Meanwhile, sugar and other refined sweeteners, fatty and oily foods, too much fruit and juice, refined grains, milk and light dairy, spices, stimulants, and other strong yin foods can contribute to overacidic urine, lead to over-expansion and swelling in these organs, or clog the fine network of cells in the kidney with fat or mucus.

14. Hysteria, excitement, hypersensitivity, nervousness, and similar conditions are caused by underlying heart and small intestine disorders. In traditional Oriental medicine, healthy conditions of these organs contribute to a calm, peaceful mind, gentleness, and an amused, humorous expression. Imbalances in these two organs can lead to hyperactivity, excessive laughter, nervousness, oversensitivity, and other manifestations of mental and emotional excess. Too much talking, nonstop talking, and other speech problems are also related to the heart and circulatory function and often show an overactive heart, high blood pressure, or heart murmur. Extreme yin foods such as sugar, chocolate, honey, and other refined sweeteners; milk, ice cream, and other dairy products; refined grains; tropical foods; herbs and spices; too much fruit and juice; stimulants; too many beverages or fluid; and other predominantly expansive items are the principal cause of these conditions. Garlic in particular can overly stimulate the heart and should ordinarily be used very infrequently and in small amounts.

15. Prejudice, discrimination, hatred, and violence are a hallmark of modern times. They are commonly seen as social or cultural problems entirely separate from physical, mental, or emotional health. However, from a macrobiotic perspective, they arise from an imbalanced way of life, especially an imbalanced way of eating. The basic underlying cause of prejudice and ha-

tred is hardening of the arteries, which contributes to a narrow, constricted view of life, especially of other people, sexes, ages, races, religions, and cultures. Heart disease is the number one degenerative disease in modern society, including the developing world. Meat, poultry, eggs, cheese, fish and seafood, and other animal products are the number one cause of atherosclerosis and hardening of the arteries, including those leading to and nourishing the brain and its functions. In addition to foods high in saturated fat and cholesterol, excessive salt, hard baked foods, and other contractive foods may contribute to this process. This includes frozen, cold, and iced foods and foods that are baked, grilled, roasted, or cooked in a very yang manner. Though primarily yang in origin, these conditions are often enhanced by overconsumption of strong yin foods, including sugar and other sweets, milk and dairy, spices, alcohol, and other expansive foods, that are commonly eaten with animal products and which can cause the accumulated yang to be discharged explosively and chaotically in the form of anger, hatred, prejudicial speech or behavior, and violence. Usually yang factors by themselves will not cause violence. They may lead to meanness, cruelty, and other tight, overly contractive conditions. But to release the stored, or accumulated, yang energy, strong yin is needed. Milk, sugar, alcohol, and drugs are the primary foods that spark this metabolic discharge. In addition to the heart and circulatory system, prejudice and discrimination can arise from disorders in other organs. Liver and gallbladder problems can harden the liver and give rise to anger and violence. Pancreas, spleen, and stomach problems can lead to hypoglycemia and violent mood swings. Lung and large intestine problems can produce labored breathing and constipation, leading to feelings of insecurity and confinement. Disorders in the kidneys and bladder can produce fear and mistrust of others.

Instead of seeing these feelings, thoughts, and emotions as arising from an inner conflict, we project them onto the external environment, including other people. There is also a yin form of prejudice and discrimination in which anger, hatred, and prejudice are internalized. Instead of finding outward, violent expression, these emotions turn inward. In some cases, the person may develop self-hatred, loathing, and ultimately suicidal tendencies. In other cases, the person begins to see himself as superior (more spiritual, long-suffering, or righteous) to those who are targeting him. He takes refuge in the thought that he will ultimately triumph, in this world or the next, and that the oppressor will get his just reward. In macrobiotics, we call this condition *yin arrogance*. It is the opposite of *yang arrogance* and equally destructive. Oppression is an unfortunate legacy of modern civilization. But we don't have to let it dehumanize us or other people. Gandhi, Martin Luther King Jr., and other prophets of peace and nonviolence, as well as many concentration camp survivors and survivors of torture and brutality, have shown that we can uphold the common humanity of all people under the most adverse circumstances.

FORMS

Bipolar Disorder. Bioporal disorder, or manic-depression, is characterized by periodic mood swings oscillating between extreme ela-

tion and melancholy. About 1–2 percent of the U.S. population is believed to suffer from this disorder, and 1 in 5 patients commits suicide. Symptoms of bipolar disorder differ widely and commonly manifest in dramatic and unpredictable behavior, including eating or drinking binges, wild shopping sprees, impulsive travel, euphoria and excessive talking, depression and self-destructive thoughts and tendencies, hallucinations, and excessive use of recreational or prescription drugs, especially amphetamines and other psychostimulants. From the macrobiotic perspective, the principal cause of bipolar disorder is long-term consumption of extreme yin and yang foods, including meat, poultry, eggs, cheese, seafood, and other animal products, too much bread and flour products, and too much salt and salty foods, in combination with sugar, chocolate, and other refined sweeteners, refined grains, tropical foods, oily and greasy foods, chemicalized foods, spices, stimulants, drugs, alcohol, and other expansive items. In many cases, hypoglycemia is an underlying condition for bipolar disease, and stabilizing blood sugar levels will substantially reduce mood swings. In addition to discontinuing all extreme foods and eating a diet centered on whole grains and vegetables, the entire way of life may need to be reoriented in a simpler, more harmonious direction. Generally, observe the dietary recommendations for Diet #3. *For further information, please see "Hypoglycemia" in "Pancreatic Problems."*

Existential Despair. Existential despair arises from a deep-rooted belief or overwhelming feeling that life is meaningless and absurd. It takes many forms, including nihilism, hedonism, angst, and ennui. Existential despair is especially common (indeed fashionable) among modern writers, poets, painters, philosophers, and musicians. It is celebrated in art, literature, and music. This kind of depression is also frequently found among biologists, chemists, physicists, historians, and other scientists, academics, or professionals.

From a cultural, social, and historical view, existential despair arose in the West following the collapse of the medieval church and the triumph of modern science and medicine. Newtonian physics, Darwinian evolution, Freudian psychoanalysis, the periodic table of elements, and the big bang hypothesis left no room for God or a creator in the design of the universe. Following social upheavals, famine, poverty, epidemics, and colonialism and imperial wars that accompanied the industrial revolution, authors such as Dostoevski, Kierkegaard, Conrad, Kafka, and Sartre, as well as Picasso in the world of art and Stravinsky in the world of music, articulated the absurdity and meaninglessness of modern life.

From an energetic perspective, the view that existence is meaningless is directly connected with the loss of order in daily life, including day-to-day cooking, eating, and flexible adaptation to the natural world. Lack of principal food in the diet—whole grains, the traditional staff of life especially—separates modern people from their evolutionary past, cultural roots, and parental heritage. The result has been the rise of an artificial, fragmented society that mirrors the artificial, fragmented modern way of eating. Return to a more natural way of eating, respect for the natural environment, and healthy lifestyle practices will help restore a feeling of order and purpose to life.

Phobias, Obsessions, and Compulsions. Phobias and compulsive and obsessive behavior take many forms, including fear of dirt, persistent anxiety over past conduct, chronic washing of the hands, voluntary or involuntary repetition of other routine acts, sounds, or thoughts, and irrational fears of heights, enclosed spaces, or other locations or situations that normally arise from time to time in daily life. In the past, some societies considered symptoms such as these as evidence of demonic possession. Modern psychiatry holds that these behaviors are the result of unconscious desires and wishes and arrested childhood development. Brain researchers and many psychologists today look at *obsessive compulsive-disorder* (clinically referred to as OCD) as a biochemical imbalance, especially reduced levels of serotonin or other neurotransmitters.

From the macrobiotic view, obsessive and compulsive behaviors are largely caused by faulty diet. In each case, the precise foods or combinations of foods that are largely giving rise to the symptoms must be discovered. Yin and yang can help diagnose the underlying cause. Heights, for example, are classified as yin because yin energy from the center of the earth rises and becomes stronger as it ascends. Fear of heights can be caused by either an overly yin condition (which is repelled by flying, mountain climbing, or visiting tall buildings) or an overly yang condition (which is too hard, rigid, and contracted to adjust to its opposite). Similarly, fear of depths, including going down in the ocean in a submarine, going into a cave, or even going into the basement, can be produced by an overly yang condition (which is repelled by yang, descending energy) or by an extreme yin condition that is too weak, timid, or insecure to adjust to its opposite. Other phobias include fear of small rooms and tight spaces (an overly yang environment) or fear of large rooms and wide-open spaces (an overly yin environment). Other yang fears include fire, light, and heat, and other yin fears include water, dark, and cold, though again both types of conditions can be affected. Fear overall, as noted in the section on fear and paranoia above, is related to the kidneys, so kidney or bladder malfunction is generally involved in phobias. Changing one's diet and condition can quickly eliminate fears and phobias. For a more yin condition, observe the dietary guidelines for Diet #1. For a more yang condition, observe the guidelines for Diet #2. And for conditions arising from a combination of extremes, follow the guidelines for Diet #3.

OCD commonly arises from food that has been artificially treated, processed, or modified, including chemically grown or treated foods, canned or bottled foods, and genetically altered foods. Compulsive washing of the hands often arises from eating a diet consisting primarily of canned, bottled, or frozen food that has been sterilized, pasteurized, or otherwise treated with chemicals or processing methods designed to kill germs. Compulsive washing is a repetitive action corresponding with this mechanical process. The hands, in this case, also correspond with the liver (right hand) and spleen (left hand), and compulsive washing is an unconscious way to stimulate these two organs and try to cleanse the blood (governed by the liver) and the lymph (governed by the spleen) of impurities (including pesticides, herbicides, and preservatives). A balanced diet centered on whole, fresh, predominantly organically grown foods will quickly eliminate compulsive behaviors, especially a

fear of dirt, germs, and contamination of all kinds. Generally observe the guidelines for Diet #1 for more yin conditions. However, if animal food is a major factor and is still being eaten, follow Diet #3 for conditions arising from a combination of yin and yang.

Other repetitive actions, including acts, sounds, and unpleasant thoughts, may also arise from taking too many sticky foods. Sticky foods cause "stuck" behavior, and these include oily, greasy foods of all kinds, such as too many fried and deep-fried foods, nuts and nut and seed butters, mayonnaise, dressings, milk, ice cream, yogurt, and other dairy foods, avocado, and especially chocolate. In addition to interrupting the smooth flow of energy in the organs, glands, meridians, and chakras, giving rise to these quirky blockages (like a stuck needle on a phonograph), sticky foods also create attachment to the past. They are the principal cause of retaining unpleasant memories and guilt over past actions. So long as we continue to eat fatty, oily, sticky foods like this, we cannot let go of dark, unhappy thoughts and feelings and learn to forgive ourselves or others. Eliminating these foods and observing the standard macrobiotic way of eating is essential to overcome stuck behavior as well as deeply rooted feelings of guilt and inadequacy. In general, observe the guidelines for Diet #3.

Post-traumatic Stress Disorder. Experiencing or reliving past traumas is known as post-traumatic stress disorder (PTSD). It primarily affects people who have been involved in a war either as soldiers or civilians, those who have suffered rape or sexual abuse, and those who have witnessed shocking or horrifying events. Previously known as *shell shock* and *battle fa-*

tigue, PTSD can be accompanied by flashbacks or recurrent dreams of the traumatic event, suspicion and paranoia, numbness and apathy, angry outbursts, and a pervasive sense of hopelessness. Headaches, pain, digestive and bowel problems, and trouble sleeping are common and may become chronic. About 1 in every 3 Vietnam War veterans experienced PTSD, and many continue to suffer decades later. Eighty-four percent of battered women have symptoms of the disorder shortly after being abused, and about half of them still experience trauma a year later. Children are vulnerable, especially if they have witnessed family violence or abuse. Modern medicine treats PTSD as a form of depression and prescribes SSRIs (selective serotonin reuptake inhibitors) and other antidepressants. Psychotherapy, relaxation and stress-reduction techniques, biofeedback, and other therapeutic methods are also frequently employed. Eye movement desensitization and reprocessing (EMDR), a simple visualization technique in which the patient focuses on distressing images while tracking the fingers of a therapist moving rapidly in front of the eyes, has produced promising results. Rather like hypnosis, it helps to break the spell or fixation on blocked images.

From an energetic perspective, PTSD results from a breakdown in neurological functioning and an inability to process and discharge old memories and images. Normally, people get over horrible events after a suitable period of grief and mourning. Of course, the understanding and support of family and friends is important, but eventually they learn to adjust and move on with their lives. The main reason why some people fail to complete this natural healing cycle is underlying dietary imbalance. Fo-

cusing on the past shows that the condition is too yang. This arises from excessive consumption of meat, poultry, eggs, salted cheese, fish and seafood, and other animal products, as well as too much bread and hard baked flour products and too much salt. These narrow and harden the arteries and vessels, including those in the brain. Meanwhile, oily and greasy foods coat the blood cells, nerve cells, and other cells and tissues with fat and mucus. The end result is that unhappy memories become trapped inside. Flashbacks and recurrent dreams are something like a VCR that is stuck playing the same images over and over again. Sticky foods create stuck images and behavior. To relieve this disorder, it is essential that all animal foods be discontinued and that all oily and greasy foods (including hamburgers, cheeseburgers, pizza, french fries, salad dressings, and mayonnaise) and other sticky foods and beverages be stopped. Depending on the symptoms, other organs and functions may be impaired. Depression usually results from pancreatic disorders, especially hypoglycemia, and from fat and mucus buildup in the lungs, large intestine, and kidneys. Fear and paranoia as well as sleeping troubles result from tight kidneys. Anger and irritability result from liver and gallbladder imbalances. Suspicion may accompany stomach and spleen troubles. For more yang conditions, observe the guidelines for Diet #2 and for conditions arising from a combination of both extremes follow Diet #3. Further adjustments can be made for the organs and functions affected. CARROT-DAIKON DRINK will help eliminate old fat and oil from the body and may be taken 3 to 4 times a week for 1 month and then less frequently for another month. SHIITAKE TEA is helpful to calm down an overly stressful condition. SWEET VEGETABLE DRINK will reduce cravings for sweets and help stabilize blood sugar levels and reduce mood swings.

MEDITATION, VISUALIZATION (including the special exercises noted above), singing a happy song every day, and light to moderate exercise and activity, as well as walking and spending time in nature, are also beneficial. In the event that the person experiencing PTSD has committed or participated in violent acts and is feeling guilt and remorse, spiritual practices may also be necessary, including prayer, chanting, and setting up an altar for the spirits of those killed. These will help lift the dark aura that surrounds many soldiers and people who have committed violent acts. Through proper diet and lifestyle practices, PTSD can be relieved and a new life of enduring health and happiness begun.

Reactive Depression and Grief. Reactive depression may arise from a severe reaction to difficulties, shock, accident, illness, or loss, and almost everyone experiences this form of extreme sadness and unhappiness at some time in their life. Death of a child, spouse, parent, or other close relative or friend can lead to this kind of depression. Having an accident, being fired from a job, divorcing or breaking up with a romantic partner, failing to achieve a desired goal or objective, or being diagnosed with a life-threatening disease may also trigger symptoms. While often severe, this form of depression is usually temporary. Most people recover in a matter of weeks, months, or occasionally a few years following traumatic events. A good example of reactive depression is the terrorist attacks

on September 11, 2001. According to surveys, 80 percent of the American people experienced depression after the tragic events. The nation as a whole was generally immobilized for the rest of the year and through the winter, with many individuals, families, and businesses virtually paralyzed. But by spring 2002, the mood of despair and helplessness began to lift, and life gradually began to return to normal.

Modern medicine and psychiatry offer counseling for this kind of depression, and sedatives, tranquilizers, and other drugs are sometimes prescribed to calm the nerves.

From a dietary view, a balanced natural way of eating, based on whole grains, vegetables, and other fresh foods will also help individuals and families through hard times, calm the mind and emotions, and eventually restore clarity, focus, and meaning. During this time, it is particularly important to avoid or reduce heavy animal food consumption (including dairy food), as well as sugar and other refined sweeteners, alcohol, and other high-energy foods. Following the death of a family member or close friend, people traditionally ate very simply for the next several weeks or months during the period of grieving.

Schizophrenia. Schizophrenia or "split mind" refers to a range of psychotic symptoms and strange behaviors, including disassociated personality, delusions, hallucinations, bizarre speech, irrational acts, catatonia, and isolation from others. It ranges from mild, episodic cases to chronic, full-blown ones. Teenage men and young women in their twenties are most likely to become schizophrenic. About 1 percent of the modern population will be treated for this affliction at some point in their lives. Conventional medicine treats schizophrenia with chlorpromazine, clozapine, risperidone, and other tranquilizers, as well as psychotherapy. However, there are serious side effects to these drugs, and counseling may provide a support environment but rarely results in a cure.

From the macrobiotic perspective, schizophrenia is an extreme yin condition. Absence of strong yang energy manifests as loss of the ego or will. The personality becomes dispersed as delusions, hallucinations, and imaginary voices replace the central self. Apathy, stupor, floppy limbs, and other overly expansive symptoms may then arise. The principal dietary cause of schizophrenia is chronic consumption of sugar, chocolate, honey, molasses, and other refined sweeteners, sugar-treated foods, and aspartame, saccharin, and other sugar substitutes. The energy of refined sugar is extremely disintegrating. As little as ¼ teaspoon of sugar can cause loss of alertness, focus, and clear thinking. In modern society, sugar consumption forms a rough balance to animal food intake. The strong dispersing energy of sugar and other simple sweets serves to offset the intense condensing energy of meat, eggs, poultry, cheese, and other animal foods. As a result, most people eating the modern diet do not experience dissociated thinking (though sugar is a main cause of heart disease, certain cancers, diabetes, and other degenerative conditions). However, if the relative balance of animal foods and simple sugars becomes tipped in favor of the latter, mental illness easily arises. Young people eating a lacto-ovo-vegetarian diet, including plenty of salads, fruit, sweets, desserts, and beverages, are particularly susceptible.

In many cases, schizophrenia can be completely reversed following the standard macrobiotic way of eating. Observe the dietary guidelines for Diet #1 for more extreme yin conditions. In addition to discontinuing sugar in all forms, other extreme yin should also be avoided, including polished grains and white flour, tropical foods, herbs and spices, stimulants, alcohol, and drugs. Fresh salad and other raw foods, fruit and juice, and other supplemental foods in the standard way of eating may also need to be temporarily avoided until the condition improves. Garlic, raw onions or scallions, spices, and other high-energy foods can also contribute to this condition and should be avoided or minimized. Whole grains, especially brown rice, should form the center of the diet, accompanied by strong MISO SOUP daily, plenty of vegetables, including proportionately more root vegetables, beans and bean products, sea vegetables, and occasional white-meat fish 2 to 3 times a week, if desired. UME-SHO KUZU may be taken 2 to 3 times a week. Salt-based seasonings and condiments can be slightly stronger than usual.

This approach is also helpful for mild to moderate yin imbalances, including forgetfulness, memory loss, confusion, and scattered thinking, and for extreme cases of multiple personality disorder. *For paranoid schizophrenia, which is more yang, see the section on fear and paranoia above in "Causes."*

Seasonal Affective Disorder. Seasonal affective disorder (SAD) is marked by an extreme change in mood or functioning at different seasons, especially in autumn and winter compared to spring and summer. People with SAD typically experience the onset of depression, loss of vitality, irritability, increased appetite, and problems coping at home or work during these times. Sufferers crave sugar, sweets, and refined carbohydrates, gain up to 20 pounds, and may sleep up to 4 hours longer than usual. In severe cases they avoid others and become disabled and even suicidal. Symptoms tend to appear in late August or early September and a dark, pessimistic or apathetic mood prevails until the following March or early April. Eleven million people in the United States suffer from this disorder. The "winter blues," a milder form, affect about 25 million others. Women are four times as likely to have SAD, and children and adolescents tend to get it when school starts in the fall. Modern medicine treats SAD as a clinical form of depression, and current research is focused on investigating the role of serotonin, a neurotransmitter that reaches its lowest levels in the brain in winter. SSRIs (selective serotonin reuptake inhibitors) and other antidepressants are commonly prescribed to alleviate depression. Light therapy is also widely used to create a brighter environment and stimulate the optical nerve. Winter vacations to sunnier climes are also recommended. People in southern or tropical latitudes are eight times less likely to have SAD than those in colder, northern regions.

From a macrobiotic perspective, the cause of SAD is the standard American diet, with its excessive consumption of foods high in fat, protein, sugar, and salt and a chaotic way of eating, especially a failure to adjust to the changing seasons. In the spring, the energy of the earth starts to rise and become active after the long cold winter and reaches a peak of growth in the midsummer. At these times, we eat lighter, more ex-

pansive food, including more fresh greens, garden vegetables, and fresh fruits, as well as use lighter cooking methods, less salt and other seasoning, and drink more liquid. This helps balance the warm, dry environment and sunny atmosphere. In the fall and winter, the energy changes and begins to contract. The trees lose their leaves, the animals hibernate, and snow and ice cover the ground. At these times, we eat stronger, more contractive food, including heartier grains, root vegetables, and dried foods; use slightly heavier cooking methods and more salt and seasoning; and drink less liquid. This helps balance the cold, moist environment and dark atmosphere.

The modern way of eating no longer respects the orderly change of seasons and includes foods from radically different climates and environments. In winter, people eat pineapples, mangoes, and other tropical foods. In the summer, they eat steaks, cheeseburgers, and other heavy animal products. Supermarkets and natural food stores provide an endless selection of foods to choose from all year round. Naturally, when people no longer eat according to their local environment, they quickly grow out of harmony and experience imbalances at many levels. SAD arises from a combination of dietary extremes, especially excessive consumption of meat, poultry, eggs, and other high-fat, high-cholesterol animal foods; cheese, ice cream, and other dairy food; pizza, crackers, cookies, chips, and other hard baked flour products; oily and greasy foods of all kinds, including mayonnaise and salad dressings; and tropical fruits and vegetables. In many cases of SAD, metabolism decreases, extra weight is gained, sex drive dulls, and the person withdraws from contact with others. This is something like hibernation among bears and other slower, larger, more yin animals. Such tendencies arise from excessive consumption of fat from both animal and vegetable sources, as well as too much hard baked flour products and too much salt. Too much yang creates a craving for sweets and simple sugars, which is a hallmark of SAD.

To relieve this disorder, observe the guidelines for Diet #3, for conditions arising from a combination of excessive yin and yang factors. Whole grains and cooked vegetables, especially sweet fall- and winter-season squashes, onions, and cabbages, will reduce cravings for sugar and simple carbohydrates. SWEET VEGETABLE DRINK can be taken daily for 1 month and then every other day for a second month to help stabilize blood sugar levels. CARROT-DAIKON DRINK or DRIED DAIKON TEA may be taken several times a week for several weeks to help eliminate excessive fat and oil that have accumulated. GRATED DAIKON with a little shoyu is also helpful.

Feeling a part of nature is essential for recovery. Eat locally grown foods as much as possible. Walk every day outdoors for a half hour or more. Learn to identify the trees, flowers, and plants in your region and the songs of birds. Garden, hike, and visit local mountains and lakes in all kinds of weather. Take up photography as a hobby. All of these will help you adapt to your surroundings and get through the long winter. Then, if you like, you can take a short vacation to a sunnier locale and return renewed, refreshed, and appreciative of your home environment.

Stress. Stress is a hallmark of modern society. Stress at work, pressure at home or school,

relationships, and other forms of tension and anxiety are blamed for a multitude of physical and psychological ills. A feeling of helplessness or resignation may arise from the pace of modern life, especially keeping up with information and new technologies and the magnitude of the nuclear threat, the environmental crisis, and the spread of drugs, alcohol, and crime. There is also existential or spiritual stress arising out of anxieties about the purpose of life, life after death, karma, and other philosophical issues. Common symptoms include headache, fatigue, digestive problems, backache, neck and shoulder pain, worry, irritability, inability to focus, loss of appetite, overeating, or cravings. Conventional medicine treats stress with diazepam and other antianxiety drugs, antidepressants, and other medications and with psychotherapy, group therapy, and other types of counseling. *See also "Post-traumatic Stress Disorder."*

From the macrobiotic perspective, stress comes from the inside, not the outside. When someone has low blood sugar, for example, a stimulus from the outside, such as a deadline, causes her to feel stress. This feeling is coming from an internal physical condition, stress on inner organs, from pancreatic troubles, liver troubles, or troubles with other organs and functions. Normally, a healthy person can function under pressure. In fact, her alertness, efficiency, and productivity may actually go up. Her judgment becomes very acute and she intuitively makes the right decision. She works tirelessly from early morning to late at night without complaining or feeling fatigued. She may take a brief rest from time to time, but she is steady, dependable, and puts tremendous energy into whatever she does. Despite adverse conditions, such as war, natural disasters, and difficulties at home and work, she perseveres and draws upon hidden resources and strength. In contrast, people today are largely sedentary, soft, and comfortable. They are dependent on cars, telephones, computers, and other modern technology to such an extent that they can hardly function when something doesn't work. They fall to pieces over the slightest criticism. They cannot cope with the simplest things.

In many cases, people who experience stress in their daily life are too yin. Their blood quality is declining, their internal organs are weak, and they simply lack the energy and vitality to function. This kind of stress results from outward pressure caused by overexpansion of internal organs. External pressure on tissues, vessels, and organs causes them to become stretched and taut, like an inflated balloon, leading to a lack of flexibility and adaptability. In other cases, especially for those who suffer from hypoglycemia, their condition arises from excessive yang factors. Excessive consumption of animal food, baked flour, or salt causes the pancreas to become tight and harden. This inward and downward force and pressure restricts the release of glucagon, the hormone that elevates blood sugar. For the first type of stress, observe the guidelines for Diet #1 for conditions arising from excessively expansive factors. For the second type, follow the recommendations for Diet #3, for conditions resulting from a combination of too much extreme yin and yang foods and beverages.

For stress arising from more yin factors, slightly stronger dishes and cooking is recommended. MOCHI is especially good, pan-fried, baked, or added to MISO SOUP. Seitan stew with root vegetables and HIJIKI with root vege-

tables may also be taken often. UME-SHO BAN-CHA may also be taken several times a week to help restore energy and vitality. For stress arising from more yang factors, slightly lighter dishes and cooking are recommended. Barley and corn, for example, may be taken more often, as well as green leafy vegetables. People experiencing stress of either type can take SWEET VEGETABLE DRINK daily for 1 month and then every other day for a second month to stabilize their blood sugar, reduce complaining and mood swings, and ease the pressure on the pancreas and inner organs. Depending on other symptoms and the overall condition, external remedies may also be helpful, including periodic GINGER COMPRESSES, a LOTUS ROOT PLASTER, or a DAIKON HIP BATH. Walking, singing a happy song each day, and other light to moderate physical and mental activities will also help reduce feelings of stress and tension. Through these dietary and lifestyle adjustments, optimal health can gradually be recovered. Life can once again be full of excitement, challenge, and adventure. Whatever difficulties may come, we pursue our endless dream.

SOLUTION

DIET
Observe the dietary suggestions noted above.

LIFESTYLE
Follow the standard way-of-life suggestions, emphasizing the following:

I. Stagnation leading to mental and emotional problems can be released through meditation, singing, or chanting. These will stimulate the autonomic nervous system and help discharge excess.

2. Light to moderate exercise, especially walking a half hour every day, will be helpful. DO-IN, SHIATSU, YOGA, tai chi, dancing, and other activities may also be beneficial. In most cases, people with mental and emotional problems need to be more physically active.

3. Eat 2 to 3 meals a day, at regular times. Avoid chaotic eating habits, including eating while standing up, eating in front of the television, and eating convenience or fast foods.

4. Avoid unnatural environments, such as those with high electromagnetic radiation. Avoid excessive use of air conditioners or heaters, and avoid stagnated air.

5. Keep your personal things clean and in order, using natural fabrics and materials as much as possible.

6. Avoid relationships that cause you stress.

7. Spend time in nature as often as possible.

8. Meditation, prayer, and other spiritual practices may be helpful if part of a comprehensive approach. Palm healing is especially beneficial for quieting the mind and emotions.

HOME REMEDIES

1. The following special dishes may be given. For talkativeness and a scattered mind, give rice or buckwheat stew. For anger, give millet or rice stew. For worry, give barley or buckwheat stew. For sadness, give barley or corn stew. For fear, give corn stew. Take every day for 5 to 10 days. These foods will also help to normalize the organs associated with the emotions. For multiple emotions, prepare vegetable nabe, served with udon noodles and a variety of vegetables, tofu,

seitan, and other foods. HOTO, a related dish, may also be taken and is a little stronger.

2. UME-SHO KUZU will help steady the mind and emotions. Take once a day for 3 days and then several times a week as needed.

3. A teaspoon of GOMASHIO, an UMEBOSHI PLUM, a teaspoon of TEKKA, or other salt-based condiment can help focus the mind. These are especially good to counteract scattered thinking and other effects of too much sugar or other strong yin.

4. In cases of mental or emotional conditions caused by extreme yin, including such accompanying symptoms as anemia, stronger foods may be given, such as mugwort mochi; BROWN RICE MOCHI IN MISO SOUP; KIMPIRA-STYLE BURDOCK; JINENJO; tempeh or seitan cooked nabe-style with mochi, fish (if desired), greens, and ginger; KINPIRA SOUP; and in extreme cases KOI-KOKU.

5. LEAFY GREENS JUICE may be taken to nourish the liver and reduce anger, impatience, or other aggressive behavior. Take daily until improvement is experienced.

6. LOTUS ROOT TEA is good to help eliminate fat and mucus from the lungs and large intestine and thereby reduce melancholy and depression.

7. ADZUKI BEAN TEA is helpful for restoring normal kidney and bladder functions and relieving timidity, fear, and general insecurity.

8. SWEET VEGETABLE DRINK will reduce the desire for sugar, sweets, and other cravings, relax the pancreas, and help prevent mood swings. It is especially helpful for overcoming anxiety, doubt, jealousy, and envy. Take daily for 2 to 4 weeks, every other day for a comparable period, and then occasionally as desired.

9. A GINGER COMPRESS on the skin over the kidneys will help restore self-confidence and self-esteem, as well as improve the circulation of blood, lymph, and other body fluids. Apply several times a week as strength permits and then less often or as needed.

10. A HOT FOOT BATH, especially one with salt added to hot water, will help bring down the energy in the body and relax the mind and emotions, including hyperactive conditions.

11. Many other specific dishes, remedies, and exercises can be recommended for each mental or emotional condition depending on the symptoms and individual needs. See a macrobiotic counselor or other professional for specific advice and guidance.

CAUTION

1. For serious mental or emotional disorders, a medical doctor, psychiatrist, or other specialist may need to be contacted. In many cases, they will support the elements of a macrobiotic approach, including a balanced diet, proper exercise, and a more natural lifestyle, as part of a comprehensive mind-body approach.

2. Decisions regarding medication or other conventional therapy should be left up to the individual, family, and medical professional involved. The macrobiotic approach will complement and support whatever decision is made, including that to continue medication or therapy. In the event that the patient decides to eliminate medication, she should do it gradually and under a physician's guidance, especially as improvement is observed in the new way of eating.

MEDICAL EVIDENCE

FAULTY DIET LINKED TO SCHIZOPHRENIA

Free radicals, highly reactive chemicals produced in the body by incomplete metabolism, are associated with the development of schizophrenia. Researchers at the University of Pittsburgh Medical Center and Western Psychiatric Institute and Clinic reported that free radicals are involved in membrane pathology associated with this mental disorder. Too much fatty and oily food, as well as smoking and air pollution, enhances their production. Whole grains, vegetables, fresh fruits, and other foods high in vitamins A, C, and E help reduce the formation of free radicals.

Source: R. D. Reddy and J. K. Yao, "Free Radical Pathology in Schizophrenia: A Review," *Prostaglandins Leukot Essential Fatty Acids* 55(1–2):33–43, 1996.

HEALTHY DIET MAY HELP LIFT DEPRESSION

A diet high in complex carbohydrates and low in fat may help lift depression and decrease aggressive hostility. In a study of 300 men and women, the *Annals of Internal Medicine* reported that depression and hostility dropped sharply in those who went on a cholesterol-reduced diet and led to greater feelings of self-efficacy and enhanced psychological well-being.

Source: *One Peaceful World Journal* 14, spring 1993.

SUGAR AND REFINED FLOUR ASSOCIATED WITH MENTAL ILLNESS

"Regarding mental disease in the people of the Transkei," a South African doctor observed, "I can say that in the past 11 years I have not diagnosed a single case of schizophrenia in a tribal African living on an unrefined carbohydrate diet, whereas this disease is the commonest psychosis among the urbanized Africans." Dr. G. Daynes associated the rise in mental illness to the widespread consumption of white sugar and refined corn flour.

Source: T. L. Cleave, *The Saccharine Disease* (Bristol: John Wright & Sons, 1974), p. 25.

EMOTIONAL INSTABILITY MAY BE CAUSED BY EXCESS SUGAR INTAKE

In a study of the effects of sugar on the development of mental and psychological disorders, nutritionist Paul Pitchford observed, "It weakens the mind, causing: loss of memory and concentration, nervousness, shyness, violence, excessive or no talking, negative thought, paranoia, and emotional upsets such as self-pity, arguments, irritability, and the desire for only sweet things in life." He said that people who stop eating sugar "nearly always experience higher spirits, emotional stability, improved memory and speech, restful sleep and dreams, fewer colds and dental problems, more endurance and concentration, and better health in general."

Source: Paul Pitchford, *Healing with Whole Foods: Oriental Traditions and Modern Nutrition* (Berkeley: North Atlantic Books, 1993), p. 150.

WHOLE GRAINS LOWER DEPRESSION

Depression is associated with deficiency in omega-3 oils that arises from not eating enough whole grains, beans, nuts, and other seeds, according to recent medical studies. Deep-water fish are also high in this substance. Omega-3 oils lower brain levels of serotonin, which contribute to depression. Depression, for example,

is sixty times more frequent in New Zealand than in Japan, affecting 6 percent and 0.12 percent of the populations respectively. The Japanese eat more whole grains, fresh vegetables, and fish, while New Zealanders eat more refined grains and dairy food.

Sources: C. B. Nemeroff et al., *Archives of General Psychiatry* 56:381, 1999, and M. Maes et al., "Fatty Acid Composition in Major Depression: Decreased Omega-3 Fractions in Cholesteryl Esters and Increased C20:4 Omega-6/C20:5 Omega-3 Ratio in Cholesteryl Esters and Phospholipids," *Journal of Affective Disorders:* 38:35–46, 1996.

PSYCHIATRIST SUCCESSFULLY TREATS HIS PATIENTS WITH MACROBIOTIC DIET

Macrobiotics has benefited many of his patients with chronic and severe mental illness, reports Dr. Stephen Harnish, a New Hampshire psychiatrist. For example, a young woman with severe depression who had been in a state hospital for two years and treated with antidepressants and antipsychotic medication recovered after discontinuing sugar and animal foods and starting a macrobiotic diet. She gradually reduced medication, returned to normal functioning, and was inspired to return to school and resume a normal life. Dr. Harnish said he believed hundreds of other psychiatric patients would benefit from this approach and called for the establishment of group homes with macrobiotic cooks and counselors and psychiatric care providers to provide the best possible integrated approach.

Source: Stephen Harnish, M.D., "On My Awakening to the Macrobiotic Way," in Edward Esko, editor, *Doctors Look at Macrobiotics* (Tokyo and New York: Japan Publications, 1988), pp. 151–68.

TABLE 29. MENTAL AND EMOTIONAL CONDITIONS AND DISORDERS

1. More Yin Cause	2. More Yang Cause	3. Yin and Yang Combined
Typical Symptoms		
Scattered nervousness	Tense, wired nervousness	Edgy nervousness
Lack of focus	Excessive focus	Pickiness
Laxity	Strictness	Obsessive and compulsive behavior
Laughter	Seriousness	
Some frustration	Some frustration	General frustration
Some excitability	Some excitability	
Fragmented view	Narrow view	Strange or erratic view
Conditions and Disorders		
Sadness, melancholy	Boredom, mental fatigue	Apathy
Some depression	Some depression	Some depression
Mania and euphoria	Contained or suppressed emotions	Hypoglycemia and mood swings
Complaining	Short temper, irritability	Hatred, violence
Overly talkative	Noncommunicative	Combination of extremes
Hesitation, apprehensiveness	Recklessness	Insecurity
Overly generous nature	Stingy nature	Calculating nature
Anxiety, worry	Suspicion, doubt	Skepticism, cynicism, jealousy
Hypersensitivity	Insensitivity	Resentment
Apprehension	Fearlessness	Recklessness
Forgetfulness, loss of memory	Preoccupation, fixation	Vengeance
Hysteria	Catatonia (some cases)	Bipolar disease
Low self-esteem	Psychosis	Multiple personality
Masochism	Meanness, cruelty	Sadomasochism
Verbal abuse	Physical abuse	Psychological abuse
Carelessness	Neglect	Irresponsibility
Slothfulness	Pride	Greed
Fear	Anger	Envy
Schizophrenia	Paranoia	Schizophrenic paranoia
Suicidal tendency	Destructive tendency	Homicidal tendency
Living in a world of illusions	Living in a world of delusions	Living in a fantasy world

CASE HISTORIES

YOUNG MAN WITH SCHIZOPHRENIA
RECOVERS WITH MACROBIOTICS

As a child, David Briscoe loved candy, cookies, ice cream, and other sugary foods. He also enjoyed steak and french fries, salty chips and crackers, and other extreme foods. In high school, he had frequent sore throats, digestive problems, fevers, a duodenal ulcer, and kidney problems. As he grew up, he became moody and withdrawn. Psychiatrists diagnosed schizophrenia, and he was on Thorazine, a tranquilizer, for six years. As his illness progressed, he went to many specialists, took many medications, and was in many mental health hospitals. With the help of his mother, Charlotte Mahoney-Briscoe, he began a macrobiotic diet. After changing to a diet based on brown rice and other whole grains, fresh vegetables, and good-quality seasonings such as shoyu, he made a complete recovery. He went on to become a macrobiotic teacher, counselor, and center director. He is the father of four children and today works as a macrobiotic dietary counselor in a community hospital in northern California, helping others heal their mental and physical problems.

Source: David Briscoe and Charlotte Mahoney-Briscoe, *A Personal Peace: Macrobiotic Reflections on Mental and Emotional Recovery* (Tokyo and New York: Japan Publications, 1989).

◎ MUSCLE PROBLEMS

Muscle conditions include swelling, inflammation, stiffness, constriction, hardening, general weakness, tension, cramps, and pains. These are most common in the back or neck but can appear in any part of the body. Muscle disorders include charley horse, spasms, dystonia, myalgia, tetanus, myotonia, tetany, atrophy, muscular dystrophy, and cerebral palsy. In today's society, stiffness, swelling, tightening, and tension in the muscles are considered a natural part of aging, and millions of people experience these symptoms. More serious disorders affecting the muscles are also increasingly common. A battery of relaxants and other drugs are used to relieve muscle problems. A more natural approach, centered on a diet of whole grains and vegetables, will contribute to healthy muscles and relief from muscle conditions and disorders. *See also "Bone and Joint Disorders" and "Nervous Conditions and Disorders" for related conditions.*

SYMPTOMS

The following symptoms may accompany muscle disorders:

1. Swelling, inflammation, or pain
2. Stiffness, hardness, and tightness
3. Softness, loosening, or redness
4. Strain or difficulty walking, stretching, or performing normal physical activities

CAUSES

1. Overall, the muscles are more dense and compact than many organs, glands, and tissues in the body. They are not as dense as bones or joints and are classified as moderate or in between in terms of their overall balance of yin

and yang energy. Healthy muscles are formed by whole grains, beans, vegetables from land and sea, and other strengthening foods, especially those that are high in plant-quality protein. The muscles are especially weakened by animal-quality protein such as that in beef, pork, eggs, chicken, and dairy food, as well as sugar, oily and greasy food, stimulants, spices, alcohol, and other expansive items.

2. In traditional Oriental medicine and philosophy, the muscles are governed by the liver and its related functions. Dietary items that particularly nourish the liver and muscles are whole grains (especially wheat and barley), leafy green vegetables, fermented foods such as miso and tempeh, and foods with a sour taste.

3. Inflammation or general muscle weakness can be caused by either strong yin factors (such as sugar, ice cream, tomatoes) or by a combination of strong yin and yang factors (also including meat, poultry, eggs, and too much salt or baked goods).

4. Swelling and softening of the muscles is caused by strong yin factors, while hardening and tightening is caused by strong yang factors.

5. Immobility of the muscles can be caused by extreme yang factors or a combination of extreme yang and yin factors.

6. Sudden paralysis of the muscles is caused by excessive yin factors, while gradual paralysis of the muscles is caused by overly yang factors.

7. Muscle pain and tension is primarily caused by extreme yin factors.

FORMS

Backache. Backache is the most common health problem among adults in modern society. It comes primarily from muscle strain around the spine, especially the curve of the lower back, and the base of the neck. The main symptoms are aching or stiffness, sharp pain in the upper or lower back or neck, especially after physical activity such as heavy lifting, or chronic aches and pains in the middle or lower back after standing or sitting for prolonged periods. Anti-inflammatory drugs, painkillers, and muscle relaxants are commonly prescribed to control the symptoms of backache. Sports medicine specialists often treat athletes with an electrotherapy known as *transcutaneous electrical nerve stimulator* (TENS), which uses an electrical current to relieve pain. In severe cases, surgery will be used to sever a nerve and eliminate excruciating pain.

A sedentary lifestyle, lack of exercise, poor posture, stress and tension, and lack of sleep are contributing factors to ordinary backache, as most physicians are aware. However, the main cause of backache and muscle strains is long-term consumption of extreme foods that produce acidic effects, especially the buildup of lactic acid, which can weaken the muscles. Animal protein is especially damaging, and all meat, eggs, poultry, and dairy foods are to be avoided to relieve this condition. However, sugar, chocolate, and other refined sweeteners; refined grains; excessive fruit and juice; tropical foods; stimulants; spices; and alcohol and drugs can produce overly expansive effects, resulting in muscle swelling, inflammation, strain, tension, and pain. Discontinuing these items and observing a balanced macrobiotic way of eating will help restore normal muscle tone and gradually eliminate symptoms. Throughout our life, from childhood to old age, we should be able to walk, bend, stretch, play, and keep active without any stiffness, aches, or pain. A centrally balanced diet, adjusted slightly according to the condition, will help eliminate the underlying cause of the ache or pain. A GINGER COMPRESS on the lower back will provide immediate relief. Apply for about 20 minutes at a time until the condition improves and then several times a week to help general circulation and to dissolve stagnation.

Backaches may also arise from other serious disorders. *See "Ankylosing Spondylotis," "Osteoarthritis," and "Osteoporosis" in "Bone and Joint Disorders"; "Spinal Cord Disorders" in "Nervous Conditions and Disorders"; "Kidney or Bladder Infections" in "Kidney and Bladder Problems"; and "Bone Cancer" in "Cancer."*

Cerebral Palsy. Cerebral palsy (CP) is a neuromuscular disorder accompanied by loss of muscle control, spasticity, and paralysis. It arises from a brain injury in embryo, infancy, or early childhood and affects the nervous impulses that govern muscle movements. About 1 or 2 in every 1,000 babies is born with or develops CP, especially premature infants. The most common type is *spastic cerebral palsy,* in which the muscles are underdeveloped, stiff, and weak. The arms and legs may be affected, only the legs, or only the arm and leg on one side of the body. Seventy percent of those with CP have this type. Another type, *choreoathetoid CP,* involves slow, jerky, uncontrollable movements, and *ataxic CP* is characterized by poor coordination and shaky movements. Speech problems commonly arise, with loss of control over the muscles in the voice box, and seizures are frequent with children with spastic CP. About 40 percent of children with this disorder have normal intelligence, while the others are below normal and, in some cases, severely retarded. CP is treated with physical therapy, braces, orthopedic surgery, speech therapy, and anticonvulsant drugs. About 50 percent of children with this disorder live into adulthood, though they require care and assistance for the rest of their lives.

From a macrobiotic perspective, CP is caused by exposure to strong expansive and contractive factors in embryo and infancy. The quality of the parents' egg and sperm may be extremely weak, the mother's diet during pregnancy may be very yin, or the foods given the developing baby may result in brain damage. A main cause is eating chicken, which contributes to overall tightening and, in extreme cases, withering or wasting away of the muscles. Strong yin is also usually involved, especially sugar, chocolate, honey, and other sweets; milk, ice cream, yogurt, and other light dairy foods; pastries and flour products; tomatoes, potatoes, and other vegetables of tropical origin; oily and greasy food; spices and herbs; coffee, black tea and other stimulants; alcohol and drugs; and infant formula. These contribute to loss of central contractive power and weakening of normal brain functioning. Exposure to X rays, CT scans, MRIs, computers, television, and other forms of radiation, as well as chemicals and toxins in food or the environment, may be contributing factors. While some brain damage may be irreversible, CP can be slowed or controlled to some extent and in some cases substantially relieved by a balanced whole-foods diet. In general, follow the dietary guidelines for Diet #3 arising out of a combination of extreme dietary factors. In addition, a daily BODY

SCRUB, PALM HEALING, SHIATSU massage, and other home remedies, healing methods, and gentle exercises will be helpful.

Cramps and Spasms. A *cramp* is a painful spasmodic contraction of muscles, most commonly in the arms and legs, but also the stomach, back, and calf (where it is known as a charley horse). A *spasm* is an involuntary, uncontrollable contraction of a muscle or of a hollow organ with a muscular wall. The onset of these conditions can produce sharp, strong pain and discomfort. From a macrobiotic perspective, cramping is caused by overconsumption of extreme yin foods and beverages, including sugar, chocolate, honey, and other refined sweeteners; milk, ice cream, and other light dairy; light pastries and other refined flour products; too many fruits and juice; tropical foods and spices; stimulants; and alcohol and drugs. Consuming too many expansive foods expands the tissues and exerts pressure on the nerves, producing a cramp or spasm. Compared to a cramp, a spasm is even more yin, resulting in comparatively greater loss of contractive ability.

For temporary relief, take a teaspoon of GOMASHIO, eat an UMEBOSHI PLUM or drink a small volume of UMEBOSHI JUICE, or take BANCHA TWIG TEA with several drops of shoyu. This will immediately yangize the body and help reduce the cramping or spasm. In the case of stomach cramps, a GINGER COMPRESS, roasted SALT PACK, or other hot application applied to the affected area may also be helpful. For leg cramps, MASSAGE may provide relief, but do not massage on the area of the cramp that is tender and painful. Massage instead toward and immediately above the cramp-ing area. Squeeze firmly the area above the cramp. Alternating towels soaked first in hot and then in cold water may also be applied.

Generally observe the dietary guidelines for Diet #1, with a slight emphasis on yang factors such as stronger MISO SOUP, a little more salt and other seasonings, and proportionately more root vegetables and sea vegetables, to prevent future cramping and the onset of a spasm.

Muscular Dystrophy. Muscular dystrophy is an inherited disease that involves weakness and progressive atrophy of the muscles in the central part of the body. *Duchenne's muscular dystrophy* affects young boys and manifests as weakness in the pelvis, shoulders, and heart. Children with this condition have difficulty moving, climbing, and getting up from a sitting position. The muscles around the joints in the arms and legs contract to the point that the elbows and knees will not extend fully. Scoliosis, or curvature of the back, usually develops by early adolescence and patients are bound to a wheelchair. Death from pneumonia or other illness usually comes by age 20. *Becker's muscular dystrophy,* another form of the disease, strikes older adolescent males, who rarely require wheelchairs and have a longer life expectancy.

From the medical view, muscular dystrophy is genetically transmitted because it is confined to males. All boys who have the defective X chromosome lack the ability to produce dystrophin, a muscle protein necessary for the maintenance of muscle cells, or else the protein is too large and malfunctions. From the macrobiotic perspective, inherited or constitutional tendencies arise from past ways of life, especially the past way of eating, of parents, grandparents, and ancestors. While dystrophin may be lacking or insufficient in males with this tendency, susceptibility to clinical manifestations of muscular dystrophy depend largely on the child's diet. It can arise from extreme dietary factors, including too much chicken, eggs, meat, and other yang, contractive foods or from sugar, chocolate, honey, and other refined sweeteners; milk, ice cream, and other light dairy; light pastries and other refined flour products; too many fruits and juice; tropical foods and spices; too much beverages and fluids; and other overly expansive items. Intake of animal protein and fat, especially poultry, can cause the muscles of the arms and legs to contract and accelerate the spread of the disease. Chicken in particular leads to contraction and weakness in the arms, shoulders, and legs and should be strictly avoided. Muscular dystrophy that begins from the leg is more yang in origin, while that which begins in the hand or upper limbs is more yin.

While muscular dystrophy may not be completely reversed, symptoms can be reduced or controlled to a large extent through proper diet. The standard recommendations will greatly help alleviate this condition. Follow Diet #1 for conditions caused by extreme yin factors or Diet #2 for conditions caused by extreme yang factors. A daily BODY SCRUB will help promote energy circulation and dissolve stagnation. A HOT TOWEL COMPRESS or a GINGER COMPRESS on the weakened muscles will also help provide relief and speed healing. In the event of swelling or inflammation, a cooling application should be used instead such as a TOFU PLASTER or LEAFY GREENS PLASTER.

Myasthenia Gravis. Myasthenia gravis (MG) is a degenerative neuromuscular disease in which the body produces antibodies that damage receptors that carry nerve impulses. This leads to progressive weakening of muscles, especially in the eyelids (drooping eyelids), eyes, vocal region, mouth, arms, and legs. Typically, MG manifests in bouts, and the ability to perform ordinary tasks and activities weakens in the space of several hours or days. Paralysis results in some cases, and about 10 percent of patients become too weak to breathe. Women are more likely to develop MG than men, and it frequently arises between the ages of 20 and 40. Pregnant women with this disease can pass it along to their babies, but symptoms disappear shortly after birth.

Conventional medicine treats MG with drugs that increase the level of acetylcholine, a neurotransmitter that strengthens the muscles. However, the most commonly prescribed drugs cause abdominal cramps, diarrhea, and other side effects that may require further medications to control. Also, over time the drugs lose their effectiveness. Crisis intervention for potentially fatal breathing complications and surgical removal of the thymus are resorted to in severe cases.

From the macrobiotic perspective, MG arises from a combination of extreme dietary factors. Overconsumption of both strong yin and yang foods and beverages eventually causes the muscles to lose their contractive ability and produce antibodies that attack the nervous system. To prevent or relieve this condition, it is essential to discontinue all animal foods high in saturated fat and cholesterol, as well as refined flour and flour products; sugar and other sweets; tropical foods; stimulants; spices; alcohol; and drugs. Oil, fruit, juice, nuts, and good-quality sweets should also be limited until the condition improves. Follow Diet #3 for conditions arising from a combination of extreme yin and yang factors. A daily BODY SCRUB will help promote energy circulation and dissolve stagnation. A HOT TOWEL COMPRESS or a GINGER COMPRESS on the weakened muscles will also help provide relief and speed healing. In the event of swelling or inflammation, a cooling application should be used instead, such as a TOFU PLASTER or LEAFY GREENS PLASTER.

Sprains and Strains. Moving a muscle beyond its normal range of movement can produce a sprain or a strain. The foot, hand, and shoulder are common sites of sprains and strains. For temporary relief, apply a TARO PLASTER or a TOFU PLASTER. If these are not available, use a LEAFY GREENS PLASTER. These external applications will help reduce the swelling and inflammation and quicken healing. If swelling has already started, apply a BUCKWHEAT PLASTER or GINGER COMPRESS followed by a TARO PLASTER or LEAFY GREENS PLASTER. Other traditional home remedies for these conditions include a plaster made of wheat flour mixed with willow leaves or a cool compress made with the liquid from boiled willow leaves. Susceptibility to sprains and strains depends on our daily health. A balanced natural way of eating will create strength and flexibility, so that most sprains and strains are avoided or harmless.

Tetanus. Tetanus is a serious, potentially fatal disorder in which the muscles of the neck, jaw, or other region seize up. Known as *lockjaw*, this condition is accompanied by grimacing, uncontrollable spasms of the muscles in the jaw and neck, and pain and spasms in other muscles. Tetanus is associated with *Clostridium tetani*, a bacterium that typically enters a wound and produces a toxin that gets in the bloodstream. It progressively damages the nerves, blocking the muscles from relaxing. Over the course of several weeks, as the microbe spreads, spasms in the facial muscles and jaw appear and progress to the back and extremities. Physicians treat tetanus with antibiotics and injection of tetanus antitoxin. An artificial respirator may be needed if breathing is impaired. Slightly more than half the patients with tetanus survive. Tetanus immunization is one of the most common vaccines. It is commonly given to infants and children in the form of DPT vaccine—diphtheria, pertussis (whooping cough), and tetanus—and booster shots are recommended every 10 years.

From an energetic view, the symptoms of tetanus are extremely yang, resulting in over-contraction of the muscles and a locking of the jaws. The bacterium associated with tetanus is a common microbe, found in the human colon as well as in the soil. Susceptibility to tetanus depends on our overall health and immune function, especially the quality of our blood, lymph, and other bodily fluids. A person in optimal health who is eating whole grains and vegetables as his or her principal food will have naturally strong blood and lymph and will be able to neutralize the effects of virulent strains of microorganisms that may enter a wound. However, if we are eating in the modern way, taking dietary extremes that produce acidic effects, the blood and lymph will not be strong enough to neutralize the microbe. For people eating in the modern way, vaccination will help protect against the onset of tetanus and other infectious diseases, but it will contribute to the overall weakening of the body and there may be serious side effects to the vaccine itself. In the event that tetanus is suspected or symptoms appear, immediate medical attention is required. A standard diet will help reduce the spread of the microbe, especially strong MISO SOUP regularly, UMEBOSHI PLUMS, sea vegetables, and good-quality salt and other seasonings in cooking. For tetanus, observe Diet #2 for more overly contracted conditions.

SOLUTION

DIET

Follow the dietary recommendations noted above with emphasis on the following:

1. Eat whole grains, not refined grains, as the main dish of every meal. Whole wheat and barley are particularly strengthening for the muscles and may be eaten regularly along with brown rice, millet, and other whole grains.

2. Reduce hard baked flour products as much as possible. Noodles may be taken several times a week, especially udon or somen noodles.

3. Avoid simple sugars (refined sugar, honey, and chocolate).

4. Avoid animal food with the exception of fish or seafood, preferably freshwater fish such as perch or trout, once or twice a week.

5. Beans provide good quality protein for muscle development. Select among a variety of beans, particularly the smaller beans such

as adzuki beans, lentils, chickpeas, and black soybeans. Bean products may also be eaten regularly, especially tofu, tempeh, and natto.

6. Eat plenty of vegetables every day, especially green leafy vegetables.

7. Cooked onions are particularly soothing for the muscles. They are excellent for heavy muscle labor and the prevention of muscle tiredness or tension.

8. Sea vegetables are strengthening and may be taken in small, regular amounts daily.

9. The amount of salt (miso, shoyu, and sea salt) should be moderate, adjusting slightly for a more expanded or contracted condition.

10. As a rule, fruit and fruit juices should be limited or avoided, except in the case of overly contracted conditions in which case a small volume may be taken.

11. Limit nuts and nut and seed butters until the condition improves. However, chestnuts and dark sesame seeds may be taken.

12. Use condiments moderately, especially those with a sour taste such as UMEBOSHI PLUMS.

13. Cut down on water to a moderate level, but do not reduce it too much. Besides BANCHA TWIG TEA, teas that nourish the kidney include KOMBU TEA and MU TEA.

14. Reduce the total volume of food and chew more.

15. Avoid late-night eating.

LIFESTYLE
Follow the standard way of life suggestions.

HOME REMEDIES
1. CARROT-DAIKON DRINK will help eliminate fat and oil accumulation that accom-

TABLE 30. MUSCLE CONDITIONS AND DISORDERS

1. More Yin Cause	2. More Yang Cause	3. Yin and Yang Combined
Typical Symptoms		
Swelling	Constriction	Constriction
Inflammation	Hardening	Inflammation
General weakness		General weakness
Pains		Immobility
Tension		
Some backache	Some backache	Some backache
Cramp		
Spasm		
Sudden paralysis	Gradual paralysis	
Diseases		
Tetany	Tetanus	Stiffness of neck and shoulder
Some hernia		Some hernia
Dystonia (writer's cramp, yips, and others)	Myotonia	Torticolis
Some muscular dystrophy	Some muscular dystrophy	Myasthenia gravis
		Cerebral palsy

panies stagnated conditions. Take 1 small cup every day for 5 days and then every second or third day for several weeks.

2. SHIITAKE-DAIKON TEA is also good to help eliminate the accumulation of fat. Take 1 small cup once every third day for 1 month.

3. To help dissolve heavy, stagnated protein that accumulates in the muscles, every day take LEAFY GREENS JUICE, made from kale, collard greens, dandelion, daikon or turnip leaves, or Chinese cabbage.

4. A BODY SCRUB every day or twice a day with a towel dipped in hot water or hot ginger water, including over the spinal region, will pro-

mote better circulation and activate physical and mental energies.

5. A hot GINGER COMPRESS may be applied over the kidneys, lower back, or region of muscle tension or pain two or three times a week to reduce stagnation and improve blood and energy flow.

6. In the event of swelling or inflammation, a TOFU PLASTER, LEAFY GREENS PLASTER, or other cooling application should be used instead of a hot towel compress, a ginger compress, or other hot application.

CAUTION

1. Prompt medical attention should be sought for any severe muscle condition, including spasm or seizure, that does not respond to the dietary and home remedies recommendations listed above.

2. If tetanus is suspected, seek immediate medical attention.

MEDICAL EVIDENCE

DIET MAY HELP TREAT MUSCULAR DYSTROPHY

In a laboratory experiment, German researchers reported that adding whole wheat kernels to the diet of mice helped prevent the progression of muscle weakness and weight loss. The study was designed to test the possible use of diet in treating muscular dystrophy.

Source: C. Hubner, "Wheat Kernel Ingestion Protects from Progression of Muscle Weakness in MDX Mice, an Animal Model of Duchenne Muscular Dystrophy," *Pediatric Research* 40(3):444–49, 1996.

WHOLE GRAINS REDUCE RISK OF CEREBRAL PALSY

In a study of the effects of diet on the development of cerebral palsy, medical researchers at the Athens University Medical School reported that the consumption of cereal grains and fish by mothers of over 300 children were associated with lower risk of cerebral palsy, while consumption of meat was associated with increased risk.

Source: E. Petridou, "Diet During Pregnancy and the Risk of Cerebral Palsy," *British Journal of Nutrition* 79(5):407–12, 1998.

◎ NAUSEA AND VOMITING

Nausea and vomiting may accompany many ailments and disorders, including indigestion, anxiety or distress, motion sickness, gastritis and other stomach ills, hiatal hernia, migraine headache, Menière's disease and inner ear problems, gallbladder problems, jaundice and liver problems, alcohol or drug abuse, diabetes, allergies, morning sickness and other complications of pregnancy, concussion, and brain tumors. The home remedies below will help relieve these symptoms.

CAUSE

1. There is no single cause for nausea or vomiting. However, in most cases there is an overly acidic condition from eating extreme foods, including meat, eggs, poultry, and other animal foods; dairy products; sugar, chocolate, and concentrated sweeteners; tropical foods and beverages; stimulants; spices; alcohol and drugs.

2. The intestines are usually weak or stagnated. Throwing up is a strong contractive discharge, often a protective mechanism against the intake of too much strong yin, or strong yin and yang combined.

SOLUTION

DIET

1. For a more yin condition, observe Diet #1; for a more yang condition Diet #2; and for one combining both factors, follow Diet #3.

2. Generally, use a little more salt, shoyu,

miso, UMEBOSHI PLUM, and salt-based condiments to help counterbalance the strong, upward energy represented by vomiting.

LIFESTYLE
Follow the standard way-of-life recommendations.

1. Soaking the feet in salty water, cold or room temperature, will help bring the energy in the body down.

2. MASSAGE, PALM HEALING, and other gentle applications may also be helpful.

HOME REMEDIES
1. Prepare SHOYU BANCHA TEA or BANCHA TWIG TEA WITH GOMASHIO. Take 1 to 3 cups every day for 1 to 3 days.

2. Take GOMASHIO, up to 3 teaspoons a day, for several days.

3. Take UMEBOSHI PLUM, UME-SHO BANCHA, or ume concentrate. Umeboshi plums will neutralize both extreme acid and alkaline conditions and improve the blood and body fluid circulation.

4. Eat sauerkraut cooked with umeboshi or soft rice with umeboshi.

5. Prepare a special remedy using salt to counteract the outward and upward energy of vomiting. Grate a piece of fresh gingerroot, mix it with salt, and bake the mixture in an oven until it becomes hard and black. Boil the powder into a tea. Drink this tea after cooling, as hot tea will make the body's energy go up, which will counteract its intended effect. If ginger is not available, use garlic or the white part and roots of scallion. These need to be baked only a short time, unlike ginger, which takes longer.

CAUTION
A physician should be consulted for persistent vomiting and nausea.

◎ NERVOUS CONDITIONS AND DISORDERS

Nervous conditions and disorders range from dizziness and numbness to pinched nerve, vertigo, epilepsy, multiple sclerosis, Alzheimer's disease, amyotrophic lateral sclerosis, neuralgia, Parkinson's disease, Huntington's disease, spinal cord disorders such as herniated disk, peripheral nerve disorders, and Tourette's syndrome. *See also "Brain Disorders," "Headaches," and "Muscle Problems."*

According to modern science and medicine, nervous conditions and disorders have an underlying physical cause or organic basis, in contrast to mental and emotional disorders, which are considered primarily psychological in origin. In many cases, the cause of organic nervous disorders is not known, and there is no cure, though medication may help slow or control their effects. From the macrobiotic perspective, there is no sharp distinction between the physical and the psychological or between nervous disorders and mental and emotional disorders. Each cell of the body receives constant nourishment and consciousness from an intricate network of nerves, blood vessels, and meridian endings. Overall health or sickness, including behavior, thoughts, emotions, and other forms of consciousness, is the product of all of these influences. Hence the nervous, circulatory, digestive, and respiratory systems are integrally related and involved in every condition and disorder. For the sake of convenience we have followed the modern classification and will look at the most commonly regarded nervous conditions in this section. However, we will show how the entire body is governed by antagonistic yet complementary systems of nervous control. In most cases, proper diet, exercise, and lifestyle practices will help prevent and alleviate nervous system problems.

CAUSES

1. The nervous system is complementary to the digestive system. Compared to each other, the tighter, more compact nervous system is yang, while the looser, more expanded digestive system is yin. The nervous system digests and processes energy in the form of waves and vibrations (yin), while the digestive system processes energy in the form of material food (yang). According to the principles of complementarity/antagonism, the nervous system is more likely to gather yang excess in the form of animal foods, salt, and baked flour, while the digestive system is more likely to gather yin excess in the form of sugar, oil, fruit, spices, alcohol, and drugs. However, as extreme yin attracts yang and vice versa, strong yin can also gather in the nervous system (e.g., drugs scrambling the brain) and strong yang can damage the digestive system (e.g., meat causing cancer in the pancreas or large intestine).

2. The nervous system consists of the brain, spinal cord, and nerves throughout the body. Functionally the nervous system can be divided into the central nervous system (yang) and the peripheral nervous system (yin). The central nervous system consists of the brain (yang) and the spine (yin). As a general rule, the central nervous system is more affected by yang and the peripheral system more affected by yin. Also, excess yin will more likely gather in the brain, while excess yang will gather in the spine, though once again the opposite tendency may occur in some cases.

3. The peripheral nervous system governs sensory judgment and response and is divided into the parasympathetic branch (yang) and the autonomic or orthosympathetic branch (yin). The parasympathetic consists of 12 pairs of cranial nerves and 31 pairs of spinal nerves. These are more peripherally located in the body (yin). The orthosympathetic consists of corresponding cranial and spinal nerves, but these are located deeper within the body (yang). The autonomic nervous system governs unconscious or automatic processes, including adjustment to the internal environment, climate, atmosphere, electrical charge, and other stimuli. As a rule, animal foods (yang) strengthen the senses and lead to keen vision, hearing, smell, taste, and other sensory abilities. Plant foods (yin) develop the autonomic nerves, leading to reception of shorter waves, higher and more subtle vibrations, stronger intuition, and extrasensory or spiritual abilities.

4. In almost all organs, tissues, and smooth muscles, there are pairs of autonomic nerves, one orthosympathetic and one parasympathetic, which act in opposite ways. For example, parasympathetic nerves cause the blood vessels to dilate, the bronchi to constrict, the iris to dilate, and the digestive sphincter to relax. Orthosympathetic nerves cause the blood vessels to constrict, the bronchi to dilate, the iris to contract, and the digestive sphincter to constrict. The response of the autonomic nervous system can be summarized as follows: When the parasympathetic nerves act on expanded organs, contraction results; on compact organs expansion or dilation is brought about. Conversely, the orthosympathetic nerves inhibit hollow, yin organs and stimulate yang, compact ones. As a rule, the parasympathetic system is especially affected by the consumption of strong yin, especially drugs and medications, while the orthosympathetic is affected by strong yang, especially meat, eggs, and salt. For example, drugs will cause the pupils of the eyes to contract and the blood vessels to dilate. However, after prolonged drug use, the parasympathetic nerves become exhausted, losing their contractive force; then the pupils dilate and the vessels contract.

5. At the cellular level, neurons, or nerve cells, consist of the more compact, central dendrite (yang) and the longer, more peripheral axon (yin). These specialized cells receive and transmit impulses. Incoming impulses are more yin structurally (expanded) but yang energetically (centripetal). Outgoing impulses are more yang structurally (contracted) but yin energetically (centrifugal). Dietary excess will affect these respective cellular structures and functions according to complementary/antagonistic principles. For example, Alzheimer's disease, characterized by deterioration of brain cells, represents a loss of central yang gathering energy in the dendrites. This symptom arises primarily from past consumption of past yin, especially sugar and sweets.

6. In general, cramping and spasms involving nerve cells and muscle tissues are yang contractions that arise in the body to offset the intake of extreme yin foods and beverages. Jerking and twitching are yin symptoms arising chiefly from loss of contractive power and also are caused by too much yin. Numbing and tingling can be produced by dietary excess of either kind. Degeneration of nerve cells and wasting away of muscle tissue arise primarily from overconsumption of yang items. Nerve pain that is mild, dull, diffuse, or long-lasting tends to be caused by taking too much yin, while nerve pain that is severe, penetrating, acute, localized, or of short duration tends to be caused by too much yang.

7. From the systemic to the cellular levels, meat, poultry, eggs, cheese, fish, seafood, and other animal products, as well as too much salt and hard baked flour products, tighten, narrow, and harden the nerves, contributing to rigid thinking and behavior.

8. From the systemic to the cellular levels, sugar, chocolate, and other refined sweeteners; milk, ice cream, and other light dairy products; refined grains; tropical foods; excessive fruit and juice; excessive oil and raw foods; stimulants; spices; alcohol; drugs; and other extremely expansive substances loosen, expand, and weaken the nerves, contributing to loss of focus and concentration, memory loss, indecision, and other yin symptoms.

FORMS

Alzheimer's Disease. Alzheimer's is a degenerative brain disease in which nerve fibers become tangled, protein deposits or plaque build up in the brain tissue, and normal mental functioning declines. Characterized by memory loss, disorientation, and confusion, Alzheimer's is commonly accompanied by frustration, bewilderment, dramatic mood swings, and gradual loss of physical and mental abilities. In the end, the persons grow noncommunicative, incontinent, and physically unable to care for themselves. Death follows from within several years to more than 20 years, with the average about 7 years. In the United States, Alzheimer's is the fourth leading cause of death after heart disease, cancer, and stroke among adults. Women are twice as likely as men to have the disease, whites are four times as susceptible as blacks, and one out of three elderly persons over 80 has Alzheimer's. The disease is considered incurable, and modern medicine uses several medications to slow down its spread, control mood swings, and other symptoms. Family support is a major concern, as caring for an Alzheimer's patient puts tremendous stress on other family members.

From the macrobiotic view, Alzheimer's is caused by long-term dietary excess. When food becomes one-sided, either too yin or yang, it affects thinking, the emotions, and mental functioning. If the nerves, neurological centers, and brain cells and tissues are too tight or too loose, thinking becomes impaired. The primary cause of Alzheimer's disease is chronic consumption of excessive animal fat and protein from meat, dairy, chicken, and eggs, which affect the nerves and capillaries. The secondary cause is excessive intake of simple sugars, especially sugar, chocolate, and honey. Sugar affects the synthesis of the B vitamins in the intestines and consequently brain functioning. Too much oily, greasy food; refined flour from bread and pasta; and hot spices, including mustard and garlic, are contributing factors. Overeating may also be involved.

If organic structural and functional changes in the brain and nerves have taken place, it may be difficult to recover completely. However, in the early stages, the onset of Alzheimer's can often be halted, and in later stages it can be controlled and sometimes reversed. The standard macrobiotic way of eating should be observed, consuming whole grains as the center of each meal. Observe the dietary guidelines for Diet #3, for conditions arising from a combination of dietary extremes. No flour products, including noodles, pasta, bread, or baked goods, should be taken until the condition improves. Take MISO SOUP, a variety of fresh vegetables prepared in different styles, a small portion of beans and bean products, and sea vegetables daily. Avoid oily, greasy food, including all nuts and nut butters. Avoid spices, stimulants, alcohol, and other high-energy foods that can accelerate the condition. Be especially careful not to eat food that has been cooked on an electric stove or microwaved. The following home remedies are especially recommended for Alzheimer's disease:

1. Sweet vegetables are especially good, and SWEET VEGETABLE DRINK may be taken daily, 1 small cup for the first month, and then every other day for the next month, and then occasionally.

2. KINPIRA SOUP is very good for this condition; take 2 or 3 times a week.

3. As a special dish, prepare the following: 3 parts dried daikon, 1 part kombu (or arame or hijiki), and 1 part carrot. Cook ingredients together, adding a light shoyu taste at the end of cooking. Take one small dish every day or every other day at mealtimes. As a substitute, add

4 times as much water to the mixture, bring to a boil, and simmer for 20 minutes, adding a light salt or shoyu taste at the end of cooking. Drink and eat every day for 10 days, then 2–3 times per week for 2 months.

4. Take ½ to 1 UMEBOSHI PLUM, finely chopped. Put in a small cup, add ½ sheet of toasted nori broken in pieces, and 3–4 drops of shoyu. Then pour hot bancha tea over the mixture, stir, and drink. Take every day for 5 days, then every other day for 10 days, and then 2–3 times per week for 1–2 months.

5. Externally, a hot towel soaked in ginger water may be applied to the neck and face to improve circulation. A FOOT BATH with ginger and a BODY SCRUB should be done once or twice a day.

Medical studies have associated exposure to aluminum and zinc with higher risks of Alzheimer's disease. While these are not primary factors, cookware should be made of stainless steel, cast iron, ceramic, or other natural material, not aluminum. Similarly, natural spring water, well water, or filtered water should be used for drinking and cooking. Avoid municipal tap water, which may contain chemicals and be high in aluminum, zinc, and other metals.

Amyotrophic Lateral Sclerosis. ALS is a progressive neurological disorder that is also called *Lou Gehrig's disease,* named after the famous New York Yankees baseball player who died in 1941. Weakness in the muscles or one limb appears in the early stages, often accompanied by problems in walking, speech, and hand coordination. As the condition spreads, other limbs may become weakened, and muscle cramps, nervous

twitching, and problems with breathing, swallowing, and chewing arise. Intellectual and sensory functioning remain normal through the course of the disease and pain rarely occurs. As the nerve cells in the brain and spinal cord deteriorate, paralysis sets in, followed by death in 2 to 5 years. Modern medicine considers ALS an incurable disease arising from unknown causes. Physical therapy helps prolong muscle use, and drugs can ease cramps.

From the macrobiotic perspective, ALS arises from a combination of dietary extremes, especially chicken, eggs, spices, and fruits, including citrus fruit, and vinegar and other sour-tasting foods. Long-term consumption of beef, pork, chicken, eggs, and other foods high in saturated fat and cholesterol lead to the degeneration of nerve cells in the brain and spinal cord that control muscle movement. Chicken and eggs are especially debilitating and contribute to ALS's characteristic overcontraction or wasting of muscles and tissues. Lemon, lime, orange, grapefruit, and other citrus fruit make the brain sharp, contributing to continued mental functioning during the course of the disease. ALS patients usually do not eat much sugar or tropical fruits such as banana that disperse and dull the mind, contributing to memory loss, sensory decline, and other extreme yin symptoms, as in the case of Alzheimer's disease and other brain and neurological disorders.

Some medical studies indicate that the neuromuscular symptoms of ALS can be relieved by administration of vitamin E and thiamin. These vitamins are naturally abundant in whole grains and other plant foods, and a balanced natural-foods diet may help prevent or relieve this condition. Of course, all animal food and strong spices should be discontinued. Observe the dietary guidelines for Diet #3, for conditions arising from a combination of dietary extremes, and the following special home remedies:

1. Prepare KINPIRA SOUP, adding daikon greens, turnip greens, or mustard greens, chopped very finely. These can constitute about 50 percent of the total mixture. Cook with onions, squash, and the other ingredients. Very occasionally, a small amount of grated ginger may be added toward the end of cooking (2–3 minutes), but generally this is not needed. Take 1 cup or bowl of this soup daily or every other day for the first month; then take twice a week for 2–3 months.

2. Prepare a special stew consisting of 5 parts soybeans soaked overnight, 1 part carrot, 1 part lotus root, 1 part daikon, 1 part onion, 1 part cabbage, 1 part squash. Add twice as much water and boil for a long time, adding a light miso, shoyu, or salt taste at the end of cooking. Take every other day or three times a week for 2–3 months. This dish will keep for 1 day and may be reheated and used the following day.

3. Hard, leafy green vegetables high in fiber are good for this condition and may be taken daily, steamed or lightly boiled.

4. Apply a HOT TOWEL COMPRESS soaked in ginger water on the arms, hands, fingers and on the legs, feet, and toes every day, once or twice a day.

In addition to diet, CHANTING, PALM HEALING, MEDITATION, and other gentle activities can also help release blockages, improve blood circulation and energy flow, and stimulate the regeneration of damaged nerve cells.

Dizziness and Vertigo. Dizziness involves feeling light-headed, faint, spaced out, or off-balance. Dizziness may also accompany other disorders related to the nervous system, including stroke or heart attack, multiple sclerosis, brain tumor or bleeding, osteoarthritis in the neck, an inflamed inner ear and/or nerve damage to the ear, Menière's disease, or motion sickness. Vertigo is a more intense form of dizziness, involving feelings of spinning or movement. It is sometimes brought on by a fear of heights or a fear of falling. For simple dizziness, physicians recommend that the person close her eyes, bow her head, and breathe deeply. Antibiotics, antihypertensives, anti-inflammatory drugs, and other medications can bring on dizziness, and these may need to be changed or discontinued. For vertigo that accompanies more serious disorders, doctors may recommend a neck collar, medication, or physical therapy.

Dizziness is generally a more yin disorder in which strong upward energy predominates over downward, contracting energy. The simple procedures noted above—closing the eyes, bowing the head, and breathing deeply—are all contractive, yang exercises designed to steady, focus, and ground the person. Often there is a lack of salt in the diet. Simple foods may also be taken to prevent or relieve dizzy spells. Take a teaspoon of GOMASHIO, eat an UMEBOSHI PLUM, or take a small cup of SHOYU BANCHA TEA. This will yangize you and provide immediate relief. Liver imbalances are a common cause of dizziness, since rising earth's force is carried up to the neck and head by the liver meridian. Yin dietary extremes, such as sugar, alcohol, or drugs, are especially taxing to this organ and can bring on dizziness. Anemia, or overall weakening of the blood, can also produce dizziness. Pancreatic problems are a frequent cause of dizziness or vertigo as blood sugar levels fluctuate. ADZUKI BEAN, SQUASH, AND KOMBU DISH may be taken frequently for this condition to stabilize the pancreas.

For dizziness caused by underlying conditions, see the specific disorder involved—for example, "Ear and Hearing Problems" for information on imbalances arising from troubles in the inner ear. True vertigo is generally more chronic. It may also be caused by extreme yin intake. However, the type of vertigo that manifests as fear of heights, including fear of flying, is commonly yang in origin. Birds and other creatures that fly are very yang, and when we get yang we tend to walk with the heels of our feet elevated. People who are afraid of heights are generally too yang from consuming too much animal food, salt, baked food, or other contractive fare. As a result, they are repelled by ascending to high places or flying in planes. Of course, there are also very yin people who are afraid of flying and high places, too, as well as new situations and experiences of any kind. Both of these types of vertigo show developing kidney problems. A GINGER COMPRESS on the lower back several times a week until the condition improves may be helpful in both cases. The standard way of eating will eliminate most types of dizziness and vertigo. For conditions arising from too much yin, observe the guidelines for Diet #1. For conditions arising from too much yang, observe the guidelines for Diet

#2. In most cases, the blood quality is weak and lacking in minerals. To strengthen the blood, cook MISO-ZOSUI. Avoid spices, including ginger for the time being. Also, sweets should be avoided or reduced until the condition improves. HOTO, another special dish, will help create stability. A special drink can be made from 3 parts adzuki beans, 1 part dried shiitake, 1 part dried daikon, 1 part kombu, and 1 part fresh daikon. Cook together for about 20 minutes and drink the liquid.

Epilepsy. Epilepsy involves brain and muscle seizures. Convulsive fits are divided into two main types: the generalized type, which affects the entire brain, and the partial type, which is confined to one area of the brain. The most common forms of seizure are generalized: a *petit mal seizure* may involve staring or swallowing motions and can take place repeatedly during the day, and a *grand mal seizure* starts with a cry, loss of consciousness, and a fall and is characterized by rigid, jerky movements and confusion, often followed by deep sleep. Partial types include temporal lobe seizures that may be accompanied by hallucinations, déjà vu and other unusual perceptions, and abdominal discomfort and Jacksonian seizures that involve twitching of specific muscles that can spread to the entire body. Epilepsy often arises in childhood, and it strikes males more than females. Modern medicine treats epilepsy with anticonvulsants that can control seizures when they occur. Epileptics are encouraged to wear a Medic Alert bracelet to alert others when they suffer an attack.

From the macrobiotic view, epilepsy is an extreme yin disorder, resulting from the overexpansion of the cells of the brain. When the brain tissue swells, it pinches the delicate network of nerve cells within the brain to the point where it interferes with the firing of neurons. A breakdown in the electrical firing of nerve cells causes temporary loss of consciousness and a seizure. The primary dietary cause of epilepsy is overconsumption of fluids, including too much water in drinking or cooking, juice, soft drinks, mineral water, coffee, tea, alcohol, and other beverages. Strong yin foods that contain a lot of liquid, such sugary foods and sweets and tropical fruits and vegetables, are contributing factors.

Men are more likely to become epileptic because they tend to consume more liquid, such as beer, than women and are not able to handle excessive yin energy as well as women. However, women who have taken birth control pills are at higher risk than women not using oral contraceptives. Exposure to certain chemicals, some prescription and over-the-counter medications, and other substances can also trigger an epileptic attack.

Epileptics can usually sense when a seizure is coming. To reduce the severity of the attack or prevent it altogether, a yang condiment should repeatedly be taken, such as UMEBOSHI PLUM, TEKKA, or GOMASHIO, at 5- to 10-minute intervals. It is recommended that someone with epilepsy carry these at all times for emergency use.

In addition to controlling liquid, eliminating sugar, alcohol, and dairy, the standard diet should be observed, including slightly stronger cooking, frequent MISO SOUP, more root vegetables, and slightly more salt and shoyu. Observe the guidelines for Diet #1.

To minimize the effects of an epileptic seizure, place a chopstick, spatula, or other small piece of wood between the person's teeth to prevent biting of the tongue. A cold towel applied to the forehead will reduce expansion of the brain cells. The cold application may also be placed on the back of the neck, as well as the hands and feet, to reduce energy to the upper body and head. Deep pressure applied directly beneath the toenail on the big toe on each foot can also reduce the severity of epileptic seizures, sometimes by half or more.

Gulf War Syndrome. Thousands of American veterans of the 1990–91 war against Iraq suffer from a constellation of symptoms known as Gulf War syndrome. Symptoms generally include fatigue, skin rash, headache, muscle and joint pain, and memory loss. In extreme cases, some former soldiers have suffered serious neurological problems and became disabled. Studies by the U.S. Department of Defense and Department of Veterans Affairs have documented the existence of such a disorder, but they have been unable to identify the cause. The four most likely causes are: (1) *exposure to sarin,* a deadly nerve gas that was used in Iraqi chemical weapons and destroyed by American forces, exposing troops to small doses, (2) *pyridostigmine bromide,* a drug given to some GIs to help counter the effects of nerve gas, (3) *depleted uranium,* a low-yielding form of uranium used in some ammunition rounds and as a protective layer in tank armor, and (4) *vaccinations against anthrax and botulinum toxin,* two deadly biochemical war agents, that American troops were given prior to being sent to Iraq in case those weapons were used in the conflict.

The most recent study by the Institute of

Medicine said these four suspected causes warranted further study but that insufficient information was available on the long-term consequences of these agents and how much exposure soldiers may have received. Whatever the ultimate agent responsible for spreading Gulf War syndrome, the underlying cause lies in the susceptibility of any given veteran to disease. All of the four factors described above produce extreme yin effects, contributing to dispersing, rapidly decomposing, and degenerative tendencies. Soldiers whose immune function was already weakened by the modern way of eating, especially those whose condition was compromised by excessive sugar, alcohol, drugs, and medications, would be at higher risk. In the future, scientists should study the military diet—then and now—and determine to what extent it reduces natural immunity to disease. The biological, chemical, and nuclear materials noted above are undoubtedly harmful and should not be employed. However, the fact that veterans in the same unit and exposed to the same stimuli have different reactions shows that deeper, more fundamental issues relating to basic health and immunity are involved. To help relieve the symptoms of Gulf War syndrome, observe the guidelines for Diet #1 if the condition is too yin or Diet #3 if the condition appears to be a combination of both extreme yin and yang factors. Slightly stronger cooking and seasoning will be beneficial. Also UME-SHO BANCHA can be taken 2–3 times a week to help reduce fatigue, restore energy, and improve memory and nervous functions. A GINGER COMPRESS on the kidneys several times a week may also help circulation and dissolve stagnation.

Huntington's Disease. Huntington's disease is a degenerative nervous disorder characterized by periodic jerks or spasms and progressive loss of brain cells. Thinking and behavior gradually decline, and sufferers commonly lose interest in their ordinary activities, wander aimlessly, and grow impulsive and sometimes promiscuous. Memory loss, irrationality, depression, and suicidal tendencies develop as the condition progresses. Symptoms typically appear between ages 35 and 40, and death usually results 13 to 15 years after onset of the disorder. The medical profession regards Huntington's disease as an inherited disorder, and studies show that children who have a parent with this affliction have a 50 percent risk of contracting it. Although this disease is considered incurable, drugs can help control symptoms and behavior.

From the macrobiotic view, Huntington's disease arises from a combination of dietary extremes, especially animal food and sugar. Chronic intake of improper food leads to gradual deterioration of the nervous system. The principal symptoms of this disorder—jerky, spasmodic movements, memory loss, and prolonged shaking—are yin, arising from exhaustion of the body's yang, contractive power. However, some yang tendencies are still present in many patients, such as the tendency to wander and uninhibited sexual desire, showing that animal foods, salty foods, and baked foods have been consumed, and may continue to be consumed, in excess. Follow the guidelines for Diet #3, for conditions arising from a combination of dietary extremes.

Huntington's disease appears to be genetic, but what is passed along is not so much genes that trigger its onset as families sharing a similar way of eating. So long as children whose parent has this disorder follow a balanced way of eating, they should have no fear of contracting this disease or passing it on to their own children. Unless the nerves have been permanently damaged, a macrobiotic diet can greatly help relieve the symptoms of Huntington's disease.

Multiple Sclerosis. Multiple sclerosis is a progressive neurological disorder in which the myelin sheaths that insulate the nerves degenerate. This results in the disruption of electrical impulses and consequent loss of muscular coordination, tremors, and weakness, stiffness, or numbness in the arms or legs and vision or speech problems. Among sufferers, mild symptoms of numbness or tingling in the limbs and balance and coordination problems often begin in the teenage years and recur sporadically or remain dormant till early adulthood or middle age. Then inflammation and scarring of the nerves becomes more pronounced, tremors may appear, and attacks grow more frequent. In some cases, severe attacks are followed by periods without any symptoms. In other cases, MS becomes chronic and debilitating. About 25 percent of sufferers are confined to wheelchairs. Women come down with MS about twice as much as men, and whites are twice as susceptible as blacks. Medically, there is no cure for multiple sclerosis, and symptoms are commonly treated with drugs or physical therapy. Experimental treatments, including replacing the lost nerve tissue with myelin from cows, are also being tried.

From an energetic point of view, MS occurs when the meridian along the spine becomes too tight (or occasionally too loose). This affects the central nervous system, the muscles, and leads to difficulty walking, impaired speech and eyesight, and loss of other body functions. In a majority of cases, the main cause is too much beef, pork, chicken, eggs, cheese, and other strong animal foods. MS is more prevalent in northern climates where these foods are eaten in greater volume and frequency than in southern climates. Also more salt and hard baked flour products are also usually consumed. For example, the incidence of MS in Canada is twice that of the United States. In addition to these foods, cold contributes to hardness and contraction. Both the colder northern climate and atmosphere and the intake of cold foods and beverages, especially ice water and mineral water, is a contributing factor. Though generally classified as more yang, MS usually arises from continued overconsumption of both dietary extremes. Sugar, chocolate, and honey; refined grains; tropical foods; too much fruit and juice; stimulants; spices; and alcohol can enhance the primary type of MS. In the absence or infrequent intake of animal food, these foods can cause a more yin type of MS in which the central energy channel becomes too loose, resulting in decreased flow of natural electromagnetic energy and loss of nervous functioning.

If the legs are the first region to be affected, the area around the intestines is stagnated or weak. This is caused primarily by excess yang. If the arms are stricken first, the heart and throat regions are blocked. This is caused primarily by excess yin. To further help determine the type, press the center of the palm and the center of the spiral on the head. If these regions are very hard, the MS arises from too much yang. If they are loose or soft, the cause is yin.

Lifestyle factors that can increase susceptibility to the more yin type of MS are abortion, appendectomy, removal of the ovaries, removal of tonsils or adenoids, long hot baths or showers (which cause the body to lose minerals), loss of contact with nature, and a sedentary way of life.

To help relieve MS, the standard diet should be observed, with all foods to be cooked. For MS arising from more yin causes, observe Diet #1; for MS arising from more yang causes, observe Diet #2; and for MS arising from a combination of extremes, observe Diet #3. The grain can be a little softer than usual. No animal food or raw salad is to be eaten, and if fruit is taken, it should be cooked. Salt and other seasonings are to be moderate. Sea vegetables should also be moderate, as they are high in minerals and can cause further contraction if overconsumed.

As a home remedy, apply a GINGER COMPRESS on the spine, every day or every other day, for 15 to 20 minutes. This makes blood circulation active. Do a BODY SCRUB or GINGER BODY SCRUB on the whole body once or twice a day. MOXIBUSTION can be applied on the back of the spine to reduce pain and hardness. Push between the vertebrae until pain comes and then hold a stick of moxa about a quarter inch over each spot for several seconds to allow the heat to penetrate. For yang MS, start at the bottom of the spine and move upward. For yin MS, start at the top of the spine and move downward. The moxa may be applied for 15 to 20 minutes several times a week until the condition improves. A hot FOOT BATH every night is also beneficial. Rubbing grated ginger into the center of the palm will also help stimulate energy flow. CHANTING can also help dissolve hardening and stiffness. Sit in a straight position, breathe deeply, and chant *aum* or *su* repeatedly for 5 to 10 minutes.

Using a natural approach, many cases of multiple sclerosis can be reversed completely. In other cases, the symptoms can be reduced or controlled from spreading further. Some people have healed after only three to four months, and others have taken one or two years or more.

Neuralgia. Neuralgia or nerve pain takes many forms. It ranges from mild, transient episodes that last for a few seconds or minutes to sharp, shooting, or burning pain that lasts for days or weeks. The most common type is facial pain resulting from irritation or inflammation of the cranial nerve. Women are three times as likely to experience this type of neuralgia as men, and it primarily affects people 50 or older. Neuralgia in the large nerves of the buttocks and legs is called *sciatica*. Doctors treat neuralgia with analgesics, anti-inflammatory drugs, and sedatives. Chiropractors and osteopaths employ manipulation of the spine and soft tissues to provide relief in some cases of neuralgia.

Nerve pain arises from long-term dietary imbalance. An overly yin condition causes expansion and swelling of cells and tissues, pressing on adjacent nerves and causing inflammation and pain. Facial neuralgia generally falls in this category. An overly yang condition can constrict and narrow cells and tissues, also resulting in irritation, pain, and nerve damage. Sciatica, which occurs near the bladder meridian extending down the buttocks and back of the legs, arises from a combination of excessive yin and yang factors, including too much animal food and sugar, eggs and spices, bread and jam, salt and oil. Eliminating dietary extremes and following a balanced macrobiotic way of eating will help prevent and relieve neuralgia. Observe Diets #1, 2, or 3, depending on the underlying cause. A HOT TOWEL COMPRESS or a GINGER COMPRESS on the affected area may help to ease pain and ache. However, if swelling or inflammation is present, use a cooling compress instead such as a TOFU PLASTER or LEAFY GREENS PLASTER.

Numbness and Tingling. Numbness and tingling frequently arise in the hands or feet but can occur in any part of the body. They most commonly accompany an underlying disorder such as stroke or heart attack, herniated or prolapsed disk, carpal tunnel syndrome, multiple sclerosis, Raynaud's syndrome, or panic attack. Exposure to environmental irritants and toxins and certain drugs and chemicals can also produce these effects. Numbness or tingling in the fingers or toes may arise after sleeping in one position or prolonged sitting. In most cases of poor circulation, numbness and tingling arise from an overly yin condition, in which the over-expansion of cells and tissues stretches or exerts slight pressure on a nerve. Sugar, chocolate, and other sweets; milk, yogurt, ice cream, and light dairy foods; refined flour; oily and greasy foods; fruit and juices; tropical foods; stimulants; spices; and other expansive items may contribute to poor circulation and weakened blood. Numbness and tingling can also arise from an overly contracted condition. In this case, the blood and circulation of bodily fluids and energy is stagnated or obstructed by the buildup of saturated fat and cholesterol from meat, poultry, eggs, hard cheese, and other animal foods. Excessive salt and hard baked flour products also

contribute to this type of poor circulation and subsequent numbness and tingling. A balanced macrobiotic way of eating, avoiding extreme foods of all kinds, will gradually restore proper circulation and clear up related nervous symptoms. For more yin conditions, observe Diet #1. For more yang conditions, observe Diet #2. A HOT TOWEL COMPRESS or a GINGER COMPRESS on the affected area will help improve circulation and ease symptoms.

Parkinson's Disease. Parkinson's disease is a degenerative nervous disorder that is accompanied by tremors of the head or hands, speech impediments, and deterioration of coordination and balance. It tends to arise in late middle age and spread slowly. Men are slightly more likely to get Parkinson's than women. Dopamine-like drugs are commonly prescribed, which control the symptoms in the early stages, but will not cure the disease. Though debilitating and often accompanied by depression, Parkinson's is not fatal.

From the macrobiotic view, there are two major types of Parkinson's: a yang type in which the shaking motion is large or very quick, and a yin type in which the tremors are slower and smaller. The yang type is caused by excessive intake of meat, eggs, poultry, and other animal products, while the yin type results from excessive intake of sugar and other sweets, refined grains, tropical foods, too much fruit and juice, stimulants, spices, and other expansive items. In many cases, Parkinson's disease may be relieved, or the symptoms substantially reduced, in 6 months to a year by discontinuing the foods that are causing the underlying nervous imbalance and observing a standard macrobiotic diet. Observe Diet #1 for Parkinson's disease arising from more yin factors. Observe Diet #2 for Parkinson's arising from more yang factors. A hot towel immersed in ginger water and applied to the spine, or a GINGER COMPRESS several times a week, is also helpful to stimulate circulation and energy flow and dissolve stagnation.

Peripheral Nerve Disorders. The peripheral nervous system includes all the nerves in the body outside of the brain and spinal cord. A wide variety of disorders can arise, including damage of the nerve fiber, the nerve cell, the myelin sheath, and other structures and functions. Peripheral disorders are generally classified into *disorders of muscle stimulation*, such as ALS; *disorders of the neuromuscular junction*, such as myasthenia gravis; *plexus disorders*, in which electrical activity is impaired; *thoracic outlet syndromes*, involving unusual sensations in the hand, neck, shoulder, or arm; *peripheral neuropathy*, or malfunction of the peripheral nerves such as carpal tunnel syndrome; and *Guillain-Barré syndrome*, an autoimmune disorder in which the myelin sheath is destroyed, leading to progressive muscle weakness, paralysis, and sometimes death.

Peripheral nervous disease can arise from a wide variety of factors, and each case must be evaluated according to its location in the body, symptoms, and diet and lifestyle of the person affected. Guillain-Barré syndrome, for example, begins in the legs and progresses upward to the arms, showing that it is primarily yang in origin. Excessive consumption of beef, pork, poultry, eggs, and other animal foods, as well as too much salt and bread and other hard baked

foods, appear to be the underlying cause. Sugar, milk, spices, stimulants, and other strong yin may accelerate its spread. Observe the dietary guidelines for Diet #2. A hot application, such as a HOT TOWEL COMPRESS or a GINGER COMPRESS, may help improve circulation and energy flow and dissolve stagnation. However, in the event of inflammation or swelling, use a cool application instead, such as a TOFU PLASTER, a LEAFY GREENS PLASTER, or several large green leaves placed over the affected area.

Pinched Nerve. A pinched nerve arises when pressure is applied to a nerve or its adjacent muscle tissue, resulting in irritation, tenderness, tingling, numbness, ache, or pain. This condition most commonly occurs in the *median, ulnar, and radial nerves*, extending from the shoulders to the arms; in the *femoral nerve*, extending from the pelvis to the knee; the *plantar nerves*, in the feet; the *spinal nerves*, between the disks in the back; the *peroneal nerve*, running along the inside of the leg; and the *sciatic nerve*, running from the base of the spine to each foot. Pinched nerves can be caused by injury, repetitive motions *(see "Carpal Tunnel Syndrome")*, a damaged spinal disk, heavy lifting, and other activities. Modern medicine advises physical therapy to strengthen surrounding muscles and may prescribe anti-inflammatory drugs or corticosteroids to relieve symptoms.

From an energetic view, pinched nerves commonly arise along or near meridians. For example, the lung, heart, and intestinal meridians run along the arms as well as the meridians comprehensively governing heat and body energy. The peroneal nerve on the side of the leg follows the gallbladder meridian, and the sciatic nerve from the spine to the feet follows the bladder meridian. In this way, we can identify which organ is involved and through dietary adjustments correct its underlying stagnation or weakness. In most cases, this will automatically relieve pressure on the related nerve and its functioning. In addition to observing the standard way of eating, external applications such as a GINGER COMPRESS applied to the sore or painful area can help provide immediate relief.

Spinal Cord Disorders. The spinal column contains bundles of nerves. *Motor nerves* carry impulses to the muscles and stimulate movement. *Sensory nerves* transmit impulses to the brain with information about heat, cold, pressure, and pain. Injuries, infections, circulatory problems, and degenerative diseases can cause damage to the spinal cord and its nervous structures and functions. Modern physiology and anatomy divides the spinal column into four areas: the cervical or neck, the thoracic or chest, the lumbar or lower back, and the sacral or tailbone. Vertebrae in each area are numbered from the top down, e.g., C1 to C8, T1 to T12, L1 to L5, and S1 to S5. Nerves in each vertebrae extend to specific areas of the body, and damage to them can cause weakness, paralysis, or loss of nervous control. For example, damage to C5 and C6 in the cervical area of the neck can cause the legs to become paralyzed and interfere with the ability to flex the arms. Neurologists can identify what part of the spinal cord is not functioning by tracing the nerves back from the part of the body affected.

Spinal cord disorders include accident-related injuries, spinal cord compression, cervical spon-

dylosis (degeneration of the disks and vertebrae in the neck), cysts, acute transverse myelitis (blockage of nerve impulses at one or more points along the spinal cord), interruption of the blood supply, spinal hematomas (hemorrhaging), nerve root disorders, and disk problems.

Disk problems are among the most common spinal cord disorders. The disks are flat, round pieces of cartilage with a fibrous outer membrane and elastic core that serve as a cushion between the bones in the spinal column. In early childhood, the disks are filled with gel or fluid, but over time they start to solidify. By adulthood, they are often hard and inflexible. Through injury, overexertion, or disease, the inner part of the disk can bulge or rupture, pushing through the outer membrane. The ruptured disk can damage surrounding nerves, leading to numbness or tingling, difficulty moving or bending, and sharp, sometimes unbearable pain. The lumbar region of the lower back is the site of most disk problems, with a small percentage occurring in the neck and shoulders. Men under 50 are most susceptible to herniated disks, especially those who are sedentary. Women and children, as well as young adults, may also rupture their disks, while the elderly experience fewer problems overall than other groups. Unless the nerves are deteriorated, rest, exercises, and physical therapy will heal most cases. A supportive collar is used for disk problems in the neck. Aspirin, analgesics, and muscle relaxants may be prescribed to reduce pain and control other symptoms. Surgery is performed in severe cases, including partial removal of the inner core that has broken through the outer wall and is pressing on a nerve. In other cases, drugs and enzymes are injected into the disk to relieve pain and inflammation and to dissolve material impinging on the nerve. Synthetic disks are expected to be introduced in the future.

From a macrobiotic perspective, herniation is an overexpansive condition in which the wall of an organ or tissue weakens and ruptures. A ruptured spinal disk is caused primarily by long-term consumption of excessive yin foods and beverages, including sugar, chocolate, and other sweets; fruits and juices; white flour and other refined flour products; tropical foods; oily and greasy foods; stimulants; spices; alcohol; and drugs and medications. Cold sweets, including good-quality sweeteners, should be avoided.

To help heal this condition, the standard way of eating should be observed, with a slightly more yang style of cooking. Observe Diet #1. Whole grains and cooked vegetables should serve as the principal foods. BROWN RICE MOCHI IN MISO SOUP may be taken regularly, and HIJIKI WITH ROOT VEGETABLES will help strengthen the spine and restore flexibility. Further insight into the underlying cause of the rupture can be gained by determining which chakras and points are located near the damaged disk. The Governing Vessel meridian runs along the center of the spine and helps distribute the overall flow of energy to the other meridians, chakras, and organs. For example, the space between the vertebrae Lumbar 4 and 5 corresponds with the Yang Gate (Yo-Kan), point 3 along the Governing Vessel meridian and the hara chakra, or intestinal energy center, in Far Eastern medicine and philosophy. The space between Thoracic 11 and 12 corresponds with the Central Metropolis (Chu-Su), point 7

along the Governing Vessel meridian and in the stomach chakra. The area between Thoracic 3 and 4 corresponds with the Body Pillar (Shin-Chu), point 12 along the Governing Vessel meridian and the center of the heart chakra.

External treatments along the Governing Vessel, spine, and corresponding chakras can help dissolve blockages, stimulate natural healing energy, and provide relief of symptoms. A cold TOFU PLASTER or LEAFY GREENS PLASTER applied over the affected region is especially effective in bringing down the inflammation and eliminating pain. Gentle exercises, including YOGA, tai chi, reflexology, chiropractic, the Feldenkrais method, and the Alexander technique may also be beneficial. In most cases, dietary and lifestyle practices will restore flexibility and movement to the spine and prevent recurrences without the need for surgery, drugs, or injections.

Tourette's Syndrome. Tourette's syndrome comprises a cluster of nervous symptoms, including repetitive grimacing, violent jerking of the head, neck, arms, or legs, and involuntary sounds. People with this condition also frequently swear and engage in inappropriate speech and other outbursts. Typically, symptoms come on for several minutes periodically throughout the day. In between fits, the person is perfectly normal and can carry out usual activities or work. In the past, the social stigma of Tourette's occasioned sufferers to be shunned or live in isolation. However, today there are many patients, including a large number of professionals, who have successfully learned to cope with the disease with the understanding and support of their families and associates. From the medical view, Tourette's is incurable and of unknown origin. Antipsychotic drugs may be prescribed to help control some symptoms.

From the macrobiotic view, Tourette's syndrome arises from dietary imbalance. The principal cause is eating too much chicken, especially in combination with hot spices. Other combinations of extreme yin and yang foods and beverages may also be involved, including other types of animal food and sugar, spices, stimulants, and other expansive items that can accelerate the progression of the disease. By taking too much chicken and poultry, an individual's natural quality begins to transmute into chicken quality. The typical medical textbook description of symptoms reads just like the behavior of a barnyard fowl: "A child with Tourette's syndrome may repeatedly move the head from side to side, blink the eyes, open the mouth, and stretch the neck. More complex tics include hitting and kicking, grunting, snorting, and humming."

A further clue to Tourette's extreme yang foundation is that males are three times more likely to get this disorder than females. Boys and men tend to eat more animal food, including more chicken and eggs, than women. Other types of animal food can also contribute to this syndrome. The characteristic barking, grunting, and snorting noises associated with Tourette's are simply discharges of excess metabolic energy that arise from eating poultry, beef, pork, and dairy. Strong spices quickly release this energy, explaining why frequent daily outbursts arise as the disease progresses. Calling out obscenities indicates underlying problems with the large intestine, the organ that discharges feces, and the kidneys, which also release solid and liquid waste and govern sexual functioning.

Discontinuing extreme foods and adopting a macrobiotic way of eating can usually eliminate the most extreme symptoms of Tourette's disease within several days. A complete recovery may take 3 to 4 months or longer. Observe the guidelines for Diet #3, for conditions arising from a combination of dietary extremes.

SOLUTION

DIET

Follow the guidelines recommended above with emphasis on the following to help prevent or relieve nervous conditions and disorders:

1. Eat whole grains as the principal dish of every meal, especially brown rice, millet, and barley often, and other grains from time to time. For more yang nervous disorders, avoid or limit buckwheat, soba, and seitan.

2. Avoid hard baked flour products, including bread and baked goods, as much as possible. Noodles may be taken, but only a few times a week.

3. Avoid simple sugars (refined sugar, honey, and chocolate).

4. For more yin conditions, fish or seafood, especially white-meat fish, may be eaten a few times a week for strength, energy, and mental focus. For yang conditions, generally avoid animal food altogether until the condition improves.

5. Minimize fat consumption, and also reduce vegetable-quality oil. Do not take raw oil, such as in the form of salad dressings.

6. Take MISO SOUP once a day, with slightly more miso for yin conditions and slightly less for yang conditions. Prepare with miso that has aged 2 to 3 years and add wakame or kombu and 1 or 2 vegetables that may change daily.

7. Take daily hard leafy greens that are high in fiber (such as daikon greens and carrot tops), round, sweet vegetables (such as fall- and winter-season squashes, cabbage, and onions), and root vegetables (daikon, carrot, burdock), adjusting slightly for season, condition, and availability.

8. Onions are particularly good for calming and soothing the nerves. They may be prepared in a variety of ways, including cooked whole and seasoned with miso, cooked with other vegetables, added to miso or other soup, and made into onion butter.

9. Eat beans or bean products such as tofu, tempeh, and natto regularly in small volume.

10. Take sea vegetables daily in small volume, either as wakame in miso soup, as a square of kombu used to season whole grains or beans, as a sheet or half-sheet of nori, and as a small side dish of arame, hiziki, or other sea vegetable 2 to 3 times a week.

11. The amount of salt (miso, shoyu, and sea salt) should be moderate.

12. Leeks and scallions are very soothing for the nervous system. They may be used in regular cooking, as well as made into a special condiment. Sauté leeks or scallions with miso for a few minutes. A small volume of BROWN RICE SYRUP may be added for tight, yang conditions.

13. Avoid or limit fruits for more yin nervous conditions. If cravings arise, a small volume of fruit may be eaten cooked with a pinch of sea salt.

14. Avoid or limit sweets and desserts (except for tight, yang conditions). However, if cravings arise, a small volume of AMASAKE, BROWN RICE SYRUP, or BARLEY MALT may

be taken. Soft desserts such as kanten, puddings, and MOCHI are preferable to baked desserts.

15. Cut down on water to a moderate level but do not take too many fluids. Use BANCHA TWIG TEA or other traditional tea as the main beverage.

16. Reduce the total volume of food, and chew thoroughly, at least 50 and preferably 100 times per mouthful.

17. Avoid late-night eating.

LIFESTYLE
Follow the standard way-of-life suggestions.

1. In most cases, people with nervous disorders need to be more physically active. Light to moderate exercise, especially walking a half hour every day, will be helpful. DO-IN, SHIATSU, YOGA, tai chi, dancing, and other aerobic activities may also be beneficial.

2. MEDITATION, PRAYER, CHANTING, and other spiritual practices may be helpful if part of a comprehensive approach. PALM HEALING is especially beneficial for calming and soothing the nerves.

HOME REMEDIES
1. UME-SHO KUZU drink will help steady the nerves and give strength and vitality. Take once a day for 3 days and then several times a week as needed.

2. A teaspoon of GOMASHIO, an UMEBOSHI PLUM, a teaspoon of TEKKA, or other salt-based condiment can help offset numbness, tingling, and tremors.

3. For extreme yin conditions, stronger foods may be given such as mugwort mochi; MISO SOUP WITH BROWN RICE MOCHI;

KINPIRA-STYLE BURDOCK; JINENJO; tempeh or seitan cooked nabe-style with mochi, fish (if desired), greens, and ginger; KINPIRA SOUP; and for extreme cases KOI-KOKU.

4. SWEET VEGETABLE DRINK will reduce the desire for sugar, sweets, and other cravings, relax the pancreas, and help steady the nerves. Take daily for 2 to 4 weeks, every other day for a comparable period, and then occasionally as desired.

5. A GINGER COMPRESS on the lower back and kidneys will help improve the circulation of blood, lymph, and other body fluids and relieve pain and discomfort. Apply several times a week as strength permits and then less often or as needed. However, do not apply in the case of swelling, inflammation, or fever. Generally apply for about 20 minutes.

6. A TOFU PLASTER, LEAFY GREENS PLASTER, or other cool application can be used to bring down fever, swelling, or inflammation. Apply for several hours and repeat as necessary.

7. A hot FOOT BATH will bring down the energy in the body and is helpful for more yin nervous conditions.

8. Many other specific dishes, remedies, and exercises can be recommended for each type of nervous condition depending on the symptoms and individual needs. See a macrobiotic counselor or other professional for specific advice and guidance.

CAUTION

1. A physician should be consulted for any condition that does not clear up quickly using the home remedies recommended above.

2. For accident, emergency, or any potentially life-threatening condition accompanied by loss of consciousness, emergency medical treatment is essential.

MEDICAL EVIDENCE

WHOLE GRAINS AID BRAIN AND NERVOUS FUNCTIONING

Whole grains and other foods high in complex carbohydrates have the ability to increase the intake of tryptophan, an amino acid that aids in relief of pain and contributes to the smooth functioning of the brain and other parts of the nervous system. MIT researchers reported that in contrast with whole grains and vegetables, meals high in animal protein lowered levels of tryptophan reaching the brain.

Source: Cited in Michio Kushi et al., *Crime and Diet* (Tokyo and New York: Japan Publications, 1987), pp. 146–47.

ALZHEIMER'S LINKED TO HIGH ANIMAL FOOD CONSUMPTION

Alzheimer's disease is associated with increased consumption of meat, eggs, poultry, and other high-fat foods and with total caloric intake, according to survey of its prevalence in 11 countries. "Diets high in total calories including acidic drinks, alcohol, fat, salt and sugars promote trace mineral imbalances and elevated free radical production in the body," the researcher reported. Foods high in antioxidants (including most plant foods) and fish helped reduce the risk of developing the disease.

Source: William B. Grant, Ph.D., "Dietary Links to Alzheimer's Disease," *Alzheimer's Disease Review* 2:42–55, 1997.

GRAINS AND VEGETABLES MAY HELP PREVENT ALZHEIMER'S

A folic-acid-rich diet high in whole grains and leafy green vegetables may help prevent Alzheimer's disease and dementia, according to a study published in the *New England Journal of Medicine*. People with elevated levels of plasma homocysteine, scientists at Boston University discovered, were at higher risk of developing Alzheimer's. Folic acid, found in abundance in whole grains and green vegetables, helps reduce homocysteine levels. The modern diet, high in meat and dairy products and low in plant foods, produces high homocysteine levels and was cited as a probable cause of the brain-wasting disease. Higher homocysteine levels earlier have been identified as a risk factor in heart attack, stroke, and other vascular diseases. The new study examined 1,092 people with no initial signs of dementia. Within 8 years, 111 had developed symptoms and this group, on average, had higher homocysteine levels than those who remained free of the disease.

Source: Raja Mishra, "Study Cites Folic Acid Role in Dementia," *Boston Globe*, February 14, 2002.

PLANT-BASED DIET RELIEVES MULTIPLE SCLEROSIS

For over 20 years, Roy L. Swank, M.D., of the Division of Neurology, University of Oregon Medical School, has used a predominantly plant-based diet to help his patients recover from multiple sclerosis. He reported that in a study of 146 patients eating mostly vegetable-quality foods and fish instead of meat, there was a 70 percent decrease in the relapse rate of mul-tiple sclerosis the first year and 25 percent in the next 5 years compared to patients eating meat and other high-fat foods. The mortality rate among meat-eaters was also 3 to 4 times higher.

Source: R. L. Swank, "Multiple Sclerosis: Twenty Years on Low Fat Diet," *Archives of Neurology* 23:460–74, 1970.

MULTIPLE SCLEROSIS LINKED WITH MEAT, SUGAR, AND DAIRY

In a review of epidemiological and clinical studies around the world, a German medical doctor reported that multiple sclerosis was associated with higher consumption of meat, eggs, butter, sugar, and milk. Conversely, vegetable and plant foods, as well as fish, were protective. "From a therapeutic, and perhaps preventive, perspective, epidemiologic, experimental, and clinical data justify the present dietary recommendations to patients to reduce animal fat and to increase intake of both vegetable fat and seafood," the researcher concluded.

Source: K. Laurer, "Diet and Multiple Sclerosis," *Neurology* 49(2 Suppl. 2):S55–61, 1997.

DIET HIGH IN VEGETABLES PROTECTS AGAINST PARKINSON'S DISEASE

In an experiment at Yale University, 11 patients with Parkinson's disease who followed a diet high in whole grains, green and yellow vegetables, and fresh fruit and low in protein from animal and vegetable sources experienced reduced movement fluctuations and less need for drugs than patients following the standard modern way of eating. All meats, egg white, gelatin, and dairy food were avoided during the experiment, as well as beans and nuts, chocolate, and pastries. "On this diet, patients can predictably expect daytime mobility, thus permitting near-normal function and independence at home or on the job," the researchers concluded.

Source: J. H. Pincus and K. Barry, "Influence of Dietary Protein on Motor Fluctuation in Parkinson's Disease," *Archives of Neurology* 44:270–72, 1987.

CASE HISTORIES

MACROBIOTICS HELPS EPILEPTIC MAN UNTIL TRAGEDY STRIKES

One day a young man in his early twenties came to see Michio Kushi and began macrobiotics after having epilepsy for seven years. After two months on the diet, he was able to discontinue medication to control his seizures. The seizures stopped altogether after the third month. Gratified at the return of his health, he went to a summer camp about six months later, and while he was there Michio Kushi received a telegram informing him that the young man had died. The weather had been very hot, and one night the young man, while visiting a nearby town with several friends, consumed three cans of beer. Back at camp, he drank several more beers before going to sleep. The next morning, he rose for an early morning swim and had a fatal seizure while swimming. Unfortunately, he did not understand that he had to continue to limit his liquid intake after his initial recovery or the epileptic seizures might recur.

Source: Michio Kushi, *The Macrobiotic Way of Natural Healing* (Tokyo and New York: Japan Publications, 1979), pp. 162–63.

ATHLETE WITH TOURETTE'S SYNDROME RECOVERS ON MACROBIOTIC DIET

In Japan, a famous baseball player introduced himself to Michio Kushi during one of his health seminars. The man suffered from Tourette's syndrome and was constantly moving and holding his head. For four years, he explained, his condition had been getting worse, and he was worried that he could no longer play professional sports. Michio explained to him that the main cause of his tremors and shaking was eating too much chicken and hot spices. He said that the nervous symptoms would stop in four days if he started eating the standard macrobiotic diet, emphasizing quick cooking and light-to-moderate use of salt and other seasonings. Amazed at the diagnosis, the man confirmed that he enjoyed eating grilled chicken teriyaki with peppers and spices almost every day. Michio suggested that he should also take sweet vegetable drink, including fresh daikon and shiitake mushroom, to speed his recovery. The ballplayer eliminated chicken, started eating a balanced, whole-grain-centered diet, and on the fourth day, his symptoms stopped completely.

Source: Michio Kushi, Macrobiotic Teachers Conference, Becket, Mass., Summer 2000.

◎ PANCREATIC PROBLEMS

The pancreas, a centrally located leaf-shaped gland that is about 5 to 8 inches in length and weighs about 3 ounces, is the site of several major disorders, including diabetes, hypoglycemia, and pancreatic cancer (*see "Cancer"*). Diabetes, the sixth leading cause of death by

TABLE 31. NERVOUS CONDITIONS AND DISORDERS

1. More Yin Cause	2. More Yang Cause	3. Yin and Yang Combined
Typical Symptoms		
Swelling	Constriction and hardening	Expansion and constriction
Inflammation	Inflammation	Inflammation
Nervousness		General weakness
Dizziness, vertigo (most cases)		
Neuralgia	Neuralgia	Neuralgia
Pinched nerve		
Numbness, tingling	Cold body temperature	
Trembling, tremors		
Tics, twitches		
Hiccups		
Less movement	Greater movement	
Diseases		
Epilepsy	Grinding of teeth	Sciatica
Gulf War syndrome	Guillain-Barré syndrome	Tourette's syndrome
Some Parkinson's disease: small trembling	Some Parkinson's disease: greater shaking	Huntington's disease
Some multiple sclerosis	Some multiple sclerosis	
Meningitis		ALS (Lou Gehrig's disease)
Some brain tumors: periphery of brain	Some brain tumors: inner part of brain	Alzheimer's disease
		Mad cow disease (variant Creutzfeldt-Jakob disease)

disease in the United States, is on the increase. Between 1990 and 1998, overall incidence increased 33 percent. Rates of diabetes among people in their thirties shot up 70 percent. Though not as acute or life-threatening, hypoglycemia may actually affect even more Americans, and underlies many emotional, family, and social problems today. Pancreatic disorders are directly related to blood sugar imbalances or digestive problems that a macrobiotic way of eating can successfully prevent or relieve.

SYMPTOMS

1. Swelling, tightening, hardening, or other abnormalities in the upper center of the abdomen

2. Hunger, weakness, nervousness, sweating, trembling, tingling in the hands or feet, dizziness, and cravings for sweets, especially in the midafternoon

3. Mood swings, anger, inability to concentrate, emotional outbursts, and a tendency toward aggressive, violent behavior

4. Excessive thirst and appetite, frequent urination, weight loss, fatigue, nausea (often including vomiting), blurred vision, excessive heartbeat, yeast infections, and impotence (in men) or vaginal infections and temporary cessation of menstruation in women

In traditional Oriental medicine, pancreatic troubles are reflected in the following signs:

1. Swellings, discolorations, or other abnormalities on the upper bridge of the nose or the outside of the temples. For example, a dark color shows the pancreas is overburdened by excessive sugar, sweets, juice, and fruits. Whitish yellow pimples are produced by fats and oils, from dairy or other animal food or from excessive vegetable oils. Dark patches and pimples result from too much sweets or salt and flour products. Moles in these regions show excess animal protein and fat and burdened pancreas and spleen.

2. A transparent or pale white color in the eyes often correspond to the development of cysts, abscesses, and tumors in the pancreas.

3. Hair growing between the eyebrows shows that during pregnancy the person's mother ate a large amount of dairy food and fatty animal food. Such markings indicate a tendency to pancreatic, spleen, and liver problems.

4. Oily or dry skin shows imbalances in fat metabolism, including pancreatic problems. A yellowish tinge to the skin indicates bile disorders and often pancreatic troubles.

5. Swellings, markings, or other abnormalities along the spleen meridian show pancreatic problems, especially the area of the foot beneath the ankle bone extending to the outside of the big toe on each foot.

CAUSES

1. Situated behind the stomach, the pancreas is connected to the duodenum through a common bile duct with the liver and gallbladder. The sections of the pancreas are known as the *head, body,* and *tail.* The head secretes pancreatic juice, which aids in the digestion of carbohydrates, fats, and protein. The body and tail of the pancreas produce enzymes and hormones, including insulin and glucagon, which regulate sugar levels in the blood. These hormones are secreted by the *islets of Langerhans,* a network of cells scattered throughout the pancreas that vary in number from 200,000 to 1.8 million; they are most numerous in the tail portion of the pancreas, which touches the spleen. The pancreas also secretes large quantities of bicarbonate into the duodenum, which neutralizes the acid coming from the stomach. Dietary imbalances can affect both the structure and the function of the pancreas, creating major health problems.

2. In the normal digestive process, complex sugars are decomposed gradually and at a nearly even rate by various enzymes in the mouth, stomach, pancreas, and intestines. Complex sugars enter the bloodstream slowly after being

broken down into small saccharide units. During the process, the pH of the blood remains slightly alkaline. In contrast, simple and double sugars are metabolized quickly, causing the blood to become overly acidic. To compensate for this extreme yin condition, the pancreas secretes a yang hormone, insulin, which allows excess sugar in the blood to be removed and enter the cells of the body. This produces a burst of energy as the glucose (the end product of all sugar metabolism) is oxidized and carbon dioxide and water are given off as wastes. Consuming too many extreme foods causes the pancreas to lose its natural ability to regulate glucose. As a result, the blood sugar becomes either chronically too high (diabetes) or too low (hypoglycemia).

3. Consumption of too much beef, pork, chicken, eggs, salted cheese, tuna, salmon, shrimp, lobster, crab, and other animal foods high in fat or cholesterol create hardness in the pancreas, causing chronic low blood sugar or hypoglycemia.

4. Consumption of too much sugar, honey, chocolate, and other concentrated sweeteners; milk, ice cream, butter, yogurt, and other light dairy foods; light, refined pastries and flour products; tropical vegetables and fruits; spices; stimulants; alcohol; drugs; and other excessive yin substances can cause the pancreas to grow soft, loosen, or swell, contributing to diabetes, pancreatitis, and other ills.

5. Eating late at night or just before bed puts an extra burden on the pancreas, as it must work to digest food during the night rather than rest and be fully energized for the next day.

FORMS

Diabetes. Diabetes is one of the major chronic diseases in modern society. In America alone, up to 20 million people suffer from this disorder. *Type 1 diabetes*, also called *insulin-dependent diabetes mellitus (IDDM), juvenile diabetes,* or *juvenile-onset diabetes*, is caused by a lack of insulin. *Type 2 diabetes*, also called *non-insulin-dependent diabetes mellitus (NIDDM), adult-onset diabetes*, or *stable diabetes*, occurs when the pancreas loses its ability to process insulin effectively. Nine out of ten cases are type 2 diabetes, which develops primarily in adults over 40 and is strongly associated with obesity. Type 1 diabetes typically appears in young people under 30.

Normally, the pancreas produces sufficient insulin to neutralize excess blood sugar. However, after years of excessive consumption of refined sugar, fruit, dairy, chemicals, and other highly yin substances, the islet cells in the pancreas become expanded and lose their ability to secrete insulin. Sugar begins to appear in the urine, the body loses water, and reserve minerals are depleted. The overproduction of insulin attracts fatty acids and may coagulate into tumors in the bile duct or the islets of Langerhans.

Type 1 diabetes is frequently accompanied by hyperglycemia, or high blood sugar. This can lead to ketoacidosis, or extreme acidity in the blood. Injections of artificial insulin and intravenous salt solutions are commonly given to prevent this complication. But as a result of injury, accident, or sudden shock, the person may go into a coma and even die.

Cataracts, glaucoma, and other vision problems are another common complication, and diabetes is the main cause of blindness among adults in the country. Nervous system problems, renal problems, and heart disease may also develop as the disease progresses. Thrush (a yeast infection in the mouth), gum problems, urinary tract infections, and lowered resistance to infection are also common.

Type 1 diabetes is treated with insulin injections, usually twice or more a day. Type 2 diabetes is often controlled with diet and exercise alone. Other cases are given drug therapy, sometimes including insulin, or an oral medication for hypoglycemia.

Diabetes may be treated and relieved by adopting a slightly more yang standard macrobiotic diet focusing on whole grains, beans, vegetables, and sea vegetables, prepared with a slightly longer cooking time and heavier taste. Follow the guidelines for Diet #1 and the dietary recommendations at the end of the chapter. In many cases of type 2 diabetes, the need for insulin or drug therapy can be reduced between 75 and 100 percent with a high-fiber diet high in complex carbohydrates. Type 1 also responds to dietary intervention but is much more difficult to relieve because of constitutional weaknesses (the mother's way of eating during pregnancy was usually very yin); insulin may gradually be reduced, usually 30 to 40 percent, as the condition improves, but achieving a complete remission in people under 20 is difficult. In addition, the following home remedies may be helpful:

1. Take SWEET VEGETABLE DRINK, 1 to 2 cups every day for 3 to 4 weeks.

2. Take UME-SHO BANCHA or UME-SHO KUZU, 1 cup every other day for 3 weeks.

3. Take a small amount of KINPIRA-STYLE BURDOCK, prepared with a small volume of sesame oil, every day.

4. Do a BODY SCRUB daily to increase circulation of the whole body.

Hyperinsulinism. This condition results when the pancreas secretes too much insulin. Its symptoms are opposite those of diabetes and include hypoglycemia, fatigue, muscular weakness, excessive thirst and perspiration, anxiety, and nervous irritability. In extreme cases, convulsions and coma may follow. An overdose of insulin, known as *insulin shock*, or tumors in the pancreas may bring on this condition.

From the macrobiotic view, hyperinsulinism is an overly yang condition, and to relieve it, the way of eating should be slightly more yin. Follow the guidelines for Diet #2. Brown rice cooked with millet should be the principal food, and grains should be cooked without salt. Vegetables should be seasoned lightly and include proportionately more leafy greens. Two servings of soup a day are recommended, with miso or shoyu very mild. Lentils, soybeans, black beans, and other more yin beans can be taken.

Hypoglycemia. Chronic low blood sugar or hypoglycemia results when the pancreas loses the ability to secrete *glucagon* or *anti-insulin* and raise blood sugar levels. This is a common condition in modern society, with up to 80 percent of the population experiencing some degree of hypoglycemia. Emotional outbursts and mood swings are common, as fluctuating blood sugar levels cause the person to be alternately manic and depressed.

People who desire sweets a couple of times a day are often hypoglycemic. After 2:00 in the afternoon and through the evening, as the sun and atmosphere descend, these people strongly crave sweets. If sweets are unavailable, they experience fatigue, insomnia, decline of energy and efficiency, frustration, depression, and dissatisfaction. Their emotional ups and downs become extreme and their human relations unstable. In the evening, they sometimes cannot even eat dinner and must lie down to rest. At night, their whole body becomes cold, especially the hands and feet. They do not sleep well, so they need to sleep longer. In the morning, when the sun and atmosphere are rising and their blood sugar is going up, their stamina returns and they feel normal or revitalized. But in the afternoon, as the energy of the day and their blood sugar sink, they are annoyed and irritated again, and the same symptoms recur. Relationship problems between men and women and parents and children easily arise. Most people with this condition do not realize that they have chronic low blood sugar or that it is the underlying cause of their relationship problems. In extreme cases, hypoglycemia can cause dizziness, fainting, and trembling through the entire body, and even unconsciousness, coma, or convulsions. Young and middle-aged women tend to be hypoglycemic more than men.

Symptoms of hypoglycemia include ruddy face, irregular pulse, allergy and dermatitis, constipation and diarrhea, muscle paralysis, headache, enteritis, candida, tendency to develop cancer or viral diseases (including AIDS and hepatitis), rheumatism, frigidity, sterility and miscarriage, anemia and dizziness, trembling of the whole body, and mental and psychological instability, including fatigue, depression, stress, irritation, emotional ups and downs, excitability, nervousness, irregular meals, suicidal tendencies, lack of dream or goals in life, doubt, fear, and autism or isolation.

Hypoglycemia is commonly treated with dietary therapy in modern society. A high-fiber, high–complex carbohydrate diet consisting of six small meals a day is now standard, and sugars, fruit, and alcohol are limited.

From the macrobiotic view, the underlying cause of hypoglycemia is not sugar or sweets, but eggs; chicken; cheese; beef, pork, and other meat; dairy products; fish and seafood, especially shrimp, lobster, crabmeat, scallops, roe, salmon, and tuna; and other strong animal food. Hard baked flour products, including bread, crackers, cookies, muffins, and rice cakes, and intake of salty or mineral-rich foods, including salty nuts, will also contribute to this condition. These strong yang items harden and stiffen the pancreas and prevent it from secreting glycogen. Any of the above foods sautéed in butter or vegetable oil is especially damaging. As blood sugar levels drop, the person craves yin in the form of sugar, honey, soft drinks, and other sweets. The hypoglycemic individual feels an immediate release when the glucose in these foods raises her blood sugar and temporarily relaxes the pancreas. Other strong yin in the form of tropical vegetables, especially nightshades, excessive fruit and juice, spices, stimulants, and other expansive foods is also craved or eaten in large volume to help relax the pancreas. Wine, beer, sake, and other alcoholic drinks may also be craved, as well as coffee, green tea, mint tea, and other beverages containing caffeine or having stimulant, aromatic effects. Tension and stress can also contribute to hypoglycemia and create a desire for sweets and alcohol. Some kinds of medicines, such as anti-cancer drugs and steroidal drugs, tend to promote hypoglycemia. Late-night snacking also puts additional stress on the pancreas and contributes to this disorder.

For hypoglycemia, follow the dietary guidelines for Diet #3, for conditions arising from a combination of extreme yin and yang factors. Chronic low blood sugar can often be relieved in 4 to 5 months by observing the following guidelines.

1. As the main food, take whole grains, especially brown rice, sweet brown rice, and millet. Cook grains soft to make them easy to digest.

2. Avoid flour products (bread, muffins, crackers, and cookies), including noodles, as much as possible.

3. A variety of ingredients can be used in MISO SOUP, especially millet, mochi, and sweet vegetables (winter squash, pumpkin, onion, and carrot) with wakame or kombu.

4. A variety of vegetables may be used for cooking. Frequent use of winter squash, pumpkin, carrot, and daikon, as in NISHIME-STYLE ROOT VEGETABLES, NISHIME-STYLE SWEET VEGETABLES, and ADZUKI BEAN, SQUASH, AND KOMBU DISH, is recommended. Avoid nightshade vegetables such as tomatoes, potatoes, eggplant, and green peppers.

5. Follow the standard guidelines for beans and bean products, as well as sea vegetables.

6. Avoid fruit or fruit juice as much as possible. If craved, stew fruit with a pinch of salt and eat a small amount.

7. Be careful not to take too much salt, including miso, shoyu, or sea salt.

8. A small volume of vegetable oil, especially sesame oil, can be used for cooking.

9. As condiments, use black sesame GO-MASHIO (16 or 18 parts sesame to 1 part sea salt), UMEBOSHI PLUMS, shiso leaf powder, TEKKA, green nori flakes, and others.

10. Avoid sugary or sweetened beverages, cola, coffee, alcohol, or distilled water as much as possible.

11. White-meat fish that is low in fat can be taken in small volume 1 to 2 times per week.

12. As sweeteners, BARLEY MALT, BROWN RICE SYRUP, AMASAKE, amacha, or mirin can be used in moderation. Cooked sweet vegetables (winter squash, pumpkin, onion, carrot, or cabbage) provide a natural sweet taste.

13. As seasonings, use miso and shoyu that have fermented for more than 2 years, sea salt with reduced magnesium compounds (nigari), mirin, brown rice vinegar and umeboshi vinegar, and ginger. Stimulant seasonings such as mustard, pepper, and curry should be avoided as much as possible.

14. Food, especially grains, must be chewed well (between 50 and 100 times per mouthful).

The following way-of-life guidelines may also be observed:

1. Go to bed early and rise early.

2. Be active mentally and physically.

3. Every day do light exercise or take a walk outside for half an hour.

4. Until the condition improves, you may take a small amount of food 4 to 5 times a day instead of 2 to 3 times a day, but have it at regular times.

5. Avoid artificial environments, including exposure to high-voltage lines, excessive air-conditioning, stagnant air, dampness or high humidity, and chemicals (including cosmetics and other body care products).

6. Keep your living area clean and in good order.

7. Avoid stressful human relations.

8. Try to keep in touch with nature.

9. Live simply.

10. Use cotton for underwear, bedsheets, pillowcases, and comforter covers.

11. Try to avoid using television, computers, microwaves, fluorescent lamps, and other devices and equipment that emit strong electromagnetic fields.

12. Sing a happy song or recite out loud every day.

The following home remedies are recommended for hypoglycemia:

1. Drink SWEET VEGETABLE DRINK, at least 1 small cup every morning and every evening for 3 to 4 weeks.

2. If the intestines are not working well, take 1 small cup of UME-SHO BANCHA or UME-SHO KUZU every other day for 3 weeks.

3. Take SWEET KUZU DRINK with barley malt or brown rice syrup when depressed, stressed, and irritated. Warm AMASAKE may be taken instead or for variety.

4. Do a BODY SCRUB every day to improve circulation.

5. Warm the pancreas or feet with a HOT WATER BOTTLE when the body is too cold to sleep.

Finally, please observe these cautions for hypoglycemia:

1. Take 1 small cup of SWEET KUZU DRINK with barley malt or brown rice syrup for 5 to 10 days when blood sugar levels are low from excessive intake of chemicals (e.g., insulin), anticancer drugs, or chemotherapy.

2. CHINESE MEDICINE, acupuncture or homeopathy may be helpful to help control some of the symptoms of hypoglycemia. See an experienced practitioner if necessary.

Pancreatitis. Pancreatitis refers to inflammation of the pancreas, often accompanied by swelling, hemorrhage, and blood vessel damage. It may be acute or chronic, mild or life-threatening. Gallstones and alcoholism account for almost 80 percent of cases. *Acute pancreatitis* produces pain that is steady and severe, has a penetrating quality, radiates to the back and chest, and persists for days. It may be accompanied by nausea, vomiting, and distention of the abdomen and may lead to cysts, abscesses, and the leaking of fluid into the abdomen. Treatment usually includes avoiding all food and water by mouth, as these stimulate the pancreas to produce more enzymes. The person is fed intravenously and given nothing by mouth for at least 2 weeks and as long as 6 weeks.

Chronic pancreatitis involves persistent pain in the middle abdomen that varies in intensity, lasting several hours or several days. It may be accompanied by weight loss and smelly bowel movements and lead to diabetes or the development of calcium deposits in the pancreas. Alcohol abuse is the primary cause. Medical treatment usually involves eating four or five meals a day consisting of food low in fat and protein and high in carbohydrates, and abstaining from alcohol.

Observe the guidelines for Diet #1 for chronic pancreatitis or Diet #2 for acute pancreatitis, also keeping in mind the suggestions listed below.

SOLUTION

DIET

In addition to the above dietary guidelines for diabetes and hypoglycemia, note the following for pancreatic conditions in general:

1. Eat whole grains as the principal food, especially millet, which is beneficial for the pancreas. It can be prepared boiled, combined and pressure-cooked with rice, prepared with vegetables such as squash, carrots, or other sweet-tasting foods, or served in soups or as a soft breakfast cereal. Brown rice cooked together with millet (about 80 percent rice and 20 percent millet) may also be prepared frequently.

2. Round vegetables are sweet-tasting and particularly nourishing and soothing to the pancreas. These include fall- or winter-season squash, onions, and cabbage. These may be served as NISHIME-STYLE ROOT VEGETABLES, NISHIME-STYLE SWEET VEGETABLES, in soups (especially MILLET SQUASH SOUP), or stews.

3. Take UMEBOSHI PLUMS, sauerkraut, or sour pickles (such as those made with umeboshi vinegar) to quiet an overactive pancreas.

4. Avoid animal foods, especially chicken, eggs, hard cheese, and shellfish such as shrimp, crabmeat, and lobster, which gradually gather in the pancreas and create hardness.

5. Avoid or limit hard baked flour products, salty food, and roasted food.

6. Avoid sugar, sugar-treated foods, honey, molasses, and other refined sweeteners.

7. Avoid or limit fruit and fruit juices, especially tropical fruits, until the condition improves.

8. Avoid or limit alcohol of all kinds.

9. Avoid spices, stimulants, chemically grown or treated foods, and genetically engineered foods.

10. Avoid or limit white rice, white flour, and other refined grains and grain products, including crackers, cookies, muffins, etc.

11. Follow the standard dietary guidelines for each condition as noted above.

12. Proper chewing is essential for pancreatic conditions. Chew each mouthful a minimum of 50 times, preferably 100 to 200 times.

13. Avoid overeating and overdrinking, especially before sleeping, which puts added stress on the pancreas at night.

LIFESTYLE

Follow the standard way-of-life suggestions and emphasize the following:

1. Since anxiety and upset commonly accompany pancreatic problems, it is important to maintain a calm, peaceful environment.

2. A BODY SCRUB with a warm towel or towel soaked in warm ginger water is beneficial. The towels may be placed on the pancreatic region for 10 to 15 minutes. A HOT WATER BOTTLE or hot SALT PACK may be used instead.

3. SHIATSU, DO-IN, PALM HEALING, and other peaceful, gentle healing practices may be helpful.

4. Physical activity is important, especially

for a person with diabetes, but do not exercise too strenuously.

5. Avoid long, hot baths and frequent showers that may deplete the body of minerals.

HOME REMEDIES

1. For pancreatic disorders, especially diabetes but also hypoglycemia, prepare ADZUKI BEAN, SQUASH, AND KOMBU DISH often. This preparation is very sweet, and a moderate to large portion (½ to 1 cup) may be eaten at every meal for 2 to 4 weeks and then less frequently.

2. Take SWEET VEGETABLE DRINK, 1 to 1½ cups, every day for 1 month, then every other day for a second month, and then occasionally.

3. Take CARROT-DAIKON DRINK, 1 to 1½ cups, every day for 2 to 4 weeks, then once every third or fourth day for a similar period, and then occasionally.

4. Fresh carrot juice, taken at room temperature or warmed, will help relax the pancreas, especially in case of pain, for 4 to 5 days.

5. Prepare fresh GRATED DAIKON, adding a few drops of shoyu to ½ cup. Take two to three times a week to help eliminate the accumulation of fat and oil in the pancreas.

6. To relieve pain in the pancreas and assist recovery, apply a hot GINGER COMPRESS over the affected area for 3 to 5 minutes followed by a cold compress, such as a TARO PLASTER or regular POTATO PLASTER, for 3 to 5 hours. Repeat as needed and continue for 1 to 2 weeks, if necessary.

CAUTION

1. Pancreatic disorders, especially pancreatic cancer, may have no outward symptoms and are commonly overlooked or misdiagnosed in routine hospital checkups. While a macrobiotic approach will benefit almost all pancreatic problems, please seek medical attention if you have reason to believe that you have a serious condition.

2. If you are diabetic and are taking insulin or other drug therapy, please consult your physician about reducing injections. In many cases, insulin can be substantially and even completely eliminated as the pancreas regains its ability to naturally secrete insulin. However, it is best to continue regular medication for at least two weeks after starting macrobiotics and then reduce it gradually, ideally under professional medical supervision.

MEDICAL EVIDENCE

MODERN DIET LINKED WITH INCREASED DIABETES AMONG NATIVE AMERICANS

The Pima native people of Arizona have one of the highest rates of diabetes in the world. Medical researchers who investigated their diet found that those who ate a modern diet high in potatoes, white bread, fatty foods, and processed foods had a 38 percent rate of the disease, while those who ate a traditional diet of corn tortillas, tepary beans, lima beans, and mesquite pods had a 6 percent rate.

Source: R. Cowen, "Seeds of Protection," *Science News* 137:350–51, 1990.

POTATOES, WHITE FLOUR, AND WHITE RICE INCREASE RISK OF DIABETES

Potatoes, white bread, and white rice contribute to diabetes, according to Boston scientists. A large study of 65,173 women found that those who ate a high-starch diet low in fiber and high in soft drinks had 2.5 times more diabetes than those who ate less of these foods and more whole grains and high-fiber foods. Dr. Walter Willett, professor of epidemiology and nutrition at the Harvard School of Public Health, said that carbohydrates in refined grains and potatoes are digested and absorbed rapidly, causing the blood sugar to go up and large amounts of insulin to be released.

Source: Denise Grady, "Diet-Diabetes Link Reported," *New York Times,* February 12, 1997.

WHOLE GRAIN DIET PROTECTS AGAINST DIABETES

A whole-grain diet can control diabetes, according to California researchers. In a study of 4,587 patients with adult-onset diabetes, scientists found that a diet high in complex carbohydrates and low in fat, combined with walking and other aerobic exercise, effectively controlled diabetes and reduced coronary heart disease risk.

Source: R. James Barnard et al., "Diet and Exercise in the Treatment of NIDDM," *Diabetes Care* 17(12):1–4, 1994.

DIET AND EXERCISE EFFECTIVE FOR ADULTS AT HIGH RISK FOR DIABETES

A Scandinavian case control study of 522 Finns found that adults at high risk for diabetes could reduce the chance of developing this disease by 60 percent by making dietary changes, losing 10 pounds, and exercising more. Both groups received advice about the importance of a healthy diet and regular exercise, but only the experimental group, which received intensive instruction from a dietitian and from fitness professionals, experienced reduced risk.

Source: "Lifestyle Can Prevent Diabetes ... Maybe," *Science News,* July 1, 2000.

◎ REPETITIVE STRESS INJURIES

Repetitive stress injuries include carpal tunnel syndrome, a painful, potentially debilitating condition that can affect the thumb and fingers and often the wrists, elbows, and other joints, and tarsal tunnel syndrome, a similar condition in the feet, ankles, and lower legs. These conditions are also referred to as occupational neuritis. Symptoms can range from mild and inconveniencing to severe and debilitating. Physical therapy and drugs are commonly prescribed, but from a medical view there is no known cause or cure. A holistic approach, focused on diet and lifestyle, often leads to marked, if not complete, recovery.

SYMPTOMS

The following symptoms may accompany carpal or tarsal tunnel syndrome:

1. Tingling or numbness in the fingers or hand or feet and toes
2. Shooting pains in the wrist or forearms and sometimes other parts of the body
3. Difficulty handling small objects or gripping things

CAUSE

1. From an energetic view, repetitive motions sometimes can lead to physical imbal-

ances. Many features of modern life, from the modern workplace to the sports field, emphasize specific limbs or functions and neglect others, sometimes with little or no movement of the joints and bones. However, if we use only certain fingers, one hand or foot, or one side of the body, the other organs, functions, and opposite side of the body will suffer. For our health and vitality, it is preferable to engage in activities that engage a large number of muscles and actively move the joints and bones. Aerobic exercise such as dancing, YOGA, and tai chi, which involve the body as a whole, are healthier than static or isometric activities such as weight lifting, water skiing, or football, which involve a limited number of muscles and movements.

2. Aside from balancing our daily activities, our daily way of eating will directly affect our tolerance of repetitive stress. In most cases of carpal tunnel syndrome, the problem is not due to repetitive activities at all. Individuals in good health who engage in long periods of typing, playing a musical instrument, and assembly line activities will usually experience no ill effects.

3. Excessive intake of hard baked flour products, especially bread, crackers, cookies, doughnuts, bagels, and baked desserts, eggs, chicken, meat, and heavy dairy food, are the main causes of stiffening of the fingers, hands, and wrists.

4. Though not primary causes, excessive intake of sugar, milk, fruit, raw salad, oil, and other expansive items will loosen and soften nerves and muscle tissue, contributing to numbness, tingling, and swelling.

5. Together, combinations of extreme yin and yang foods cause fat to accumulate around the joints, leading to pain, swelling, inflammation, osteoarthritis or rheumatoid arthritis, hardening of the arteries, and other chronic conditions. Avoiding dietary extremes and adopting a centrally balanced macrobiotic way of eating will help relieve the symptoms of carpal or tarsal tunnel syndrome.

FORMS

Carpal Tunnel Syndrome. Carpal tunnel syndrome occurs most frequently among computer users, typists, musicians, assembly line workers, and others whose work involves repetitive hand movements. It can be disabling and result in permanent damage to nerves and muscles. Conventional treatment includes hand and arm exercises to relax and stretch overworked nerves and muscles, physical therapy in more serious cases, and various anti-inflammatory drugs, cortisone creams, and injections to control pain.

Tarsal Tunnel Syndrome. Tarsal tunnel syndrome, affecting the feet and lower legs, tends to arise from the intake of proportionately stronger yang factors that cause contractive energy to gather and collect in the lower part of the body. A diet emphasizing slightly more good quality yin factors, such as more leafy green vegetables and overall less salt and seasoning, can help relieve this condition. Follow Diet #2 for tarsal tunnel syndrome.

SOLUTION

DIET

Generally, observe the guidelines for Diet #3, arising from a combination of both dietary extremes. The following special dishes are helpful for this condition:

1. Eat soba noodles with vegetables and a slight shoyu taste several times a week.

2. Take KINPIRA SOUP 2–3 times a week for general strengthening and circulation.

3. As a special dish, take lotus root, carrot, and daikon (including the tops and connecting parts). Chop very finely in equal amounts. Combine, bring to a boil, and simmer for 25 minutes in 3 to 5 times as much water. Drink the liquid, 1 cup a day, until the condition improves. Alternatively, add a little less water to the mixture and add a shoyu taste at the end of cooking. Eat one medium dish daily.

LIFESTYLE

1. Follow the standard way-of-life suggestions, including a BODY SCRUB daily on the arms, hands, and fingers and on the legs, feet, and toes.

2. MASSAGE, DO-IN, YOGA, martial arts, gardening, playing a musical instrument, and other practices and activities can help open the energy channels and improve energy flow in the extremeties.

HOME REMEDIES

Use a GINGER COMPRESS on the affected region for 10 minutes. Then apply a COLD TOWEL COMPRESS on the region for 3 minutes. Repeat this twice a day.

◎ SINUS PROBLEMS

Sinus congestion, or *sinusitis*, is one of the most common ailments in modern society. In the United States, an estimated 50 million people suffer from inflammation or infection of the si-nuses, and almost 1 in 8 has chronic sinus blockage. The 4 sinus pockets are located on the front of the face, one pair on the sides of the nose and the other pair above the eyes leading down to the inner part of the bridge of the nose. Normally, mucus on the linings of these organs traps particles in the air that is breathed in and drains them through tiny openings in the nasal cavity. However, too much mucus causes swelling and congestion, and infection may set in. *Nasal polyps,* or small benign growths, may also develop, interfering with breathing and causing other complications. Sinus problems are usually treated with antibiotics for periods of 1 to 3 weeks. Decongestants, steroid inhalants, and other medications may also be prescribed. Antihistamines are not generally recommended because they tend to increase the mucus. A natural approach to sinusitis, centered on a balanced macrobiotic diet, usually provides immediate relief and prevents future congestion.

SYMPTOMS

1. Pressure behind the eyes

2. Obstructed nasal passages and trouble breathing

3. Heaviness in the face

4. Dripping nose

5. Bad odor in the nasal passages

6. Occasional fever

7. Occasional toothache

CAUSES

1. The main cause of sinus problems is mucus-producing foods, especially milk, cream, butter, ice cream, yogurt, cheese, and other dairy foods; sugar, chocolate, and other concentrated sweeteners; fruit and juices; oily and greasy foods; and bread, crackers, cookies, and other flour products, especially those made with white flour. Such items create mucus in the sinuses, intestines, and other areas of the body, leading to blockages, inflammation, and infection.

2. Too much oats can also create mucus, especially rolled oats or ordinary oatmeal.

3. Congestion on the left side of the face, including a blocked left nostril and sore left eye, is usually caused by excessive intake of sugar, sweets, fruit, alcohol, or other strong yin foods or beverages.

4. Congestion on the right side of the face, including a blocked right nostril and sore right eye, is generally caused by taking too much bread, baked food, or floury desserts, and sometimes by too much salt, soy sauce, or other contractive food.

5. Congestion in both nostrils and inflammation of both eyes is caused by dietary extremes of both types.

SOLUTION

DIET

Observe the standard macrobiotic way of eating, balancing slightly according to the condition. For more serious or chronic cases, observe Diet #3 with the following focus:

1. Eat whole grains, not refined grains, as the main dish of every meal. Eat grains in whole form, not as rolled grain, flaked grain, made into grits, or processed in other ways, until the condition improves.

2. Avoid oats, including whole oats, until the condition improves.

3. Reduce flour products to as little as possible, including good-quality whole-wheat bread, crackers, cookies, and pastries. Noodles may be taken, but only a few times a week.

4. Avoid simple sugars (refined sugar, honey, and chocolate).

5. Avoid dairy food. Avoid soy milk, soy cheese, soy yogurt, soy ice cream, and other highly processed soy products. (Miso, tofu, tempeh, and natto are fine.)

6. Avoid animal foods with the exception of fish or seafood once or twice a week if desired.

7. Minimize fat consumption, and also reduce vegetable-quality oil. Do not take raw oil such as in the form of salad dressings, sauces, and dips.

8. Avoid vegetables that originated in tropical regions, such as tomatoes, eggplants, and peppers.

9. Take daily hard leafy greens that are high in fiber (such as collard greens, kale, and turnip greens); round, sweet vegetables such as fall- and winter-season squash, cabbage, and onion; and root vegetables such as daikon, carrot, and burdock.

10. The amount of salt (miso, shoyu, and sea salt) should be moderate.

11. Cut down on water to a moderate level, but do not reduce it too much.

12. Take a small amount of sea vegetables on a daily basis.

13. Reduce the total volume of food and chew more.

14. Avoid late-night eating.

LIFESTYLE

Follow the standard way-of-life guidelines, noting the following:

1. Take a walk every day for 20 to 30 minutes. Fresh air will help invigorate you and improve breathing.

2. Avoid unnatural environments, such as those with high electromagnetic radiation. Avoid excessive use of air conditioners or heaters, and avoid stagnated air.

3. Keep plants in your home or office to create oxygen and improve breathing.

4. Avoid or limit decongestants, antibiotics, and other strong medications as much as possible. Even many herbal remedies and natural sprays may have strong aromatic or fragrant effects and overstimulate the body.

HOME REMEDIES

1. A daily BODY SCRUB will help improve blood and energy circulation.

2. A LOTUS ROOT PLASTER will help relieve sinus congestion, including eliminating the buildup of mucus and calcified stones that have accumulated in the sinuses for years. Before applying this plaster, apply a GINGER COMPRESS or HOT TOWEL COMPRESS to the sinus region. When the skin turns red, apply the lotus root plaster to a thickness of about ⅔ inch, covering the entire region of the sinuses, including the forehead and around the nose. Hold the plaster in place with a cotton bandage wrapped around the head. Apply the plaster just before going to sleep at night and leave it on until the following morning. Then wash it off. Repeat this for 7 to 10 days or sometimes 2 to 3 weeks, until a large quantity of mucus starts to discharge. Calcified stones may also be eliminated through sneezing.

Note: A mask can be made to hold the plaster on while sleeping. Sew two layers of gauze together with cutouts for eyes and nose, something like a Halloween mask. Place the lotus paste between the two layers of gauze, above and/or next to the nose. Then attach the mask to the face. It should stay in place for several hours. In the morning, rinse the nose out with salty BANCHA TWIG TEA.

3. LOTUS ROOT JUICE TEA may also help disperse congestion and improve the condition. Take a small cup once a day for several days.

4. Take UME-SHO KUZU 2 to 3 times a week to strengthen the blood.

5. Lotus seeds cooked with kombu can also help to clear up stagnated mucus. Fresh or dried lotus root may be used instead of the seeds.

6. Acupressure or MOXIBUSTION applied to the pressure points on the sinus region will help loosen mucus deposits. Apply pressure or moxa twice a day for several days.

◉ SPLEEN PROBLEMS

The spleen, a spongy, soft, purplish organ about as big as a fist, is located in the upper part of the abdominal cavity, just under the rib cage on the left side. It is the major organ of the lymphatic system. Unlike the bloodstream, the lymphatic system has no central organ to pump the lymph fluid. The flow of lymph is maintained by several factors such as activity, contraction of the lungs and diaphragm during breathing, and the movements of the villi and the contractions of the small intestine.

The spleen filters substances such as bacteria and worn-out red blood cells from the lymph and body fluid. The spleen also contributes to the formation of white blood cells, especially lymphocytes, which protect against infection. It stores blood and minerals, particularly iron, produces antibodies, and contributes to the production of bile.

A healthy spleen contributes to warmth, vitality, natural resistance to disease, and proper formation of cells, tissues, and organs. It is associated with balance, sympathy, understanding, and compassion. An unhealthy spleen contributes to circulatory and lymphatic problems, especially a loss of natural immunity and susceptibility to infection. An impaired spleen also contributes to skepticism, envy, jealousy, and other negative emotions.

Common spleen disorders are discussed below. *See also "Lymphoma and Hodgkin's Disease" in "Cancer."*

SYMPTOMS

1. Swelling, pain, or other abnormality in the spleen region
2. Swelling of lymph nodes in the neck, armpits, or groin
3. General weakness, fatigue, and susceptibility to infection
4. Complaining, doubt, anxiety, skepticism, envy, jealousy, and similar emotions

Spleen troubles are traditionally evaluated in Far Eastern medicine according to the following diagnostic signs:

1. Redness in the outer layer of the ear, except during strong exercise or outdoor activity in cold weather, shows developing spleen and lymphatic disorders.
2. Swellings, hardness, discolorations, and other abnormalities along the spleen meridian running from the outside of the big toe up along the foot, around the ankle, and up the inside of the leg to the spleen, heart, and other middle organs.
3. A pronounced bulge on the outside of the big toe along the spleen meridian shows a fondness for sugar, fruit, desserts, and other sweets.
4. If the first toe curves abnormally toward the second toe, spleen and lymphatic functions are overactive from intake of too much fats and oils of both animal or vegetable quality and extreme yin foods in general.
5. On the head, swollen temples signify developing spleen and lymphatic problems.
6. The left eye corresponds with the spleen and lymphatic functions. Vision or eye problems often correspond with underlying spleen or lymph problems.

CAUSES

1. The spleen and liver are complementary. The spleen is more expansive, governing the lymphatic system, white-blood cells, and other more yin functions. The liver is more compact, regulating the circulatory system, red blood cells, and other more yang functions. As a result, sugar and sweets, dairy food, oily and fatty food of all kinds, refined grains, tropical foods, spices, soft drinks and carbonated beverages, and other extreme yin foods especially affect the spleen and other lymphatic organs.
2. While spleen problems are often caused

by yin factors, excessive yang in the form of meat, poultry, eggs, shellfish, and other strong animal foods, as well as baked flour and too much salt, can contract the spleen and harden lymph nodes, organs, ducts, and capillaries.

FORMS

Enlarged Spleen. An enlarged spleen can reduce the number of red and white blood cells and platelets in circulation. When too many blood cells are removed, a variety of problems can develop, including anemia, frequent infections, and bleeding problems. In some cases, the spleen is removed surgically by modern medicine, in which case the liver usually takes over the functions of this organ. Many conditions can enlarge the spleen, especially overeating. To relieve this condition, simplify the diet for several days, eating primarily millet or brown rice cooked together with barley, MISO SOUP, and a special side dish of half dried daikon and half daikon leaves pickled for several months with sea salt and rice bran. SAUTÉED VEGETABLES, including onions, carrots, cabbage, and other sweet vegetables cooked in sesame oil, may also be taken. The main beverage should be BANCHA TWIG TEA. To alleviate the underlying condition, observe the guidelines for Diet #3, for conditions caused by both yin and yang dietary extremes. A HOT TOWEL COMPRESS or a GINGER COMPRESS on the spleen can help reduce pain and promote better circulation. However, if the spleen is swollen or inflamed, use a cool compress instead, such as a LEAFY GREENS PLASTER or CABBAGE LEAF PLASTER. As a special drink for an enlarged spleen, combine 1 part burdock, 1 part carrots, 2 parts dried daikon. Chop finely, add four times as much water, and bring to a boil and simmer for 15 to 20 minutes, adding a pinch of sea salt toward the latter part of cooking. Drink the liquid and eat the vegetables, 1 cup daily, for several days or until the condition improves. UME-SHO KUZU or BANCHA TWIG TEA poured over a small volume of GOMASHIO in a teacup is also beneficial. As a frequent snack or as part of the meal, take BROWN RICE BALLS prepared with GOMASHIO around the outside instead of nori.

Ruptured Spleen. A ruptured spleen results from a severe blow to the stomach area. It commonly results from car accidents, athletic mishaps, or beatings. Surgery is usually required to prevent life-threatening loss of blood. Meanwhile, the bleeding can be minimized by taking DENTIE, 1/3 teaspoon mixed in a little hot or cold water, every 20 minutes, but only several times. The dentie will thicken the blood, enabling it to clot more easily and slow the bleeding. Refrain as much as possible from taking tea, water, or other liquid until the bleeding has stopped. Instead of dentie, GOMASHIO may be taken, 1 teaspoon mixed in a little hot or cold water. A cold compress or plaster, such as a TOFU PLASTER or an ice pack, may be placed on the stomach region until medical help arrives or the person gets to the hospital.

SOLUTION

DIET

1. Eat whole grains as the principal foods, especially millet, which is beneficial for the spleen. It can be prepared boiled, combined and pressure-cooked with rice, prepared with vegetables such as squash, carrots, or other sweet-tasting foods, or served in soups or as a soft breakfast cereal.

2. Round vegetables are sweet-tasting and particularly nourishing and soothing to the spleen. These include fall- or winter-season squash, onions, and cabbage. These may be served nishime-style, in soups (especially MILLET SQUASH SOUP), or stews.

3. Take UMEBOSHI PLUMS, sauerkraut, or sour pickles (such as those made with umeboshi vinegar) to quiet an overactive spleen.

LIFESTYLE

Follow the standard way-of-life suggestions.

I. Since anxiety, suspicion, jealousy, envy, and a critical mentality commonly accompany spleen problems, it is important to maintain a calm, peaceful environment.

2. A BODY SCRUB with a warm towel or towel soaked in warm ginger water is beneficial. The towels may be placed on the spleen region for 10 to 15 minutes. A HOT WATER BOTTLE or hot SALT PACK may be used instead.

3. SHIATSU, DO-IN, PALM HEALING, and other peaceful, gentle healing practices may be helpful.

MEDICAL EVIDENCE

SEA VEGETABLES ENHANCE SPLEEN FUNCTIONS

Hijiki and other sea vegetables stimulated spleen cells to proliferate and boosted the immune function in human and animal experiments conducted by scientists at Hiroshima University School of Medicine. The sea vegetables also enhanced Ig production by B cells, increased tumor necrosis factor by macrophages, and stimulated human lymphocytes to multiply. "These results suggest that seaweed extracts have stimulating activity on B cells and macrophages and this ability could be used clinically for the modulation of immune responses," the scientists noted.

Source: J. N. Lieu et al., "B Cell Stimulating Activity of Seaweed Extracts," *International Journal of Immunopharmacology* 19(3):135–42, 1997.

@ STOMACH PROBLEMS

Gastritis, gastroenteritis, heartburn, ulcers, and other digestive problems are associated with the stomach, a hollow gourd-shaped organ located in the upper left of the abdominal cavity between the esophagus and the small intestine. The interior lining of the stomach, the mucosa, contains millions of tubular glands that secrete hydrochloric acid, pepsin, and small amounts of mucin, anti-anemia materials, and inorganic salts. The stomach acids primarily break down protein into its various amino acids. Together with muscular peristalsis, enzymatic actions convert solid food into semiliquid chyme, which passes from the stomach to the duodenum, the first section of the small intestine.

A healthy stomach contributes to good appetite and digestion, as well as overall balance, sympathy, compassion, and understanding. Stomach upsets and disorders cause not only poor appetite and digestive problems but also anxiety, doubt, jealousy, and other negative emotions. Common stomach ailments will be looked at below. *See also "Stomach Cancer" in "Cancer" and "Digestive Problems."*

SYMPTOMS

Stomach ailments and disorders may be accompanied by some of the following symptoms:

1. Weak digestion or digestive problems
2. Poor appetite
3. Nausea
4. Dull sense of taste
5. Abdominal bloating
6. Pain in the upper abdomen
7. Blood sugar imbalances
8. Weight problems
9. Sallow complexion
10. Ulcers

Stomach troubles are traditionally evaluated in Far Eastern medicine according to the following diagnostic signs:

1. The top half of the upper lip corresponds to the stomach. Puffiness, tightness, discolorations, or other abnormalities indicate developing stomach problems.

2. The bridge of the nose corresponds to the stomach. Swellings, darkness, and other abnormalities here point to stomach ills and disorders.

3. The main branch of the stomach meridian runs from the corner of the nose, enters the body and descends to the stomach, and continues down the trunk to the outside of the lower leg. From here it continues to run over the top of the foot to the second and third toes. Pain, tightness, and soreness along the meridian show developing stomach problems.

4. Anxiety, upset, envy, jealousy, doubt, skepticism, and other emotions show disorders in the stomach (as well as spleen and pancreas).

CAUSES

1. Most stomach ills are associated with the modern way of eating, high in foods and beverages that overtax the stomach, causing the repeated oversecretion of stomach acids and leading to inflammation, irritation, ulcerations, and ultimately tumors.

2. Whole grains mostly pass through the stomach and are digested primarily in the small intestine. There they are absorbed in the villi and transformed into red blood cells and other strengthening fluids. In contrast, refined grains, flour, sugar and other sweets, soda and ice-cold drinks, alcohol, aromatic and stimulant beverages, chemicals, and drugs start to be absorbed directly in the stomach and enter the blood and body fluids prematurely, producing a thinner, more acidic quality of blood, lymph, and bodily fluids.

3. White rice, MSG, and chemically grown and treated food are particularly irritating to the upper part of the stomach, known as the body or fundus.

4. Meat, poultry, eggs, fish, shellfish, and other animal-quality foods, as well as too much baked food and salt, can cause problems in the lower stomach, known as the pylorus.

5. Ice cream, yogurt, soy milk, and other soy dairy products can lead to abdominal lumps, cysts, tumors, and cramps.

6. Liver and gallbladder problems may spill over and weaken the stomach.

FORMS

Gastritis. Gastritis is a generic term for the inflammation of the stomach lining. It encompasses a variety of symptoms such as pain or discomfort, nausea, vomiting, diarrhea, and loss of appetite. It may be mild or severe. *Acute gastritis* lasts for short periods, while *chronic gastritis* may persist for days, weeks, or longer. The chronic form can lead to pernicious anemia. The stomach lining may be irritated by many factors, including prescription drugs, aspirin and other over-the-counter medications, severe illness or injury, and viral or fungal infection. Gastritis may progress into ulcer, which may enlarge and start bleeding. Medical researchers have recently singled out a bacillus, *Helicobacter pylori,* which grows in the mucus-secreting cells of the stomach lining, as a primary cause of gastritis and ulcers. Gastritis is often treated with antibiotics.

From the macrobiotic view, overly acidic foods are the main cause of gastritis, especially refined grains and flour products, sugar and sweets, dairy food, meat, poultry, and other heavy animal foods, including too much fish and seafood. The combination of these foods cause excessive stomach acids to be released, irritating and inflaming the lining of the stomach as well as creating the kind of interior environment in which harmful bacteria and viruses thrive.

To relieve gastritis, follow the dietary guidelines for Diet #1, noting further the recommendations below.

Gastroenteritis. Gastroenteritis is a general inflammation of the stomach and digestive tract, frequently accompanied by painful cramps, fever, weakness, vomiting, and diarrhea. Medically, this condition is associated with a variety of causes, including viruses, bacteria, parasites, and food poisoning. Traveler's diarrhea is a common form of gastroenteritis and is associated with contaminated water, excessive chemicals and toxins, and in some cases taking certain medications or pills. To relieve gastroenteritis, follow the dietary guidelines for Diet #1, for more yin conditions. UMEBOSHI PLUMS, MISO SOUP (including instant miso), TEKKA, and other strong, salt-based foods and condiments are often useful to neutralize many of these symptoms, especially when sudden stomach ills come while traveling. *See also "Motion Sickness" in "Digestive Problems."*

Heartburn. Heartburn is felt as a burning sensation behind the sternum. It generally occurs after eating and may last from several minutes to several hours. Other symptoms include a burning in the throat, chest pain after bending over or lying down, and belching. Though named after the heart, this condition occurs when excessive stomach acid refluxes, or seeps, into the esophagus. The cause is excessive yin foods, especially oily and fatty foods, milk and light dairy foods, sugar and sweets, soft drinks and carbonated beverages, tropical foods (especially tomatoes), citrus fruits, stimulants, herbs and spices, and alcohol. All of these foods relax the lower esophageal sphincter, which normally prevents stomach acid from backing up into the esophagus. Medically this condition is treated with antacids or strong drugs. To relieve heartburn, discontinue all these strong expansive foods, follow the guidelines for Diet #1, and take

UME-SHO BANCHA or UME-SHO KUZU once or at most twice a day for several days.

Stomach Ulcers. There are two types of stomach ulcer. A *peptic ulcer* consists of a round or oval sore where the lining of the stomach or duodenum has been eaten away by stomach acid and digestive juices. Most commonly these occur in the *duodenum*, the first few inches of the small intestine.

Gastric ulcers are less common and occur in the upper curve of the stomach. Ulcers develop when the process of producing acid breaks down or when the amount of mucus production changes. Gastric ulcers are more common in later life and are associated with aspirin, ibuprofen, and other anti-inflammatory drugs given to the elderly.

Symptoms of ulcer include gnawing, burning, aching, soreness, an empty feeling, and hunger. For peptic ulcers, the pain tends to occur when the stomach is empty, and it is steady and mild or moderately severe and localized, almost always just below the breastbone. Modern medicine treats this type of ulcer with milk, antacids, and other mild substances. In gastric ulcers, eating can cause pain rather than relieve it. Gastric ulcers cause swelling of the tissues leading into the small intestine, which may prevent food from easily passing out of the stomach. This may cause bloating, nausea, or vomiting after eating.

Compared to each other, peptic ulcers are more yang, gastric ulcers more yin. Peptic ulcers are caused by the intake of proportionately more animal foods, baked food, and salt, which cause pepsin to be oversecreted in the lower stomach, leading to irritation and rupture. Gastric ulcers are caused by consuming more flour and other refined grains, sugar, dairy, and other expansive foods and beverages that cause excessive hydrochloric acid to be released in the upper stomach, producing inflammation and injury.

Fasting is often recommended to cure ulcers, but this is unnecessary. Proper chewing, up to 200 times per mouthful, is essential. To relieve ulcerous conditions, observe the recommendations for Diet #1 for gastric ulcers and Diet #2 for peptic ulcers. Emphasize whole grains and cooked vegetables, especially root vegetables for gastric ulcers and green leafy vegetables for peptic ulcers. Seasoning, condiments, and cooking styles may also be adjusted according to the type of ulcer, with milder seasoning and lighter cooking for peptic ulcers and stronger seasoning and longer cooking for gastric ulcers. Hot applications such as a GINGER COMPRESS or hot SALT PACK are beneficial for gastric ulcers, while cool applications such as a LEAFY GREENS PLASTER or TOFU PLASTER are effective for duodenal ulcers. (A GINGER COMPRESS may be applied for duodenal ulcers too for a few minutes prior to putting the cool compress over the affected area.)

SOLUTION

DIET

Observe the dietary suggestions noted above, with the following adjustments:

1. Eat whole grains as principal foods, especially millet, which is beneficial for the stomach. It can be prepared boiled, combined and pressure-cooked with rice, prepared with vegetables such as squash, carrots, or other sweet-tasting foods, or served in soups or as a soft breakfast cereal.

2. Round vegetables are sweet-tasting and particularly nourishing and soothing to the stomach. These include fall- or winter-season squash, onions, and cabbage. These may be served nishime-style, in soups (especially MILLET SQUASH SOUP), or stews.

3. Take UMEBOSHI PLUMS, sauerkraut, or sour pickles (such as those made with umeboshi vinegar) to quiet an overactive stomach.

LIFESTYLE

Follow the standard way-of-life suggestions.

HOME REMEDIES

1. Take ½ to 1 UMEBOSHI PLUM to neutralize acidity in the stomach.

2. Take 1 small cup of UME-SHO BANCHA or UME-SHO KUZU every day for up to 5 days to overcome the effects of acid-producing foods, to promote digestion, and to restore energy.

3. Take KINPIRA SOUP 2–3 times a week to strengthen the blood and increase vitality.

4. Since anxiety and upset commonly accompany stomach problems, it is important to maintain a calm, peaceful environment.

5. A BODY SCRUB with a warm towel or towel soaked in warm ginger water is beneficial. The towels may be placed on the abdomen for 10 to 15 minutes. A HOT WATER BOTTLE or hot SALT PACK may be used instead.

6. SHIATSU, DO-IN, PALM HEALING, and other peaceful, gentle healing practices may be helpful.

CAUTION

Stomach bleeding is usually serious and requires medical attention. Meanwhile, the bleeding can be minimized by taking DENTIE, ⅓ teaspoon mixed in a little hot or cold water, every 20 minutes, but only several times. The dentie will thicken the blood, enabling it to clot more easily and slow the bleeding. Refrain as much as possible from taking tea, water, or other liquid until the bleeding has stopped. Instead of dentie, GOMASHIO may be taken, 1 teaspoon mixed in a little hot or cold water. A cold compress or plaster, such as a TOFU PLASTER or an ice pack, may be placed on the stomach region until medical help arrives or the person reaches the hospital.

MEDICAL EVIDENCE

WHOLE GRAINS PROTECT AGAINST DUODENAL ULCER

Harvard researchers reported that in a large study of 47,806 men, higher intakes of whole grains and other foods high in fiber reduced the risk of duodenal ulcer by up to two-thirds. Vegetables and fruits high in vitamin A also lowered the risk by one-third.

Source: W. H. Aldoori et al., "Prospective Study of Diet and the Risk of Duodenal Ulcer in Men," *American Journal of Epidemiology* 145(1):42–50, 1997.

◎ TMJ AND RELATED PROBLEMS

TMJ or *temporomandibular joint syndrome* refers to pain or discomfort in the jaw region. Symptoms range from mild and moderate to severe and debilitating. Severe cases, involving chronic pain and disability, are treated with painkillers and muscle relaxants, eating soft foods or a liquid diet, physical therapy, or dental surgery. The underlying cause of TMJ is usually dietary imbalance. Return to a more natural way of eating can ease and help relieve this condition.

SYMPTOMS

A variety of symptoms may accompany teeth disorders, including the following:

1. Facial pain
2. Jaw popping when eating or yawning
3. Difficulty opening the mouth
4. Rigidity or a locked feeling in the jaw region
5. Pain in the neck and shoulders
6. Chronic pain and disability

CAUSES

1. The structure of the teeth reflects natural order and millions of years of biological evolution. Adult humans have 32 teeth, including 20 molars that are used primarily for grinding grains, 8 incisors that are effective for cutting vegetables and other plant-quality foods, and 4 canine teeth that may be used to tear flesh or animal foods. The ratio of teeth used for digesting vegetable food compared to animal food is 7:1. This suggests that seven-eighths of the human diet should consist of plant foods, especially whole cereal grains and their products, and one-eighth can be animal food. When we depart from this ratio, many health problems begin to arise, including teeth problems.

2. Healthy saliva is slightly alkaline and produces many types of bacteria that are beneficial to the teeth. Unhealthy saliva is acidic and fosters the growth of bacteria that attack and weaken the teeth, leading to tooth decay. A grain- and vegetable-centered diet creates slightly alkaline blood, lymph, and saliva, while a modern diet high in meat, sugar, refined flour, fruits, spices, and stimulants leads to acid conditions in body fluids, tooth decay, tooth loss, and gum disease.

3. Large teeth indicate a predominantly yin past way of eating, including a diet rich in protein and fat.

4. Small teeth show that the formative diet was rich in carbohydrates and minerals.

5. The teeth correlate to major systems and functions in the body. Problems in certain types of teeth show corresponding problems in internal organs. The incisors correspond to respiratory and circulatory organs and functions. Canines correspond to the liver, gallbladder, spleen, pancreas, and stomach. Premolars correspond to the upper intestinal region and excretory region. The molars correspond to the lower digestive tract, including the small and large intestines, and to the reproductive organs.

6. Crooked teeth result from a lack of whole grains, beans, and vegetables and a diet high in meat, poultry, eggs, dairy, sugar, and other highly processed foods.

7. From an energetic view, TMJ arises from one of two primary causes: (1) chronic intake of sugar and other sweets, fruit and juice, tropical vegetables, milk and ice cream, soft drinks, coffee and other stimulants, and other excessive yin foods that causes the jaw to gradually expand, or (2) chronic intake of meat, poultry, and other animal products, salty cheese, bread and

other baked flour products, salt and salty foods, and other excessive yang foods that cause the bones and muscles in this region to contract. If there is an overbite and the teeth push out, the condition is more yin. If there is an underbite and the teeth push in, the condition is too yang.

8. Beside an improper diet, environmental and lifestyle factors can contribute to teeth and gum problems. These include chemicalized toothpastes, mouth rinses, and other body care products; unclean, chemicalized, or toxic water; exposure to artificial electromagnetic energy, including dental X rays; and overmedication, including tooth extractions and other surgery.

SOLUTION

DIET

For TMJ and related teeth conditions, discontinue dietary extremes and follow the standard macrobiotic way of eating, paying special attention to the following:

1. Observing the dietary guidelines for Diet #1 for conditions caused by more yin factors, Diet #2 for those caused by more yang factors, or Diet #3 for combined conditions will gradually improve the overall alignment of the jaw, reduce muscle tension, and allow the joint to move smoothly.

2. Eat whole grains as the principal food at every meal. Take whole grains primarily in whole form, with cracked and processed grains and flour products such as noodles, pasta, unyeasted sourdough bread, and seitan taken occasionally.

3. Whole brown rice contains natural fluoride that is associated with reduced cavities and tooth decay. Other fluoride-rich natural foods include rye, parsley, cabbage, sea vegetables, and BANCHA TWIG TEA.

4. Avoid simple sugars (refined sugar, honey, and chocolate).

5. If you desire to eat animal food, it is best to choose white-meat fish, and then to consume it only occasionally.

6. Minimize fat consumption, including vegetable-quality oil. Do not take raw oil, such as in the form of salad dressings, sauces, and dips. Sesame oil is most recommended.

7. Avoid vegetables that originated in tropical regions, such as tomatoes, eggplants, and peppers. These are very acid-producing.

8. Take daily hard leafy greens that are high in calcium (such as collard greens and kale), round vegetables (such as fall- and winter-season squashes, cabbages, and onions), and root vegetables (daikon, carrot, burdock).

9. Consume a small volume of beans or bean products (tofu, tempeh, natto) regularly. These are high in calcium and will benefit the teeth and gums.

10. Take a small amount of sea vegetables on a daily basis. These are also high in calcium and minerals and will benefit the teeth and gums.

11. The amount of salt (miso, shoyu, and sea salt) should be moderate or, in the case of yang teeth conditions, very light.

12. Follow the standard guidelines in respect to supplemental foods, including fruit, juice, seeds, nuts, snacks and desserts. While recovering from tooth or gum problems, these items may temporarily be avoided or limited until the condition improves. However, for some yang conditions, a little fruit or juice may be advisable.

13. For a concentrated sweet taste, use natural grain-based sweeteners as much as possible, including BARLEY MALT, AMASAKE, and BROWN RICE SYRUP. While recovering from teeth problems, these may need to be limited, unless cravings arise. In this case, rice syrup is generally preferable, as it has a slightly more downward energy than barley malt or amasake and will be less likely to enhance the condition.

14. Cook and drink with natural water, including spring water, well water, or filtered water. Avoid chemicalized water, including fluoridated water.

15. Reduce the total volume of food and chew very well, at least 50 times per mouthful and ideally 100 times or more. Chewing will alkalinize the saliva, mouth, and digestive tract, help to neutralize any harmful bacteria, and contribute to overall health of the teeth and gums.

16. Avoid late-night eating and snacking.

LIFESTYLE

1. Proper dental hygiene is recommended, including brushing regularly.

2. Use a toothbrush made of natural materials and bristles instead of plastic or synthetic materials. Similarly, if you floss, use a natural floss.

3. In most cases, use DENTIE or a light salt-based toothpaste to brush the teeth and gums and keep the mouth clean. This is particularly good for people who have been eating modern food for many years and have overly acidic conditions, including teeth loss and gum disease.

4. For people whose teeth are more contracted, including some long-time macrobiotic persons, DENTIE or a salt-based toothpaste may be too yangizing and cause irritation. In this case, a natural herbal toothpaste may be

used, especially one without strong stimulant or aromatic ingredients.

5. Avoid fluoridated water and toothpastes containing fluoride. Fluoride is a trace mineral that will help to prevent cavities and bone loss, but it can produce other overall debilitating and weakening effects.

6. As much as possible, avoid having teeth extracted, especially if the roots are in good condition. Similarly, cavities may not necessarily need to be filled if a healthy diet is being eaten. Extraction, fillings, root canals, and other dental procedures may cause long-lasting vibrational effects. The energy pathways in the meridians that pass through the mouth may be disturbed, leading to physical, mental, or emotional imbalances. Anesthesia may also provoke adverse reactions. On the other hand, emergency cases may need dental treatment or surgery *(see "Caution," below)*.

7. The adverse effects of mercury amalgams have been widely publicized in recent years. As fillings are lost, it is advisable to avoid refilling them with mercury or other substances that can produce an imbalanced energy or abnormal charge. One by one, mercury fillings can be taken out or replaced as they naturally deteriorate. However, it is generally not recommended that existing mercury amalgam fillings be taken out, especially all at once if there are many, as some people have. Mass extractions may have an even stronger vibrational effect than leaving them in. Over time, they will naturally begin to decay. Eating a balanced diet is the most important change to make, and daily consumption of whole grains and vegetables will usually neutralize any harmful effects of existing fillings in the teeth. In the event that mercury is dislodged and swallowed, take salt added to strong BAN-CHA TWIG TEA or UMEBOSHI PLUM added to BANCHA TWIG TEA to help neutralize its effects. Strong MISO SOUP and/or sea vegetables are also good to help detoxify the body from the effects of mercury or other heavy metals.

8. If dentures are worn, select natural materials as much as possible, avoiding plastic or other synthetic materials.

9. Listening to tranquil sounds and music can help reduce tooth pain. Singing, toning, and humming may also be effective. Generally, peaceful, harmonious music is best, or intuitively make sounds that resonate and soothe the tooth or region of the mouth affected.

HOME REMEDIES

1. The pressure point in the indented region of the jaw can be used to relieve problems with the teeth. Apply pressure to these points on either side of the neck to help relieve tooth pain.

2. Warm salt water has a cleansing and antiseptic effect. Dissolve a small amount of salt in water and use to brush the teeth and cleanse the mouth. Cold salt water can be used as a mouthwash.

3. Salted BANCHA TWIG TEA may be used as a mouthwash or remedy in case of aches and pains. Add 1 teaspoon of salt for 4 cups of tea.

4. DENTIE can be used for all teeth and gum problems with a yin cause. For aches, rub the dentie into the gums around the affected area for 5 minutes. It may also be used as a toothpaste, but as a black powder, it is somewhat messy and abrasive. A variety of commercial dentie toothpastes are available that include natural whiteners and have a creamy texture. For healing, the black powder is recommended.

5. Apply a cooling compress or plaster such as grated daikon, radish, or onion on the region for aches or pains caused by acute inflammation. This type of ache is accompanied by heat and swelling.

6. Apply a hot compress or plaster such as a GINGER COMPRESS or a SALT PACK on the affected region for pains and aches not accompanied by inflammation.

CAUTION

1. It is advisable to see a dentist periodically, especially for serious teeth problems, emergency cases, or cases of chronic pain where the home remedies recommended in this section are not effective or when it is too painful or uncomfortable to do nothing. By nature, the teeth are very yang (small, compact) and tooth pain can be excruciating. If natural home remedies fail, it may be advisable to take antibiotics to relieve the suffering. However, you may reduce the amount to half strength depending on the case and your sensitivity to medication.

2. When seeking professional advice, seek a macrobiotic or holistic-oriented dentist whose own condition is well balanced, who is familiar with a dietary approach, and who is aware of the hazards of X rays, anesthesia, and other procedures and assists his or her patients in minimizing these risks.

MEDICAL EVIDENCE

MERCURY AMALGAMS LINKED TO SERIOUS DISORDERS

Mercury amalgams and fillings have been linked to amyotrophic lateral sclerosis, Alzheimer's disease, Parkinson's disease, and multiple sclerosis. They have been banned or restricted in Germany and Sweden.

Source: Gregory Dennis, "Holistic Dentistry," *New Age Journal*, April 1997.

FLUORIDE MAY WEAKEN BONES

Fluoride was added to many water systems after World War II. Today an estimated two-thirds of Americans live in communities with municipally fluoridated water. In a review of the scientific literature, scientists reported "a consistent pattern of evidence" showing that fluoridation damages bones, leading to hip fractures, skeletal fluorosis, osteosarcomas, and other disorders. The researchers also called into question the benefits of fluoride for teeth.

Source: M. Diesendorf et al., "New Evidence on Fluoridation," *Australian and New Zealand Journal of Public Health* 21(2):187–90, 1997.

FLUORIDE ASSOCIATED WITH ALZHEIMER'S-LIKE SYMPTOMS

Rats exposed to lower levels of fluoride (similar to levels in municipal tap water) developed neurological changes similar to Alzheimer's disease or dementia.

Source: J. A. Verner et al., "Chronic Administration of Aluminum-Fluoride or Sodium Fluoride to Rats in the Drinking Water," *Journal of Brain Research* 784(1–2):284–98, 1998.

MUSIC HELPS MASK DENTAL PAIN

Listening to sound and music at the dentist's office can help suppress pain. Dr. Wallace J. Gardner, a Boston dentist, reported that this approach was "fully effective" in 65 percent of 1,000 patients who had formerly required nitrous oxide or a local anesthetic. The patients listened to a variety of recordings, including a waterfall, on headphones.

Source: Dr. Wallace J. Gardner, "Suppression of Pain by Sound," *Science* 132:32–33, 1960.

HUMMING RELIEVES PAINFUL TOOTH ABSCESS

One winter Alex Jack, a teacher at the Kushi Institute, developed a painful abscess above his top left front tooth. The dietary remedies that he had used successfully before didn't work. While driving his car, he started humming to a cassette of traditional Christmas carols and after fifteen minutes the level of pain dropped sharply, affording him the first relief in several days. "Through a combination of sound diet and nutritious sounds, the abscess proceeded to clear up," he reported.

Source: Don Campbell, *The Mozart Effect* (New York: Avon Books, 1997), p. 278.

PART **III**

MANAGING YOUR HEALTH

The Standard Macrobiotic Way of Eating

Part III includes comprehensive dietary guidelines, three healing diets that form the basis for many of the conditions and disorders in Part II, basic recipes, special drinks, and other home remedies that will allow you to get started immediately.

The guidelines in this chapter are the standard macrobiotic dietary guidelines for persons in general good health, including those beginning the macrobiotic way of eating. They may also be used by those with fatigue, cuts and nicks, bruises and scrapes, light aches and pains, and other minor ailments, especially in conjunction with some of the specific home remedies recommended in Part II. For someone with a moderate to serious imbalance or disorder, it is recommended that a special diet be observed. Please see one of the three healing diets that follow in the next chapter. However, the standard guidelines present an overview of the full scope and variety of the macrobiotic way of eating, including lists of foods for regular use, occasional use, and infrequent use. *Regular use* means suitable for daily use or 5 or more times a week. *Occasional use* indicates that the food or

beverage may be taken 2 to 3 times a week. *Infrequent use* means 1 to 3 times a month.

For those on a healing diet, once the condition has improved (typically after 3 to 4 months), wider guidelines may gradually be observed. The guidelines that follow are for a temperate climate, including most of the United States, Canada, Europe, Russia, China, Japan, and temperate parts of Africa, South America, and Australia. Please review Table 2 in Part I of this book for a summary of adjustments for other climates and environments. Table 32 summarizes modifications for men, women, and children, while Table 33 presents those for age, activity level, and spiritual development.

Whole Cereal Grains

Whole grains are the principal food, comprising from 40 to 60 percent of the total percent of daily intake by weight. Ideally, whole grains prepared in whole form are the center of each meal, especially brown rice, millet, and barley. Other grains may be used occasionally, including

TABLE 32. ADJUSTMENTS FOR WOMEN, MEN, AND CHILDREN*

Kind of Food	For Women	For Men	For Children
General cooking	Less salty, lighter cooking	Slightly saltier, stronger cooking	Slightly sweeter, less salty, more dynamic cooking
Whole grains	Slightly less volume and seasoning; lighter grains; more boiling and shorter cooking	Slightly more volume and seasoning; stronger grains; more pressure-cooking and longer cooking	Slightly less volume and seasoning; lighter grains; more boiling and shorter cooking
Soup (1–2 servings a day)	Slightly lighter flavor (slightly less miso, shoyu, or sea salt)	Stronger flavor (more miso, shoyu, or sea salt)	Milder flavor (less miso, shoyu, or sea salt)
Vegetables (25–30 percent of daily volume)	Balance of green leafy, round, and root vegetables daily, but emphasize more leafy green varieties, fresh salads, and lighter sauces and dressings	Balance of green leafy, round, and root vegetables daily, but emphasize more root varieties, less fresh salads, and stronger sauces and dressings	Balance of green leafy, round, and root vegetables daily, but emphasize more sweet, round varieties, fresh salad, and lighter sauces and dressings
Beans and bean products (5 percent daily)	A little less strongly seasoned, use less regularly; sweetened occasionally	Slightly more seasoned, use more regularly	A little less strongly seasoned, use less regularly; sweetened occasionally
Sea vegetables (about 2 percent daily volume)	Quicker cooking, lighter taste	Longer cooking, stronger taste	Quicker cooker, lighter taste
Pickles (small volume daily)	More short-time, lighter pickles	More long-time, stronger pickles	More short-time, lighter pickles
Salt and seasonings	Slightly less salty, lighter seasoning	More salty, stronger seasoning	Much less salty, lighter seasoning, about a third to half that for adults depending on the child's age; avoid shoyu at the table
Oil	Slightly more oil, lighter cooking, and more stir-fries and other quick dishes	Slightly less oil, stronger cooking, and more deep-fried or tempura dishes	Slightly more oil, lighter cooking, and a balance of light, quick dishes and strong, rich-tasting ones
Condiments	Lighter use; gomashio 18:1	Stronger use; gomashio 16:1	Very light use; gomashio 20:1

Kind of Food	For Women	For Men	For Children
Beverages	Lighter tasting bancha tea and other beverages	Stronger tasting bancha tea and other beverages	Lighter tasting bancha tea and other beverages
Cooking fire	Gas, wood, or natural flame; avoid microwave and electric	Gas, wood, or natural flame; avoid microwave and electric	Gas, wood, or natural flame; avoid microwave and electric
Supplemental Foods			
Animal food	Less fish; avoid or minimize tuna, salmon, shrimp, and strong varieties	Slightly more fish; occasional strong fish or seafood	Occasional fish and seafood (optional)
Fruit and juice	Slightly more occasional use of fruits and juice	Slightly less occasional use of fruits and juice	Slightly more occasional use of fruits and juice
Seeds and nuts	Standard amount; limit nut and seed butters	Standard amount	Standard amount
Snacks and desserts	Slightly more sweets and desserts, but limit hard baked flour products	Slightly less sweets and desserts, but limit hard baked flour products, puffed, and dried snacks	Plenty of good-quality snacks, sweets, and desserts

*These are general or standard recommendations. The guidelines for any person will differ according to his or her specific condition, climate, environment, sex, age, activity level, personal needs, and other factors.

TABLE 33. MODIFICATIONS FOR AGE, ACTIVITY LEVEL, AND SPIRITUAL DEVELOPMENT*

Kind of Food	For Aging and Longevity	For a More Physically Active Way of Life	For a More Spiritually Oriented Way of Life
General cooking	Well-balanced and varied; less salty, lighter, softer cooking; smaller volume of food and drink	Slightly saltier, stronger cooking and greater volume of food	Simpler cooking, all grain and vegetable-quality; no animal food; and smaller volume of food
Whole grains	Slightly less volume and seasoning; lighter grains; softer grains	More volume and seasoning; stronger grains; more pressure cooking and longer cooking; rice, millet, and barley may be used regularly; whole oats are very warming; buckwheat and soba give strength	Slightly less volume and moderate seasoning, brown rice to be main grain; slightly more barley and corn, less cracked grains; avoid or minimize bread and baked goods
Soup (1–2 servings a day)	Slightly lighter flavor (slightly less miso, shoyu, or sea salt)	Stronger flavor (more miso, shoyu, or sea salt)	Light to moderate flavor and seasoning (miso, shoyu, or sea salt)
Vegetables (25–30 percent of daily volume)	Balance of green leafy, round, and root vegetables daily, but emphasize more leafy green varieties, fresh salads, and lighter sauces and dressings	Balance of green leafy, round, and root vegetables daily, but emphasize more root varieties, more nishime-style dishes, less fresh salads, and stronger sauces and dressings	Balance of green leafy, round, and root vegetables daily, especially in soup, more kinpira and nabe-style dishes, less sauces and dressings; smaller portions; avoid garlic
Beans and bean products (5 percent daily)	Less beans and slightly more tofu and natto; more simply seasoned; sweetened occasionally	More regular use, greater volume, and more highly seasoned; more tempeh	Less regular use, light to moderately seasoned; slightly more tofu
Sea vegetables (about 2 percent of daily volume)	Quicker cooking, lighter taste	Longer cooking, stronger taste	Light to moderate use, especially in soup
Pickles (small volume daily)	More short-time, lighter pickles	More long-time, stronger pickles	Various pickles, more frequent use
Salt and seasonings	Slightly less salty, lighter seasoning	More salty, stronger seasoning	Light to moderate seasoning; avoid spices and pungent foods

Kind of Food	For Aging and Longevity	For a More Physically Active Way of Life	For a More Spiritually Oriented Way of Life
Oil	More oil, including 1 or 2 sautéed vegetable dishes daily, if desired	Moderate use of oil, stronger cooking, and more deep-fried or tempura dishes	Light to moderate use of oil
Condiments	Lighter use; gomashio 18:1 to 20:1	Standard use; gomashio 16:1	Average use; gomashio 18:1
Beverages	Lighter-tasting bancha tea and other beverages	Stronger-tasting bancha tea and other beverages	Light- to moderate-tasting bancha tea and other beverages; avoid stimulants and alcohol
Cooking fire	Gas, wood, or natural flame; avoid microwave and electric	Gas, wood, or natural flame; avoid microwave and electric	Gas, wood, or natural flame; avoid microwave and electric
Supplemental Foods			
Animal food	Less fish, once every 10–21 days; minimize strong varieties	More fish; occasional strong fish or seafood, if desired	Avoid or minimize
Fruit and juice	Occasional use of fruits and juice	Occasional use of fruits and juice	Light use of fruits and juice
Seeds and nuts	More seeds than usual; standard amount of nuts	Standard amount	More seeds than usual; standard amount of nuts
Snacks and desserts	Slightly more soft sweets and desserts, less hard baked flour products, puffed and dried snacks	Standard amount of sweets and desserts, moderate use of hard baked flour products, puffed and dried snacks	Slightly less sweets and desserts; avoid baked foods; occasional kanten, amasake pudding, and other soft foods
Other	Overall, food may be softer and easier to digest, using more oil and liquid to offset drying of cells and tissues; more calcium-rich foods such as tofu, collards, kale, and other leafy greens, and hijiki, arame, and other sea vegetables to offset bone loss and thinning	Strong, dynamic foods and cooking styles may be used be used more often; wider variety; more frequent use of ginger, lemon, mustard, and other seasonings, condiments, and garnishes; over time whole grains and beans provide greater strength and endurance than animal food	Chew each mouthful thoroughly, 100–200 times, especially whole grains; occasionally eat wild foods, including wild grasses, roots, pine nuts, berries, reishi and maitake mushrooms; periodic fasting for 1 day a week, or several days a month: just rice, soup, pickles, and tea

*These are general modifications. The guidelines for any person will differ according to his or her specific condition, climate, environment, sex, age, activity level, personal needs, and other factors.

whole wheat berries, rye, corn, whole oats, and buckwheat. Whole-grain noodles or pasta, including udon, soba, and somen, may be eaten 2 or 3 times a week. Whole-grain bread, muffins, or other baked goods, especially unyeasted sourdough wheat or rye bread, may be taken two to three times a week. Seitan (wheat gluten), fu, grits, rolled oats, bulgur, couscous, rice cakes, and other grain products may be taken occasionally as part of the whole-grain portion. Whole grains and grain products include:

Regular Use
Short-grain brown rice
Medium-grain brown rice
Long-grain brown rice (for hotter climates and in hotter weather)
Millet
Whole barley
Whole wheat berries
Corn (on the cob or corn kernels)
Whole oats
Rye
Buckwheat

Occasional Use
Sweet brown rice
Wild rice
Mochi (pounded sweet rice)
Hato mugi (pearl barley)
Spelt
Cracked wheat (bulgur)
Couscous
Steel-cut oats
Rolled oats
Corn grits
Cornmeal
Rye flakes

Quinoa
Amaranth
Teff
Basmati rice
White rice
Other traditionally used or commonly consumed whole grains

Occasional Use: Flour Products
Whole-wheat noodles and pasta (udon, somen, spaghetti)
Buckwheat noodles (soba)
Whole-wheat chapatis
Whole-wheat bread, unyeasted (sourdough)
Whole-rye bread, unyeasted
Wheat gluten (seitan)
Wheat gluten, puffed (fu)
Corn tortilla or arepa (masa)
Corn pasta
Rice pasta
Spelt pasta
Rice kayu bread
Other traditionally used or commonly consumed whole grain products

Infrequent Use
Muffins
Biscuits
Crackers
Pancakes
Pastries
Puffed cereals
Popcorn
Rice cakes
Chips
Cookies

- Grains may constitute about half the meal by weight (50 percent) or one-third (35 percent) by volume.

- Pressure-cooked or boiled brown rice is the staple in most macrobiotic households, being cooked freshly once a day.

- Among the many variations and combinations, brown rice may be cooked with 10 to 20 percent millet, barley, pearl barley, whole wheat berries, fresh corn, whole oats, etc.

- Brown rice may be cooked with 10–20 percent adzuki beans, lentils, black soybeans, chickpeas, etc.

- In pressure-cooking, the ratio of grain to water should be 1:2. Boiling may be substituted for pressure-cooking occasionally.

- For seasoning, use a pinch of sea salt per cup of uncooked grain.

- A delicious morning porridge can be made by taking leftover rice or other grain, adding a little more water to soften, simmering for 2–3 minutes more, and seasoning with a ½ to 1 teaspoon of miso per cup of grain at the end of cooking.

- Other popular dishes include fried rice with vegetables, fried noodles with vegetables, rice with sweet rice, rice with lotus seeds, rice with sesame seeds, rice with presoaked dried chestnuts, rice and vegetable sushi, barley and sweet vegetable stew, millet and sweet vegetable stew, and porridge made from leftover grain for breakfast.

- Whole grains will keep for about 24 hours and may be used the next day as porridge, steamed or reheated, added to soups, or fried.

◎ Soup

One or 2 servings of soup, either a cup or bowl, seasoned with miso, shoyu, or sea salt is recommended, making up about 5 percent of daily intake. Soups may be prepared with a variety of ingredients, including vegetables from sea and land, seasonal vegetables, beans, and grains.

- Miso soup with wakame and seasonal vegetables is usually eaten once a day or more in most macrobiotic households. Use barley, brown rice, or all soybean miso that has aged 2 to 3 years.

- Shoyu broth is also eaten frequently.

- Squash soup, millet soup with sweet vegetables, carrot soup, and other sweet vegetable soups are delicious and may be made often.

- Other popular vegetable soups include broccoli soup, cauliflower soup, onion soup, celery soup, mushroom soup, and others.

- Barley soup with vegetables is very satisfying, as are other grain and vegetable soups.

- Bean soups are thick and filling, including black bean soup, navy bean soup, pinto bean soup, kidney bean soup, lentil soup, adzuki bean soup, and split pea soup.

- Other good combinations are tofu and vegetable soup, daikon and green vegetable soup, noodle soup with vegetables, and pasta soup with vegetables.

- Fish chowder made with white-meat fish and vegetables (and without dairy) may be taken occasionally by those who eat animal food.

◎ Vegetables

Twenty to 30 percent of daily food includes fresh vegetables prepared in a variety of ways, including steaming, boiling, or sautéing (with a small amount of sesame or other unrefined oil). A balance of green leafy, round, and root vegetables is recommended, with the major portion cooked and a smaller portion taken in the form of salad or pickles.

Regular Use: Leafy Vegetables
Kale
Collard greens
Watercress
Leeks
Mustard greens
Chinese cabbage (napa)
Carrot tops
Daikon tops
Turnip greens
Parsley
Scallions
Mizuma
Dandelion greens
Broccoli rabe
Arugula
Bok choy
Pak choy

Regular Use: Round or Ground Vegetables
Broccoli
Cauliflower
Onion
Cabbage
Acorn squash
Butternut squash
Buttercup squash

Hubbard squash
Pumpkin
Hokkaido pumpkin
Delicata squash
Rutabaga
Turnip
Brussels sprouts
Celeriac
String beans

Regular Use: Root Vegetables
Carrots
Burdock
Parsnip
Daikon
Red radish
Lotus root
Dandelion root
Jinenjo (mountain potato)

Occasional Use Vegetables
Beets
Celery
Chicory
Chives
Coltsfoot
Cucumber
Endive
Escarole
Garlic
Green peas
Iceberg lettuce
Jerusalem artichoke
Kohlrabi
Lamb's quarters
Mushrooms
Pattypan squash
Red cabbage

Romaine lettuce
Salsify
Shiitake
Snap beans
Snowpeas
Spaghetti squash
Sprouts
Summer squash
Wax beans
Zucchini

Infrequent Use Vegetables (or Avoid)
Artichoke
Asparagus
Avocado
Bamboo shoots
Curly dock
Eggplant
Fennel
Ferns
Ginseng
New Zealand spinach
Okra
Peppers (green or red)
Plantain
Potato
Purslane
Shepherd's purse
Sorrel
Spinach
Sweet potato
Swiss chard
Taro potato (albi)
Tomato
Yams

- Use organically grown vegetables as much as possible.

- If vegetables are sprayed with chemicals or waxed, rinse lightly in salted water and peel off the skin.

- When cooking vegetables, pressure cooking is not recommended.

- Use fresh vegetables as much as possible rather than frozen or canned.

- Cook vegetables fresh every day and try to use them up the same day, as they lose their freshness and energy if kept overnight.

- Prepare steamed leafy greens daily or regularly.

- Prepare nishime-style dishes two to three times a week with various combinations of root and round vegetables such as carrot, parsnip, and cabbage; squash, onion, and daikon; cabbage and onion; turnip, shiitake mushroom, and cabbage cooked with a little kombu.

- Prepare squash with adzuki beans and kombu 1 to 3 times a week.

- Other occasional dishes may include dried daikon with kombu; daikon and daikon leaves; carrots and carrot tops; turnip and turnip tops, or dandelion roots and leaves.

- Boiled salad (blanched vegetables) may be eaten regularly.

- Pressed salad (quick pickling) may be eaten regularly.

- For those in good health, fresh salad may be eaten once or twice a week with natural dressings, including those made with umeboshi plum, miso, shoyu and lemon juice, rice vinegar, umeboshi vinegar, tofu, pumpkin seeds, sesame seeds, scallions, and parsley.

- Sautéed vegetables may be taken 2 or 3 times a week.
- Kinpira-style vegetables may be taken once or twice a week.
- A stew may be made once or twice a week consisting of dried or fresh tofu, tempeh, or seitan with vegetables.
- Vegetable nabe, consisting of lightly boiled vegetables, tofu, mochi, tempeh, and noodles cooked homestyle on the table, may be enjoyed several times a week as a special festive dish.

◎ Beans

Five percent of daily intake may be taken as beans, such as adzuki beans, lentils, chickpeas, or black soybeans. These are usually cooked together with kombu or other sea vegetable or with a small volume of onions and carrots. Other beans may be used occasionally, 2 to 3 times a month. For seasoning, a small volume of unrefined sea salt or shoyu or miso can be used, and occasionally beans may be sweetened with barley malt. Bean products, such as tempeh, natto, and dried or cooked tofu, may be used regularly but in moderate volume.

Regular Use Beans
Adzuki beans
Chickpeas (garbanzo beans)
Lentils (green or brown)
Black soybeans

Regular Use Bean Products
Tofu (fresh or dried)

Tempeh
Natto (fermented soybeans)

Occasional Use Beans
Anasazi beans
Black-eyed peas
Black beans (turtle beans)
Great northern beans
Kidney beans
Lentils (red)
Lima beans
Mung beans
Navy beans
Pinto beans
Soybeans (yellow)
Split peas and whole dried peas
Other traditionally used or commonly consumed beans

Occasional Use Bean Products
Okara (residue from making tofu)
Soy milk (homemade)
Yuba (skin from soy milk)

- Except for soft beans such as lentils and split peas, most beans are hard and require soaking for several hours or overnight to improve their digestibility.
- Beans are traditionally seasoned with sea salt, miso, shoyu, or a 1-inch square of kombu, which may or may not be eaten.
- Beans may be boiled, pressure-cooked, or very occasionally baked.
- Recommended combinations include beans cooked with kombu; beans with carrots and onions (20 percent); beans with acorn, butternut, or buttercup squash (30–50 per-

cent), adzuki beans or black soybeans (70–90 percent) with chestnuts (10–30 percent); beans in soup with other vegetables; beans (90 percent) combined with grains (10 percent).

- Try to use up bean dishes within 24 hours.

⊚ Sea Vegetables

A small portion of sea vegetables is eaten daily, about 2 percent of total volume, including wakame and kombu cooked in daily grain, soup, or other regular dishes. A sheet or half sheet of toasted nori may also be taken daily. A small side dish of hijiki or arame should be prepared 2 times a week. All other sea vegetables are optional. Sea vegetables may also be taken in the form of condiments.

Regular use
Toasted nori sheet
Wakame
Kombu

Occasional Use
Arame
Hijiki

Optional Use
Agar-agar
Dulse
Irish moss
Mekabu
Ocean ribbons
Sea palm
Other traditionally used or commonly consumed sea vegetables

- Wakame and kombu are used regularly in soups, beans, and vegetable dishes.
- Nori sheets may be toasted over an open flame and eaten plain, sprinkled on grains, used to make sushi or rice balls, or made into nori flakes or cooked nori condiment.
- Flavorful combinations for side dishes include arame or hijiki with onions; arame or hijiki with sweet corn; arame or hijiki with dried tofu and carrots; arame or hijiki with tempeh and lotus root; arame or hijiki with dried daikon and onions.
- Agar-agar may be used to make a kanten or aspic, a delicious gelatin that can be prepared with fruit, juice, vegetables, broth, or beans.

⊚ Condiments

Condiments provide a specific taste or flavor, give color, and help balance the meal as a whole. Condiments should be available on the table for optional use. Regular use condiments include gomashio (on the average made with 1 part salt to 16 parts sesame seeds); kombu, kelp, or wakame powder; umeboshi plum; and tekka. These condiments may be used daily on grains and vegetables, but the volume should be moderate to suit individual appetite and taste, about 1 teaspoon altogether per day.

Main Use
Green nori flakes
Gomashio
Seaweed powder with or without toasted sesame seeds

Shiso leaf powder

Tekka

Umeboshi plums

Other Condiments

Brown rice vinegar

Cooked miso with scallion

Nori condiment

Shio kombu

Shiso leaf powder with toasted sesame
seeds

Umeboshi plum with scallions

Umeboshi vinegar

Other traditionally and commonly used
condiments

• Homemade gomashio is highly recommended in a ratio of 16 to 18 parts roasted
sesame seeds to 1 part sea salt. The gomashio in the natural foods store is usually
very salty and may not be fresh.

◎ Seasonings

Principal seasonings include unrefined sea salt,
miso, and shoyu. Only naturally processed,
nonchemicalized seasonings should be used. In
general, seasonings are used in cooking, not
added at the table. The taste should be moderate, neither too strong, nor too bland. White sea
salt that flows freely is the standard. Avoid gray
sea salt or high-mineral-content white sea salt,
which can cause yang, contractive effects. For
daily miso soup, use barley, brown rice, or all
soybean miso that has aged 2–3 years. White,
red, yellow, and other lighter and quicker-aged
misos may be used occasionally for sauces,

dressings, or special dishes. Ginger, umeboshi
vinegar, brown rice vinegar, tamari (wheat-free
soy sauce), lemon, orange peel, and other seasonings may be used occasionally, as well as
mirin (a sweet cooking wine).

Regular Use

Barley miso

Brown rice miso

Soybean miso (hatcho miso)

Shoyu (natural soy sauce)

Unrefined white sea salt

Occasional Use

Ginger

Horseradish

Mirin

Rice vinegar

Umeboshi paste

Umeboshi plum

Umeboshi vinegar

Garlic

Lemon

Red miso

White miso

Yellow miso

Tamari (wheat-free soy sauce)

Other traditionally and commonly used
seasonings

◎ Cooking Oil

For cooking, naturally processed, cold-pressed
unrefined vegetable oil is recommended. It is
used for frying rice and other grains, noodles,
and sautéing vegetables, on average about 2 to
3 times per week. It may also be used in deep-

frying foods or to make tempura. It is always eaten cooked, not raw or added at the table.

Regular Use
Sesame oil (dark or light)
Corn oil (preferably non-GMO or organic)
Mustard seed oil

Occasional Use
Safflower oil
Sunflower oil
Soybean oil
Olive oil
Peanut oil
Other traditionally used or commonly consumed vegetable oils

◎ Pickles

Pickles aid in digestion and are eaten in small volume, about 1 tablespoon or less a day.

Regular Use (Types)
Bran
Brine
Miso
Miso bran
Pressed
Sauerkraut
Takuan
Shoyu
Umeboshi
Other traditionally and commonly consumed pickles

◎ Beverages

Bancha twig tea is the principal beverage. Barley tea, brown rice tea, and other traditional, non-stimulant, nonaromatic teas may also be taken regularly. Use good-quality spring, well, or filtered water, avoiding chemicalized tap water, distilled water, or mineral water (even as a beverage on social occasions). Two to 3 cups of fresh carrot juice or other vegetable juice may be taken each week. Grain coffee, green tea, and other "occasional use" beverages may be taken several times a week. Beer, sake, and other "infrequent use" beverages may be taken a few times a month.

Regular Use
Bancha twig tea (kukicha)
Bancha stem tea
Roasted barley tea
Roasted brown rice tea
Spring water
Well water
Filtered water

Occasional Use
Carrot juice
Celery juice
Apple juice, apple cider, or other temperate-climate fruit juice
Dandelion tea
Grain coffee (without figs, dates, or tropical sweeteners)
Kombu tea
Mu tea
Sweet vegetable drink
Green tea
Umeboshi tea

Other traditionally or commonly consumed non-stimulant, non-aromatic beverages

Infrequent Use
Herbal teas
Beer
Sake
Wine
Other alcoholic beverages
Soy milk (with kombu or other ingredients), rice milk, or other highly processed commercial beverages
Sprouted barley powder tea
Spritzers and other sugar-free carbonated beverages
Other beverages

◎ Supplemental Foods for People in Good Health

In addition to the daily food groups described above, those in good health may wish to supplement their diet with occasional animal food, fruits, seeds and nuts, and snacks and desserts.

ANIMAL FOOD

Animal food is optional and not necessary for daily health or vitality. If desired, fish and seafood are the best quality of animal food for consumption in a temperate climate. White-meat fish may be eaten once or twice a week in small volume. The fish should generally be prepared steamed, boiled, or poached, only very occasionally prepared by broiling, grilling, and baking. Limit tuna, salmon, shrimp, and other blue-meat and red-meat fish or shellfish to in-frequent use, once or twice a month. Fish and seafood should always be taken with grated daikon, lemon, horseradish, or other garnish to help digest the fat and oil. It should ideally also be taken with plenty of fresh vegetables and whole grains as part of a balanced meal.

Occasional Use
Cod
Flounder
Haddock
Halibut
Scrod
Red snapper
Smelt
Sole
Trout
Other white-meat fish

Infrequent Use Fish
Bluefish
Chirimen iriko (tiny dried fish)
Eel
Iriko (small dried fish)
Salmon
Sea bass
Swordfish
Tuna
Other strong fish

Infrequent Use Shellfish
Clams
Crab
Lobster
Oysters
Scallops
Shrimp
Other shellfish

FRUIT

Temperate-climate fruits may be enjoyed 2–3 times per week, including apples, pears, apricots, berries, and melons. These may be eaten fresh in season, cooked, or dried. Avoid tropical fruits as much as possible. Juice or cider may be taken occasionally.

Occasional Use
Apples
Apricots
Blackberries
Blueberries
Cantaloupe
Cherries
Cranberries
Currants
Grapefruit
Grapes
Honeydew melon
Oranges
Peaches
Pears
Plums
Prunes
Raspberries
Raisins
Strawberries
Tangerines
Watermelon
Other temperate-climate fruits

NUTS AND SEEDS

A small volume of nuts and seeds may be taken, about 1 small cup a week, unsalted, lightly blanched, boiled, or roasted. Select among the less fatty and oily nuts, such as almonds, peanuts, walnuts, and pecans. Avoid tropical nuts as much as possible. Sesame seeds, pumpkin seeds, squash seeds, and sunflower seeds may be taken and are less fatty and oily than nuts. A small amount of nut or seed butters may also be taken occasionally, but be careful not to overconsume.

Occasional Use
Sesame seeds
Sunflower seeds
Pumpkin seeds
Chestnuts
Almonds
Filberts
Peanuts
Pecans
Walnuts
Other temperate-climate nuts and seeds

SNACKS AND DESSERTS

Macrobiotic cooking includes an assortment of delicious, satisfying snacks and desserts made with all-natural ingredients that can be enjoyed from time to time.

To satisfy cravings for a sweet taste, use sweet vegetables every day in cooking, drink sweet vegetable drink occasionally, and prepare sweet vegetable jam. Mochi, rice balls, sushi, and other grain-based snacks may be eaten regularly. Rice cakes, popcorn, and other dry or baked snacks may be enjoyed occasionally, but they can cause tightness, so don't take too many. A small volume of grain-based sweeteners such as amasake, barley malt, or brown rice syrup may be used occasionally for a concentrated sweet taste. Cakes, pies, cookies, pastries, and other hard baked desserts may be enjoyed several times a week, provided they are made with all-natural ingredients. Avoid too many baked foods, as they can produce tightness, mucus, and other strong effects.

Sweet Foods for Regular Use
Cabbage
Carrots
Chestnuts
Daikon
Onions
Parsnips
Squash (acorn, butternut, buttercup, delicata, kabocha, and others)
Pumpkin
Sweet vegetable jam

Occasional Use Snacks
Mochi
Noodles
Popcorn (homemade and unbuttered)
Puffed whole grains
Rice balls
Rice cakes
Seeds and nuts
Sweet vegetable drink
Vegetable sushi (homemade)

Other Sweets for Occasional Use
Amasake (sweet rice beverage or sweetener)
Barley malt
Brown rice syrup
Hot apple juice
Hot apple cider

Infrequent Use
Maple syrup

◎ Way-of-Eating Suggestions

- Eat 2 to 3 meals at regular times each day.

- Eat in a calm, peaceful environment, sitting down at the table. Avoid eating while standing or moving.

- Eat comfortably, as much as you like, provided the general proportions and guidelines are observed. There is no need to count calories or calculate nutrients.

- Drink when thirsty, but do not overconsume or underconsume liquids.

- Chew very well, at least 50 times, preferably 100 times per mouthful. Ideally, after each mouthful, put down the utensils and chew thoroughly. Then pick up the utensils and take another bite.

- Avoid overeating and overdrinking. Ideally, leave the table satisfied but only about 80 percent full.

- Express appreciation to God, the universe, or nature for the food you have received and the energy it is dedicated to creating. This may take the form of grace, prayer, meditation, or a moment of silence before and after the meal.

- Avoid or limit all ice-cold foods and drinks served with ice cubes, which may be harmful to the intestines and kidneys.

- Avoid or limit eating food cooked on an electric stove or microwave oven as much as possible. Ideally, food is prepared with gas, wood, or other natural flame.

- Avoid or limit all chemicalized, irradiated, genetically altered, and other artificially produced and treated foods and beverages. As much as possible, use organically grown food, especially for whole grains, beans and bean products, vegetables, fruits, seasonings, oil, and condiments. Corn and soybeans are the two most widely available genetically altered crops at the current time. Laboratory tests indicate that the majority of foods in the supermarket and natural foods store containing these products are genetically altered. Be careful to use only organic or natural corn tortillas, corn chips, corn oil, tofu, tempeh, miso, and similar products.

- Avoid or limit late-night snacks and eating within 3 hours of sleeping. Eating before sleep can overwork the intestines, stress the pancreas, and burden the kidneys and bladder.

◎ Foods to Avoid for Better Health

The following foods are customarily avoided, minimized, or reduced in the modern macrobiotic way of eating in a temperate climate:

Animal Products
Beef (hamburger, steak, ribs, corned beef, etc.)
Lamb
Pork (chops, hot dogs, etc.)
Ham
Bacon
Salami
Veal
Eggs
Chicken
Turkey
Goose
Duck
Sausage
Wild game (venison, rabbit, squirrel, etc.)
Other red meat and poultry

Dairy Products
Butter
Cheese
Cream
Ice cream
Kefir
Milk (whole, skim, buttermilk, raw, etc.)
Sour cream
Whipped cream
Yogurt
Other dairy

Tropical Vegetables and Wild Vegetables
Asparagus
Avocado
Curly dock
Eggplant
Fennel
Ferns
Green and red pepper
Plantain
Potato
Purslane
Shepherd's purse
Sorrel
Spinach
Sweet potato
Taro (albi)
Tomato
Yam
Other tropical vegetables

Tropical Fruits
Banana
Coconut
Date
Fig
Kiwi
Mango
Papaya
Pineapple
Other tropical fruits

Tropical Nuts
Brazil nuts
Cashews
Macadamia nuts
Pistachios
Other tropical nuts

Sugar and Concentrated Sweeteners
Sugar (white sugar, raw sugar, brown sugar, turbinado sugar)
Molasses
Honey
Carob
Corn syrup
Saccharin
NutraSweet
Fructose and high-fructose corn syrup
Sucanat
Stevia
Other highly refined sweeteners

Seasonings and Oils
Refined salt (iodized salt, rock salt, table salt, chemically processed salt)
Gray sea salt
High-mineral-content white sea salt
Canola oil

Margarine
Coconut oil
Lard, shortening, and all animal fats
Palm oil
Soybean oil
Refined, chemically processed vegetable oils
Herbs
Spices
Ginseng
Others that produce extreme effects

Highly Processed Soy Products
In contrast to traditionally or naturally processed soy foods, many highly processed soy products are now available in the natural foods store. These are not recommended and may produce extreme effects. They also may be made with genetically modified soybeans.
Soy milk (sweetened with sugar, sucanat, crystals, etc.)
Soy margarine
Soy mayonnaise
Soy ice cream
Soy yogurt
Soy cheese
Soy protein isolate
Textured soy protein
Defatted soybean meal
Genistein
Lecithin
Soy infant formula
Other highly processed soy products or derivatives

Other Processed Foods
Polished rice (nonorganic white rice)
Bleached white flour
Canned foods

Dyed foods

Frozen foods

Genetically engineered foods

Instant foods

Irradiated foods

Sprayed foods

Foods processed with:

    Additives

    Artificial coloring

    Artificial flavoring

    Chemicals

    Emulsifiers

    Preservatives

    Stabilizers

    Other highly processed foods

Vitamins and Supplements

Vitamin pills (natural or synthetic)

    B complex

    B_1

    B_2

    B_6

    B_{12}

    Biotin

    C

    Choline

    E

    Folic acid

    Inositol

    Niacin

    Niacinamide

    PABA

    Pantothenic acid

    Other vitamins

Mineral supplements

    Bone meal

    Calcium

    Dolomite

    Iron

    Selenium

    Zinc

    Other minerals

Bee pollen

Shark cartilage

Bran tables

Brewer's yeast

Dessicated liver

Diet pills

Ginseng tablets or pills

Herbal tablets

Papaya tablets

Psyllium

Other similar products

◎ Dietary Guidelines for People in General Good Health

The following dietary guidelines may be followed for people in usual good health. They may need to be adjusted slightly for each person according to climate, environment, age, sex, activity level, personal condition and needs, and other factors. Please see the previous section for a comprehensive list of recommended macrobiotic-quality foods in a temperate climate and foods to avoid for better health.

1. Avoid extreme yang animal foods, including beef, pork, lamb, chicken, turkey, eggs, salted cheese, and other meat, poultry, and heavy dairy products.

2. Avoid extreme yin foods and beverages including sugar, chocolate, honey, and other concentrated sweeteners; milk, butter, cream, ice cream, yogurt, and other light dairy foods;

white rice, white flour, and other polished or refined grains in bread, crackers, cookies, pastries, and other baked goods; excessive fruits and juices; foods of tropical or subtropical origin, including tomatoes, potatoes, and peppers; herbs and spices; coffee, black tea, and other stimulants; alcohol; and drugs and medication.

3. Avoid all chemicalized, irradiated, genetically engineered, and other artificially produced and treated foods and beverages. As much as possible use organically grown food, especially for whole grains, beans and bean products, vegetables, oil, and condiments.

4. Avoid or limit all ice-cold foods and drinks served with ice cubes.

5. Avoid or limit food cooked on an electric stove or microwave oven. Prepare food as much as possible with gas, wood, or other natural flame.

6. Eat whole grains in whole form as the main portion of the diet. Fifty to 60 percent of daily consumption, by weight, should consist of whole cereal grains. The first day prepare pressure-cooked short-grain brown rice. The next day prepare brown rice pressure-cooked together in the same pot with 10 to 20 percent millet. The third day prepare brown rice with 10 to 20 percent barley. The fourth day prepare brown rice with 10 to 20 percent adzuki beans or lentils. The fifth day prepare plain brown rice again. Then repeat this pattern. Boiling may be substituted for pressure-cooking occasionally. Fried rice or grain croquettes may be enjoyed several times a week. A delicious morning porridge can be made by taking leftover rice, adding a little more water to soften, simmering for 2–3 minutes more, and seasoning with a half to 1 teaspoon of miso per cup of grain at the end of cooking. Morning porridge may be soft and

creamy, but otherwise the grain should be on the firm side. In pressure-cooking, the ratio of grain to water should be about 1:2. For seasoning, use a pinch of sea salt per cup of uncooked grain. Other grains may be used occasionally, including whole wheat berries, rye, corn, whole oats, and buckwheat. Whole-grain noodles or pasta, including udon, soba, somen, and spaghetti, may be eaten two or three times a week. Whole-grain bread, biscuits, muffins, or other baked goods, especially unyeasted sourdough wheat or rye, may be taken two to three times a week. Seitan (wheat gluten), grits, rolled oats, bulgur, couscous, rice cakes, and other grain products may be taken occasionally as part of the whole-grain portion.

7. One to 2 servings of soup, constituting of about 5 to 10 percent of the diet, is recommended each day, cooked with wakame and various land vegetables such as onions and carrots and seasoned with miso, shoyu, or sea salt. Grain soups, bean soups, vegetable soups, and other soups may be taken from time to time.

8. Twenty-five to 30 percent of daily food should be taken as vegetables, cooked in a variety of ways. These include a balance of green leafy vegetables such as broccoli, collards, and kale, round vegetables such as fall- and winter-season squash, cabbage, and onions, and root vegetables such as carrots, daikon, and burdock. Generally, prepare the following, though amounts and frequencies will vary according to the individual: nishime-style (long-time stewed) vegetables, 2 to 3 times a week; adzuki bean, squash, and kombu dish, 2 times a week; dried daikon, 1 cup, 1 time a week; carrots and carrot tops or daikon and daikon tops, 1 time a week; boiled salad, 3 to 5 times a week; pressed salad, 3 to 5 times a week; raw salad 1 to 2 times a week;

steamed greens, 5 to 7 times a week; sautéed vegetables, 2 to 3 times a week; kinpira-style (matchsticks), 1 to 2 times a week; dried tofu, tofu, tempeh, or seitan with vegetables, 1 to 2 times a week. Vegetable nabe (lightly boiled vegetables, tofu, mochi, tempeh, and noodles cooked homestyle at the table) may be enjoyed several times a week as a special side dish.

9. Five percent of daily intake may be taken as beans, such as adzuki beans, lentils, chickpeas, or black soybeans. These are usually cooked together with kombu or other sea vegetable or with a small volume of onions and carrots. Other beans may be used occasionally, 2 to 3 times a month. For seasoning, a small volume of unrefined sea salt or shoyu or miso can be used, and occasionally beans may be sweetened with barley malt. Bean products, such as tempeh, natto, and dried or cooked tofu, may be used occasionally but in moderate volume.

10. Five percent or less of daily intake may be in the form of sea vegetables, including wakame and kombu daily when cooking grain, in soup, or in other regular dishes. A sheet or half sheet of toasted nori may also be taken daily. A small side dish of hijiki or arame should be prepared 2 times a week. All other sea vegetables are optional.

11. Condiments should be available on the table and may be used in small volume, if desired. Regular use condiments include gomashio (on the average made with 1 part salt to 16 parts sesame seeds), kombu, kelp, or wakame powder; umeboshi plum; and tekka. These condiments may be used daily on grains and vegetables, but the volume should be moderate to suit individual appetite and taste, about 1 teaspoon altogether per day.

12. Pickles, made at home in a variety of ways, should be eaten daily, in small volume (1 tablespoon total), to aid in digestion.

13. For those who wish animal food, white-meat fish may be eaten once every 7 to 10 days in small volume. The fish should generally be prepared steamed, boiled, or poached and be garnished with fresh grated daikon or ginger and occasionally, if desired, prepared by broiling, grilling, and baking. Limit tuna, salmon, shrimp, and other blue-meat and red-meat fish or shellfish to infrequent use, once or twice a month.

14. Temperate-climate fruits may be enjoyed 2 to 3 times per week, including apples, pears, apricots, berries, and melons. These may be eaten fresh in season, cooked, or dried. Avoid tropical fruits as much as possible. Juice or cider may be taken occasionally.

15. To satisfy cravings for a sweet taste, use sweet vegetables every day in cooking, drink sweet vegetable drink, and prepare sweet vegetable jam. Mochi, rice balls, sushi, and other grain-based snacks may be eaten regularly. Rice cakes, popcorn, and other dry or baked snacks may be enjoy occasionally, but they can cause tightness, so don't take too many. A small volume of grain-based sweeteners such as amasake, barley malt, or brown rice syrup may be taken for a stronger sweet taste and used occasionally. Cakes, pies, cookies, pastries, and other hard baked desserts may be enjoyed several times a week, provided they are made with all-natural ingredients. Avoid too many baked foods, as they can produce tightness, mucus, and other strong effects.

16. A small volume of nuts and seeds may be taken, about 1 small cup a week, unsalted, lightly blanched, boiled, or roasted. Select from the less fatty and oily nuts, such as almonds, peanuts, walnuts, and pecans. Avoid tropical nuts as much as possible. Sesame seeds, pumpkin seeds, squash seeds, and sunflower seeds may be taken and are less fatty and oily than nuts. A small amount of nut or seed butters may also be taken occasionally, but be careful not to overconsume.

17. Seasonings for regular use include unrefined white sea salt, shoyu, and miso. For daily miso soup, use barley, brown rice, or all-soybean miso that has aged 2–3 years. White, red, yellow, and other lighter and quicker-aged misos may be used occasionally for sauces, dressings, or special dishes. Ginger, umeboshi vinegar, brown rice vinegar, tamari (wheat-free soy sauce), lemon, orange peel, and other seasonings may be used occasionally, as well as mirin (a sweet cooking wine).

18. Drink bancha twig tea or other traditional tea as the main beverage. Barley tea, brown rice tea, and other traditional, nonstimulant, nonaromatic teas may also be taken regularly. Use good-quality spring, well, or filtered water, avoiding chemicalized tap water, distilled water, or mineral water (even as a beverage on social occasions). Two to 3 cups of fresh carrot juice or other vegetable juice may be taken each week. Grain coffee, green tea, and other "occasional use" beverages may be taken several times a week. Beer, sake, and other "infrequent use" beverages may be taken several times a month.

19. Chew very well, at least 50 times and preferably 100 times per mouthful.

20. Avoid overeating and overdrinking.

21. Avoid late-night snacks and eating within 3 hours of sleeping.

Healing Diets

◉ Diet #1 for More Yin Conditions and Disorders

The following dietary guidelines may be followed for an ailment, condition, or disorder arising from predominantly extreme yin factors. They may need to be adjusted slightly for each person according to climate, environment, age, sex, activity level, personal condition and needs, and other factors. Refer to further modifications under each specific condition or disease. The use of oil and supplementary foods such as fruit, nuts and seeds, and sweets may differ significantly according to the specific condition. Special drinks and dishes, as well as home remedies, may also be recommended. Please see Chapter 9 for comprehensive lists of recommended macrobiotic-quality foods and foods to avoid, and Chapters 13 and 14 for how to prepare special drinks, dishes, compresses, and other home remedies. For moderate to serious cases, follow this diet for three to four months or until the condition improves. Then the standard macrobiotic way of eating for persons in usual

good health may gradually be implemented, offering a much wider scope and variety.

1. Avoid all extreme yin foods and beverages, including sugar, chocolate, honey, and other concentrated sweeteners; milk, butter, cream, ice cream, yogurt, and other light dairy foods; white rice, white flour, and other polished or refined grains; excessive fruits and juices; foods of tropical origin, including tomatoes, potatoes, and peppers; herbs and spices; coffee, black tea, and other stimulants; alcohol; and drugs and medication.

2. Avoid all extreme yang animal foods, including beef, pork, lamb, chicken, turkey, eggs, salted cheese, tuna, salmon, shellfish, and other meat, poultry, and seafood.

3. Avoid or reduce all hard baked flour products such as bread, crackers, cookies, and pastries, except for the occasional consumption of unyeasted, unsweetened whole-grain sourdough bread, if craved, once or twice a week. In serious cases, even sourdough bread may need to be completely avoided for several months until the condition improves.

4. Eliminate all chemicalized, irradiated, genetically engineered, and other artificially produced and treated foods and beverages. As much as possible use organically grown food, especially for whole grains, beans and bean products, vegetables, fruits, oils and other seasonings, and condiments.

5. Avoid or limit food cooked on an electric stove or in a microwave oven. Prepare food as much as possible with gas, wood, or other natural flame.

6. Unless otherwise indicated, miminize oil for a 1- to 2-month period, even good-quality vegetable oil, and then use only a small amount of sesame oil in cooking, preferably brushed on the skillet, once or twice a week.

7. Avoid raw salads temporarily for 1 month or more until the condition improves.

8. Avoid all ice-cold foods and drinks served with ice cubes.

9. In general, the cooking for a yin condition may be slightly stronger than usual and use a little more sea salt, miso, or shoyu in cooking.

10. Eat whole grains in whole form as the main portion of the diet. Fifty to 60 percent of daily consumption, by weight, should consist of whole cereal grains or whole-grain products. The first day prepare pressure-cooked short-grain brown rice. The next day prepare brown rice pressure-cooked together in the same pot with 20 to 30 percent millet. The third day prepare brown rice with 20 to 30 percent barley. The fourth day prepare brown rice with 20 to 30 percent adzuki beans or lentils. The fifth day prepare plain brown rice again. Then repeat this pattern. Boiling may be substituted or alternated for pressure-cooking. A delicious morning porridge can be made by taking leftover rice, adding a little more water to soften, simmering for 2–3 minutes more, and seasoning with ½ to 1 teaspoon of miso per cup of grain at the end of cooking. Morning porridge may be soft and creamy, but otherwise the grain should be on the firm side. In pressure-cooking, the ratio of grain to water should be about 1:2. For seasoning, cook with a small piece of kombu the size of a postage stamp, though in some cases sea salt may be used depending on the person's condition. Other grains may be used occasionally, cooked by themselves or with brown rice, including whole wheat berries, rye, corn, and whole oats, though oats should be avoided for the first month. Buckwheat and seitan are very strengthening and in some cases will be helpful. In other cases, they should be avoided or minimized because they may cause too rapid a discharge. Good-quality sourdough bread, preferably steamed, may be enjoyed 2–3 times a week if craved, though in some cases even this should be avoided for 1 month or more until the condition improves. Both udon and soba, or other whole-grain noodles or pasta, may be taken 2–3 times a week. Avoid all hard baked products until the condition improves, including cookies, cake, pie, crackers, muffins, and pastries. Avoid or limit cracked or processed grains such as bulgur, couscous, oatmeal, rye flakes, and puffed grains, until the condition improves, in which case they may be used occasionally.

11. Eat 1–2 servings of soup each day, constituting about 5 to 10 percent of the daily diet. The principal soup should consist of wakame and onions, carrots, or other land vegetables cooked together and seasoned with miso and occasionally shoyu. A small volume of shiitake may be added to the soup several times a week. The miso may be barley miso, brown rice miso, or soybean (hatcho) miso and should be naturally aged 2 to 3 years. Grain soups, bean soups, vegetable soups (especially made with sweet vegetables), and other soups may be taken from time to time. Soup may be slightly stronger in flavor than usual, but avoid a salty taste. Several times a week, kinpira soup may be taken for strength and vitality.

12. Twenty-five to 30 percent of daily food should be taken as vegetables, cooked in a variety of ways. All temperate-climate types may be taken daily, including hard green leafy vegetables such as collards, kale, or turnip greens, sweet round vegetables such as squash, onions, and cabbage, and root vegetables such as carrot, burdock, and daikon. Slightly emphasize more root varieties to help strengthen overly yin conditions. Generally, prepare the following, though amounts and frequencies will vary according to the individual: nishime-style (long-time stewed) vegetables, 3 to 4 times a week; adzuki bean, squash, and kombu dish, 3 times a week; dried daikon, 1 cup 3 times a week; carrots and carrot tops or daikon and daikon tops, 3 times a week; boiled salad, 5 to 7 times a week; pressed salad, 5 to 7 times a week; raw salad and salad dressing, avoid; steamed greens, 5 to 7 times a week; sautéed vegetables, using water the first month instead of oil, then occasionally (2 to 3 times a week) a small volume of sesame oil brushed on the skillet; kinpira-style (matchsticks) sautéed in water, ⅔ cup 2 times a week, then oil may be used brushed on the skillet after 1 month; dried tofu, tofu, tempeh, or seitan with vegetables, 2 times a week. Vegetable nabe (lightly boiled vegetables and noodles cooked homestyle at the table with sliced vegetables, tofu, tempeh, and mochi) may be eaten several times a week as a special side dish.

13. Five percent of daily intake may be taken as beans, such as adzuki beans, lentils, chickpeas, or black soybeans, cooked together with kombu or other sea vegetables or with a small volume of onions and carrots. Other beans may be used occasionally, 2 to 3 times a month. For seasoning, a small volume of unrefined sea salt or shoyu or miso can be used. Bean products such as tempeh, natto, and dried or cooked tofu may be used occasionally but in moderate volume. Use firm rather than soft tofu as much as possible.

14. Two percent or less of daily intake may be in the form of sea vegetables with slightly longer cooking and a thicker taste than usual. This includes wakame and kombu taken daily when cooking grain, in soup, or other dishes. A sheet or half sheet of toasted nori may also be taken daily. A small dish of hijiki or arame should be prepared about twice a week. All other sea vegetables are optional.

15. Condiments to be available on the table may include gomashio (on the average made with 1 part salt to 18 parts sesame seeds, reduced to 1:16 after 2 months); kombu, kelp, or wakame powder; umeboshi plum; and tekka. These condiments may be used daily on grains and vegetables, but the volume should be moderate to suit individual appetite and taste, about 1 teaspoon combined per day. Umeboshi (½ to 1 plum a day) and tekka (¼ to ⅓ teaspoon a day) are helpful in neutralizing infection and restoring digestive ability and may be taken several times a week or more for expansive conditions.

16. Pickles, made at home in a variety of

ways, should be eaten daily, in small volume (1 tablespoon total), with a slight emphasis on long-time, stronger pickles (but rinse thoroughly to avoid too much salt).

17. Animal food is to be avoided. However, white-meat fish may be eaten once every week or 2 weeks in small volume, if craved. The fish should be prepared steamed, boiled, or poached and be garnished with fresh grated daikon or ginger to facilitate digestion. After 2 months, the fish may be eaten once or twice a week and may be prepared occasionally with other cooking styles such as broiling, grilling, and baking. Completely avoid tuna, salmon, and other blue-meat and red-meat fish and all shellfish until the condition improves.

18. Unless otherwise indicated, avoid fruit and juice as much as possible, including temperate-climate as well as tropical fruit, until the condition improves. If cravings develop, a small volume of dried fruit or cooked temperate-climate fruit, especially apples, with a pinch of salt may be taken. Avoid raisins, which have a high concentration of simple sugars.

19. In general, avoid or limit all desserts and sweets, including good-quality desserts, until the condition improves. Even a small volume of sugar, chocolate, carob, honey, maple syrup, or soy milk may worsen an overly expanded condition and produce new symptoms. To satisfy cravings for a sweet taste, use sweet vegetables every day in cooking, drink sweet vegetable drink, and prepare sweet vegetable jam. Mochi, rice balls, sushi, and other grain-based snacks may be eaten regularly. Rice cakes, popcorn, and other dry or baked snacks should be minimized, as they may cause tightening. A small volume of grain-based sweeteners such as amasake, barley malt, or brown rice syrup may be taken in the event of cravings.

20. Avoid nuts and nut and seed butters on account of their high fat and protein content, except for chestnuts, which are high in complex carbohydrates, until the condition improves. Unsalted, lightly blanched, boiled, or roasted seeds such as squash seeds and pumpkin seeds may be consumed as a snack, up to 1 cup altogether per week. Avoid sunflower and larger seeds, except in the summer or hot weather, until recovery is experienced.

21. Seasonings, such as unrefined sea salt, shoyu, and miso, are to be used moderately in order to avoid unnecessary thirst and cravings for sweets. If you become thirsty after a meal or between meals, cut back on these seasonings. Avoid mirin (a sweet cooking wine) and garlic, which may make the condition more active. In cases of inflammation, avoid ginger, horseradish, umeboshi vinegar, and brown rice vinegar until the condition improves.

22. Drink bancha twig tea as the main beverage. Strictly avoid all aromatic, stimulant beverages, and do not drink grain coffee for the first 2 to 3 months. Use good-quality spring, well, or filtered water, avoiding chemicalized tap water, distilled water, and carbonated or mineral water (even as a beverage on social occasions). Other traditional, nonstimulant beverages, such as barley or rice tea, may be taken. One to 2 cups of fresh carrot juice or other vegetable juice may be taken a week.

23. Chew very well, at least 50 times and preferably 100 times per mouthful.

24. Avoid overeating and overdrinking.

25. Avoid late-night snacks and eating within 3 hours of sleeping.

◎ Diet #2 for More Yang Conditions and Disorders

The following dietary guidelines may be followed for an ailment or disorder caused by predominantly yang factors. They may need to be adjusted slightly for each person according to climate, environment, age, sex, activity level, personal condition and needs, and other factors. Refer to further modifications under each specific condition or disease. The use of oil and supplementary foods such as animal food, fruit, nuts and seeds, and sweets may differ significantly according to the specific condition. Special drinks and dishes, as well as home remedies, may also be recommended. Please see Chapter 9 for comprehensive lists of recommended macrobiotic-quality foods and foods to avoid, and Chapters 13 and 14 for how to prepare special drinks, dishes, compresses, and other home remedies. For moderate to serious cases, follow this diet for 3 to 4 months or until the condition improves. Then the standard macrobiotic way of eating for persons in usual good health may gradually be implemented, offering a much wider scope and variety.

1. Avoid all extreme yang animal foods, including beef, pork, lamb, chicken, turkey, eggs, salted cheese, tuna, salmon, shellfish, and other meat, poultry, and seafood.

2. Avoid all extreme yin foods and beverages, including sugar, chocolate, honey, and other concentrated sweeteners; milk, butter, cream, ice cream, yogurt, and other light dairy foods; white rice, white flour, and other polished or refined grains; excessive fruits and juices; foods of tropical origin, including tomatoes, potatoes, and peppers; herbs and spices; coffee, black tea, and other stimulants; alcohol; and drugs and medication.

3. Avoid or reduce all hard baked flour products, such as bread, crackers, cookies, and pastries, except for the occasional consumption of unyeasted, unsweetened whole-grain sourdough bread, if craved, once or twice a week. In serious cases, even sourdough bread may need to be completely avoided for several months until the condition improves.

4. Eliminate all chemicalized, irradiated, genetically engineered, and other artificially produced and treated foods and beverages. As much as possible, use organically grown food, especially for whole grains, beans and bean products, vegetables, fruits, oils and other seasonings, and condiments.

5. Avoid or limit food cooked on an electric stove or in a microwave oven. Prepare food as much as possible with gas, wood, or other natural flame.

6. Unless otherwise indicated, miminize oil for a 1- to 2-month period, even good-quality vegetable oil, and then use only a small amount of sesame oil in cooking, preferably brushed on the skillet, once or twice a week.

7. Avoid raw salads temporarily for 1 month or more until the condition improves.

8. Avoid all ice-cold foods and drinks served with ice cubes.

9. In general, the cooking for a yang condition may be slightly lighter than usual and use a little less sea salt, miso, or shoyu in cooking.

10. Eat whole grains in whole form as the main portion of the diet. Fifty to 60 percent of daily consumption, by weight, should consist of whole cereal grains or whole grain products. The first day prepare pressure-cooked short-grain brown rice. The next day prepare brown rice pressure-cooked together in the same pot with 20 to 30 percent millet. The third day prepare brown rice with 20 to 30 percent barley. The fourth day prepare brown rice with 20 to 30 percent adzuki beans or lentils. The fifth day prepare plain brown rice again. Then repeat this pattern. Boiling may be substituted for pressure-cooking occasionally. A delicious morning porridge can be made by taking leftover rice, adding a little more water to soften, and simmering for 2–3 minutes more, seasoning with ½ to 1 teaspoon of miso per cup of grain at the end of cooking. Morning porridge may be soft and creamy, but otherwise the grain should be on the firm side. In pressure-cooking, the ratio of grain to water should be about 1:2. For seasoning, cook with a small piece of kombu the size of a postage stamp, though in some cases sea salt may be used depending on the person's condition. Other grains may be used occasionally, cooked by themselves or with brown rice, including whole wheat berries, rye, corn, and whole oats, though oats should be avoided for the first month. Buckwheat and seitan should be avoided because they are too contractive. Good-quality sourdough bread, preferably steamed, may be enjoyed 2–3 times a week if craved, though in some cases even this should be avoided for several months until the condition improves. Udon, somen, or other whole-wheat noodles or pasta, may be taken 2–3 times a week, but minimize soba, which includes buckwheat flour and may be too contracting. Avoid all hard baked products until the condition improves, including cookies, cake,

pie, crackers, muffins, and pastries. Avoid or limit cracked or processed grains, such as bulgur, couscous, oatmeal, rye flakes, and puffed grains, until the condition improves, in which case they may be used occasionally.

11. Eat 1–2 servings of soup each day, constituting about 5 to 10 percent of the daily diet. The principal soup should consist of wakame and onions, carrots, or other land vegetables cooked together and seasoned with miso and occasionally shoyu. A small volume of shiitake may be added to the soup several times a week. The miso may be barley miso, brown rice miso, or soybean (hatcho) miso and should be naturally aged 2 to 3 years. Grain soups, bean soups, vegetable soups (especially made with sweet vegetables), and other soups may be taken from time to time. Soup may be slightly lighter in taste and flavor than usual.

12. Twenty-five to 30 percent of daily food should be taken as vegetables, cooked in a variety of ways. All temperate-climate types may be taken daily, including hard green leafy vegetables such as collards, kale, or turnip greens; sweet round vegetables such as squash, onions, and cabbage; and root vegetables such as carrot, burdock, and daikon. Slightly emphasize more hard green leafy varieties to help offset overly yang conditions. Generally, prepare the following, though amounts and frequencies will vary according to the individual: nishime-style (long-time stewed) vegetables, 2 to 3 times a week; adzuki bean, squash, and kombu dish, 2 to 3 times a week; dried daikon, 1 cup 3 times a week; carrots and carrot tops or daikon and daikon tops, 3 times a week; boiled salad, 5 to 7 times a week; pressed salad, 5 to 7 times a week; raw salad and salad dressing, unless otherwise indicated, 1 to 2 times a week; steamed greens, 5 to 7 times a week; sautéed vegetables, unless otherwise indicated, cooked in a little sesame or other unrefined oil, 2 times a week; kinpira-style (matchsticks), ⅔ cup 2 times a week; dried tofu, tofu, tempeh, or seitan with vegetables, 2 times a week. Vegetable nabe (lightly boiled vegetables and noodles cooked homestyle at the table with sliced vegetables, tofu, tempeh, and mochi) may be eaten several times a week as a special side dish.

13. Five percent of daily or regular intake (5 to 7 times a week) may be taken as beans, such as adzuki beans, lentils, chickpeas, or black soybeans, a little more lightly seasoned than usual. These are usually cooked together with kombu or other sea vegetable or with a small volume of onions and carrots. Other beans may be used occasionally, 2 to 3 times a month. For seasoning, a small volume of unrefined sea salt or shoyu or miso can be used and occasionally barley malt or other natural sweetener for a sweet taste. Bean products, such as tempeh, natto, and dried or cooked tofu may be used occasionally but in moderate volume.

14. Two percent or less of daily intake may be in the form of sea vegetables with slightly shorter cooking and a lighter taste than usual. This includes wakame taken daily when cooking grain, in soup, or other dishes. A sheet or half sheet of toasted nori may also be taken daily. A small dish of hijiki or arame should be prepared 2 times a week. Minimize kombu, as this may be too contracting. All other sea vegetables are optional.

15. Use condiments slightly lighter than usual and in small volume, including gomashio (on the average made with 1 part salt to 18 parts sesame seeds, reduced to 1:16 after 2 months); kombu, kelp, or wakame powder; umeboshi plum; and tekka. These condiments may be used daily on grains and vegetables, but the volume should be moderate to suit individual appetite and taste.

16. Pickles, made at home in a variety of ways, should be eaten daily, in small volume (1 teaspoon total), with an emphasis on short-time, lighter pickles (but rinse thoroughly to avoid too much salt).

17. Avoid all animal foods for several months until the condition improves. However, if cravings arise, a small volume of white-meat fish may be eaten every 10 to 14 days in small volume if desired. The fish should be prepared steamed, boiled, or poached and be garnished with fresh grated daikon or ginger to aid digestion. Completely avoid tuna, salmon, and other blue-meat and red-meat fish and all shellfish until the condition improves.

18. Unless otherwise indicated, a small amount of fruit and juice, especially temperate-climate fruit such as apples, pears, or apricots, may be taken several times a week, preferably stewed or cooked but occasionally fresh in hot weather. Avoid raisins, which have a high concentration of simple sugars.

19. Avoid all desserts and sweets, including good-quality macrobiotic desserts, until the condition improves. To satisfy cravings for a sweet taste, use sweet vegetables every day in cooking, drink sweet vegetable drink occasionally, and prepare sweet vegetable jam. Mochi, rice balls, sushi, and other grain-based snacks may be eaten regularly. Rice cakes, popcorn, chips, and other dry or baked snacks should be minimized, as they may cause tightening. A small volume of grain-based sweeteners such as amasake, barley malt, or rice syrup may be taken if cravings arise. As the condition improves, a small volume of softly prepared desserts may be taken, such as puddings, kantens, and stewed fruit. Avoid hard baked desserts such as cakes, pies, and cookies.

20. Avoid nuts and nut and seed butters on account of their high fat and protein content, except for chestnuts, which are high in complex carbohydrates, until the condition improves. Unsalted, lightly blanched or boiled seeds such as squash seeds and pumpkin seeds may be consumed as a snack, up to 1 cup altogether per week.

21. Unrefined sea salt, shoyu, miso, and other seasonings may be used in cooking, but seasoning should be lighter than usual.

22. Drink bancha twig tea as the main beverage, steeped for slightly less time and tasting slightly lighter than usual. Strictly avoid all aromatic, stimulant beverages, and do not drink grain coffee for the first 2 to 3 months. Use good-quality spring, well, or filtered water, avoiding chemicalized tap water, distilled water, or mineral water (even as a beverage on social occasions). Other traditional, nonstimulant beverages may be taken, such as barley or rice tea. One to 2 cups of carrot or other vegetable juice may be taken a week.

23. Chew very well, at least 50 times and preferably 100 times per mouthful.

24. Avoid overeating and overdrinking.

25. Avoid late-night snacks and eating within 3 hours of sleeping.

☺ Diet #3 for More Yang and Yin Conditions and Disorders

The following dietary guidelines may be followed for an ailment or disorder caused by a combination of yang and yin dietary extremes. They may need to be adjusted slightly for each person according to climate, environment, age, sex, activity level, personal condition and needs, and other factors. Refer to further modifications under each specific condition or disease. The use of oil and supplementary foods such as animal food, fruit, nuts and seeds, and sweets may differ significantly according to the specific condition. Special drinks and dishes, as well as home remedies, may also be recommended. Please see Chapter 9 for comprehensive lists of recommended macrobiotic-quality foods and foods to avoid, and Chapters 13 and 14 for how to prepare special drinks, dishes, compresses, and other home remedies. For moderate to serious cases, follow this diet for 3 to 4 months or until the condition improves. Then the standard macrobiotic way of eating for persons in usual good health may gradually be implemented, offering a much wider scope and variety.

1. Avoid all extreme yang animal foods, including beef, pork, lamb, chicken, turkey, eggs, salted cheese, tuna, salmon, shellfish, and other meat, poultry, and seafood.

2. Avoid all extreme yin foods and beverages, including sugar, chocolate, honey, and other concentrated sweeteners; milk, butter, cream, ice cream, yogurt, and other light dairy foods; white rice, white flour, and other polished or refined grains; excessive fruits and juices; foods of tropical origin, including tomatoes, potatoes, and peppers; herbs and spices; coffee, black tea, and other stimulants; alcohol; and drugs and medication.

3. Avoid or reduce all hard baked flour products such as bread, crackers, cookies, and pastries, except for the occasional consumption of unyeasted, unsweetened whole-grain sourdough bread, if craved, once or twice a week. In serious cases, even sourdough bread may need to be completely avoided for several months until the condition improves.

4. Eliminate all chemicalized, irradiated, genetically engineered, and other artificially produced and treated foods and beverages. As much as possible, use organically grown food, especially for whole grains, beans and bean products, vegetables, fruits, oils and other seasonings, and condiments.

5. Avoid or limit food cooked on an electric stove or in a microwave oven. Prepare food as much as possible with gas, wood, or other natural flame.

6. Unless otherwise indicated, miminize oil for a 1- to 2-month period, even good-quality vegetable oil, and then use only a small amount of sesame oil in cooking, preferably brushed on the skillet, once or twice a week.

7. Avoid raw salads temporarily for 1 month or more until the condition improves.

8. Avoid all ice-cold foods and drinks served with ice cubes.

9. In general, the cooking for a condition arising from both more yang and more yin factors should be moderate and use an in-between amount of sea salt, miso, or shoyu in cooking.

10. Eat whole grains in whole form as the main portion of the diet. Fifty to 60 percent of daily consumption, by weight, should consist of whole cereal grains or whole grain products. The first day prepare pressure-cooked short-grain brown rice. The next day prepare brown rice pressure-cooked together in the same pot with 20 to 30 percent millet. The third day prepare brown rice with 20 to 30 percent barley. The fourth day prepare brown rice with 20 to 30 percent adzuki beans or lentils. The fifth day prepare plain brown rice again. Then repeat this pattern. Boiling may be substituted for pressure-cooking occasionally. A delicious morning porridge can be made by taking leftover rice, adding a little more water to soften, and simmering for 2–3 minutes more, seasoning with ½ to 1 teaspoon of miso per cup of grain at the end of cooking. Morning porridge may be soft and creamy, but otherwise the grain should be on the firm side. In pressure-cooking, the ratio of grain to water should be about 1:2. For seasoning, cook with a small piece of kombu the size of a postage stamp, though in some cases sea salt may be used depending on the person's condition. Other grains may be used occasionally, cooked by themselves or with brown rice, including whole wheat berries, rye, corn, and whole oats, though oats should be avoided for the first month. Buckwheat and seitan should be avoided because they are too contractive. Good-quality sourdough bread, preferably steamed, may be enjoyed 2–3 times a week if craved, though in some cases even this should be avoided for several months until the condition improves. Udon, somen, or other whole-wheat noodles or pasta may be taken 2–3 times a week, but minimize soba, which includes buckwheat flour and may be too contracting. Avoid all hard baked products until the condition improves, including cookies, cake, pie, crackers, muffins, and pastries. Avoid or limit cracked or processed grains, such as bulgur, couscous, oatmeal, rye flakes, and puffed grains, until the condition improves, in which case they may be used occasionally.

11. Eat 1–2 servings of soup each day, constituting about 5 to 10 percent of the daily diet. The principal soup should consist of wakame and onions, carrots, or other land vegetables cooked together and seasoned with miso and occasionally shoyu. A small volume of shiitake may be added to the soup several times a week. The miso may be barley miso, brown rice miso, or soybean (hatcho) miso and should be naturally aged 2 to 3 years. Seasoning should be moderate, neither too mild nor too salty. Grain soups, bean soups, vegetable soups (especially made with sweet vegetables), and other soups may be taken from time to time.

12. Twenty-five to 30 percent of daily food should be taken as vegetables, cooked in a variety of ways. All temperate-climate types may be taken daily, but emphasize round varieties such as squash, onions, and cabbage with a moderate amount of leafy green vegetables such as collards, kale, and mustard greens and a moderate amount of root vegetables such as carrots and daikon. Generally, prepare the following, though amounts and frequencies will vary according to the individual: nishime-style (long-time stewed) vegetables, 2 to 3 times a week; adzuki bean, squash, and kombu dish, 2 times a week; dried daikon, 1 cup 3 times a week; carrots and carrot tops or daikon and daikon tops, 3 times a week; boiled salad, 5 to 7 times a week; pressed salad, 5 to 7 times a week; raw salad and salad dressing, avoid; steamed greens, 5 to 7

times a week; unless otherwise indicated, sautéed vegetables, using water the first month instead of oil, then occasionally (2 to 3 times a week) a small volume of sesame oil brushed on the skillet; kinpira-style (matchsticks) sautéed in water, ⅔ cup 2 times a week, then oil may be used after 3 weeks; dried tofu, tofu, tempeh, or seitan with vegetables, 2 times a week. Vegetable nabe (lightly boiled vegetables and noodles cooked homestyle at the table with sliced vegetables, tofu, tempeh, and mochi) may be eaten several times a week as a special side dish.

13. Five percent of daily intake may be taken as beans, such as adzuki beans, lentils, chickpeas, or black soybeans, moderately seasoned and in moderate volume. These are usually cooked together with kombu or other sea vegetable or with a small volume of onions and carrots. Other beans may be used occasionally, 2 to 3 times a month. For seasoning, a small volume of unrefined sea salt or shoyu or miso can be used. Bean products such as tempeh, natto, and dried or cooked tofu may be used occasionally but in moderate volume.

14. Two percent or less of daily intake may be in the form of sea vegetables with moderate cooking and a medium taste. This includes wakame and kombu taken daily when cooking grain, in soup, or in other dishes. A sheet or half sheet of toasted nori may also be taken daily. A small dish of hijiki or arame should be prepared 2 times a week. All other sea vegetables are optional.

15. Condiments may be used moderately, including gomashio (on the average made with 1 part salt to 18 parts sesame seeds, reduced to 1:16 after 2 months); kombu, kelp, or wakame powder; umeboshi plum; and tekka. These condiments may be used daily on grains and vegetables, but the volume should be moderate to suit individual appetite and taste.

16. Pickles, made at home in a variety of ways, should be eaten daily, in small volume (1 teaspoon total), with an emphasis on medium-strength pickles (but rinse thoroughly to avoid too much salt).

17. Avoid all animal food until the condition improves. However, white-meat fish may be eaten once every 10–14 days in small volume if cravings arise. The fish should be prepared steamed, boiled, or poached and be garnished with fresh grated daikon or ginger to aid in digestion. Completely avoid tuna, salmon, shrimp, and other blue-meat and red-meat fish and all shellfish until the condition improves.

18. Avoid or minimize fruit and juice until the condition improves. However, if cravings arise, a small amount of fruit may be taken, provided it is grown in a temperate climate and taken in season. Generally, it may be cooked with a pinch of salt. A little dried fruit may be taken, but avoid raisins, which are high in concentrated simple sugars.

19. Avoid or limit desserts and sweets, including good-quality macrobiotic desserts, until the condition improves. To satisfy cravings for a sweet taste, use sweet vegetables every day in cooking, drink sweet vegetable drink, and prepare sweet vegetable jam. Mochi, rice balls, sushi, and other grain-based snacks may be eaten regularly. Rice cakes, popcorn, and other dry or baked snacks should be minimized, as they may cause tightening. A small volume of grain-based sweeteners such as amasake, barley malt, or brown rice syrup may be taken in the event of cravings.

20. Limit nuts and nut and seed butters on account of their high fat and protein content, except for chestnuts, which are high in complex carbohydrates, until the condition improves. Unsalted, lightly blanched or boiled seeds such as sesame seeds and pumpkin seeds may be consumed as a snack, up to 1 cup altogether per week.

21. Unrefined sea salt, shoyu, miso, and other seasonings may be used in cooking, but these should have a moderate flavor and taste, neither too salty nor too bland. Avoid mirin (a sweet cooking wine) and garlic until the condition improves. In cases of inflammation, avoid ginger, horseradish, umeboshi vinegar, and brown rice vinegar until the condition improves.

22. Drink bancha twig tea as the main beverage prepared with medium strength. Strictly avoid coffee, black tea, soft drinks, and all aromatic, stimulant beverages, and do not drink grain coffee for the first 2 to 3 months. Use good-quality spring, well, or filtered water, avoiding chemicalized tap water, distilled water, or carbonated or mineral water (even as a beverage on social occasions). Other traditional, non-stimulant beverages may be taken, such as barley or rice tea. One to 2 cups of fresh carrot juice or other vegetable juice may be taken a week.

23. Chew very well, at least 50 times and preferably 100 times per mouthful.

24. Avoid overeating and overdrinking.

25. Avoid late-night snacks and eating within 3 hours of sleeping.

TABLE 34. SUMMARY OF MACROBIOTIC HEALING DIETS*

Kind of Food	1. More Yin Condition	2. More Yang Condition	3. More Yin and Yang Condition
General cooking	Slightly more salty, stronger cooking	Less salt, lighter cooking	Moderate cooking
Whole grains (40–60 percent) of daily volume	Brown rice, millet, barley, whole wheat, corn regularly; other grains occasionally; avoid baked flour, taking sourdough bread, if craved; noodles/pasta occasionally; buckwheat, soba, and seitan will depend on the individual case	Brown rice, millet, barley, corn, whole wheat regularly; other grains occasionally; avoid baked flour, taking sourdough bread, if craved; noodles/pasta occasionally; avoid or minimize buckwheat, soba, and seitan	Brown rice, millet, barley, corn, whole wheat regularly; other grains occasionally; avoid baked flour, taking sourdough bread, if craved; noodles/pasta occasionally; avoid or minimize buckwheat, soba, and seitan
Soup (1–2 servings a day)	Slightly stronger flavor (slight more miso, shoyu, or sea salt)	Milder flavor (less miso, shoyu, or sea salt)	Moderate flavor
Vegetables (25–30 percent of daily volume)	Balance of green leafy, round, and root vegetables daily, but emphasize more root varieties; avoid raw salad; occasional boiled or pressed salad	Balance of green leafy, round, and root vegetables daily, but emphasize more leafy green varieties; occasional raw salad; frequent boiled or pressed salad	Balance of green leafy, round, and root vegetables daily, but emphasize more round varieties; avoid raw salad; frequent boiled or pressed salad
Beans and bean products (5 percent daily)	A little more strongly seasoned, use less regularly	Lightly seasoned, use more regularly; occasionally sweetened	Moderately seasoned and moderate volume
Sea vegetables (about 2 percent daily volume)	Longer cooking, slightly thicker taste	Quicker cooking, lighter taste	Moderate cooking, medium taste
Pickles (small volume daily)	More long-term, stronger pickles	More short-term, lighter pickles	Either type in moderation
Salt and seasonings	Slightly more salty, stronger seasoning; use unrefined white sea salt; barley, brown rice, or soybean miso aged at least 2 years; and shoyu	Less salty, lighter seasoning; use unrefined white sea salt; barley, brown rice, or soybean miso aged at least 2 years; and shoyu	Moderate seasoning; use unrefined white sea salt; barley, brown rice, or soybean miso aged at least 2 years; and shoyu

Kind of Food	1. More Yin Condition	2. More Yang Condition	3. More Yin and Yang Condition
Oil	Depending on the case, may need to avoid for 1 month or apply with brush as little as possible; sesame only; no raw oil; from second month, occasional use	Depending on the case, may need to avoid for 1 month or apply with brush as little as possible; sesame only; no raw oil; from second month, regular use	Depending on the case, may need to avoid for 1 month or apply with brush as little as possible; sesame only; no raw oil; from second month, occasional use
Condiments	Stronger use; gomashio 16:1	Lighter use; gomashio 18:1	Moderate use; gomashio 18:1
Beverages	Longer-cooked, stronger-tasting bancha or other traditional tea; use spring, well, or filtered water; carrot juice occasionally	Shorter-cooked, lighter-tasting bancha or other traditional tea; use spring, well, or filtered water; carrot juice, apple cider, and other juice occasionally	Medium-cooked, medium-tasting bancha or other traditional tea; use spring, well, or filtered water; carrot juice and other juice or cider infrequently
Cooking fire	Gas, wood, or natural flame; avoid microwave and electric	Gas, wood, or natural flame; avoid microwave and electric	Gas, wood, or natural flame; avoid microwave and electric
Supplemental Foods			
Animal food	Occasional small volume of white-meat fish, steamed, boiled, or poached, and properly garnished	Avoid or minimize fish or seafood	Minimize fish or seafood
Fruit and juice	Avoid or minimize; cooked temperate-climate fruit only if craved; fresh berries or melons in the summer only if craved	Occasional temperate-climate fruit cooked with a pinch of sea salt, dried, or fresh with a pinch of salt	Small amounts of temperate-climate fruit cooked with a pinch of sea salt, dried, or fresh with a pinch of salt
Seeds and nuts	Avoid nuts and nut butters; occasional seeds blanched or lightly roasted (unsalted); sunflower seeds only in the summer	Minimize nuts and nut butters; occasional seeds blanched or lightly roasted (unsalted)	Minimize nuts and nut butters; occasional seeds blanched or lightly roasted (unsalted); sunflower seeds only in the summer

Kind of Food	1. More Yin Condition	2. More Yang Condition	3. More Yin and Yang Condition
Snacks and desserts	Sushi, mochi, kanten, pudding, and other soft snacks; avoid hard baked, puffed, or dried snacks; small volume of amasake, barley malt, or rice syrup only if craved	Sushi, mochi, kanten, pudding, and other soft snacks; avoid hard baked, puffed, or dried snacks; small volume of amasake, barley malt, or rice syrup occasionally	Sushi, mochi, kanten, pudding, and other soft snacks; avoid hard baked, puffed, or dried snacks; small volume of amasake, barley malt, or rice syrup infrequently

*These are general or standard recommendations. The guidelines for any person will differ according to his or her specific condition, climate, environment, sex, age, activity level, personal needs, and other factors.

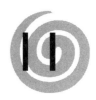

Way-of-Life Suggestions

Observing the following suggestions will contribute to a healthy, peaceful, orderly life:

1. Maintain the dream and image of health, happiness, and peace for yourself, others, and the planet.

2. Live each day happily, without being preoccupied with your health, and stay mentally and physically alert and active.

3. View everything and everyone you meet with gratitude. Offer thanks before and after each meal.

4. It is best to retire before midnight and get up early in the morning, especially with the sunrise.

5. It is best to avoid wearing synthetic or woolen clothing directly against the skin. Wear cotton (preferably non-GMO or organic) as much as possible, especially for undergarments. Avoid excessive metallic accessories on the fingers, wrists, or neck. Keep such ornaments simple and graceful.

6. If your strength permits, go outdoors in simple clothing. Walk up to half an hour every day, preferably on the grass, beach, or soil.

7. Keep your home and other surroundings in good order.

8. Initiate and maintain an active correspondence with your family and friends, extending best wishes to them. Also initiate and maintain good relationships with everyone else around you.

9. Avoid taking long, hot baths or showers unless you have been consuming too much salt or animal food.

10. Scrub your entire body with a hot, damp towel until the skin becomes red, every morning or every night before retiring. If that is not possible, at least scrub your hands, feet, fingers, and toes.

11. Avoid chemically perfumed cosmetics. For care of the teeth, brush with natural preparations or sea salt.

12. If your condition permits, keep physically active as part of your daily life, including household chores such as scrubbing floors and cleaning windows and activities such as yoga, dance, martial arts, or sports.

13. Avoid using electric cooking devices (ovens or ranges) or microwave ovens. Convert

TABLE 35. BENEFITS OF PHYSICAL AND MENTAL ACTIVITY

Walking, Yoga, Tai Chi, Dancing, and Light to Moderate Physical Activity	Meditation, Visualization, Singing, and Other Mental and Aesthetic Activities
Stimulates circulation	Relaxes the autonomic nerves
Improves breathing	Lowers blood pressure
Tones the muscles	Relieves stress on internal organs
Increases appetite	Improves control over digestive, respiratory, and circulatory functions
Clears the mind	Dissolves negative thoughts and emotions
Dissolves stress	Creates positive thoughts and feelings
Increases bowel motility	Releases endorphins and enhances feelings of wholeness and well-being
Improves energy flow to chakras, meridians, organs, functions, tissues, and cells	Improves energy flow to chakras, meridians, organs, functions, tissues, and cells

to a gas or wood stove at the earliest opportunity.

14. It is best to minimize the frequent use of television, computers, cell phones, and other electronic equipment that emits artificial electromagnetic energy.

15. Include some large green plants in your house to freshen and enrich the oxygen content of the air.

16. Everyone is encouraged to learn how to cook basic, healthy meals. Participate in some aspect of food preparation, including gardening, shopping, cooking, food processing, or washing the dishes.

17. Sing a happy song each day.

Menus

The following menus provide a typical week of dishes for each of the four seasons. They offer both a theme (whole grains at every meal, miso soup or other soup once or twice daily, cooked vegetable dishes, regular bean and sea vegetable dishes, pickles, and beverages) and variation (use of different ingredients, occasional noodle dishes, bread and baked goods, and occasional snacks, desserts, and special drinks).

The menus are intended for generally healthy individuals and families living in a temperate climate. They present a dynamic, centrally balanced macrobiotic way of eating for active people. Of course, those who are healing, live in other climates and environments, or have other special requirements or metabolisms will need to modify these menus and recipes. On a healing diet, the use of oil, salt and other seasonings, bread and flour products, fish and seafood, fruit and juice, and snacks and desserts may be limited or temporarily avoided until the condition improves. Please refer to the specific recommendations in Part II for any given condition or disorder.

In many instances, even for those in usual good health, the menus may be simplified, especially by those who are single, live alone, and the elderly. Often just a bowl of rice or millet, a cup of soup, steamed greens, and a cup of tea are completely satisfying, especially if they are thoroughly chewed. Also, please keep in mind that babies, infants, and children require special foods, condiments, and seasonings. Please see our forthcoming book on a macrobiotic approach to family health for guidelines for different family members.

The recipe section includes most of the basic dishes listed in the menus. Others may be found in one of the macrobiotic cookbooks listed in the Recommended Reading section. As noted earlier, every member of the family should learn how to cook and take cooking classes with an experienced macrobiotic cooking teacher. Many simple mistakes can be avoided and a truly satisfying and delicious cuisine readily learned. Macrobiotic cooking is an endless adventure, with new foods and dishes regularly being introduced, old ones rediscovered, and subtle changes constantly being made to balance the climate and environment and changing atmospheric and celestial conditions. The menus, recipes, and home remedies in this book should help get you started on the way to better health, greater happiness, and the abiding peace that comes with eating in harmony with nature.

SPRING WEEKLY MENU

	Monday	Tuesday	Wednesday	Thursday	Friday	Saturday	Sunday
Breakfast	*Breakfast*	*Breakfast*	*Breakfast*	*Breakfast*	*Breakfast*	*Breakfast*	*Breakfast*
Soft Grain Miso Soup Steamed Greens Beverage	Soft Millet & Onions Miso Soup w/ Leek, Corn & Broccoli Steamed Kale	Soft Rice Miso Soup w/ Daikon & Shiitake Boiled Cabbage	Soft Rice & Barley Miso Soup w/ Carrot & Parsley Steamed Chinese Cabbage & Scallion	Rice Porridge w/ Daikon, Celery, Watercress & Miso Boiled Cabbage & Carrot	Soft Rice & Whole Oats Miso Soup w/ Cauliflower, Leek & Dulse Steamed Watercress	Soft Rice & Wheat Berries Miso Soup w/ Squash, Onion & Parsely L.O. Pressed Salad	Whole Oat Porridge Boiled Salad w/ Broccoli & Carrots Whole-Grain Pancakes w/ Barley Malt
Lunch	*Lunch*	*Lunch*	*Lunch*	*Lunch*	*Lunch*	*Lunch*	*Lunch*
Grain L.O. Beans L.O. Seaweed Quickly Cooked Vegetable or Salad Beverage	Rice Balls Carrots & Tops w/ Toasted Sesame Seeds Pressed Salad w/ Chinese Cabbage & Radish	Rice & Wheat Loaf Slices (plain or pan-fried) L.O. Sweet & Sour Chickpea Purée	Rice & Barley Stew w/ Vegetables Fresh Salad	Vegetable Sushi L.O. Nabe Steamed Watercress	L.O. Tofu Stew w/ Udon L.O. Nishime Steamed Celery	Rice & Hato Mugi Salad w/ Blanched Veggies L.O. Lentil Pâté Spread L.O. Dried Daikon & Kombu	Rice & Chickpea Balls Udon in Broth L.O. Nishime Pressed Salad w/ Bok Choy & Carrots
Snack	*Snack*	*Snack*	*Snack*	*Snack*	*Snack*	*Snack*	*Snack*
Snack Sweet Vegetable Drink or Special Drink	Steamed Sourdough Bread w/ Parsnip Jam Sweet Vegetable Drink	Mochi with Nori Fresh Carrot Juice	Corn on the Cob (boiled or steamed) Sweet Vegetable Drink	Rice Cakes with Hummus L.O. Pressed Salad Green Tea	Amasake Kanten with Grated Lemon Rind	Fresh Carrot Juice Steamed Rice Kayu Bread	Blanched Celery w/ Tofu-Ume Dip Sweet Vegetable Drink

	Monday	Tuesday	Wednesday	Thursday	Friday	Saturday	Sunday
Dinner	*Dinner*	*Dinner*	*Dinner*	*Dinner*	*Dinner*	*Dinner*	*Dinner*
Rice Dish *Second* *Soup* *Bean/Sea-* *weed* *Long &* *Quickly* *Cooked* *Vege-* *table* *Dishes* *Salad* *Pickle* *Dessert* *Beverage*	Rice Clear Broth w/ Tofu & Chives Sweet & Sour Chick- peas w/ Ume Vinegar & Squash Arame Salad with String Beans, Daikon, and Cauli- flower Shoyu & Ginger Dressing Quick Sautéed Dande- lion Greens	Rice & Barley Udon & Summer Squash in Broth w/ Shoyu & Shiitake Natto w/ Nori & Scallions Blanched Collard Green Rolls w/ Sauer- kraut Strawberry Couscous Cake	Rice Vegetable Nabe Miso-Scallion Condiment Puréed Broccoli Soup Dandelion & Dandelion Roots Pressed Salad w/ Red Cabbage & Watercress	Rice & Millet Split Pea Soup w/ Onion, Dakion & Squash Stewed Tofu, Fu, Chinese Cabbage, Shiitake & Fish (optional) Raw Salad Steamed Green Apple w/ Rice Syrup & Kuzu Glaze	Rice & Wheat Berries Lentils w/ Leeks & Corn Dried Daikon & Kombu Creamy Onion Soup Quick Sauté with Chinese Cabbage, Broccoli & Celery Pressed Salad with Cucum- bers, Wakame, Chives & Ume Vinegar	Rice & Chick- peas Miso Soup w/ Onion, Parsley & Cabbage Nishime w/ Onion, Cauli- flower & Carrot Quick Sauté Cucum- bers, Leeks & Sauer- kraut Turnips & Turnip Tops	Barley Stew w/ Corn, Daikon, Shiitake & Miso Hijiki- Tofu Rolls w/ Scallions Steamed Kale with Lemon Juice & Toasted Sun- flower Seeds

Key: L.O. = Leftover; Salad = Boiled, Pressed, or Fresh. Bancha twig tea may be taken at every meal, with roasted barley tea, brown rice or millet tea, or grain coffee as an occasional substitute

SUMMER WEEKLY MENU

	Monday	Tuesday	Wednesday	Thursday	Friday	Saturday	Sunday
Breakfast	*Breakfast*	*Breakfast*	*Breakfast*	*Breakfast*	*Breakfast*	*Breakfast*	*Breakfast*
Soft Grain Miso Soup Steamed Greens Beverage	Barley Porridge Boiled Salad w/ Cauliflower & Green Beans	Rice Porridge (Short & Long-Grain) Miso Soup w/ Nori & Scallion Boiled Watercress	Soft Rice & Corn Miso Soup w/ Shiitake & Daikon	Soft Miso Rice w/ Peas, Onions, & Parsley Garnish Miso Soup w/ Celery & Carrot Steamed Cabbage & Scallion	Whole Oats w/ Rice Syrup Miso Soup w/ Leek, Daikon & Wakame Steamed Bok Choy	Soft Rice & Hato Mugi Steamed Chinese Cabbage	Mochi Waffles w/ Strawberries Miso Soup w/ L.O. Rice & Watercress
Lunch	*Lunch*	*Lunch*	*Lunch*	*Lunch*	*Lunch*	*Lunch*	*Lunch*
Grain L.O. Beans L.O. Seaweed Quickly Cooked Vegetable or Salad Beverage	Rice Balls Dipped in Toasted Sunflower Seeds Miso Soup w/ Dulse & Broccoli Steamed Collards w/ Grated Carrots	L.O. Rice & Corn Sushi w/ Takuan Pickle L.O. Adzuki Beans L.O. Dried Daikon Fresh Salad	Quick Steamed Long-grain Rice w/ Scallion & Shiso L.O. Arame Salad Boiled Salad w/ Broccoli & Squash	Rice Chickpea Salad w/ Blanched Onion, Broccoli, Scallion & Parsley-Ume Dressing	Rice & Black Soybean Sushi w/ Ginger Pickle L.O. Nishime Fresh Salad	Noodle Salad w/ Pressed Veggies L.O. Fu Stew	Sushi w/ Cucumber and also w/ Natto Scrambled Tofu w/ Corn & Scallions L.O. Nishime
Snack	*Snack*	*Snack*	*Snack*	*Snack*	*Snack*	*Snack*	*Snack*
Snack Sweet Vegetable Drink or Special Drink	Mochi w/ Grated Daikon, Shoyu, Ginger & Scallions Sweet Vegetable Drink	Rice Cakes with Almond Butter Green Tea	Rice Cake w/ Carrot Butter Sweet Vegetable Drink	Steamed Bread w/ Puréed Chickpea (from Salad) Cool Barley Tea	Corn on the Cob w/ Ume Paste Sweet Vegetable Drink	Fresh Cantaloupe w/ a Pinch of Salt Fresh Carrot Juice	Popcorn Hot Amasake w/ Ginger

	Monday	Tuesday	Wednesday	Thursday	Friday	Saturday	Sunday
Dinner	*Dinner*	*Dinner*	*Dinner*	*Dinner*	*Dinner*	*Dinner*	*Dinner*
Rice Dish *Second* *Soup* *Bean/Sea-* *weed* *Long &* *Quickly* *Cooked* *Vege-* *table* *Dishes* *Salad* *Pickle* *Dessert* *Beverage*	Rice (Short & Long-Grain) Somen in Cool Broth Adzuki, Squash & Kombu Dried Daikon w/ Onion & Kombu Quick-Sautéed Dande-lion, Mung Bean Sprouts & Mush-rooms Pressed Salad w/ Lettuce, Radish & Cucum-ber Strawberry Shortcake	Rice & Corn Lima Bean Soup w/ Carrots, Peas, Corn & Onion Arame Salad w/ Corn, Broccoli & Ume-Tofu Dressing Nishime w/ Cauli-flower & Carrots Radishes & Tops Water-melon w/ Pinch of Salt	Rice Vegetable Nabe Corn Chowder Steamed Mustard Greens Amasake Kanten w/ Grated Lemon Rind	Rice & Black Soybeans Puréed Soup w/ Cucum-ber & Onion Lightly Steamed Tofu, Daikon, Shiitake, Chinese Cabbage & Dipping Sauce Quick Sauté w/ Bok Choy & Snow Peas Pressed Radish Peach Pie w/ Ama-sake Topping	Rice & Hato Mugi Nori Paste Condi-ment Split Pea Aspic w/ Red Onion Carrots & Tops Fu Stew w/ Water-cress, Shiitake & Summer Squash Pressed Salad w/ Cabbage, Sprouts & Shiso Leaves	Boiled Rice Steamed Filet of Sole w/ Lemon (optional) or Tempeh Cutlets Nishime w/ Daikon & Shiitake Quick Sauté w/ Chinese Cabbage, Celery, Onion, Carrot & Ginger Fresh Salad w/ Toasted Sun-flower Seed Dressing	Barley Salad w/ Red Radish, Green Peas & Summer Squash Adzuki Bean & Squash Cool Soup Dried Daikon & Kombu Kinpira w/ Lotus and Onion Boiled Collards w/ Tan-gerine, Soy Sauce Dressing

Key: L.O. = Leftover; Salad = Boiled, Pressed, or Fresh. Bancha twig tea may be taken at every meal, with roasted barley tea, brown rice or millet tea, or grain coffee as an occasional substitute

AUTUMN WEEKLY MENU

	Monday	Tuesday	Wednesday	Thursday	Friday	Saturday	Sunday
Breakfast	*Breakfast*	*Breakfast*	*Breakfast*	*Breakfast*	*Breakfast*	*Breakfast*	*Breakfast*
Soft Grain *Miso Soup* *Steamed* *Greens* *Beverage*	Soft Millet w/ Toasted Pumpkin Seeds Miso Soup w/ Chinese Cabbage & Shiitake Steamed Kale	Soft L.O. Rice Umeboshi Plum Boiled Salad w/ Cabbage & Carrots	Soft L.O. Rice & Millet w/ Shiso Powder Miso Soup w/ Leek & Shiitake Steamed Sourdough Bread with Sweet Vegetable Jam	Soft L.O. Rice & Barley w/ Greens & Miso Boiled Salad w/ Chinese Cabbage & Red Radish	Pan-fried Mochi wrapped in Nori Miso Soup w/ Water-cress & Shiitake Steamed Collards	Soft L.O. Rice Whole Grain Pancakes w/ Rice Syrup & Apple Topping Boiled Salad w/ Bok Choy & Red Cabbage	Soft Whole Oats w/ Gomasio Miso Soup w/ Corn, Shiitake & Tofu Cubes Steamed Scallions
Lunch	*Lunch*	*Lunch*	*Lunch*	*Lunch*	*Lunch*	*Lunch*	*Lunch*
Grain *L.O. Beans* *L.O.* *Seaweed* *Quickly* *Cooked* *Salad* *Beverage*	Barley Stew w/ Veggies Arame w/ Onions & Corn Kernels Boiled Salad w/ Onions, Carrots, Cabbage & Radish	Sushi Nori Roll w/ Takuan & Carrot L.O. Nishime L.O. Chick-peas Pressed Salad w/ Lettuce, Carrot & Celery	Udon Noodles w/ Kombu, Shoyu & Ginger Broth Boiled Salad w/ Broccoli, Carrot, & Cauliflower	Fried L.O. Rice & Barley w/ Sautéed Veggies & Tofu Toasted Nori L.O. Dried Daikon Pressed Salad w/ Red Cabbage	Millet & Squash L.O. Kinpira Boiled Salad w/ Onions, Celery, Mush-room & Carrots	Udon & Tofu w/ Kombu, Shoyu & Ginger Broth Pressed Salad w/ Bok Choy, Red Radish, Onions & Tofu-Ume Scallion Dressing	Rice Balls Steamed Bread w/ Squash Butter L.O. Arame & Veggies Boiled Salad w/ Onion, Cabbage, Seeds & Sauer-kraut

	Monday	Tuesday	Wednesday	Thursday	Friday	Saturday	Sunday
Snack	*Snack*	*Snack*	*Snack*	*Snack*	*Snack*	*Snack*	*Snack*
Snack *Sweet* *Vegetable* *Drink or* *Special* *Drink*	Pan-Toasted Mochi Sweet Vegetable Drink	Roasted Seeds Fresh Carrot Juice or Apple Cider	Dried Fruit & Nuts Sweet Vegetable Drink	Rice Cakes w/ Onion or Apple Butter Hot Amasake	Rice & Black Soybean Balls Rolled in Sesame Seeds Sweet Vegetable Drink	Toasted Nori Sheet Fresh Carrot Juice or Apple Cider	Pudding from L.O. Rice & Chestnuts Green Tea
Dinner	*Dinner*	*Dinner*	*Dinner*	*Dinner*	*Dinner*	*Dinner*	*Dinner*
Rice Dish *Second* *Soup* *Bean/Sea-* *weed* *Long &* *Quickly* *Cooked* *Vege-* *table* *Dishes* *Salad* *Pickle* *Dessert* *Beverage*	Rice Chickpea Soup w/ Onions & Squash Nori Condiment Nishime w/ Lotus Root, Daikon & Kombu Carrot & Tops Pressed Salad w/ Chinese Cabbage & Red Radish	Rice & Millet w/ Black Gomashio Miso Soup w/ Daikon & Tops Squash & Adzuki Beans w/ Kombu Steamed Mustard Greens w/ Pumpkin Seed Dressing Steamed Pears w/ Tofu Glaze	Rice & Barley w/ Green Nori Flakes Millet & Squash Soup Dried Daikon w/ Kombu Sautéed Greens & Tofu Pressed Salad w/ Daikon & Carrot Ume Pickle	Rice & Black Soybeans Puréed Broccoli Soup Kinpira Daikon & Tops Steamed Bok Choy Quick Shoyu Pickles Pumpkin Pie Garnished w/ Pecans	Short & Medium Grain Rice w/ Tekka Dried Tofu or Steamed Fish (optional) & Veggie Stew w/ Ginger & Shoyu Sautéed Yellow Squash & Onions Pressed Salad w/ Cucumbers	Rice & Chestnuts Lentil Soup w/ Broccoli & Shoyu Arame w/ Dried Tofu, Carrots & Onions Steamed Brussel Sprouts Salt Pickles	Sweet Rice & Adzuki Beans Puréed Soup w/ Cauliflower Nishime w/ Daikon & Tops, Kombu & Tempeh Pressed Salad w/ Radish & Tops & Ume Vinegar Takuan Pickle Squash Pudding w/ Walnuts, Barley Malt & Kuzu

Key: L.O. = Leftover; Salad = Boiled, Pressed, or Fresh. Bancha twig tea may be taken at every meal, with roasted barley tea, brown rice or millet tea, or grain coffee as an occasional substitute

WINTER WEEKLY MENU

	Monday	Tuesday	Wednesday	Thursday	Friday	Saturday	Sunday
Breakfast	*Breakfast*	*Breakfast*	*Breakfast*	*Breakfast*	*Breakfast*	*Breakfast*	*Breakfast*
Soft Grain Miso Soup Steamed Greens Beverage	Barley Porridge Miso Soup w/ Squash Steamed Bok Choy	Soft Whole Oats Miso Soup w/ Cauliflower, Fu & Parsley Steamed Cabbage & Scallions	Soft Rice w/ Umeboshi Boiled Salad w/ Cauliflower, Parsnips, & Watercress	Mochi Steamed in Chinese Cabbage w/ Shoyu-Daikon Dipping Sauce Miso Soup w/ Kale	Soft Whole Oats Miso Soup w/ Daikon, Shiitake & Snow Peas Steamed Bok Choy & Grated Carrot	Soft Millet with Squash Steamed Leeks & Kale	Soft Rice & Rye Miso Soup w/ Daikon, Shiitake & Bok Choy Steamed Radish & Radish Tops
Lunch	*Lunch*	*Lunch*	*Lunch*	*Lunch*	*Lunch*	*Lunch*	*Lunch*
Grain L.O. Beans L.O. Seaweed Quickly Cooked Salad Beverage	Sushi w/ L.O. Rice Carrot Sticks & Sesame Seeds Boiled Salad w/ Daikon, Broccoli & Creamy Ume-Tofu Dressing	Gomoku Rice Croquettes with L.O. Rice L.O. Nishime Steamed Turnip Greens	Fried Rice L.O. Adzuki Beans L.O. Hijiki Steamed Collards	L.O. Hato Mugi Stew Fresh Salad w/ Tofu Dressing	Rice & Black Soybean Balls L.O. Dried Daikon L.O. Kinpira Boiled Salad w/ Cabbage & Onion	Soba or Udon Noodles in Broth w/ Scallions L.O. Pressed Salad	Millet w/ Parsnips L.O. Nishime Squash Pressed Red Cabbage, Carrot & Ume Vinegar
Snack	*Snack*	*Snack*	*Snack*	*Snack*	*Snack*	*Snack*	*Snack*
Snack Sweet Vegetable Drink or Special Drink	Pan-Fried Mochi w/ Brown Rice Syrup Hot Carrot Juice	L.O. Chestnut Pudding Sweet Vegetable Drink	Popcorn Hot Carrot Juice or Apple Cider	Steamed Sourdough Bread w/ Apricot Jam Sweet Vegetable Drink	Dried Mulberries & Walnuts Green Tea	Steamed Rice Kayu Bread w/ Apple or Onion Butter Sweet Vegetable Drink	Rice Cakes w/ Hummus Hot Carrot Juice or Apple Cider

	Monday	Tuesday	Wednesday	Thursday	Friday	Saturday	Sunday
Dinner	*Dinner*	*Dinner*	*Dinner*	*Dinner*	*Dinner*	*Dinner*	*Dinner*
Rice Dish *Second* *Soup* *Bean/Sea-* *weed* *Long &* *Quickly* *Cooked* *Vege-* *table* *Dishes* *Salad* *Pickle* *Dessert* *Beverage*	Gomoku Rice w/ Tempeh, Onion, Burdock, Carrot & Shiitake Nishime Lotus Root & Leek Turnips & Tops Pressed Chinese Cabbage & Radish Sauerkraut Chestnut Pudding	Rice Udon in Broth w/ Shiitake & Scallion Adzuki Beans w/ Onion & Lotus Root Hijiki w/ Parsnip, Sesame & Ginger Boiled Salad w/ Kale, Carrots & String Beans Pressed Cucumber w/ Brown Rice Vinegar Brine Pickles	Hato Mugi Stew w/ Dried Daikon, Leek, Dried Tofu, Carrot & Miso Carrots & Tops Sautéed Squash, Escarole, & Onions Pressed Chinese Cabbage & Dulse Ginger Pickles Apple Pie	Rice & Black Soybeans Creamy Squash Soup Dried Daikon & Shiitake Kinpira w/ Burdock, Carrot, Scallions & Ginger Boiled Salad w/ Mustard Greens, Broccoli & Onions Brown Rice Vinegar Pickle	Millet & Cauli-flower "Mashed Potatoes" w/ Shoyu, Onion & Mush-room Gravy Dried Tofu Stew w/ Daikon, Squash, Brussels Sprouts & Fish (optional) Pressed Salad w/ Chinese Cabbage & Water-cress Miso Pickle Fruit Compote	Rice & Rye Lentil Soup w/ Onion, Burdock & Msio Nishime Squash Quick Sautéed Chinese Cabbage & Scallions Blanched Snow Peas, Mush-rooms, Cauli-flower, Onions w/ Pumpkin Seed Dressing Ume Pickles	Sweet Rice & Adzuki Beans Barley Soup w/ Celery, Squash & Wakame Dried Daikon w/ Carrot & Onion Boiled Salad w/ Collards, Onion & Cauli-flower Takuan Pickle Amasake Pudding Gar-nished w/ Almonds

Key: L.O. = Leftover; Salad = Boiled, Pressed, or Fresh. Bancha twig tea may be taken at every meal, with roasted barley tea, brown rice or millet tea, or grain coffee as an occasional substitute

Macrobiotic Recipes

This chapter includes some of the basic recipes for the dietary recommendations in this book and will help you get started. People with a serious health problem should be careful to follow the guidelines for the individual conditions and disorders in Part II and may need to restrict their use of bread and other flour products, oil, fish and seafood, fruit, nuts, seeds, salad, dessert, and other items. For a wider selection of recipes, please obtain one of the following cookbooks as soon as possible:

General Cookbooks
Aveline Kushi's Complete Guide to Macrobiotic Cooking by Aveline Kushi with Alex Jack, Warner Books, New York, 1984.
Aveline Kushi Introduces Macrobiotic Cooking by Aveline Kushi and Wendy Esko, Japan Publications, New York, 1987.
Amber Waves of Grain by Alex and Gale Jack, One Peaceful World Press, Becket, Mass., 2000.
The Changing Seasons Macrobiotic Cookbook by Aveline Kushi and Wendy Esko, Avery Publishing Group, New York, 1985.

Rice Is Nice by Wendy Esko, revised edition, Amberwaves, Becket, Mass., 2001.

Specialty cookbooks are listed in the Recommended Reading section.

General Suggestions

Macrobiotic cooking is unique. Natural and simple ingredients are best for creating delicious meals that are nutritious, tasty, and attractive. The cook has the ability to change the quality of the food. Stronger cooking, the use of greater pressure, salt, heat, and time, all make the energy of the food more concentrated and activating. Lighter cooking, the use of less pressure, salt, heat, and time, produce a lighter, more relaxing energy. A good cook manages these energies according to the ever-changing environment, climate, seasons, weather, and personal needs of those he or she cooks for and creates health and happiness by varying the selection of ingredients and cooking styles.

TABLE 36. 12 STEPS TO ENERGIZE YOUR FOOD

1. Use the highest-quality, locally grown, seasonally available, freshest ingredients.
2. Use organically grown food.
3. Cook whole grains or beans under pressure or with a heavy pot and heavy lid.
4. Cook with stainless steel, cast iron, ceramic, or other natural cookware
5. Cook with gas, wood, or natural fuel.
6. Use a slightly higher flame.
7. Use a slightly longer cooking or aging.
8. Use slightly more salt or seasoning.
9. Cook dynamically with a variety of foods, styles, colors, tastes, and other energies.
10. Cook with love and a calm, peaceful mind.
11. Chew each mouthful thoroughly.
12. Say grace, meditate, or observe a moment of silence to express your appreciation.

For variety, these aspects of day to day cooking can be changed:

1. The selection of foods within the following categories: grains, soups, vegetables, beans, sea vegetables, condiments, pickles, and beverages
2. The methods of cooking: boiling, steaming, sautéing, frying, pressure cooking, blanching, etc.
3. The ways of cutting vegetables
4. The amount of water used
5. The amount of seasoning and condiments used
6. The kind of seasoning and condiments used
7. The length of cooking time

8. The use of higher or lower flame in cooking foods
9. The combination of foods and dishes
10. The seasonal cooking adjustments
11. Adjustments in cooking for age and sex
12. Adjustments in cooking for the type of daily activity

The way of eating is as important as the food itself. Try to keep meals peaceful and relaxed. You may eat regularly two or three times a day, as much as you like, so long as the food is good quality and you chew well.

Each dish has particular flavors and effects, so it is better not to mix different foods and stir them together on the plate.

In order to gain experience and knowledge of the art of macrobiotic cooking, it is recommended that everyone attend cooking classes, read cookbooks, and learn from experienced people. This can greatly benefit you in understanding how to prepare balanced meals, including the recipes that follow.

◎ Methods of Cooking and Food Preparation

Regular Use (daily or often)
Pressure cooking
Boiling
Steaming (under 3 minutes)
Waterless
Soup
Pickling
Sautéing with oil
Sautéing with water

Pressing
Marinating
Blanching (under 3 minutes)

Occasional Use (once or twice a week)
Raw or uncooked
Stir-frying
Deep-frying
Tempura
Broiling
Baking

Note: In some cases, the above cooking methods may not be recommended for a short period of time.

◎ Whole Cereal Grains

PRESSURE-COOKED BROWN RICE

*2 cups organic brown rice (short- or
    medium-grain)
3½ to 4 cups water (more water for
    softer rice)
2 pinches sea salt*

Gently wash the rice in cold water, place the rice in a pressure cooker, and smooth the surface of the grain so it is level. Add water slowly down the side of the pressure cooker so the surface of the rice remains even and calm. Add sea salt, cover, and bring up to pressure slowly. When pressure is up, place a flame deflector underneath and turn flame to medium low, just enough to maintain pressure. (If you don't have a deflector, keep flame as low as possible.) Cook for 50 minutes from the time the pressure is up.

When rice is done, remove the pressure cooker from the burner and let the pressure come down naturally, about 5 minutes. Remove the cover, let the rice sit for a few minutes so that it will not stick to the bottom, and transfer to a serving bowl. If possible, use wooden implements such as a rice paddle or wooden spoon and serving bowl. Rice prepared in this way has a delicious, nutty taste and gives strong, peaceful energy.

- Soaking the rice for several hours or overnight will make it more digestible.
- Instead of salt, the rice may be seasoned with a small piece of kombu the size of a postage stamp.
- Each cup of uncooked rice yields about 3 cups of cooked rice. Allow about 1 cup of cooked rice per person.
- Leftover rice will usually keep about 24 hours unrefrigerated in a wooden bowl covered with a thin bamboo mat or cotton towel. If it is hot or humid, keep in the refrigerator in a closed container.
- Warm up leftover rice in a small steamer or place in a small saucepan, add a little water, cover, and heat for a few minutes.

BOILED BROWN RICE

*2 cups brown rice (short-, medium-, or long-
    grain)
4 cups water
2 pinches sea salt*

Wash rice and place in a heavy pot or saucepan. Add water and salt and cover with a lid. Bring to a boil, lower the flame, and simmer for about 45–50 minutes or until all the water has been absorbed. Remove and serve.

BROWN RICE WITH MILLET OR BARLEY

2 cups brown rice
½ cup millet or barley
4½ to 5 cups water
2 pinches sea salt

Wash the grains and place in pressure cooker. When the water is warm, add the sea salt, put on the cover, and bring up to pressure. Cook for about 45 minutes. Let sit for 5 minutes. Bring down the pressure and gently remove from the pot.

• Other grains such as whole wheat berries, whole oats, rye, and fresh corn removed from the cob may be cooked in this way.

BROWN RICE WITH BEANS

2 cups brown rice
¼ cup adzuki beans, chickpeas, lentils, or
*   other beans*
3½ to 4 cups water
2 pinches sea salt

Wash rice and beans separately. Cook beans ½ hour before cooking the rice using the basic recipes in the bean section below. Allow beans to cool. Add the beans, bean cooking water, and sea salt to rice in a pressure cooker. The bean water counts as part of the total water in the recipe. Pressure-cook for 45 to 50 minutes and serve.

BROWN RICE PORRIDGE

2 cups leftover brown rice
4 to 6 cups water

Place leftover rice in a saucepan and add the water. Bring to a gentle boil, cover with a lid, and cook until it softens to porridge-like consistency, about 10–20 minutes. Garnish with crumbled toasted nori, an umeboshi plum, gomashio, or other condiment.

• Add a variety of finely chopped vegetables to leftover rice and cook as above.
• Dilute a small volume of miso (about ½ teaspoon miso paste per cup of porridge) and add toward the end of cooking for seasoning. But be careful not to use too much miso. The porridge should not taste salty.

GENUINE BROWN RICE CREAM

1 cup brown rice
10 cups water
Pinch sea salt or ½ umeboshi plum

Dry-roast the rice in a cast-iron or stainless-steel skillet until golden brown. Place in a pot, add water and seasoning, and bring to a boil. Cover, lower heat, and place flame deflector beneath pot and turn flame to low. Cook for about 2 hours until the water is about half its original volume. Let the rice cool and place in a cheesecloth or clean unbleached muslin cloth. Tie and squeeze out the creamy liquid into a pot. Reheat the creamy liquid, adding a little more seasoning if needed. Garnish with scallions, chopped parsley, nori, gomashio, or sunflower seeds.

- Rice cream is recommended for people who are weak or who have no appetite or vitality, those who cannot chew, or for sick children.
- The remaining pulp can be saved and eaten. Make into a small ball and steam with grated carrot, lotus root, or other vegetable.
- The powdered brown rice cream sold in the natural foods store is not recommended for regular use. Its energy and vitality have been dispersed. Genuine brown rice cream retains the strong, whole energy of the grain and is freshly prepared.

FRIED RICE WITH VEGETABLES

2 cups cooked brown rice
1 celery stalk, diced
1 onion, diced
1 medium carrot, diced
Sesame oil
Several teaspoons of water
Shoyu to taste (1 teaspoon to 1 tablespoon)

Dice the vegetables. Brush the skillet with a small amount of sesame oil, let heat for a minute or less, and sauté the vegetables until crip but not overcooked. Add the rice on top of the vegetables and a few teaspoons of water. Cover the skillet and cook on low flame for 10–15 minutes. Add a little shoyu to taste and cook for another 5 minutes. Do not stir; just mix before serving.

- Vegetables may be varied. Other nice combinations include corn cut from the cob and diced nori; cabbage, carrots, and onions; fresh peas, carrots, and onions; cabbage and mushroom; daikon and daikon tops.

BROWN RICE BALLS

1 cup cooked brown rice
½ to 1 umeboshi plum
1 sheet toasted nori
Pinch of sea salt
Dish of water

Toast the nori by holding the shiny side over a burner about 10–12 inches from the flame. Rotate for 3–5 seconds until the color changes from black to green. Fold nori in half and fold again so you have four pieces that are about 3 inches square. Add a pinch of salt to the dish of water and wet your hands. Form a handful of rice into a solid ball. Press a hole in the center with the thumb and place a piece of the umeboshi plum inside. Close hole and knead rice ball again until it is compact. Cover rice ball with nori, one square at a time, until it sticks. Wet hands from time to time to prevent rice and nori from sticking to your skin, but do not use too much water.

- Rice balls make wonderful travel food because they do not require utensils and keep fresh for one or two days.
- For variety, make triangles instead of balls by cupping your hands into a V shape.
- As an outside coating instead of nori, roll the rice balls in roasted crushed sesame seeds, shiso leaves, dried wakame sheets, or green leafy vegetable leaves.

RICE KAYU BREAD

2 cups whole wheat flour
⅛ to ¼ teaspoon sea salt
2 cups softly cooked brown rice

Kayu is the Far Eastern word for "soft grain," and this bread is a favorite among macrobiotic families around the world. Actually, combining rice and wheat together in cooking is very traditional in the West as well. George Washington grew up on waffles made from whole wheat to which boiled rice had been added. (Please see recipe in Alex and Gale Jack's *Amber Waves of Grain* cookbook.)

Mix together the flour and salt. Add the softly cooked rice and form the dough into a ball. Knead the dough from 350 to 400 times, adding a little flour from time to time to prevent sticking. Oil an 8-inch-square baking pan with a little sesame oil and lightly dust the pan with flour. Shape the dough into a loaf and place it in the pan, pressing down around the edges to form a rounded loaf. With a sharp knife, make a shallow slit in the top center of the dough. Place the loaf in a warm place, such as a warm radiator or a pilot-lit oven, and let sit for 8 to 10 hours. Occasionally moisten the damp towel with warm water to prevent drying. After the dough has risen, bake in a preheated 300- to 350-degree oven for about 30 minutes. Increase the temperature to 350 degrees and bake for another hour and 15 minutes. When done, remove and place on a rack to cool.

- Add roasted seeds, nuts, or raisins into the dough for a sweeter, crunchier, or more festive bread.

MILLET AND SQUASH PORRIDGE

1 cup millet
½ cup butternut or other squash, sliced into small chunks
Pinch of sea salt
3 to 4 cups water

Wash millet in cold water and place in a saucepan. Add fresh cooking water and seasoning. Bring to a boil, lower flame, and add cut-up squash. Cover and let simmer for about 20–25 minutes. Garnish with chopped scallions, parsley, gomashio, or other condiment. This gives a sweet, delicious morning porridge and is also very strengthening.

WHOLE OATS

1 cup whole oats
Pinch sea salt
5–6 cups water

Wash oats and soak for several hours or preferably overnight. Place in a pressure cooker with water and seasoning. Bring to pressure, reduce heat, and cook for 1 hour. Use a flame deflector to prevent burning, if available. Garnish with toasted nori, chopped scallions, or gomashio.

PAN-FRIED MOCHI

8 ounces of mochi, cut into 2-inch squares

Mochi is pounded sweet rice that is traditionally eaten as a festive dish or for special occasions. It can be made at home by pounding cooked sweet rice with a heavy wooden pestle in a wooden bowl. Pound until grains are crushed and become very sticky. Wet pestle occasionally to prevent rice from sticking to it. Form rice into small balls or cakes or spread on a baking sheet that has been oiled and dusted with flour and let dry. Mochi is also now available in ready-made packages in the natural foods store.

Cut mochi into squares and place on a pre-heated skillet. No oil is necessary. Cover and cook over a low to medium flame for a few minutes until the mochi expands and puffs up. Check frequently or it will overexpand and burst. Turn over and cook the other side. Eat plain or serve with a little barley malt for a sweet taste; a few drops of shoyu for a salty taste; or wrap in toasted nori.

FRESH CORN ON THE COB

Several ears of corn
Water
Umeboshi plums or paste

Steam or boil corn in a saucepan for about 10 minutes in a small volume of water. (Use about ¼ to ½ inch water or just enough to generate steam. Do not immerse ears into a full pot of water.) Set out pieces of umeboshi plum or plum paste to rub on the corn as seasoning at the table.

UDON NOODLES IN BROTH

1 package udon noodles
2 dried shiitake mushrooms, soaked, stems
*   removed, and sliced*
1 piece kombu, 2–3 inches long
4 cups water
2–3 tablespoons shoyu

Add noodles to a pan of rapidly boiling water. No salt is needed for Oriental noodles. After about 10 minutes, check to see if they are done by breaking the end of one noodle. If the inside and outside are the same color, noodles are ready. If the inside is white or lighter, cook some more until done. Remove noodles from pot, strain, and rinse with cold water to stop from cooking and prevent clumping.

For the broth, place kombu in a saucepan and add 4 cups water and mushrooms. Bring to a boil, reduce flame, and simmer for 3–5 minutes. Remove kombu and shiitake. Add shoyu to taste and simmer for another 3–5 minutes. Serve noodles with hot broth and garnish with scallions, chives, or toasted nori.

- Grated ginger may be added to the broth.
- Soba, somen, and other noodles may be cooked in this way. However, buckwheat noodles cook faster than whole wheat, and thinner somen noodles cook more quickly than udon.
- For variety, add vegetables that are steamed or boiled separately. Nice combinations include watercress and tofu; tempeh or seitan; or dried daikon, carrots, and onions.
- Western-style whole-grain noodles and pasta may also be used occasionally, including spaghetti, shells, spirals, elbows, flat noodles, and lasagna. Add a pinch of salt in cooking.

FRIED NOODLES WITH VEGETABLES

8 ounces cooked udon or soba
2 cups cabbage, thinly sliced
½ cup scallions, sliced
1 tablespoon sesame oil
1–2 tablespoons shoyu

Oil skillet and put in cabbage. Place cooked noodles (from previous recipe) on top of vegetables. Cover and cook on a low flame for several minutes until the noodles are warm. Add shoyu and mix noodles and vegetables well, but otherwise don't stir. At the end of cooking, add scallions and cook for another minute.

- Use 2 tablespoons of water for sautéing if you cannot use oil.
- For variety, other vegetables may be used. Nice combinations include tofu and cabbage, mushrooms and scallions, and carrots and onions. Broccoli, cauliflower, napa cabbage, celery, and yellow squash are also tasty.
- Grated ginger makes a nice garnish, especially if scallions are not used.

Soups

MISO SOUP

2-inch piece dried wakame
1 cup onions, sliced thinly
1 quart water
Barley miso

Soak the wakame (about ¼ to ½ inch per person) for 5 minutes and cut into small pieces. Add the wakame to fresh, cold water and bring to a boil. Meanwhile, cut onions into small pieces. Add the onions to the boiling broth and boil all together for 3–5 minutes until the onions are soft and edible. Reduce flame to low. Dilute miso (½ to 1 teaspoon per cup of broth) in a little water, add to soup, and simmer for 3–4 minutes on a low flame. Once the miso is added, don't boil the soup; just let it simmer. Garnish with finely chopped scallions or parsley before serving.

- Be sure to simmer the soup for 3–4 minutes *after* miso paste is added to the broth. This is a very simple soup to make, but not letting the miso cook properly will reduce its effects.
- For variety, brown rice miso or all soybean (hatcho) miso may be used occasionally. However, they should be aged a minimum of 2 years. Misos may also be combined for a unique taste and flavor.
- Vary the vegetables daily. Nice combinations include onions and tofu; onions and sweet autumn or winter squash; cabbage and carrots; and daikon and daikon greens.
- Include leafy greens often in miso soup, including kale, collards, watercress, etc. Add them toward the end of cooking since they don't need to cook as long.
- A small volume of shiitake mushrooms (soaked and finely chopped beforehand) may be added and cooked with the other vegetables from time to time.
- Leftover grain or beans may be added to miso soup from time to time to make a thicker soup.
- For the most beneficial effect, miso soup should be cooked fresh each time and not reused at later meals or stored overnight.

CLEAR SHOYU BROTH

2 cakes of tofu, cubed
2 shiitake mushrooms
3-inch piece kombu
4 cups water
2–3 tablespoons shoyu
¼ cup scallions, sliced
Nori

Soak shiitake mushrooms 10–20 minutes. Place kombu and shiitake in water (including soaking water) and boil for 3–4 minutes. Take kombu and shiitake out and save for another recipe. Add tofu and boil until tofu comes to the surface. Do not boil too long or tofu will become hard. Add shoyu and simmer for 2–3 minutes. Garnish with scallions and nori.

- For variety substitute chopped watercress or other vegetables for the tofu. Shiitake is also optional.

MILLET AND SWEET VEGETABLE SOUP

1 cup millet
*½ cup butternut or other squash, finely
  chopped*
½ cup carrots, finely chopped
½ cup cabbage, finely chopped
½ onion, chopped finely
1-inch piece of wakame
Small piece of shiitake mushroom
Miso or shoyu to taste

Wash millet and chop vegetables. Combine ingredients except for seasoning and add three times as much water. Bring to a boil, reduce

flame, and let simmer for about 30 minutes or until done. Toward the end of cooking, season lightly with miso (about ½ teaspoon per person or serving) or shoyu (several drops) and simmer for another 3 to 4 minutes. Garnish with chopped scallions or parsley.

LENTIL SOUP

1 cup green or brown lentils
2 onions, diced
1 medium carrot, diced
1 quart spring water
¼ to ½ teaspoon sea salt
1 tablespoon chopped parsley

Wash lentils. Layer onions on bottom of saucepan, followed by carrots, and place lentils on top. Add water and just a pinch of sea salt. Bring to a boil, reduce flame to low, cover, and simmer for 45 minutes. Add parsley and remaining salt and simmer for 10 to 15 more minutes or until done. A little shoyu may also be added for flavor toward the end of cooking, if desired.

BARLEY STEW

½ cup barley
1 small onion or leek, sliced
½ cup corn kernels
5–6 cups water
Shoyu to taste

Layer the ingredients with the onions on the bottom, the corn in the middle, and the barley on top. Cook gently until barley is done, about 45 minutes. Add shoyu to taste toward the end of cooking. Garnish with chopped scallion or nori.

FRESH CORN CHOWDER

4 ears fresh corn
1 celery stalk, diced
2 onions, diced
5–6 cups water
¼ teaspoon sea salt
Shoyu to taste

Remove the kernels from the corn with a knife. Place celery, onions, and corn in a saucepan. Add water and a pinch of salt. Bring to a boil, lower the flame, cover, and simmer until the corn and celery are soft. Add rest of salt and shoyu to taste, if desired. Garnish with chopped parsley, watercress, or scallions and nori.

CREAMY SQUASH SOUP

1 large butternut squash
Water
Shoyu to taste

Wash and peel squash. Cut into 1-inch chunks and put in a pot. Add water to partially cover the squash. Bring to a boil, reduce heat, and simmer until tender. Remove from burner and purée in a hand food mill. Add additional water to desired thickness. Reheat, adding a small amount of shoyu (1–2 teaspoons) to taste, and simmer for a few minutes. Garnish with chopped parsley or scallions and nori.

• Broccoli or cauliflower soup may be prepared in the same way. Add a little lemon juice for a slightly different flavor.

Vegetables

NISHIME-STYLE VEGETABLES
(Waterless Cooking)

Vegetables prepared in this way are cut in large chunks and are cooked slowly for a long time over low heat. The steam in the pot allows the ingredients to cook in their own juices, so that little water is usually needed. Seasoning may be added in the beginning or toward the end of cooking. The vegetables are very juicy and may be served together with their cooking liquid. They give strong, calm energy.

Use a heavy pot with a heavy lid or cookware designed for waterless cooking. Soak a ½-inch piece of kombu per cup of vegetables. Place kombu in the bottom of the pot and add about 1 to 2 inches of water. Add sliced vegetables, usually cut in large chunks or slices. Generally two or three vegetables are cooked together, though more or less may also be used. The vegetables are layered in the pot on top of the kombu or placed in sections around the pot.

Cover the pot with a heavy lid and set the flame on high until sufficient steam is generated. Lower the flame and simmer for about 15–20 minutes. (The time needed may be as little as 10 minutes, especially in the summer when using lighter vegetables and ones cut in smaller pieces.) Add more water during cooking as needed if the liquid evaporates too quickly. When the vegetables are soft and edible, add a few drops of shoyu and shake the pot gently with the lid on (do not stir). Cook over a low flame for 3–5 minutes longer with the lid on. Remove the lid, turn off the flame, and let the vegetables sit for about 2 minutes. You may serve the remaining liquid, which is very sweet and delicious, along with the vegetables.

• Suggested combinations of vegetables include the following (all cooked with kombu): carrot, burdock, onions; carrot, parsnip, cabbage; turnip, shiitake mushroom, cabbage; burdock, leeks, lotus root; daikon or lotus root, carrot, corn; carrot, onion, cabbage; squash, onion, daikon; daikon, squash, cabbage; cabbage, onion. Carrot and daikon or carrot and turnip do not go so well.

ADZUKI BEANS, SQUASH, AND KOMBU DISH

½ cup adzuki beans
1-inch piece kombu
1 to 1½ cups butternut, acorn, buttercup, or
*   Hokkaido squash, chopped*
Water

Wash and soak the adzuki beans and kombu for several hours or overnight. Put the kombu in the bottom of a heavy pot and add chopped squash. Add adzuki beans on top of squash. Add enough water to just cover the layer of squash. Do not place a lid on the pot at the start. Bring to a boil slowly, covering after 10–15 minutes. Cook on a low flame until the beans are three-quarters done, about an hour or more. The water will evaporate as the beans expand, so gently add water along the sides of the pot to keep the water level constant and to make the beans soft. When the beans are three-quarters done, add a few pinches of sea salt. Cover and cook for another 15–30 minutes or until most of the liquid has evaporated. Turn off the flame and let the pot sit for several minutes.

• Refrain from stirring while cooking.
• If squash is not available, use carrots, onions, or parsnips.
• Lentils or chickpeas may occasionally be substituted for adzuki beans.

DRIED DAIKON WITH KOMBU

1-inch piece kombu
½ cup dried daikon
Water
Shoyu to taste

Soak a small piece of kombu for 10 minutes. Cut into ½-inch pieces and place at the bottom of a pot with a heavy lid. Soak the dried daikon for 10 minutes or until soft. Discard the soaking water if dark, or otherwise it may be used in cooking. Place the dried daikon (chopped if desired) on top of the kombu and add enough water to cover. Cover the pot with the lid, bring to a boil, and lower the flame. Simmer for 20–30 minutes, until the daikon is tender. Add a small amount of shoyu toward the end of cooking and cook away the excess liquid.

• For variety, a small volume of onions, carrots, or cabbage may be added to this dish. Add sliced vegetables on top of the daikon and proceed as above.

DAIKON AND DAIKON LEAVES

1 daikon root and leaves
Water
Pinch of sea salt or shoyu to taste

Finely chop the daikon root. Place in a pot with a small amount of water. Cover and cook in steaming water for about 5–7 minutes. Add a small pinch of salt or shoyu to taste. Place finely chopped greens on top of roots, then simmer for 2–3 minutes more.

- Red radish and radish leaves may be used if daikon is not available.
- Other variations include carrots and carrot tops, turnip and turnip tops, or dandelion roots and leaves.

HIJIKI WITH LOTUS ROOT

1 ounce hijiki
½–1 cup fresh lotus root, sliced into half moons
water
shoyu to taste

Wash and drain the hijiki. Slice the seaweed into small pieces and slice the fresh lotus root into thin half moons. (In case you are using dried lotus root, first soak it until soft.) Place a small amount of water into a frying pan. Add lotus root and water-sauté lightly for 2 to 3 minutes. Put drained hijiki on the top of the lotus root and a small amount of water to just cover the lotus root. Bring to a boil, turn the heat to low and add a small amount of shoyu. Cover and simmer on the low flame for 40 to 60 minutes, until the bitter taste of the hijiki disappears. Add a little more shoyu to taste. (Be careful not to make it too salty.) Simmer for another 5 to 10 minutes on a low flame, stirring well until the liquid evaporates.

BOILED SALAD

Assortment of fresh vegetables

When blanching vegetables, boil each vegetable separately, one at a time, in the same boiling water. Cook the mildest-tasting vegetables first so that each vegetable retains its distinctive flavor. Stronger-flavored ones such as daikon, turnips, celery, and especially watercress are preferably cooked at the end. The ingredients are usually just dipped in and out quickly, 1 minute or less. Any combination of two or three vegetables may be used. For this quick cooking style, the vegetables should be finely sliced.

Place an inch or two of water and a pinch of sea salt in a pot and bring to a boil. Drop in a small amount of vegetables at a time and boil for 1 minutes or less. Remove the vegetables quickly and place them in a strainer to drain. Repeat with each vegetable. Transfer to a serving dish when done.

- The vegetables should be fresh, brightly colored, and crispy.
- Vary the vegetables and combinations daily.
- Boiled watercress, parsley, or other greens need only to be dipped into the boiling water and taken out right away. This will brighten their color and eliminate their strong, raw, bitter, or pungent taste.
- Spreading the vegetables on a platter to expose them to the cool air will help stop the cooking and preserve their bright colors.
- Serve the vegetables plain or add a few drops of brown rice or umeboshi vinegar, a condiment, or one of the dressings described below.

PRESSED SALAD

Assortment of fresh vegetables
Sea salt

Wash and slice vegetables into very thin slices. In a large bowl, mix vegetables and add about ½ teaspoon of sea salt per cup of chopped vegetables. Mix gently by hand. Transfer to a salad press and apply pressure to the press. If a press is not available, leave in a bowl and place a small plate that fits inside the bowl, adding a weight on top of the plate. Let the vegetables sit for 30–60 minutes or more (depending on the vegetables) or until water is expelled from the vegetables. Discard the water before serving and rinse off the vegetables under fresh water so that they are not too salty. Serve plain, with lemon juice, rice vinegar, or umeboshi vinegar.

- Nice pressed salads include: mustard greens or radish greens, chopped finely and pressed for 30 minutes; cabbage leaves, finely chopped, layered with sea salt, and pressed for 30 minutes; carrots, grated, shredded, or cut into matchsticks, pressed for 30 minutes.
- Ingredients may be pressed longer, up to a couple of days, to make light pickles.
- Brown rice vinegar, umeboshi vinegar, or shoyu may be used for variety in the pressing instead of salt.

RAW SALAD

A variety of vegetables may be used in this preparation, including finely chopped cabbage, grated carrots, radishes, cucumbers, celery, watercress, and lettuce. Season with any of the following dressings.

SALAD DRESSING SUGGESTIONS

Use homemade rather than store-bought dressings that are usually high in salt, oil, herbs, and spices.

1. One umeboshi plum or 1 teaspoon of umeboshi paste, added to ½ teaspoon of miso, puréed in a suribachi.
2. Dilute miso in warm water and heat for a few minutes. Let cool and add a few drops of rice vinegar.
3. Gomashio or shio leaf powder.
4. Sprinkle a small amount of shoyu and lemon juice on the salad.
5. One umeboshi plum or 1 teaspoon of umeboshi paste may be added to ½ cup of water and puréed in a suribachi.
6. A few drops of rice vinegar (½ to 1 teaspoon) or umeboshi vinegar (¼ to ½ teaspoon) sprinked over the salad.
7. Tofu dressing.
8. Pumpkin seed dressing.
9. Sesame seed dressing.
10. Umeboshi-scallion or parsley dressing.

TOFU DRESSING

½ teaspoon puréed umeboshi plum
¼ onion, grated or diced
2 teaspoons water
8 ounces tofu
Chopped scallions or parsley

Purée umeboshi, onion, and water in a suribachi or bowl. Add tofu and purée until creamy. Add water to increase creaminess if desired. Garnish with scallions or parsley. Serve with salad.

KUZU SAUCE

1 tablespoon kuzu
1½ cups water or vegetable stock
Shoyu to taste

Dilute kuzu in a small volume of cold water and add to pot containing water or stock. Bring to a boil, lower flame, and simmer 10 to 15 minutes. Stir constantly. Add shoyu to taste. Serve over vegetables, tofu, noodles, grains, or beans.

- Arrowroot powder may be used instead of kuzu. Avoid refined thickeners such as cornstarch.

STEAMED GREENS

Kale, collards, watercress, mustard greens
Dandelion greens, carrot tops, Chinese
*   cabbage, or other greens*

Wash and slice any of the above vegetables. Place the vegetables in a small amount of water, about ½ inch, or in a stainless-steel steamer over 1 inch of boiling water. Cover and steam or boil for 2–3 minutes, depending on the texture of the vegetables. Transfer quickly to a serving dish to prevent overcooking.

- The vegetables should be a bright green color and crispy.
- Wait until the water is fully boiling before you put in the vegetables.
- You may lightly sprinkle shoyu over the greens at the end of the cooking.
- You may serve plain or occasionally add a few drops of brown rice or umeboshi vinegar.
- When boiling, do not cover the pot with a lid or the greens will lose their bright green color.

SAUTÉED VEGETABLES

Assortment of fresh vegetables
Sesame oil
Sea salt or shoyu to taste

Finely cut vegetables. Leafy greens and thickly sliced root vegetables as well as sprouts or corn kernels may all be sautéed, by themselves or in various combinations. Heat a skillet and add a small volume of sesame oil (or just brush it with oil if on an oil-restricted diet). When the sesame oil is hot, sauté the vegetables quickly for a few minutes. Gently stir the vegetables with chopsticks or another wood utensil. There is no need for vigorous stirring or constant mixing. Sprinkle with a pinch of sea salt or shoyu. Simmer for a few more minutes, adding a little water if necessary.

- The vegetables should be crispy and colorful, cooked but not overcooked.
- The cooking time may vary depending on the type, size, and thickness of the ingredients.
- For those who cannot use oil, water-sauté by adding a small volume of cold water to the skillet instead.

KINPIRA-STYLE VEGETABLES

Cut equal amounts of burdock and carrots (sliced into matchsticks or shaved). Lightly brush sesame oil in a skillet and heat on a medium-high flame. Use 1 teaspoon of oil per person if oil is allowed. When oil is hot, sauté the burdock for 2–3 minutes in the skillet and layer the carrots on top of the burdock. Lightly cover the bottom of the skillet with water, just enough to cover the burdock. Cover and cook until the vegetables are 80 percent done. This takes about 10–20 minutes or longer. Add a small volume of shoyu for a light taste. Cover again with lid. Cook until all the water has evaporated. At the very end of cooking, add a few drops of ginger juice (squeezed from grated ginger) if your condition permits it.

- Onions, turnips, or lotus root may be substituted or used together with carrots and burdock.
- When burdock is not available, you may use carrots only or substitute another vegetable.
- If oil is to be avoided for your condition, you may water-sauté instead. Use a little bit of water on the bottom of the pan, heat as you would oil, and proceed as above.
- Dried burdock may be soaked and used in place of fresh burdock if the latter is unavailable.

DRIED TOFU, TOFU, OR TEMPEH STEW WITH VEGETABLES

2-inch piece of kombu
Dried tofu, tempeh, or seitan, sliced into cubes
Daikon, burdock, lotus root, or other root
*   vegetable*
3 cups water
Sea salt or shoyu to taste
2–3 scallions

Soak kombu in 3 cups of water. Add any one of the following: soaked and sliced dried tofu, tempeh cubes, or seitan, along with sliced daikon, burdock, carrots, or lotus root. Bring to a boil and simmer for about 15 minutes. Add a pinch of sea salt or shoyu (unless you are using seitan, which may not require additional sea-

soning). Add one or a combination of the following vegetables (2 or 3): onions, cabbage, Chinese cabbage, squash or Brussels sprouts. Cook for 3–5 minutes. These vegetables take less time to cook than root vegetables and should be lightly crisp. Finely chop 2–3 scallions and add at the very end of cooking for 1 minute or less.

- If you use fresh tofu, add it toward the end of cooking.
- If you add leafy greens, add them toward the end of cooking. They should still be crisp and not soggy or overcooked.
- A small amount of ginger may be added at the very end of cooking if your condition permits.
- You may sometimes make a thicker gravy for the stew. Remove the vegetables and add diluted kuzu to the broth. Stir until the sauce thickens. Add the vegetables and cook for a few more minutes.
- A mild seasoning of miso may be added at the end of cooking, instead of shoyu or sea salt.

◎ Beans

ADZUKI BEANS

1 cup adzuki beans
2½ cups water per cup of beans
¼ teaspoon sea salt per cup of beans

Wash beans and place in pressure cooker. Add water, cover, and bring to pressure. Reduce flame to medium-low and cook 45 minutes. Remove pressure cooker from burner and run cold water over it to bring pressure down quickly. Open, add salt, and cook uncovered until liquid evaporates.

- Except for lentils, split peas, and other soft, light beans, most beans are hard and should be soaked several hours or overnight before cooking to improve their digestibility.
- Black soybeans should not be pressure-cooked because they clog up the vent.
- Instead of salt, a 1-inch square of kombu may be used to season the beans. Rinse the kombu and soak for a few minutes in cold water. Place the strip on the bottom of the pot and the beans on top. (The kombu may also be soaked together with the beans.)
- For variety cook with 30–50 percent acorn, butternut, or buttercup squash or 10–30 percent chestnuts (best with adzuki beans or black soybeans).
- Cooking time will vary depending on the type of bean and the particular batch. Sometimes another 30–60 minutes is necessary.
- Beans may be boiled, pressure cooked, or (less frequently) baked (condition permitting). Do not add the salt at the beginning of cooking, but when the beans are about 80 percent done. If you pressure cook the beans, open the pressure cooker, add the salt, miso, or shoyu, and continue gently simmering without a lid until any excess liquid has evaporated.

CHICKPEAS WITH CARROTS AND ONIONS

1 cup chickpeas
1-inch piece kombu
½ cup carrots
½ cup onions
3 cups water
Pinch of sea salt

Soak chickpeas for 6–8 hours or overnight with a little kombu. Dice carrots and onions. Layer kombu on the bottom of the pressure cooker and place chickpeas on top. Add the water, including the soaking water, if desired. Bring mixture to a boil without a lid, reduce the flame, and cook for 30 minutes. Discard any foam that rises to the surface. Cover the pressure cooker and bring to pressure on a low flame. Cook with low pressure for about 40 minutes. Allow pressure to come down completely and remove the cover. Remove the beans and layer the carrots and onions on the bottom of the pot. Place the beans on top of the vegetables. Bring to a boil, cover with a heavy regular lid (it is better not to pressure-cook the vegetables), reduce heat, and cook on a medium flame for about 1 hour until the beans are 80 percent done. Add a pinch of sea salt and continue cooking until the beans are well done, but not mushy and most of the liquid has evaporated. Transfer to a serving dish.

BLACK SOYBEANS

1 cup black soybeans
Water
Shoyu to taste

Wash the beans with cold water. Cover with about 3 cups of water and soak for 5–8 hours or overnight. Discard the soaking water. Place beans in a pot and add enough water to cover. Bring to a boil, reduce the flame to low, and simmer without a cover. Skim and discard the black foam that floats to the surface. When foam no longer appears, cover and cook for about 2½ hours or until beans are about 90 percent done. If more water is needed during the cooking time, gently add it along the sides of the pot. Remove the cover and add a small amount of shoyu, which will give the beans a shiny black color. Shake the pot gently to mix the beans with the juice and shoyu but do not mix with a spoon. Continue cooking until beans are soft and most of the remaining liquid has evaporated. Transfer to a serving dish.

SCRAMBLED TOFU

1 pound tofu
Sesame oil
½ cup scallions, sliced
1 small carrot, cut into matchsticks
½ cup mushrooms, diced
1 cup fresh corn kernels

This makes a nice breakfast or brunch dish, and children especially love it. Heat a small amount of oil in a skillet. (Water-sauté if oil must be avoided.) Add mushroom and cook 1–2 minutes. Next add the carrots and corn and finally the scallions. Crumble tofu over vegetables. Reduce flame and simmer for 5 minutes. Season with shoyu to taste or chopped umeboshi plum. Simmer again for 3–4 minutes and serve.

TEMPEH SQUASH STEW

1 onion, cut in chunks
½ buttercup squash, cut in chunks
1 pound tempeh, cut in chunks
½ cup cabbage, sliced
2 to 2½ cups water
1 teaspoon miso
1 teaspoon kuzu

This thick stew is sweet and delicious. It is especially warming in autumn or winter, but it is good all year round. Boil tempeh and vegetables together for 10–15 minutes. Add diluted miso and simmer for 3–4 minutes. Add a little kuzu diluted in cold water at the end for thickening.

◎ Sea Vegetables

ARAME WITH ONIONS

1 ounce dried arame
1 tablespoon sesame oil
1 medium onion, sliced

Wash and drain arame. Brush a skillet with light or dark sesame oil and heat it. Add the onions and sauté for 2–3 minutes. (Water-sauté if oil is to be avoided.) Place the arame on top of the onions and add enough water to just cover the onions. Bring to a boil, turn the heat down to low, and add a small amount of shoyu. Cover and simmer for about 20–25 minutes. Add shoyu to taste, but dish should not be overly salty. Simmer for another 5–10 minutes, mix, and stir until the liquid has evaporated.

- Carrot, dried daikon, rutabaga, sweet corn, or other vegetables may also be added.
- Hijiki may be cooked in the same way, but it should be cooked longer, up to 1 or 1½ hours total cooking time, in order to lose its bitterness and become sweet.

WAKAME-CUCUMBER SALAD

1 cup wakame

*1 large cucumber, quartered lengthwise and
    sliced*

¼ cup red radish, thinly sliced

1 tablespoon brown rice vinegar

¼ to ½ teaspoon sea salt

Rinse wakame, soak for 10 minutes, drain, and cut into small pieces. Place ½ inch of water in a saucepan and bring to a boil. Simmer radishes for 1 minute and remove. Simmer wakame for 1–3 minutes and remove. Mix sea salt with rice vinegar and add to wakame, cucumbers, and radish. Put in a pickle press for 1–3 hours. Remove, rinse off excess salt, and serve.

◎ Condiments and Seasonings

GOMASHIO

1 part sea salt

16 to 18 parts sesame seeds

Wash seeds in a fine-mesh strainer and allow them to dry. Dry-roast the sea salt in a stainless-steel frying pan over a medium-high flame until it turns gray. Place the salt in a suribachi or mortar and grind into a fine powder. Roast the seeds on medium heat. While roasting, push seeds back and forth gently with a wooden paddle or spoon to avoid burning. The seeds are done when they crush easily between the thumb and forefinger, about 5–10 minutes. The seeds will begin to pop when done and give off a nutty fragrance. Lower the flame toward the end and do not overcook or the seeds will have a bitter taste. Add seeds while they are still hot to the ground salt in the suribachi. Slowly and gently grind the seeds in an even circular motion with the suribachi pestle, making sure to use the grooved sides of the suribachi to grind against instead of the bottom of the bowl. Grind until each seed is crushed and thoroughly covered with salt. Allow the gomashio to cool, then transfer to an airtight container to serve.

- Use sparingly over grain or vegetables, about 1 teaspoon a day or less.
- Medicinally, gomashio is helpful to neutralize acidity in the blood, relieve tiredness, and strengthen the nervous system.
- For children, the ratio of sesame seeds to salt should be higher, 20:1 to 24:1.
- Black sesame seeds are preferable, but brown (white) may also be used.
- Ready-made gomashio is available in the natural foods store. However, the proportion of salt to sesame seeds is often 1:10 or less. This is too salty and not recommended. Also, commercial gomashio may lose its freshness more quickly than homemade.

WAKAME OR KOMBU POWDER

Roast several strips of wakame or kombu in a dry skillet over the stove (not in the oven) until dark and crisp. Cover and cook over a low flame so that the sea vegetable does not burn. Turn the strips over when needed so they roast evenly. Grind into a fine powder in a suribachi.

• For variety, add toasted sesame seeds. Toast them according to the directions in the go-mashio recipe. Add to the seaweed powder and crush them together. The ratio of seaweed to sesame seeds should be about 50-50.

UMEBOSHI PLUMS

Umeboshi are plums related to the apricot family that have been dried, pickled with sea salt, and aged from 1 to 3 years. They usually come with deep red shiso leaves. Umeboshi may be eaten by themselves (1 plum, ½ plum, or a piece of plum) or used as a seasoning instead of sea salt, shoyu, or miso in cooking. They may also be puréed for making a tart and tangy dressing, sauce, or tea. Umeboshi contain a balance of energies that strengthen the intestines, neutralize acidity in the blood, and counter the effects of alcohol, sugar, and other extreme foods. Umeboshi paste is available without the hard pits in the center of the fruit. The paste is not so strong and is used for dressings, sauces, and as a spread for fresh corn on the cob. For medicinal teas and as a healing condiment, the whole plum is preferable.

TEKKA

⅓ cup burdock, finely minced
⅓ cup carrot, finely minced
⅓ cup lotus root, finely minced
½ teaspoon grated ginger
¼ cup sesame oil
⅔ cup hatcho miso

Chop vegetables, mincing as finely as possible. Heat oil in a skillet and sauté vegetables.

Add miso. Reduce flame to low and cook 3–4 hours. Stir frequently until liquid evaporates and a dry, black mixture is left.

• Tekka is very strengthening for the blood but should be used sparingly (about ½ teaspoon or less daily). It is also available ready-made in the natural foods store.

GINGER

Fresh grated gingerroot is used in small volume as a garnish or flavoring on noodles, vegetable dishes, soups, pickled vegetables, and fish or seafood. Grate finely with gentle circular motions on a hand grater. Sometimes recipes call for ginger juice, which is made by taking a small amount of ginger gratings, compacting them with the tips of your fingers, and squeezing out the liquid directly into the pot, skillet, medicinal drink, or special dish.

SEA SALT

Natural unrefined, white sea salt is recommended for daily use. It is customarily added to foods during the cooking process and not at the table. In the natural foods store, there are a variety of sea salts. Avoid those that are high in minerals or gray or off-white in color. Usually the generic white sea salt that flows freely and does not clump is suitable.

MISO

Miso, or fermented soybean paste, is used to make miso soup and as a seasoning in other dishes. Traditionally made organic miso (barley miso, brown rice miso, or hatcho miso) that has fermented a minimum of 2 years is the standard for daily cooking. Short-time misos (red miso, yellow miso, or white miso) are used for sauces, dressings, and special dishes. Instant miso is convenient for traveling but is not for daily home use. As a general rule, about ½ teaspoon of miso paste is used per cup of soup. Miso contains enzymes that may be destroyed by boiling. After adding miso to soup, let it simmer for 3–4 minutes over a low flame.

SHOYU

Shoyu is traditional, naturally processed soy sauce made from fermented soybeans, wheat, and sea salt. The chemically processed, artificially aged soy sauce available in many supermarkets and Oriental markets is not recommended. In the natural foods store, there are many soy sauces, including genuine or real tamari, which is made without wheat. Tamari has a strong flavor and may be used occasionally for a special dish but is not recommended for daily use. Similarly, low-sodium soy sauces or those with other ingredients are usually avoided or used sparingly. In macrobiotic cooking, shoyu is added to foods during the last few minutes of the cooking process and is not added to rice or vegetables at the table. This makes it more digestible and prevents cravings for sweets or liquid that easily arise if it is eaten uncooked.

VEGETABLE OIL

Unrefined vegetable oil (sometimes labeled "cold-pressed" or "solvent-free") is used in macrobiotic cooking. The standard is sesame oil, light or dark. Other polyunsaturated oils may also be used, including corn oil, sunflower oil, and walnut oil. Safflower oil is light and is often used in making tempura. Olive oil may be used occasionally for special meals or dishes but is monosaturated and most suitable in hot climates. Corn oil may be genetically modified, so find a trustworthy supplier that uses organic or natural ingredients. Avoid canola oil, palm oil, cottonseed oil, and coconut oil. Oil is used primarily in cooking and in moderate amounts.

◎ Pickles

UMEBOSHI PICKLES

6–8 umeboshi plums
2 quarts water
1 bunch red radishes

Place umeboshi plums in a large jar. Add the water. Shake and let sit for a few hours, until the water turns pink. Place sliced vegetables in the water, cover them with a cheesecloth and place the jar in a dark, cool place. Serve after 4–5 days.

QUICK SHOYU PICKLES OR UMEBOSHI VINEGAR PICKLES

Round or root vegetables
¾ cup water
¼ cup shoyu or umeboshi vinegar

Slice vegetables ⅛ inch thick and cover with a mixture of water and shoyu or umeboshi vinegar. Cover jar with cheesecloth to keep out dust. Set aside. After 24 hours, remove cloth, place lid on jar, and refrigerate. Remove as needed. Rinse before eating.

BRINE PICKLES

3 cups water
1 teaspoon sea salt
3-inch piece of kombu
Carrot, onion, daikon, broccoli, cucumber, or other vegetables, sliced

Boil the water and salt. Let cool. Place the kombu and sliced vegetables in a jar with the cool salt water. All the vegetables should be immersed in the water. If not, place a smaller jar or cup inside in order to press the vegetables below the surface of the water. Cover with a cheesecloth and keep in a cool place for 2–3 days. Refrigerate and begin using when the vegetables have lost their raw flavor, but still retain their crunchiness.

◎ Desserts and Snacks

STEWED APPLES

1 cup apples, sliced
Pinch of sea salt
Water
1 tablespoon kuzu

Place fruit in a saucepan and add enough water to half cover. Add sea salt and bring to a boil. Cover and simmer on low flame for about 10–15 minutes or until tender. Dissolve kuzu in several tablespoons of cold water and add slowly to cooked fruit, stirring with a wooden spoon.

The fruit is done when the liquid thickens slightly and is clear. Remove from pan and serve.

- Dried apples may be used instead of fresh apples. Cook a little longer, about 20 minutes.
- Apricots, peaches, pears, or other temperate-climate fruit may be prepared in the same way.

STRAWBERRY KANTEN

1 cup strawberries, freshly sliced
⅔ cup apple juice per person
⅓ cup water per person
¼ cup amasake (optional)
2 tablespoons agar-agar flakes
1 teaspoon kuzu

Kanten is a delicious, mild gelatin. Made with agar-agar, a sea vegetable that is processed into flakes or powder, it is very light and refreshing.

Slice strawberries and set aside. Simmer liquid ingredients and agar flakes until the agar has dissolved. Dissolve kuzu in a few tablespoons of water and stir in mixture until it thickens. Pour liquid over the strawberries and serve.

- For variety, use peaches, apples, blueberries, cherries, cantaloupe, or other seasonal fruit, individually or in combination.

AMASAKE PUDDING

1 quart amasake
3 tablespoons kuzu
Pinch of sea salt
Almonds, roasted and slivered

Place amasake in a pot. Dissolve kuzu in several tablespoons of cold water and stir into the amasake. Add salt and stir gently but continually while bringing mixture to a boil over low heat. Simmer several more minutes. Pour into individual serving dishes. Garnish with 1 teaspoon of slivered almonds per serving.

SQUASH PUDDING

1 squash (3 to 4 cups puréed)
3 tablespoons agar-agar flakes
1 tablespoon barley malt
1 teaspoon tahini (optional)
⅛ teaspoon sea salt
1 tablespoon arrowroot powder

Boil squash for about 30 minutes or until done. Peel squash and purée in a handmill. Place squash in a saucepan, and add agar-agar powder, barley malt, tahini, and sea salt. While simmering, mix arrowroot in a little cold water and add to squash. Simmer 5 to 10 more minutes. Place in dessert bowls and let cool.

RICE PUDDING

2 cups long-grain rice, cooked
¾ cup apple juice
¾ cup water
2 tablespoons raisins
½ teaspoons tahini (optinal)
2 tablespoons rice syrup
Pinch of cinammon (optional)
Pinch of sea salt
1 tablespoon kuzu
Almonds or walnuts, roasted and slivered

Put the rice, raisins, sea salt, and cinnamon in a saucepan. Add apple juice, water, tahini, and rice syrup. Cook over a low flame for 25 minutes. Dissolve kuzu in cold water and add to the other ingredients and stir so it will thicken the mixture. Serve in individual dishes and let sit until ready to serve. Top with roasted, slivered almonds or walnuts.

CHESTNUT PURÉE

½ pound dried chestnuts
½ cup water
½ cup barley malt

Soak chestnuts for several hours. Combine water, barley malt, and chestnuts in a large saucepan. Bring to a boil over medium heat, lower the heat, and simmer about 30 minutes until the chestnuts are very soft and tender. Remove from the pan and let cool for a minute. Purée in a food mill while still warm.

- The purée will keep for several days in the refrigerator but should be warmed before eating.
- To make chestnut pudding, cook the purée with a little agar-agar or arrowroot powder, place in individual serving bowls, and let harden before serving.

ROASTED SEEDS

Dry-roast sesame, sunflower, pumpkin, or squash seeds by placing several cups of seeds in a skillet. Turn on flame to medium low and stir gently with a wooden utensil for 10–15 minutes. Seeds are done when they turn crisp and darker in color and give off a fragrant aroma.

- For those whose condition permits, seeds may be lightly seasoned with a pinch of sea salt or a small volume of shoyu while roasting.

SWEET VEGETABLE JAM

2 cups onions
2 cups cabbage
2 cups carrots
2 cups hard winter squash
2–2½ cups water

Finely cut vegetables. Place into a large pot and add water. Bring to a boil, reduce to a low flame, and simmer for 4–5 hours or until vegetables cook down into a jam consistency. Add more water from time to time if necessary. Add a pinch of sea salt toward end of cooking and cook another 20 minutes. Pour into a glass jar and store in a refrigerator and use as needed.

- This jam may be made from the same combination of vegetables as sweet vegetable drink. For variety, it can be made with just one vegetable in which case it is called onion butter, carrot butter, or squash butter. Parsnips may also be used.

◉ Beverages

BANCHA TWIG TEA

Bancha twig tea is served as the principal beverage in most macrobiotic households. It is usually available dry-roasted and is sometimes called kukicha. It consists of the twigs or stems of the tea plant. Green tea is made from the leaves of the tea plant, while black tea is made from leaves that have been fermented. The leaves are high in caffeine, while the twigs and stems are virtually caffeine-free.

To make tea, add a tablespoon of twigs to 1 quart of water and bring to a boil. Lower flame and simmer for several minutes. Place tea strainer in cup and pour out tea. Twigs in strainer may be returned to teapot and used several times, adding a few fresh twigs each time.

ROASTED BARLEY TEA

To melt away animal fat from the body and to reduce fever. Please refer to ROASTED BROWN RICE TEA, below. This tea can also be purchased preroasted from some Oriental markets or natural food stores.

ROASTED BROWN RICE TEA

Take a cup of uncooked brown rice and dry-roast in a skillet over a medium flame for about 10 minutes or until a fragrant aroma is released. Stir and shake pan occasionally to prevent burning. Add 2–3 tablespoons of roasted rice to 1½ quarts of water. Bring to a boil, reduce flame, and simmer for 10–15 minutes.

- Other whole grains may be used to make teas in this way. ROASTED BARLEY TEA is especially recommended to help melt animal fat from the body or reduce fever. It is also very relaxing, especially in the spring or summer.

HOME REMEDIES

The primary home remedies recommended in this book, including special dishes, drinks, and external applications, are included in this section. The major conditions and disorders for which they are used or contraindicated are listed first, followed by recipes or descriptions of how to prepare or apply. The *amount, frequency,* and *duration* for each remedy (for example, take 1 cup a day for 3 days or apply for 4 hours every day for 1 month) may vary from condition to condition and person to person. See the individual ailments for suggested use, keeping in mind that these are general recommendations and may differ in individual cases.

Please note that the frequent recommendation "take 1 small cup" refers to a small teacup-size portion (about 6 ounces). However, in preparing recipes at the stove, "1 cup rice" or "4 cups water" refers to the usual measuring cup size (8 ounces).

As much as possible, contemporary names are given for the remedies. In many cases, however, the original term in Chinese, Japanese, Sanskrit, or other language has moved into English and is commonly used.

ACUPUNCTURE

General conditions and specific ailments, including headaches, heart problems, hypoglycemia, shoulder and neck problems, sleeping problems

Contraindications: for pregnant women who have a premonition of premature birth

Acupuncture involves the use of tiny needles on the body to activate energy flow through the meridians, release stagnation, and improve the health and functioning of internal organs and systems. A specialist or qualified practitioner is advised.

ADZUKI BEANS

Kidney problems, varicose veins

See recipe for this dish in the recipe chapter.

- For tight kidneys, sweeten with a little brown rice syrup at the end of cooking.

ADZUKI BEAN, BROWN RICE, DRIED DAIKON, AND SHIITAKE TEA

Kidney ailments; rheumatoid arthritis

Mix adzuki beans (2 parts), brown rice (2 parts), chopped dried shredded daikon (2 parts), and chopped dried shiitake mushroom (1 part). Add 3 to 4 times the total volume of water. Bring to a boil, lower the flame, and simmer for about 30 minutes. Strain and keep this tea in a thermos and drink as needed.

ADZUKI BEAN, SQUASH, AND KOMBU DISH

Anemia, diabetes, dizziness, gout, hypoglycemia, pancreatic problems

See the recipe for this dish in the recipe section.

ADZUKI BEAN TEA

Bone and joint disorders, hives, kidney cancer and other kidney problems

Place 1 cup of adzuki beans in a pot with a 2-inch strip of kombu. Soak 4 hours or overnight, then finely chop the kombu. Add 4 cups of water and bring to a boil. Lower the flame, cover, and simmer for approximately 20–30 minutes. Strain out the beans and drink the liquid while hot. You may continue cooking the beans longer with additional water until soft and edible for regular consumption.

ALZHEIMER DISH

Alzheimer's disease

Prepare the following: dried daikon (3 parts), kombu (or arame or hijiki) (1 part), and carrot (1 part). Cook ingredients together, adding a light shoyu taste at the end of cooking. Take one small dish every day or every other day at meal times.

- As a substitute, add 4 times as much water to the mixture, bring to a boil, and simmer for 20 minutes, adding a light salt or shoyu taste at the end of cooking. Drink and eat every day for 10 days, then 2–3 times per week for 2 months.

ALS STEW

Amyotrophic lateral sclerosis

Prepare a special stew consisting of soybeans soaked overnight (5 parts), carrot (1 part), lotus root (1 part), daikon (1 part), onion (1 part), cabbage (1 part), squash (1 part). Add twice as much water and boil for a long time. Add a light miso, shoyu, or salt taste at the end of cooking. Take every other day or 3 times a week for 2–3 months. This dish will keep for 1 day and may be reheated and used the following day.

AMASAKE

Depression, hypoglycemia, and many conditions, to relax and satisfy cravings for a sweet taste

Made from fermented sweet rice that is cooked and processed into a liquid, amasake is a high-quality grain-based complex sugar. It may be drunk hot or cold, thickened with kuzu as a pudding (see AMASAKE PUDDING in the recipe section), or added to recipes as a sweetener.

AME KUZU TEA

Headache in the back of the head and generally to relax

Dissolve 1 heaping teaspoon of kuzu in 2–3 tablespoons of cold water. Add 1 cup cold water to the dissolved kuzu. Add 1–2 teaspoons brown rice syrup or barley malt and ½ cup apple juice or cider. Bring to a boil over medium heat and stir constantly to avoid lumping. Reduce flame to very low and continue stirring until the tea is translucent. Drink while hot.

APPLE JUICE

Gallbladder problems, headache in the back of the head or deep inside, liver cancer, and many other conditions to relax and soothe

Grate an apple and press out its juice through a cheesecloth. Drink hot, warm, or at room temperature.

- For headache in general, dip a cloth in this juice, and rub it on the forehead to reduce a headache.

ARAME

Valve disorders

See ARAME in the recipe section.

BAKED KOMBU CONDIMENT

AIDS, mad cow disease

Bake kombu in the oven until it turns black. Crush to a powder in a suribachi. Sprinkle 1 teaspoon of this preparation on porridge, grains, or vegetables as a condiment or mix it into 1 cup of hot tea or hot water and then drink it.

- The baked kombu may be mixed with baked dried shiitake mushroom and roasted black sesame seeds that have been crushed in a suribachi.

BANCHA TWIG TEA

Used as a regular daily beverage and medicinally for many conditions, including atopy, kidney stones, gallstones, and prostate cancer

Place 1½ to 2 tablespoons of roasted twigs in 1½ quarts of spring water and bring to a boil. Keep unused twigs in an airtight jar until needed. When the water boils, reduce heat to low and simmer for several minutes. For a light tea, simmer 2 to 3 minutes. For a darker, stronger tea, simmer for 10 to 15 minutes. To serve, place a small bamboo or metal tea strainer in each cup and pour out the tea. Twigs in the strainer may be returned to the teapot and reused several times. You may cool the tea to room temperature after boiling and drink it in between and after meals.

BANCHA TWIG TEA WITH GOMASHIO

Brain tumor (during seizure, if conscious), nausea and vomiting

Put a teaspoon of gomashio in a small cup. Pour hot bancha twig tea into the cup, stirring constantly. Eat and drink to calm down a seizure.

BANCHA TWIG TEA WITH TEKKA

To neutralize excess sugar

Put a teaspoon of tekka in a small cup. Pour hot bancha twig tea into the cup, stirring constantly. This will instantly strengthen the blood and help offset extreme yin effects of too much sugar.

BANCHA TEA BATH

Atopy

Make a bath using a handful of bancha twig tea or bancha stem added to the bath water. (Tea stains the bathtub, so it is better not to keep the tea in the bathtub very long. Wash the tub well after using.)

BANCHA TEA COMPRESS

Atopy and other itchy conditions; conjunctivitis, stye, and other eye problems

Boil bancha twig tea as usual, soak a cotton towel in the tea, and squeeze out the liquid. Cool to room temperature and put it on the affected part for several minutes or until relief is experienced.

BANCHA TEA AND SEA SALT ENEMA

Constipation, obstructed bowels

As an alternative to commercial enemas, mix 1 gallon of bancha twig tea with 1 teaspoon of sea salt. Pour this liquid into a refillable enema bottle and then do the enema. Consult with someone who has experience doing enemas if you haven't done it before.

BARLEY MALT

Used as a high-quality sweetener for many regular recipes and medicinally to relax and keep blood sugar levels stable; diabetes, gallbladder problems, hypoglycemia

Barley malt is a grain-based, complex carbohydrate sweetener resembling molasses.

BEET JUICE

Kidney cancer, ovarian cancer

Beet juice may help relax overly contracted conditions.

Extract the juice from red beets and drink it either room temperature or heated. If in good health, an electric juicer may be used, provided the juice is allowed to sit for 3 minutes after juicing to allow the electric charge to disperse. If not in good health, it is better to finely grate the beets, or finely mince, and then mash in a suribachi. The juice is squeezed out using a cheese cloth. Depending on the condition, the juice can be drunk lightly salted or unseasoned.

- For liver conditions, add a little lemon in case of liver stagnation.

- Another drink can be made from grated daikon (1 part), grated beets (2 parts), dried shiitake (1 part), and 3 times as much water. Bring to a boil, simmer, and add 3–4 drops of lemon juice at the end of cooking.

BLACK SOYBEANS WITH CHESTNUTS

Bone and joint disorders

Wash 2 cups of black soybeans with cold water very quickly and put them in a bowl. Cover with about 6 cups of water in total. Add ½ teaspoon of sea salt and let the beans soak for several hours or overnight. Separately soak ½ cup of dried chestnuts. Put the beans in a pot on top of the dried chestnuts and pour in the salted soaking water. Bring to a boil, reduce the heat to medium-low, and simmer until the beans and chestnuts are about 90 percent done. During the simmering, add water when necessary as the liquid evaporates. As the beans and chestnuts cook, skim off and discard any skins that float to the surface, as well as any gray foam that surfaces. When the beans are about 90 percent done, add 1¼ to 1½ tablespoons of shoyu. Shake the pot gently up and down to evenly coat the beans with the juice and shoyu. Do not mix with a spoon. Shaking gives the skins a very shiny black appearance. Total cooking time for this dish is 2½ to 3 hours.

BLACK SOYBEAN TEA

Bone and joint disorders, bronchitis, diarrhea, kidney and bladder problems, and generally to relax

Place 1 cup of black soybeans in a pot with a 2-inch strip of kombu (soaked and finely chopped). Add 4 cups of water and bring to a boil. Lower the flame and simmer for 30 to 45 minutes. Strain the beans from the water. Drink this dark, slightly sweet liquid while hot. You may continue cooking the beans longer until soft and edible.

BLACK SOYBEANS WITH KOMBU AND DRIED DAIKON

Constipation

Combine black soybeans (3 parts), kombu (1 part), and dried daikon (2 parts). Cook for a long time until all ingredients are soft, following the basic recipe for BLACK SOYBEANS in the recipe chapter. Season toward the end of cooking with a small amount of sea salt and cook for another 20 minutes until done.

BODY SCRUB

A standard way-of-life recommendation for everyone, but especially those who are weak or stagnated, and for many health conditions

A body scrub will help activate blood circulation and promote the physical and mental energy flow of the whole body. It will also help clear and clean the skin, discharge fat accumulated under the skin, and open skin pores to promote smooth and regular elimination of any excess fat and toxins to the surface of the body. Usually recommended every morning and every evening, twice a day, before or after a shower or bath, but apart from it.

Dip a small cotton towel or cloth in hot water. Wring out excess water. Scrub the whole body, dipping the towel or cloth into hot water again when cool. Include the hands and feet, each finger and toe. The skin should become pink or slightly red. This result may take a few days to achieve if the skin is clogged with accumulated fats.

• A GINGER BODY SCRUB may be more effective for certain conditions.

BOILED SALAD

A daily way of preparing vegetables; for high blood pressure and many other conditions

See BOILED SALAD in the recipe section.

BREATHING EXERCISES

Beneficial to general health and well-being as well as for fatigue, heart problems, nervous conditions, and other ailments and disorders.

Simple exercises may be learned from introductory books. More complex exercises should be studied with an experienced practitioner.

BROWN RICE AND BARLEY PORRIDGE WITH GRATED DAIKON

Liver Cancer

Wash ½ cup of brown rice and ½ cup of barley. Place in a pressure cooker and add 3 to 4 cups of spring water. Soak 4 hours or overnight for more digestible porridge; add a pinch of sea salt, cover, then turn the flame to medium high and bring it to pressure. (If not soaking, turn the initial flame to low and bring to a boil slowly. Then add sea salt, cover, and bring up

to pressure.) Lower the flame, insert a flame deflector, and pressure-cook about 50 minutes. Let the pressure come down naturally, then remove the cover. Remove 1 cup of the porridge, and put in a small saucepan. Grate 1 tablespoon of fresh daikon and add to the saucepan. Bring to a boil and simmer 2 to 3 minutes until the daikon becomes sweet. Serve in a rice bowl.

• This porridge can be boiled for about 1 hour, using 5 cups of water.

BROWN RICE AND CORN PORRIDGE

Prostate cancer

Wash ½ cup of brown rice. Add ½ cup of fresh corn cut off the cob. Place in a pressure cooker, and add 3 to 4 cups of spring water. Soak 4 hours or overnight for more digestible porridge; add a pinch of sea salt, cover, then turn the flame to medium high and bring it to pressure. (If not soaking, turn the initial flame to low and bring to a boil slowly. Then add sea salt, cover, and bring up to pressure.) Lower the flame, insert a flame deflector, and pressure cook about 50 minutes. Let the pressure come down naturally, then remove the cover. Remove about 1 cup of the porridge, and put in a small saucepan. Grate about 1 tablespoon of fresh daikon, and add to the saucepan. Bring to a boil, and simmer 2 to 3 minutes until the daikon becomes sweet. Serve in a rice bowl.

• For lighter effects, this porridge can be boiled for about 1 hour, using 5 cups of water; or the corn can be added after the rice has cooked alone; or cook 1 cup of leftover brown rice with 1½ cups of water for 15 minutes until soft, add the fresh corn, and simmer for about 5 minutes, until the corn is soft and sweet.

BROWN RICE BALLS

Travel food, quick lunches, semifasting, and some medicinal conditions and emergencies such as colitis, spleen problems, and many others

See BROWN RICE BALLS in the recipe section.

BROWN RICE BRAN COMPRESS (NUKA)

Allergies, atopy (skin allergy), and other skin problems

Put several handfuls of rice bran (nuka) in a small cotton bag or cheesecloth and tie the bag with cotton string. Bring 2 to 3 quarts of water to a boil, and drop in the rice bran, shaking the bag from time to time. The water should become milky yellow. Soak the brown rice bran bag in lukewarm water and apply it on the itchy part. Rice bran is very nutritious for the skin. Applied in this form, it quiets down skin inflammation. Do not discard the water after using it for compresses. Use it instead for washing yourself or add it to a bath.

BROWN RICE CREAM

For general vitality and strength and many medicinal conditions and disorders

Follow the recipe for GENUINE BROWN RICE CREAM in the recipe section. You may boil for 2 hours, or pressure-cook for 1 hour. Let the rice cool sufficiently to be handled. Place the rice in a cheesecloth or clean unbleached muslin cloth, tie, and squeeze out the creamy liquid.

• Sweeten it at the end with a little brown rice syrup, barley malt, amasake, or apple juice.

BROWN RICE–GINGER COMPRESS

Used to dissolve stagnation in the lungs, chest, or for coughing, colds, or flu

This compress is mild and soothing and will help open the chest or other congested region. It is also very fragrant. The brown rice–ginger compress may be made in two ways:

1. Make basic pressure-cooked brown rice (see the recipe section). Mash a small amount in a suribachi until it forms a paste. Grate an equal volume of ginger and mix it thoroughly with the rice. Place it on the affected region and cover with cotton. Leave on for up to several hours and repeat, if necessary.

2. Prepare by roasting rice in pan and add a few slices of raw gingerroot. Wrap the rice and ginger mixture in a cheesecloth or other cotton and apply it on the chest. Leave on for up to several hours and repeat, if necessary.

BROWN RICE JUICE (OMOYU)

Bone and joint disorders, kidney and bladder functions

This is the liquid that rises to the surface after cooking soft brown rice. See BROWN RICE in the recipe section.

BROWN RICE MILK (SWEETENED)

Stimulates the appetite for conditions and disorders such as bone cancer

This beverage is made from grains, beans, vegetables, and sea vegetables. In a big pot, mix the following ingredients: brown rice (40 percent), sweet brown rice (10 percent), beans (10 percent) (selecting among adzuki beans, soybeans, and others), other grains (10 percent) (which can include barley, millet, corn, and others), chopped vegetables (15 percent) (selecting among winter squash or pumpkin, onion, daikon, carrot, cabbage; daikon leaves or turnip leaves), seaweed (10 percent) (selecting among nori, wakame, arame, and others), and apple (5 percent).

Then add 5 to 7 times the total volume of water, bring to a boil, lower the flame, and cook it a long time, on a flame deflector, to make a porridge-like cream. Shut off the fire and allow it to cool to a moderate temperature.

Wrap it with gauze or cheesecloth and squeeze out the sticky cream. Add water to the cream and cook it for 2 to 3 minutes. Then sweeten the grain milk with amasake, brown rice syrup, or barley malt to taste and drink it.

BROWN RICE, MILLET, BUCKWHEAT, AND VEGETABLE PORRIDGE

Lymphoma

Make a porridge following the basic BROWN RICE PORRIDGE recipe with the following ingredients: lightly roasted brown rice (3 parts), lightly roasted millet (2 parts), lightly roasted buckwheat groats (1 part), and chopped vegetables (3 parts, which is a combination of chopped burdock, carrot, daikon, cabbage, and onion), along with a small piece of kombu, and water.

BROWN RICE–MISO PLASTER

An external application to reduce inflammation, swelling, or itching; cuts and wounds

Cook brown rice, and let it cool. Then mash it to a paste in a suribachi. Add an equal volume of miso and thoroughly mix the two together.

- The rice plaster alone can calm down inflammatory processes.
- Miso alone can be applied externally for bleeding, cuts and wounds, itchy skin diseases, or any kind of swelling.

BROWN RICE MOCHI IN MISO SOUP

Gives strength, increases energy, and strengthens the blood generally or for conditions such as anemia, mental conditions, nervous conditions, and spinal cord disorders

Prepare ½-inch squares of PAN-FRIED MOCHI with or without oil, using the basic recipe. Meanwhile, cook soup using the basic MISO SOUP recipe. When the mochi is softly melted, place it in a soup bowl. Immediately pour the hot miso soup over the mochi.

- For softer mochi, simmer it for a few minutes in the miso soup.
- Uncooked mochi may be used instead of pan-fried.
- Grate mochi into the soup for a creamy texture.

BROWN RICE MOCHI FRIED IN OIL

Anemia

Spread sesame oil on the bottom of a frying pan and heat it up. When the oil has spread out completely, add brown rice mochi that has been chopped into 1-inch squares. Cover and fry until soft. Turn the mochi over and fry for another few minutes.

- Dip the mochi in kinako (roasted soybean flour) sweetened with brown rice syrup or barley malt.
- Add the oil-fried mochi to miso soup and cook it at the same time.
- Wrap the oil-fried mochi in narrow nori strips that have been dipped in shoyu.

BROWN RICE PORRIDGE (KAYU)

A soft porridge used for general strength and vitality and many medicinal conditions and disorders, including colds, flu, fever, and others

Wash 1 cup brown rice and add 10 cups spring water. Cook with a small pinch of sea salt, following the recipe for BOILED BROWN RICE in the recipe section. Not all the water will be absorbed. The rice should be creamy, and some of the grains should still be visible after cooking. In case the water boils over while the rice is cooking, turn off the heat and allow the rice to cool off. Then turn on the heat again and continue to cook until done. The heavy liquid that rises to the top of the porridge is called *omoyu* or BROWN RICE JUICE. It is especially good for babies. The porridge itself is called *kayu*.

- To pressure-cook, use 1 cup of brown rice and 5 cups of spring water with a small pinch of sea salt. Follow the basic PRESSURE-COOKED BROWN RICE recipe above.
- Kayu can be cooked from leftover brown rice. Simply add water, bring to a boil, and simmer 10 to 15 minutes until soft.

BROWN RICE PORRIDGE WITH GRATED DAIKON

Cervical cancer

Make BROWN RICE PORRIDGE, season lightly with sea salt or miso, and add 20 to 30 percent grated daikon. Simmer for about 2 minutes.

BROWN RICE PORRIDGE WITH GRATED DAIKON AND LEMON

Ovarian cancer

Make BROWN RICE PORRIDGE and add 20 to 30 percent grated daikon. Simmer for about 2 minutes. Season with a pinch of sea salt or shoyu and squeeze in a few drops of lemon juice, then mix well.

BROWN RICE PORRIDGE WITH GRATED DAIKON AND UMEBOSHI

Colon cancer

Into BROWN RICE PORRIDGE mix grated daikon and chopped umeboshi plum (from which the pit has been removed). Simmer for 3 minutes.

BROWN RICE PORRIDGE WITH GRATED LOTUS ROOT

Lung cancer

Add 20 percent to 30 percent grated lotus root to thin brown rice porridge and stir well. Simmer on a low flame for 2 to 3 minutes.

BROWN RICE SYRUP

Used as a natural sweetener for ordinary cooking, to relax the body, and for many medicinal conditions, including dry coughs

Brown rice syrup is a grain-based, complex-carbohydrate sweetener resembling honey. Use as is; put on mochi, arepas, or rice cakes; or mix a small volume in tea and warm up for a few minutes.

BROWN RICE WITH MARINATED DRIED DAIKON

Skin cancer

Finely chop dried shredded daikon and marinate it for 1 hour in shoyu that has been diluted by adding 2 times the amount of water. Pressure-cook it together with brown rice, mak-

ing it softer. The amount of dried daikon should be 5 to 10 percent of the volume of the brown rice.

BROWN RICE WITH WATER-SAUTÉED DAIKON & DAIKON LEAVES

Stomach cancer

Finely chop dried shredded daikon and daikon leaves. Sauté with water. Season lightly with shoyu. Mix vegetables into already-cooked brown rice and set aside for 3 to 4 minutes before eating.

BUCKWHEAT PLASTER

Used to reduce swelling, including for allergies, appendicitis, liver problems, pancreatic problems, and prostate cancer

This traditional Far Eastern remedy helps to draw out water or other excess fluids that are retained by the body. It may be applied to swollen areas on the legs, arms, abdomen, etc. Buckwheat, which is a very yang, grainlike plant, attracts and draws out the more yin water or liquid. It is more effective to make fresh flour from whole buckwheat groats than to use packaged buckwheat flour. The energy is much stronger; however, if groats are not available, you may use store-bought flour.

Apply first a HOT TOWEL COMPRESS or GINGER COMPRESS to the affected region to make the area hot before applying the buckwheat plaster. The plaster should be as stiff, hot, and dry as possible.

Mix buckwheat flour with a little sesame oil and enough hot water to form a stiff, hard dough. Spread the dough on a cotton cloth, about ½ inch thick. Apply the dough side (not the cloth side) directly to the swollen area. Remove after one to two hours. As the plaster draws out the fluid, the dough will become soft and watery. When this happens, replace the plaster with a new, stiff dough.

BUCKWHEAT, SPROUTS, SHIITAKE, DAIKON, DAIKON LEAVES, AND SCALLION DRINK

Liver problems

This drink will harmonize the function of the liver. Prepare with buckwheat groats (2 parts), bean sprouts or other sprouts (2–3 parts), dried shiitake mushroom (1 part), fresh daikon (1 part), daikon leaves or any other leafy greens (2 parts), and scallions (1 part). Chop the vegetables finely and add 5 times as much water to the mixture. Boil and simmer about 30 minutes. The buckwheat absorbs water, so you may need to add more liquid during cooking.

CABBAGE AND CARROT JUICE

Breast cancer

For medicinal purposes, it is preferable to juice vegetables by hand rather than with an electric juicer, which destroys much of their vitamin C. Very finely chop or grate the cabbage and the carrot. Then squeeze out the juice by wringing out the gratings wrapped in cheesecloth. If the cabbage is still not fine enough, it may have to be mashed in a suribachi.

Combine fresh cabbage juice (2 parts) with fresh carrot juice (1 part), gently stir, and drink.

• Add a small amount of water and cook for 2 to 3 minutes before drinking.

CABBAGE JUICE

Bladder cancer

In case of pain in the abdomen, make raw CABBAGE JUICE. Very finely chop or grate raw cabbage. Mash it in a suribachi, and squeeze out the raw juice from the gratings wrapped in cheesecloth. Then simmer it slightly, for about 3 minutes.

CABBAGE LEAF COMPRESS

Ankle problems, brain tumor, breast cancer (swelling)

The leaves of large, leafy green vegetables are very helpful in cooling down fever, neutralizing inflammation, and relieving burns and bruises. Sometimes just putting leaves (either big ones or ones that grow upward) such as cabbage leaves on the head, chest, or arms will provide immediate relief. Cabbage is particularly good because it is a more yang vegetable and has drawing or contractive power. This compress is used to cool down quickly, and it can be recycled by dipping the used leaves in cold water and reusing. The CABBAGE LEAF PLASTER, on the other hand, is used for a longer time to dissolve lumps and facilitate healing.

Carefully remove whole leaves from a head of cabbage or Chinese cabbage. Flatten them slightly by scoring the spine horizontally with a vegetable knife. Then apply the leaves 2 layers thick on the hot or inflamed area. They may be held on for a short time by wrapping with a piece of cheesecloth. As the leaves become heated, they may be cooled in cold water and reused.

- For brain tumor, ice cubes cannot be used. Keep changing the leaves to cool down the affected area of the brain and reduce swelling.

CABBAGE LEAF PLASTER

Breast cancer (arm swelling after lymph node removal), rheumatoid arthritis (inflammation or redness), spleen problems, thyroid and throat cancer

The CABBAGE LEAF COMPRESS above is used in the short term to cool down, and it can be recycled by dipping the used leaves in cold water and reusing. The CABBAGE LEAF PLASTER, on the other hand, is used for a longer time to dissolve lumps and facilitate healing. Carefully remove whole leaves from a head of cabbage or Chinese cabbage. Flatten them slightly by scoring the spine horizontally with a vegetable knife. Then apply the leaves 2 layers thick on the affected area. They may be held on for 2 to 3 hours by wrapping with a piece of cheesecloth. They are generally not reuseable.

- For breast cancer arm swelling, wrap the entire swollen arm area in cabbage leaves.
- For rheumatoid arthritis, in case of inflammation or redness on the hands, fingers, heels, or other region, apply a fresh raw cabbage leaf plaster directly by cutting small pieces. Use it 2 to 3 hours a couple of times a day; or it can be applied when you go to sleep and kept on overnight.

- For thyroid and throat cancer, raw cabbage leaf can be applied directly to the throat.

CABBAGE PLASTER

Colitis, hemorrhoids, hepatitis, hernia, irritable bowel syndrome, lymphoma, rheumatoid arthritis, throat cancer

This differs from CABBAGE LEAF PLASTER in that the leaves are chopped and mashed and made into a paste with white flour. It has a more concentrated effect and may be used at once or after whole leaves have absorbed the initial heat.

Finely chop and mash fresh raw cabbage; add 10–20 percent white flour to it to make a paste. Spread it 1 inch thick on a cotton cloth and directly apply it to the affected area.

CABBAGE TEA

Lymphoma (sweating)

Finely chop cabbage leaves. Place in a pot, cover with spring water, and bring to a boil. Then lower the flame and simmer until the cabbage becomes soft and sweet. Strain off the cooking liquid as CABBAGE TEA.

- For lymphoma (sweating), cool the tea to room temperature before drinking.

CAMELLIA OIL

Atopy and other skin conditions

Apply pure camellia oil to the skin to relieve the itching, burning, and redness of this skin allergy.

CARBONIZED UMEBOSHI and CARBONIZED UMEBOSHI SEEDS

Colds, diarrhea, stomach ulcer, intestinal tuberculosis, intestinal cancer

See also BAKED KOMBU and UMEBOSHI PLUM. Bake several umeboshi in the oven under the broiler until their outer surface turns black. Crush this baked umeboshi meat to a powder. Take this powder with a tablespoon of hot water or BANCHA TWIG TEA. For CARBONIZED UMEBOSHI SEEDS, roast the seeds inside the pit in the oven at a very high temperature. Then crush them into a black powder. Store in a jar. It is a very yang preparation. Take 1 teaspoon in BANCHA TWIG TEA for stomach or intestinal troubles. It can also be sprinkled on rice or other grains as a condiment.

CARP PLASTER

Acute pneumonia with high, life-threatening fever

This plaster has traditionally been used primarily for pneumonia. Its ability to reduce fever is far stronger than that of ice or tofu. It can reduce very high fevers of any origin. It is contraindicated for mild fevers.

Obtain a carp of about 1 pound in weight. If you get a live carp, try to collect its blood before crushing the carp into a plaster. Knock it unconscious. Remove its head and collect the blood in a cup. Then wrap the carp in a cloth and crush it with a hammer as if you were crushing ice. If you have a dead carp, do not use its blood. Have the patient drink the fresh carp blood, but only in a very small quantity: ½ to 1 sake cup for an adult, and ½ or less sake cup for a child. It should be drunk as it is, before it coagulates.

Apply the plaster to the chest, if possible on the back as well as on the front, but do not cover the heart area. Do not apply the carp meat directly on the skin, because this feels too cold. Instead, leave the crushed carp in the cloth.

This plaster makes the body temperature drop very quickly. It is necessary to take the temperature every 15 to 20 minutes and to remove the plaster as soon as the temperature reaches 98 degrees Fahrenheit. It may take 1, 3, or up to 6 hours to reach this, and sometimes another fresh plaster may need to be applied before the temperature drops sufficiently.

- If a carp is not available, use any large yin fish, especially a freshwater fish.
- As an alternative, use yin meat: raw fatty hamburger while still very cold from being stored in a freezer.
- A TARO PLASTER, TOFU PLASTER, LEAFY GREENS PLASTER, or ice pack may be used if no fish or meat is available.

CARROT-DAIKON DRINK

Bone and joint disorders, high cholesterol, gallstones, kidney stones, kidney and bladder problems, kidney cancer, liver troubles, lung problems, muscle problems, pancreatic problems, post-traumatic stress disorder, and upper digestive cancers

This drink was first developed for liver troubles, to help discharge eggs, cheese, and beef fat. But it is helpful in dissolving fat deposits anywhere within the body and quickly reducing high cholesterol. It also helps dissolve calcified stones in such areas as kidneys and gallbladder. It is now recommended for many chronic conditions, including many forms of heart disease and tumors.

Daikon is relatively yin and gives a dissolving effect, while carrot is relatively yang and is added to strengthen and help move energy down in the body. However, if continuously taken together, they tend to weaken. By adding umeboshi and nori, this drink can be taken for a long time: every day for 10 days or every other day for 3 weeks.

Finely grate ½ cup each of carrots and daikon. Place in a saucepan. Do not let the gratings sit for a long time. Add 2 cups of water and bring to a gentle boil. Add ⅓ of a sheet of nori and ½ of an umeboshi plum; cook together with the grated vegetables. Simmer for about 3 minutes and add a few drops of shoyu toward the end. Eat and drink the vegetables and broth.

- Add ⅓ cup of grated lotus root, especially for lung or lymphatic conditions.
- A little scallion or ginger may be added to the basic recipe if desired.
- This drink may also be used to eliminate fat and oil that accompanies stagnated conditions.

CARROT JUICE

Used to relax the pancreas and to recover from excessive sweet consumption; pancreatic cancer

An occasional beverage, carrot juice may be taken 2 to 3 times a week, if desired. Juicing in an electric juicer destroys some vitamins; therefore, for those who are healing, it is recommended to juice by hand.

Wash 1 to 3 fresh carrots and finely grate them. Place the gratings in a cheesecloth and wring to squeeze out the juice. Collect the liquid. The gratings can be added to soups, stews, salads, and other dishes. The carrot juice may be drunk warm, cool, or at room temperature.

CHANTING

ALS, nervous disorders, and many other conditions

A traditional practice recommended for daily usage along with singing happy songs and reading aloud. It opens the chest, makes better breathing and circulation, elevates the mood, and activates body energy. Basic chants include the prolonged utterance of *su*, which contributes to peace and harmony of physical and mental functions and *aum (om)*, the traditional Sanskrit syllable that harmonizes the energy centers in the central channel from the top of the head to the midbrain, throat, heart, solar plexus, intestinal center, and reproductive region.

CHINESE MEDICINE

Bone fractures and dislocations, hypoglycemia, and many other conditions

Dating back thousands of years, Chinese medicine is based on a deep understanding of yin and yang and its application to dietary practice, environment, and way of life influences. Practitioners of Chinese medicine today tend to

focus primarily on ACUPUNCTURE, MOXI-
BUSTION, herbal medicine, and other complementary treatments. In some cases, these
methods may complement the macrobiotic
guidelines. An experienced practitioner should
be consulted.

COLD TOWEL COMPRESS

Brain tumor, headache (frontal), kidney
stone pain, tonsilitis, and throat problems

Cold towels can be used to relieve tension
and reduce pain caused by too much sugar,
sweets, soft drinks, fruit, ice cream, and other
more extreme yin foods. For example, a headache in the front of the head is usually caused by
these types of foods, and applying a COLD
TOWEL COMPRESS will help ease the ache.
In some cases, hot and cold towels may be alternated every few minutes. For example, leg
cramps (usually caused by extreme yin foods
but characterized by yang cramping) can be
treated in this way. First massage toward and
immediately above the cramping region (but
not on it directly). Then apply alternately towels
drenched in hot and cold water.

To do a cold towel compress, dip plain cotton towels in cold water, wring out, and apply to
affected areas. Remove towels as they lose their
strength, replacing them with fresh towels for
up to 7 minutes or until the area becomes pink.
See also HOT TOWEL COMPRESS.

• For brain tumor: If a seizure occurs, or consciousness is lost similar to epilepsy, cover
the whole head, including the forehead, with
a cold towel compress. Massage the toes well
(especially the first toe).

• For headache (frontal): Apply on forehead
for a frontal headache.

COOKED BLACK SESAME SEEDS

Constipation

Simmer washed black sesame seeds in water
and season with a small amount of sea salt.

CORN SOUP WITH LOTUS SEEDS

Cervical cancer

Combine 50 percent corn, 10 percent onion,
10 percent daikon, 10 percent soaked lotus seeds,
15 percent daikon leaves, and 5 percent shiitake
mushroom or nori. Add 3 times the total volume
of water, bring to a boil, and simmer until soft.
Season with miso, shoyu, or sea salt.

DAIKON AND DAIKON LEAVES QUICK PICKLES

Colon cancer

Follow the recipe for PRESSED SALAD,
using finely sliced daikon and daikon leaves and
sea salt. After pressing for ½ day or longer, rinse
the salad with water to remove the excess salt
before serving. Eat a small amount of this
preparation with your meals.

DAIKON LEAVES QUICK PICKLES

Prostate cancer

Eat light DAIKON LEAF PICKLES. These
are pickled briefly in sea salt as a PRESSED
SALAD or BRINE PICKLES. See the recipe sec-

tion. If they are salty, rinse off the excess salt before eating.

DAIKON HIP BATH

Women's reproductive organ conditions

This treatment warms the body and is good for women's reproductive organs, skin problems, drawing out excess fat and oil from the body, and discharging body odors arising from consumption of animal foods.

Dry fresh daikon leaves in a shady place until they are brown and brittle. If daikon leaves are not available, use turnip leaves or a handful of arame sea vegetable. Place about 4 or 5 bunches of dried leaves, or a handful of arame, in a large pot. Add 4 or 5 quarts of water and bring to a boil. Reduce to a medium flame and simmer until water is brown. Add approximately 1 cup of any kind of sea salt to the pot and stir well to dissolve. Pour the hot liquid into a small tub or bath. Add water until the bath level is waist-high when sitting in the tub. Keep the temperature as hot as possible and cover your upper body with a large towel to induce perspiration. Stay in the bath for 10 to 20 minutes or until the hip becomes very red and hot. Keep this hip area warm after coming out of the bath. This bath is best and most effective just before bedtime, but at least an hour after eating.

• If daikon or other leaves or arame is not available, do a salt hip bath, following the process outlined above, using a handful of any kind of sea salt in the hot bath water.

DAIKON NISHIME WITH MISO TASTE

See the recipe for NISHIME-STYLE VEGETABLES (WATERLESS COOKING) in the recipe section. Simply use daikon and kombu as ingredients, and season with diluted miso rather than shoyu.

DAIKON NORI GINGER TEA

Kidney and bladder conditions

Add 2 tablespoons of grated daikon, one roasted crushed nori sheet, and ½ teaspoon of grated ginger (seasoned with 1 teaspoon of shoyu) to several cups of water, bring to a boil, and let boil for 3 to 5 minutes. Drink 1 or 2 cups to stimulate the bladder and proper urinary passage.

DAIKON PLASTER

Ankle problems, bruises, fever, and heart disease (yang cause)

In the Orient, daikon is the most popular vegetable used in cooking, pickling, and medicinal preparations. The purpose of this plaster is to dissolve hard animal fat on the periphery of the body, such as chicken fat, dairy fat, or anything clogging the capillaries beneath the skin and blocking circulation. It is also good for bruises, surface burns, fevers, inflammations, or swellings. It helps to cool down and to clean up internal bleeding. Daikon has a pungent, stimulating effect. Use only for a short time until the skin becomes red. Although it begins to irritate if left on too long, the daikon plaster is milder than the mustard plaster. Because it is pungent, don't add grated ginger, as with some other plasters. If it becomes too hot, take it off.

The daikon plaster is a simple, quick application for local stagnation, to improve blood and energy circulation. It has a cooling effect that is about as effective as ice. Apply this plaster in particular on bruised areas. Not only will it cool down the pain, but any internal bleeding will quickly be cleared up. For a large bruise, repeat the treatment several days in a row.

Grate several ounces of daikon (or an equal amount of turnip if daikon is not available). Do not use the juice. Mix with a little flour. Apply this grated root directly on the area to be treated, and leave it on for 15 to 30 minutes. For large bruises, repeat for several days.

DENTIE

TMJ and related problems, cuts and wounds, nosebleed, ruptured spleen

Dentie can be used for all teeth and gum problems with a yin cause, as well as to eliminate mouth odor, heal cuts and wounds, stop nosebleeds, and treat other ailments. It is made from the calyx of the eggplant, or the top part, which is attached to the stem. It can be prepared at home by roasting the top parts of the eggplant slowly until they pulverize. Add 30 to 50 percent roasted sea salt. It is also available ready-made in the natural foods store as a black powder or a toothpaste combined with mint or other ingredients. The black powder is the strongest for healing purposes. It is a little messy, so be careful to wash the sink clean of black streaks and smudges.

DO-IN

For many conditions and general good health

A form of self-massage that originated in the Far East that is based on harmonizing the energy flow through the meridians. It can be practiced as little as 5 to 10 minutes daily for usual good health or modified to strengthen specific organs and functions.

DRIED DAIKON AND SHIITAKE TEA

Pancreatic cancer with swelling in abdomen, stiff shoulders, fever

Soak and finely chop dried, shredded daikon (3 parts) and dried shiitake mushroom (1 part). Place in a pot and add 3 times the total amount of water. Bring to a boil, lower the flame, and simmer for 20 to 25 minutes. Strain and save the tea in a thermos or refrigerator.

DRIED DAIKON, DAIKON LEAVES, AND SHIITAKE TEA

Prostate cancer, uterine cancer

After soaking, finely chop and combine dried shredded daikon (3 parts), daikon leaves (2 parts), and dried shiitake mushroom (1 part). Add 3 times the total volume of water, bring to a boil, and simmer for about 25 minutes. Strain and keep this broth in a thermos.

DRIED DAIKON, DAIKON LEAVES, ROASTED BROWN RICE, AND SHIITAKE TEA

Colon cancer

Combine dried shredded daikon (3 parts), daikon leaves (3 parts), lightly roasted brown rice (2 parts), and dried shiitake mushroom (1 part). Add 3 times the total volume of water, bring to a boil, and simmer on a low flame for 20 to 25 minutes. Strain the liquid and save this broth in a thermos.

DRIED DAIKON, DRIED DAIKON LEAVES AND BURDOCK TEA

Lymphoma

Finely chop soaked dried shredded daikon (3 parts), soaked dried daikon leaves (2 parts), and burdock (1 part). Add 3 times the total volume of water, bring to a boil, and simmer for 25 minutes over a low flame. Strain and put this tea in a thermos.

DRIED DAIKON, DRIED DAIKON LEAVES, BURDOCK, SHIITAKE, AND CABBAGE TEA

Ascites resulting from liver cancer

Finely chop soaked dried shredded daikon (3 parts), burdock (1 part), soaked dried shiitake mushroom (1 part), cabbage (1 part), and soaked dried daikon leaves (2 parts). Add 3 times the total volume of water, bring to a boil, and simmer for about 25 minutes. Put this tea in a thermos.

DRIED DAIKON, DRIED DAIKON LEAVES, SHIITAKE, DRIED LOTUS ROOT, AND ROASTED BROWN RICE TEA

Bladder cancer

Soak dried daikon (2 parts), dried daikon leaves (2 parts), dried shiitake mushroom (1 part), and dried lotus root (1 part). Finely chop all ingredients. Mix with 2 parts lightly roasted brown rice. Add 3 times the total volume of water, bring to a boil, and simmer for about 25 to 30 minutes. Strain and store in a thermos or refrigerator.

DRIED DAIKON LEAVES COMPRESS

Atopy, allergies

Boil dried daikon leaves in water and cool it to room temperature. Soak cotton gauze in the dried daikon water and apply it for about 2 to 3 hours. During that time, change the gauze frequently.

DRIED DAIKON, SHIITAKE, AND CABBAGE TEA

Breast cancer

Finely chop soaked dried shredded daikon (3 parts), soaked dried shiitake mushroom (1 part), and fresh cabbage (2 parts). Mix in a pot and add 3 times the total volume of water. Bring to a boil and simmer on a low flame for 20 to 25 minutes. Strain and save this broth in a thermos.

DRIED DAIKON, SHIITAKE, AND KOMBU TEA

Skin cancer, melanoma

Soak dried, shredded daikon (3 parts), dried shiitake mushroom (1 part), and kombu (1 part). Finely chop and mix in a pot. Add 3 times the total volume of water, and simmer on a low flame for 20 to 25 minutes. Strain and drink the liquid.

DRIED DAIKON, SHIITAKE, AND ONION TEA

Ovarian cancer

Finely chop and combine soaked dried shredded daikon (3 parts), soaked dried shiitake mushroom (1 part), and fresh onion (2 parts). Add 3 times the total volume of water, bring to a boil, and simmer for 20 to 25 minutes. Strain and keep this broth in a thermos or refrigerator.

DRIED DAIKON, SHIITAKE, CABBAGE, BURDOCK, AND ROASTED RICE TEA

Brain tumor, swelling with brain tumor

Combine soaked dried shredded daikon (3 parts), soaked dried shiitake mushroom (1 part), burdock or carrot (2 parts), and roasted brown rice (2 parts). Add 3 times the total volume of water, bring to a boil, and simmer for about 25 minutes. Strain and save this liquid in a thermos or refrigerator.

DRIED DAIKON, SHIITAKE, DRIED LOTUS ROOT, AND CARROT LEAF TEA

Lung cancer

Finely chop and combine soaked dried shredded daikon (3 parts), soaked dried shiitake mushroom (1 part), soaked dried lotus root (2 parts), and carrot leaves (2 parts). Add 3 times the total volume of water, bring to a boil, and simmer on a low flame for 20 to 30 minutes. Strain and save the broth in a thermos or refrigerator.

DRIED DAIKON TEA

Ear problems, fever, headache (back or sides of head) and migraines, lymphoma (sweating), and seasonal affective disorder

This tea is good for dissolving all fatty substances, and a small cup can be taken daily for 2 to 3 months. Dried daikon is stronger than fresh daikon and can be used for a longer period of time. Dried daikon can be made at home from the roots in your garden or purchased at the natural foods store. Often it is sold shredded in packages imported from Japan.

Combine soaked dried shredded daikon (1 part) to water (4 parts). Bring to a boil, reduce flame, and simmer 15 to 30 minutes. Toward the end of cooking, add a pinch of sea salt and let simmer until done.

- This drink is good for headaches in the back and sides of the head and migraines. For ear problems, give this drink and a GINGER COMPRESS on the kidney and ear. It can be used after delivery by mothers whose infants are jaundiced.

- A person needs seasoning with this drink, or the tea makes them too weak. The standard method of seasoning is with a pinch of salt or small piece of kombu.
- For liver/gallbladder conditions, you may use umeboshi plum instead.
- For lung or liver conditions, use shiso leaves.
- For lungs, add lotus root.
- The drink is already yin, so do not add sweetener.
- This tea is often prepared with lotus root, shiitake mushroom, and kombu. The shiitake helps to dissolve fat and protein deposits, while the kombu gives minerals and counters the weakening effect of daikon and shiitake.

EGG OIL

Heart failure, to increase vitality

This is the oil that is released when eggs are carbonized. Egg oil can simply be prepared in a pan. Roast 5 egg yolks in a skillet until they are completely black. Oil will appear during this process.

ENEMA

See SALT WATER ENEMA and BANCHA TEA and SEA SALT ENEMA.

FASTING

Headaches, gallbladder problems, and liver problems

It is occasionally helpful to practice fasting, but it must be limited to 1 week to 10 days.

Take water or tea at that time. See also SEMI-FASTING.

FOOT BATH

Used to create warmth, promote circulation, and move energy to different regions of the body for various conditions and disorders

A foot bath helps to stimulate blood and energy flow and warm the body. Foot baths may be divided into two major types: those with hot water and those with cold water (actually the water is at room temperature). Generally, hot foot baths are given for conditions caused by more yang, contractive factors or a combination of yin and yang, while cold foot baths are usually given for conditions caused by more yin, expansive factors. (Those with yin conditions are often weak, cold, or have poor circulation to begin with, so room-temperature water is better than cool or cold water.)

In turn, foot baths may be made with (1) plain water, (2) water to which a tiny amount of ginger juice has been added (see GINGER COMPRESS for instructions on how to make ginger juice from grated, squeezed-out gingerroot), (3) water to which a handful of salt (any kind) has been added, (4) water to which both ginger and salt have been added, and (5) water in which sea vegetables have been cooked. Each type has slightly different uses and effects.

Ordinary hot water may be used for overly tight conditions, to relax and bring the energy in the body up. For example, this is good for prostate problems, tight kidneys, and stress. Contraindication: ovarian cancer.

Ginger may be added to hot water to increase warmth and circulation and bring the energy to the periphery or outside. For example, this type of foot bath may be helpful for someone with arthritis, rheumatism, Alzheimer's disease, or other condition arising from extreme yin and yang factors. Contraindication: ovarian cancer.

Salt may be added to either hot or cold water to bring the energy down and inside. For example, a salted hot foot bath is helpful for someone with kidney tightness or insomnia (especially at night after 2 A.M.). A cold (room-temperature) saltwater foot bath is beneficial to help relieve diabetes, kidney weakness, or insomnia (especially at night before 2 A.M.).

Salt may be added to ginger water to bring the energy inside and to balance and control the activating power of the ginger. For example, a hot ginger salt water foot bath may be prepared for someone with hypoglycemia to stabilize and balance extremes of yin and yang that give rise to frequent mood swings. It may also be helpful for a hardened breast tumor on the right side of the body caused by excessive cheese, chicken, eggs, and meat consumption, in order to bring the energy up and out in a gradual manner.

The water from cooked sea vegetables (boiled, strained, and cooled to room temperature) may be used to prepare a foot bath with a slightly more strengthening effect. For example, a cold (room-temperature) foot bath with sea vegetable water may be prepared for someone with diabetes or an inflammatory breast tumor on the left side of the body to bring the energy down and inside. A hot foot bath with sea vegetables is helpful for someone with cervical, testicular, or other external reproductive organ difficulties, to bring the energy up and inside.

The foot bath is generally administered just before bed. To prepare, place a basin or tub in the bathtub or sink and fill with about 6 inches of hot or room-temperature water. Add juice from squeezed-out ginger, a handful of salt, or the liquid from cooked sea vegetables (such as kombu, wakame, hijiki, or arame), if applicable. Place basin or tub on floor and immerse the feet ankle deep in the water for 3 to 5 minutes. Dry feet with a towel and go to bed.

Ideally, the foot bath should be made fresh each time. However, ginger water or sea vegetable water will keep for up to 24 hours and may be reused, though its energy will dissipate.

- Note: the yin/yang principle is very clear and simple. However, practically, it takes time to master and apply correctly. If you are uncertain of which type of foot bath to take, generally a salt hot water foot bath moderates extremes and contributes to overall balance and harmony.
- Avoid using ginger in a foot bath if you have a swollen, inflamed, or infected condition.
- It is best to consult with an experienced macrobiotic teacher or counselor about the proper use of a foot bath for any cancerous condition.

FRESH APPLE JUICE

Heart problems (yang), jaundice

If health is good, 1 to 2 cups can be taken per week, either heated, at room temperature, or cold.

For general good health, it is acceptable to prepare the juice from fresh apples with an electric juicer (waiting about 5 to 10 minutes for the vibration to settle before drinking) or using store-bought organic apple juice. But for sickness, it is best to finely grate an apple, wrap the gratings in cheesecloth, and squeeze out the juice by hand.

For jaundice, sour green (Granny Smith) apples are used.

FRESH APPLE JUICE AND SWEET VEGETABLE DRINK

Pancreatic cancer with jaundice

Combine equal amounts of FRESH APPLE JUICE to SWEET VEGETABLE DRINK, and simmer for about 2 minutes.

FRIED BROWN RICE

Anemia, heart failure, and varicose veins

See FRIED RICE WITH VEGETABLES in the recipe section.

FRIED MISO

Diabetes, eye diseases, and tuberculosis

Fry 3½ ounces of miso in a large tablespoon of sesame oil. Add finely chopped leek or scallion and some grated orange peel. Eat 1 teaspoon of this with rice or vegetables. This is a medicinal condiment, not to be used daily by healthy people.

FRIED RICE BALLS

Bone and joint conditions

Follow the instructions for BROWN RICE BALLS in the recipe section. Form a handful of rice into a solid ball. If desired, press a hole in the center with the thumb and place a piece of umeboshi plum inside. Close hole and knead rice ball again until it is compact. Rice triangles are easier to fry because of their flat faces; cup your hands into a V-shape when forming them. Pour a small amount of sesame oil into a frying pan and pan-fry the rice balls until slightly brown. Turn over and fry the other face. Season with shoyu, and eat hot.

GENUINE BROWN RICE CREAM

Skin cancer (after surgery), stomach cancer (after surgery), stroke, and upper digestive cancers

See the recipe section.

GINGER BATH

Make a bath using a handful of BANCHA TWIG TEA added to the bath water along with a little juice (½ to 1 teaspoon) from freshly grated gingerroot. (Tea stains the bathtub, so it is better not to keep the tea in the bathtub very long. Wash the tub well after using.)

GINGER BODY SCRUB

Bone and joint disorders, diarrhea, digestive disorders, multiple sclerosis, and scoliosis

This is similar to the BODY SCRUB but stronger. The purpose is to promote better circulation and energy flow through the entire body.

Heat about 1 gallon of water until it is hot but not boiling. Meanwhile, grate enough gingerroot to equal the size of a small baseball.

When the water becomes hot, reduce the heat to low and place the ginger into a single layer of cheesecloth. Tie with a string and squeeze the ginger juice from the cheesecloth sack into the water. (The water at this point should be just below the boiling point.)

Put the sack into the pot and allow it to steep in the water without boiling for about 5 minutes. Dip a small cotton towel or cloth into the hot water. Wring out the excess water (you may need rubber gloves, or leave the ends of the towel out of the hot water to handle them).

Scrub the whole body, dipping the towel or cloth into hot water again when cool. Be sure to include the hands and feet and each finger and toe. The skin should become pink or slightly red. This result may take a few days to achieve if the skin is clogged with accumulated fat.

- Water left over from a GINGER COMPRESS may be used for a GINGER BODY SCRUB.

GINGER COMPRESS

Allergies, anemia, arm and hand problems, ankylosing spondylitis, asthma, backache, blood disorders, boils, bone and joint disorders, bunion, bursitis, bronchitis, carpal tunnel syndrome, cramps, diarrhea, digestive disorders, dizziness, ear problems, enteritis, foot and leg problems, fractures and dislocations, gallbladder problems, gout, Gulf War syndrome, jaundice, kidney stones, kidney and bladder problems, Lyme disease, muscular dystrophy, myasthenia gravis, mental disorders, multiple sclerosis, muscle problems, nervous conditions, neuralgia, numbness and tingling, osteoarthritis, Parkinson's disease, pancreatic problems, peripheral nerve disease, pinched nerve, psoriosis, rheumatoid arthritis, scoliosis, shoulder and neck problems, spleen problems, stomach cramps, stomach ulcers, stress, TMJ and teeth problems

Limited use: cancer (see important note below)

Contraindicated: The ginger compress is not recommended for use on the brain or on the head when high fever is present, on the lower abdominal area during pregnancy, for appendicitis, or for a baby or an older person.

The purpose of a hot GINGER COMPRESS is to dissolve stagnation and tension, melt blockages, and stimulate blood circulation and energy flow.

Bring about 1 gallon of water to a boil. Meanwhile, grate enough gingerroot to equal the size of a baseball. When the water comes to a boil, reduce the heat to low, and place the ginger into a double layer of cheesecloth and tie with string. The water at this point should be just below the boiling point. Also, the string should be long enough so that the other end hangs out of the pot for easy retrieval. Place the sack into the pot and allow it to steep in the water without boiling for about 5 minutes. Dip a towel into the ginger water, wring out tightly (using a long wooden cooking spoon or stick), and apply it to the desired area on the body. Cover with a second towel to hold in the heat. Change the towel every 2 to 3 minutes, replacing it with a fresh hot towel. This can be done by using 2 towels and alternating them so that the skin does not cool off between applications. Continue the applications for about 10 to 15 minutes, until the area becomes pink.

- Important: For people with a serious illness such as cancer, this remedy is sometimes used preceding a POTATO PLASTER or other plaster. But do not use a ginger compress more than once or twice, and for no more than 3 to 5 minutes each time.
- Be sure to keep the towels even on the back, not turned up at one or both ends. It is better to keep the pot on the flame in between applications of towels, so that the water remains consistently hot, rather than turn off the flame or place the pot on the floor next to the person.

GINGER TEA

Better circulation, diarrhea (yin type), and motion sickness

Take a small amount of grated ginger, place in a cheesecloth, squeeze out the ginger juice into hot water or bancha tea, heat for a few minutes, and drink. This will increase blood circulation.

GOMASHIO

Asthma, cuts and wounds, dizziness, drug allergies, epilepsy, fainting, frontal headache, mental disorders, motion sickness, nausea and vomiting, nervous conditions, nosebleed, and ruptured spleen

Gomashio is roasted sesame seeds and sea salt. In addition to its use as a condiment, it is used medicinally to strengthen the blood quickly. It provides an immediate yangizing effect and can help offset extreme yin conditions and reactions. See GOMASHIO in the recipe section.

GRATED DAIKON WITH SHOYU

Diarrhea (yin type), heart problems, irritable bowel syndrome, kidney problems, liver problems, lung problems, pancreatic problems, seasonal affective disorder, and upper digestive cancers

Fresh grated daikon is used in small volume as a garnish for tempura, deep-fried, and other oily foods; fish and other seafood; mochi; and other rich styles of cooking.

Grate a small amount of fresh daikon finely with a hand grater using gentle circular motions. Grated daikon is customarily eaten with a few drops of shoyu. It is used in many medicinal preparations, as described below.

GRATED DAIKON AND CARROT

Breast cancer

Finely grate ½ cup each of daikon and carrot. Mix well. Add a few drops of shoyu and again mix well. Then eat. If the daikon is too pungent, you may also add a small amount of water and simmer for 2 to 3 minutes, adding the shoyu near the end of cooking.

GRATED DAIKON AND CARROT WITH SCALLIONS AND SHOYU

Dissolving animal-quality fat and protein

Finely grate ½ cup each of daikon and carrot. Add 1 teaspoon of chopped scallions and a few drops of shoyu. Mix well and eat.

GRATED DAIKON AND CARROT WITH SCALLIONS AND SHOYU, COOKED

Lung cancer

Grate the same amount each of daikon and carrot and mix well. Add 1 teaspoon of finely chopped scallions and mix well. Simmer quickly with just enough water to cover the ingredients in a pan, and add a few drops of shoyu.

GRATED DAIKON AND CARROT WITH SHIITAKE TEA

Pancreatic cancer with swollen abdomen

Combine finely grated daikon (3 parts), finely grated carrot (1 part), and soaked and finely chopped dried shiitake mushroom (1 part). Add 2 times the total volume of water and simmer on a low flame for about 3 to 4 minutes.

GRATED DAIKON AND CARROT WITH UMEBOSHI, SHISO, LEMON, AND SHOYU

Cervical cancer

Combine finely grated daikon (3 parts) and finely grated carrot (1 part) to make 1 small cup of this mixture. Add ½ umeboshi plum and

1 teaspoonful of ume-shiso leaves (red leaves from pickled umeboshi, finely chopped and with the surface salt washed off). Add 1 teaspoon of lemon juice and mix well. Add a few drops of shoyu.

GRATED DAIKON AND POTATO JUICE

Colon cancer

Prepare grated daikon and squeeze the juice from it. Peel and finely grate a potato and squeeze the juice from it. Mix together equal amounts of the daikon and potato juice. Add a pinch of sea salt for seasoning, if desired. But be careful not to take too much, as excess can lead to weakness.

GRATED DAIKON WITH CARROT AND SHOYU

Brain tumor

If liquid collects around the tumor, finely grate 3 parts daikon and 2 parts carrot. Add a few drops of shoyu and mix well.

GRATED DAIKON WITH CARROT AND SHOYU, COOKED

Stomach cancer

In a saucepan combine finely grated daikon (2 parts) and finely grated carrot (1 part). Add a small amount of water and simmer for about 2 minutes. Add 1 pinch of sea salt or a few drops of shoyu.

GRATED SOUR APPLE

Fever, liver troubles, and swelling of feet and legs

Peel and grate a sour green apple (Granny Smith). Put in a small saucepan. Add a small amount of water and simmer for about 2 minutes.

HARA-MAKI

Coldness and poor circulation, and frequent diarrhea

A hara-maki is a traditional cotton or woolen stomach band worn to keep the abdomen from getting cold or to relieve frequent diarrhea. It may be purchased from some traditional or natural clothing stores.

HATO MUGI–CABBAGE PLASTER

Breast cancer

Hato mugi, also called pearl barley or Job's tears, is a grass, not a grain. It is used in macrobiotic cooking as an occasional supplemental grain. Do not confuse *pearl* barley with *pearled* barley, or polished barley. In Far Eastern medicine, hato mugi has traditionally been used to melt excess animal protein and fat and to beautify the skin. In this plaster, it is good for harmonizing body energy and drawing out and softening excess fat and protein. The cabbage in the plaster is very helpful in cooling down fever and neutralizing inflammation. Cabbage is particularly good because it is a more yang vegetable and has drawing, or contractive power. It tends to keep tumors from spreading.

Cook hato mugi following the basic recipe for PRESSURE-COOKED BROWN RICE or BOILED BROWN RICE, using slightly more water. While still warm mash it in a suribachi. Let it cool to room temperature. Then very finely chop and mash the same volume of fresh cabbage as pearl barley, and combine with the pearl barley 50-50. Mix 10 to 20 percent of the total volume of white flour into the barley mixture to make it less watery and make a paste for the plaster.

Spread the mixture about 1 inch thick on a cotton cloth. Apply the mixture directly on the breast and tie with a cotton strip or a bolt of cheesecloth. Cover if necessary with a cotton brassiere and a large cotton towel pinned together.

Leave the plaster on for 4 hours or more. Repeat once or twice every day. You may leave the plaster on overnight when you sleep.

HATO MUGI WITH CABBAGE PLASTER

Bone cancer (pain)

Follow the recipe for HATO MUGI–CABBAGE PLASTER, but change the ratio of hato mugi and cabbage from ½/½ to ⅔/⅓. Combine with 10 to 20 percent white flour, if necessary. Spread it about 1 inch thick on a cotton cloth and apply it directly to the painful part for 3 to 4 hours twice a day. You may also sleep with it overnight until the next morning.

HATO MUGI–POTATO PLASTER

Ovarian cancer

Cook hato mugi following the basic recipe for PRESSURE-COOKED BROWN RICE or BOILED BROWN RICE, using slightly more water. While still warm, mash it in a suribachi. Let it cool to room temperature. Peel and finely grate potatoes. Combine equal amounts of mashed hato mugi and potato. Add 10 to 20 percent white flour to make a paste. Spread the plaster about 1 inch thick on a cotton cloth. Apply the plaster directly on the affected part of the ovary area. Leave the plaster on for 4 hours or longer. Repeat twice a day, or leave the plaster on all night while sleeping, if possible. Continue every day for about 3 weeks.

HATO MUGI–POTATO-CABBAGE PLASTER

Liver cancer, thyroid and throat cancer

Cook hato mugi following the basic recipe for PRESSURE-COOKED BROWN RICE or BOILED BROWN RICE, using slightly more water. While still warm, mash it in a suribachi. Let it cool to room temperature. Meanwhile, peel and finely grate potatoes in the same volume as the hato mugi. Very finely chop and mash the same volume of fresh cabbage as the pearl barley or potato. Combine the pearl barley, potato, and cabbage. Add 10 to 20 percent white flour to make it less watery and to make a paste for the plaster.

Spread this about 1 inch thick over a cotton cloth and apply it directly to the affected area. Keep it on for 3 to 4 hours twice a day, or sleep with it overnight. Do this for 2 to 3 weeks.

HEART DRINK

Heart conditions

Prepare a special drink consisting of daikon greens and other hard leafy greens (2 parts), dried shiitake mushroom (1 part), corn or corn products such as grits (1 part), cabbage (1 part), and wakame or nori (1 part). Add 4 to 5 times as much water. Drink 1 cup for 3 weeks.

HIJIKI

Hernia, lung problems, stress, and valve disorders

See HIJIKI WITH LOTUS ROOT in the recipe section. Vegetables may be omitted.

HIJIKI WITH DRIED DAIKON AND SHIITAKE

Bladder cancer

Soak and chop hijiki (4 parts), dried shredded daikon (1 part), and dried shiitake mushroom (1 part). A few drops of sesame oil can be added to a fry pan. Layer shiitake on bottom, then daikon, and hijiki on top. Cook according to the recipe HIJIKI WITH LOTUS ROOT. Season with a little bit of shoyu.

HOTO

Dizziness, mental disorders, weakness, fatigue, and many other conditions

Hoto is a special noodle stew made with udon or other whole-wheat noodles, squash (always included when available), and about a half dozen other fall and winter season vegetables. Hoto is traditionally prepared in a ceramic dish, which gives a more peaceful, stable vibration than metal, especially for healing. It is very strong and energizing, especially for persons with weak, more yin conditions.

Prepare by making homemade noodles, or boiling a quart of water and cooking an 8-ounce package of ready-made udon. Set the noodles aside to be added with the vegetables later. Select among such vegetables as daikon, carrots, onions, lotus root, and burdock. Slice equal amounts of five or six vegetables and layer with the more yang (denser, harder, or firmer) on the bottom (e.g., burdock and carrot) in the ceramic pot on the stovetop. Half cover with water and cook for 20 to 30 minutes or until done. When the vegetables are almost done, add the noodles and, if desired, small pieces of mochi for further strength. To season, add miso (especially young sweet miso) to taste and several pinches of sea salt to firm up the noodles and make the vegetables sweeter. Watch the water level carefully, especially after adding the noodles, and add more when needed. Serve when done. The dish should have sufficient broth to be enjoyed as a stew or soup.

• Dried tofu may be added to this dish, but usually not fresh tofu.

HOT TOWEL COMPRESS

ALS, arm and hand problems, bone and joint disorders, bursitis, cardiovascular problems (alternated with cold compress), digestive disorders, ear problems, foot and leg problems, headache (back of head), kidney stone pain, liver problems, Lyme disease, muscular dystrophy, myasthenia gravis, neuralgia, numbness and tingling, peripheral nerve disease, rheumatoid arthritis, spleen problems, stomach cancer (before cold towel compress)

Hot towels can be used to relieve tension and reduce pain, especially on areas of the body that are tight from overconsumption of animal food, salt, or other more contractive foods. For example, a headache in the back of the head is usually caused by these foods, and applying a hot towel will ease the ache. In some cases, hot and cold towels may be alternated every few minutes. For example, leg cramps (usually caused by extreme yin foods, but characterized by yang cramping) can be treated in this way. First massage toward and immediately above the cramping region (but not on it directly). Then apply alternately towels drenched in hot and cold water.

To prepare this compress, dip plain cotton towels in hot water, wring out, and apply to affected areas. Remove towels as they lose their strength, replacing them with fresh towels for up to 7 minutes, or until the area becomes pink. See also COLD TOWEL COMPRESS.

• For cardiovascular disease, alternate hot and cold towels on the affected area for embolism, thrombus, varicose veins, and other ailments caused by a combination of extreme yin and yang factors.

HOT WATER BOTTLE

Anemia with coldness, depression, hypoglycemia (on pancreas or feet), pancreatic problems, and ovarian cancer (coldness)

Contraindicated: Do not place on swelling feet or hands

A rubber hot water bottle can be purchased at drugstores or medical supply stores. It can be filled with water (either hot or cold), and used to warm or cool the body when resting.

- For hypoglycemia, warm the pancreas or feet with a HOT WATER BOTTLE when the body is too cold to sleep.
- For ovarian cancer, if you feel your feet so cold that you cannot sleep, you may use a HOT WATER BOTTLE, (but do not do a HOT FOOT SOAK or a GINGER FOOT SOAK).

JINENJO

Mental disorders, nervous disorders, vitality

This soft Oriental potato grows deep underground, has a long shape, and may reach several feet in length. It gives a very strong energy and is especially warming in winter. Traditionally, it is also said to be good for restoring sexual vitality.

Jinenjo is usually eaten raw in very small amounts. It is sticky like natto or cheese. To prepare it, grate 1 to 2 tablespoons and add a pinch of grated fresh ginger and a couple of drops of shoyu. Serve with a few small squares of toasted nori. Jinenjo may also be sliced and eaten raw or marinated with brown rice vinegar and shoyu and served with toasted sesame seeds.

Grated and added to miso soup or shoyu broth, jinenjo alters the taste of a dish completely. Use about 1 teaspoon per cup, pouring the hot soup over the grated jinenjo in a soup bowl and garnishing with scallions. It is also very good eaten with soba noodles. Mochi pounded with a little jinenjo mixed in, about 5 percent, keeps it soft longer.

Cooked nishime-style, jinenjo may be boiled in large slices and seasoned with a little shoyu. It may also be added to oden- or nabe-style dishes and consumed from the common pot at the table.

KIDNEY DRINK

Kidney conditions and disorders

Prepare a special drink consisting of soaked adzuki beans (1 part), shredded dried daikon (1 part), dried shiitake mushroom (1 part), and kombu (1 part). Add 5 times as much water, boil, and then simmer for about 25 minutes. Take 1 cup every day for 10 days. Don't eat the kombu.

KINPIRA SOUP

AIDS, allergies, ALS, anemia, bleeding and blood disorders, bone and joint problems, brain disorders, breast cancer, carpal tunnel syndrome, congenital heart defects, constipation (yin variety), diabetes, digestive disorders, environmental illness, fatigue, hepatitis, infectious disease, leukemia, Lyme disease, mad cow disease, mental disorders, osteoarthritis, osteoporosis, skin cancer, stomach problems, swelling in the lower abdomen, and upper digestive cancers.

This strengthening soup should be like a hearty stew. It is similar in use and texture to KOI-KOKU (carp and burdock soup) but entirely vegetarian. Chop very finely equal amounts of burdock root, carrot, and lotus root (if using lotus root, either fresh or dried and soaked). Lightly brush sesame oil in the bottom of a pan (or add a small amount of water if not using oil) and heat on a medium high flame. When oil or water is hot, sauté the burdock for 2 to 3 minutes, adding a pinch of sea salt if desired.

Layer the lotus root (optional) and carrots on top of the burdock. Cover all vegetables with spring water, bring to a boil, lower the flame, cover, and simmer for a long time (30 to 40 minutes) until all vegetables are very soft. Water may need to be added from time to time.

Add very finely chopped onion and sweet winter squash, and cook further until the onion and squash become very soft. Mix sweet young white miso and dark aged barley miso 50-50 and dilute in some of the soup broth. Slowly add enough of the miso for a nice taste, gently stir, and simmer for another 5 minutes.

KINPIRA-STYLE BURDOCK

Anemia, diabetes (with oil), mental disorders, nervous disorders, and pulmonary heart disease

See KINPIRA-STYLE VEGETABLES in the recipe section, using only burdock.

KINPIRA-STYLE BURDOCK, CARROT, AND KOMBU

Lymphoma

This dish may be water-sautéed or oil-sautéed using a few drops of sesame oil. Prepare following the recipe for KINPIRA-STYLE VEGETABLES, using burdock (2 parts), carrot (2 parts), and kombu (1 part). The kombu, sliced into matchsticks, may be sautéed in the beginning along with the burdock, and the carrots layered on top. Cook as in the recipe. At the end of cooking, season it with a pinch of sea salt, or a few drops of shoyu.

KINPIRA-STYLE VEGETABLES

Ankylosing spondylitis, and constipation

See KINPIRA-STYLE VEGETABLES in the recipe section.

KOI-KOKU

AIDS, congenital heart defects, heart failure, infectious disease, leukemia, mental disorders, and nervous conditions

This is also known as carp and burdock soup and is very strengthening.

Obtain a whole carp, as fresh as possible. Ask the fish seller to remove the bitter gallbladder and thyroid and leave the rest of the fish intact, with all scales, bones, head, and fins. If you must remove them yourself, place the carp on a fish cutting board to remove the thyroid and gallbladder. If the carp has roe inside, it also must be removed. Chop the fish into large 2- to 3-inch slices, including the head, scales, fins, and bones. The eyes may be removed, if desired. Set these aside.

Wash and chop burdock into very thin slices or matchsticks. The amount of sliced burdock should be the same volume as the carp. Sauté the burdock for a few minutes in oil, or water-sauté, if needed.

Tie used bancha twigs or stems (about 1 cup) in a cotton cheesecloth to make a tea bag as big as a tennis ball. Layer the tea bag on top of the burdock and place the chopped fish on top. The tea twigs will help soften the bones while cooking. Add enough liquid to cover all ingredients. Use approximately ⅓ bancha tea and ⅔ spring water. Cover with a heavy lid or pressure cooker lid. Bring to a boil on a high flame. Reduce the heat. If boiling, simmer for 2 hours or longer; if using a pressure cooker, simmer for 1 to 1½ hours or longer.

While cooking, the burdock and carp neutralize each other and the bones of the fish become very soft. When almost cooked, bring down the pressure, if necessary, and remove the lid. Add miso dissolved in water to season to taste, as you would for regular MISO SOUP. Add 1 tablespoonful of juice from freshly grated ginger and mix well. Cover and simmer for another 5 minutes on a low flame. When seasoning with miso, you may need to add some water if the soup is too thick.

Serve with the cooking liquid. Garnish with chopped scallions and serve hot.

Have a small bowl of this preparation every day for 3 days in a row. Save leftovers in the refrigerator or freezer for future use; then cook again for 10 to 15 minutes before eating.

- If a carp and burdock are unavailable, trout or other white-meat fish may be substituted for carp, and carrot for burdock. Cook for 1 to 1½ hours. But the effectiveness of this preparation is less.
- It is better to include *used* bancha twigs, since fresh twigs lend a bitter taste to the dish.
- Koi-koku is of benefit to both males and females lacking in energy.

KOMBU

Kombu, a sea vegetable used daily in macrobiotic cooking, has many medicinal applications, and is used in teas and plasters. The *Laminaria* family of sea vegetables includes kombu, some kelps, tangle, oarweed, and other deep-ocean varieties. Japanese kombu is blackish brown in color, has wide, thick celery-like leaves, and is gathered in cold seas off southern Hokkaido. It is harvested between July and September by boatmen with long poles. It is then dried on the ground by sun and wind. After drying in a dark place for 2 to 3 years, kombu is packaged and sold in a variety of grades and forms. The city of Osaka is known for its superior kombu, and there are said to be large warehouses stocking over 100 different varieties.

Without kombu, Japanese cuisine would not exist. Its distinctive taste is the basis for *dashi*, the traditional broth used as a stock for soups and noodles. It is enjoyed as a side dish or as an accompaniment to grains, beans, and root vegetables. Kombu is also made into teas, pickles, condiments, snacks, and candy. High in vitamins A, B$_2$, C, calcium, and iodine, kombu is therapeutic and protective against degenerative disease.

KOMBU TEA

Bone and joint disorders, food allergies, gout, kidney problems

Kombu tea is good for strengthening the blood. It helps to discharge animal fats and proteins from the body. Traditionally known for its calming properties, it aids in restoring the nervous function and in promoting clear thinking.

Wipe off a 3-inch piece of dry kombu with a wet cloth. Place the kombu in 1 quart of water and bring to a boil. Reduce the heat and simmer gently (covered with a lid) until the quantity of water is reduced by half (about 10 to 15 minutes). Drink 1 cup while hot. You may reheat the remaining tea and drink.

KOMBU-LOTUS-SHIITAKE DRINK

Skin cancer, melanoma

Combine chopped kombu (20 percent), lotus root (40 percent), and shiitake (40 percent). Add 4 to 5 times as much water, cook 20 minutes or longer, and add several drops of shoyu at the end of cooking and a pinch of grated ginger, and let simmer for several minutes. Take 1 small cup for 3 weeks, then twice a week for one month, and then occasionally as needed.

KOMBU-CABBAGE PLASTER

Breast cancer (after surgery), lymphoma (swelling), and prostate cancer (swollen lymph nodes)

A kombu plaster is good for burns from radiation (such as medical X rays), skin lesions, and scars. It is also good to help relieve stagnation and tumors caused by dairy consumption. The cabbage is particularly good because it is a more yang vegetable and has a drawing or contractive power. It helps to cool down fever, neutralize inflammation, and relieve burns and bruises.

Soften strips of kombu by soaking in hot water for 10 to 15 minutes. Cut two pieces to a proper size, large enough to cover the affected part. Apply the soaked kombu 2 layers thick, directly on the skin. Then carefully separate cabbage leaves from a large cabbage and score the spine with a vegetable knife so the leaf flattens slightly. Apply a layer of cabbage leaves on top of the kombu. Hold in place with a cotton towel, cotton cloth, or cheesecloth. The cloth or towels help to soften the kombu prior to removing it.

- After breast cancer surgery, a lump of fat sometimes grows on the scar. To prevent a lump from growing, do a KOMBU AND CABBAGE PLASTER. Leave on for about 4 hours or overnight.
- For lymphoma, apply this plaster directly to the swollen area. Wrap it with bleached cotton and keep it for about 4 hours. Do this twice a day; or it is possible to keep it on while sleeping until the next morning. This can be continued until the swelling disappears.

• For prostate cancer, if the lymph nodes are swollen, apply and leave on for 6 hours or more. You may leave it on all night while sleeping. Repeat once or twice every day for 2 to 3 weeks.

KOMBU PLASTER

Allergies, atopy, burns from radiation (such as medical X rays), skin lesions, scars, heart failure, and rheumatoid arthritis (inflammation or redness)

Soften strips of kombu by soaking in hot water for 10 to 15 minutes. Cut two pieces to a proper size, large enough to cover the affected part. Apply the soaked kombu 2 layers thick, directly on the skin. Hold in place with a cotton towel, cotton cloth, or cotton cheesecloth. The cloth or towel helps to soften the kombu prior to removing it. Keep it on 2 to 3 hours a couple of times a day, or it can be applied when you go to sleep and be kept on overnight.

KUMQUAT JAM

Ovarian cancer

Finely slice kumquats. Do not peel them. Remove all seeds and stems. Add a small amount of water and a pinch of sea salt, and then simmer to make a jam.

KUMQUAT TEA

Ovarian cancer

Dissolve KUMQUAT JAM in BANCHA TWIG TEA, or hot water, and drink.

KUZU CREAM

Cholera, diarrhea (yin variety), dysentery, gas pains, and influenza

Dissolve a heaping teaspoon of kuzu in cold water. Add to a cup of cold water, stir, and bring to a boil. Continue to stir while boiling until the mixture is transparent. Add several drops of shoyu or a pinch of sea salt.

KUZU TEA

Gallbladder problems, influenza, and many other conditions

Dissolve 1 teaspoon of kuzu powder in cold water. Add the water gradually and stir well until all the kuzu pieces are dissolved. Add 1 cup of boiling water and stir well. Add a pinch of sea salt or a few drops of shoyu.

LARGE INTESTINE DRINK

Colon conditions and disorders

Prepare the following special drink: lotus root (2 parts), daikon root (1 part), daikon greens (1 part), carrot (1 part), carrot greens (1 part), and dried shiitake mushroom (1 part). Add 4 to 5 times as much water, boil, and simmer for 15 to 20 minutes. Drink 1 cup for about 3 to 5 days.

LEAFY GREENS JUICE

Gallbladder problems, liver problems, and muscle problems

This special drink was originally devised to treat liver disorders, especially yang conditions resulting from eating eggs. It helps to dissolve heavy, stagnated protein, animal fat, and cholesterol deposits. To obtain counterbalancing, light, upward energy from leafy greens, it is easier for many people to take the juice of young barley plants (sold under the name Green Magma in the natural foods store) or another preparation, but this is not as effective. This drink may be taken daily.

Very finely chop 2 or 3 kinds of large leafy green vegetables (kale, collards, dandelion, daikon or turnip leaves, or Chinese cabbage). Add twice the amount of cold water. Bring to a gentle boil and simmer for 3 to 5 minutes. Strain out the solid vegetables. Add a pinch of sea salt or a few drops of shoyu toward the end of simmering and stir. Drink hot or at room temperature.

- You may or may not reuse the leafy green vegetables.
- Heat 1 cup fresh celery or leafy green vegetable juice; add a small pinch of sea salt. Simmer for 3 to 5 minutes. Drink hot, warm, or at room temperature.

LEAFY GREENS PLASTER (CHLOROPHYLL PLASTER)

Ankle problems, arm and hand problems, bone and joint disorders, brain disorders, bronchitis, diarrhea (yin variety), digestive disorders, diverticular disease, enteritis, fever, foot and leg problems, headaches (frontal), inflammation, knee problems, liver problems, lung problems, muscular dystrophy, myasthenia gravis, muscle problems, nervous conditions, neuralgia, osteoarthritis, peripheral nerve disease, pneumonia, spinal cord

disorders, spleen problems, stomach ulcers, strains and sprains, swollen toenail, tonsillitis, and throat problems

The leaves of large, leafy green vegetables are very helpful in cooling down fever, neutralizing inflammation, and relieving burns and bruises. Sometimes just putting leaves (either big ones or ones that grow upward) such as cabbage leaves, collard greens, turnip tops, or daikon tops on the head, chest, or arms will provide immediate relief. This plaster has a more concentrated effect than just the leaves and may be used initially or after whole leaves have absorbed the initial heat.

Finely chop several green leafy vegetables such as daikon leaves, kale, collards, cabbage, or Chinese cabbage. Place in a suribachi and mash well. Add 10 to 20 percent unbleached white flour and mix into a paste. Spread the mixture about ½ inch thick on a towel or cloth and apply the greens directly to the skin (not the cloth side). Leave on for 2 to 3 hours.

LIVER TEA

Liver congestion and eye problems

Finely chop all vegetables, and mix ingredients in the following proportion: unroasted buckwheat groats (2 parts), daikon (1 part), daikon greens (2 parts, or turnip greens, radish greens, or other large greens), scallions (1 part), sprouts (2 parts, any kind, such as alfalfa, mung bean, soybean), shiitake mushroom (1 part). Add 5 times the total volume of water, bring to a boil, lower the flame, and simmer for about 30 minutes. Strain out the contents, and save the liquid.

LOTUS-DAIKON-CABBAGE JUICE

Thyroid and throat cancer

Mix ½ cup raw juice squeezed from grated lotus root, ¼ cup of juice squeezed from grated daikon, and ¼ cup of juice squeezed from finely chopped and mashed cabbage leaves. Add a small amount of water and simmer for 2 minutes.

LOTUS ROOT JUICE TEA

Lung cancer (with cough)

In case of a cough that accompanies this type of tumor, grate fresh lotus root. Wrap the grated pulp in cheesecloth and then squeeze out the juice by hand. (The pulp may be saved and added to other dishes, such as BROWN RICE PORRIDGE, MISO SOUP, or croquettes.) Drink ½ to ⅔ cup of the juice.

You may also place the juice in a saucepan with a small amount of water. Add a pinch of sea salt or a few drops of shoyu, bring to a boil, and let it simmer gently on a low flame for 2 to 3 minutes. This tea should be thick and creamy and should be drunk while hot. If your condition permits, you may also add a few drops of grated ginger juice toward the end (not for some coughs).

- For cough, it is best to drink LOTUS ROOT JUICE TEA from evening time to night when you cough.

LOTUS ROOT PLASTER

Allergies, brain tumor, cystic fibrosis, lung problems, sinus problems, and stress

Lotus root—the long, many-chambered, pale root of the lotus plant—is known traditionally for helping to dissolve excess mucus in the lungs, bronchi, throat, or sinuses. This is often caused by dairy food consumption, but lotus is good to release any kind of stagnation, such as that from chicken and egg fat, as well. This remedy is traditionally known for its effectiveness in dispersing and moving stagnated mucus in the respiratory system.

Activate the area to be treated first with a HOT TOWEL COMPRESS or GINGER COMPRESS for 5 minutes. Generally stagnation begins to loosen up and mucus starts to drain within 3 applications of this plaster. Calcified stones in the sinuses sometimes are loosened and come out with sneezing. Stubborn ones can take 3 weeks to discharge.

Grate enough lotus root to cover the area, about ½ inch thick. Mix thoroughly with 5 percent grated ginger, if using ginger, and 10 to 15 percent unbleached white flour. Spread the mixture on a cloth or paper towel and apply directly to the skin (not the cloth side). Leave on for 20 minutes to 1 hour.

- To dissolve mucus deposits in the sinuses, you may leave the plaster on for several hours or overnight. In this case, sew a gauze mask with holes for the nose and eyes. The lotus plaster should cover the area around the eyes and above the nose. This application should be repeated for 7 to 10 days, and may sometimes take up to 2 to 3 weeks to clear the sinuses. Watery or thick mucus may start to be discharged from the eyes and nose.

LOTUS ROOT TEA

Anemia, allergies, blood disorders, lung congestion, sinus problems, and chronic coughing

Usually, salt is used for seasoning with this drink. Since its purpose is to take out or neutralize excessive protein, shoyu that contains protein is not used. Also, the tea is sweeter with salt. This tea is most effective when prepared from fresh lotus root. However, if fresh is not available, dried lotus root or lotus root powder may be used.

- If using fresh lotus root, grate ½ cup of the vegetable, squeeze the juice into a pot through a cheesecloth or thin cotton cloth, and add a small volume of water. Cook for 5 to 8 minutes, add a pinch of sea salt or shoyu, and drink hot.
- If using dried lotus root, place ⅓ ounce dried lotus root in 1 cup water. Let sit for a few minutes until soft, then chop finely. Mash it in a suribachi. Return the finely chopped lotus root to the soaking water. Add a pinch of sea salt or a few drops of shoyu. Bring to a boil and allow to simmer gently for approximately 15 minutes. Strain the liquid and drink while hot. You may also add a few drops of grated ginger juice toward the end, if your condition permits. You may use the pulp in other dishes.
- If using lotus root powder, use 1 teaspoon

lotus root powder per serving. Add 1 cup of cold water per teaspoon of powder and stir to dissolve. Add a pinch of sea salt or a few drops of shoyu. You may add a couple drops of grated ginger juice, if your condition permits. Heat on a low flame but do not boil. Turn off the heat when the liquid begins to simmer. Drink while hot.

LOTUS SEEDS

Allergies, lung cancer, and lung problems

Lotus seeds are traditionally said to contribute to vitality and longevity. Lotus seeds are delicious cooked with adzuki beans and kombu, brown rice, roasted brown rice, or deep-fried seitan with carrots and scallion roots.

LOTUS SEED, SEAWEED, AND ONION TEA

Cervical cancer

Place soaked lotus seeds in a pot; add 10 percent soaked and chopped wakame or arame and 20 percent finely chopped scallion or onion. Add water, bring to a boil, and simmer to make a tea.

LUNG DRINK

Lung conditions and disorders

Prepare the following special drink, consisting of lotus root (2 parts), daikon root (1 part), daikon greens (1 part), carrot (1 part), carrot greens (1 part), and dried shiitake mushroom (1 part). Add 4 to 5 times as much water, boil, and simmer for 15 to 20 minutes. Drink 1 cup for about 3 to 5 days.

MARINATED DAIKON AND CARROT

Ovarian cancer

Finely cut 1 cup daikon and ½ cup carrots into matchsticks. Mix them together. Prepare a marinade of either 1 tablespoon brown rice vinegar and a small amount of shoyu or 1 tablespoon umeboshi vinegar and 1 tablespoon spring water. Pour on the vegetables and marinate for 30 minutes or longer.

MASSAGE

Brain tumor, cervical cancer, coma, cramps, fatigue, irritable bowel syndrome, headache, leukemia (abdomen for digestion), lung cancer, motion sickness, pancreatic cancer, ovarian cancer, stomach cancer, upper digestive cancers, and many other conditions

Massage of the fingers and toes helps stimulate various organs, systems, and functions by activating energy flow through the meridians that begin or end in the extremities. Basic books on massage are *Beginner's Guide to Shiatsu* by Patrick McCarty and *Basic Shiatsu* by Michio Kushi. More comprehensive books are *Shiatsu Handbook* by Shizuko Yamamoto and Patrick McCarty and *Barefoot Shiatsu* by the same authors. For self-massage, please see *The Book of Do-In* by Michio Kushi.

MEDITATION

ALS, heart problems, irritable bowel syndrome, post-traumatic stress disorder, and many other conditions and disorders

There are many types of meditation that can contribute to the healing process. For a dis-cussion of different styles of meditation and their respective yin or yang effects, please see *The Book of Macrobiotics* by Michio Kushi and Alex Jack.

MILLET SQUASH SOUP

Pancreatic problems, and stomach problems

See MILLET AND SWEET VEGETABLE SOUP in the recipe section.

MILLET AND SWEET VEGETABLE PORRIDGE

Headache

Wash 1 cup millet (regular, kibi or sweet millet, or awa) in cold water. Add 1½ cups sweet vegetables (Hokkaido pumpkin, kabocha squash, buttercup squash, butternut squash, sweet dumpling squash, delicata squash, cabbage, carrot, onion, sweet corn, or parsnip), cut into small chunks, to the bottom of a large saucepan or pressure cooker. For the sweetest porridge, layer the vegetables with the most yin on the bottom and the most yang on top (bottom has onion, sweet corn, cabbage; middle has squash; top has carrot or parsnip, etc.) Place the millet on top, and gently pour 3 to 4 cups water down the sides so not to disturb the layering. Slowly bring to a boil, scooping off any foam that rises to the top. Lower the flame and add 1 pinch sea salt. Cover and bring to pressure, if using a pressure cooker. Place a flame deflector underneath and let it simmer for about 20–25 minutes, or pressure-cook for 15–20 minutes. Remove from the heat and let pressure reduce naturally, if necessary. Place in serving bowls, and garnish with chopped scallions, parsley, gomashio, or other condiment. This gives a sweet, delicious morning porridge and is also very strengthening.

- Pressure-cooking gives the porridge a creamier texture.
- If this is difficult to eat, you may add miso and a little water, if necessary, and make MILLET AND SWEET VEGETABLE SOUP.

MILLET AND SWEET VEGETABLE SOUP

Stomach cancer, hypoglycemia and other pancreatic disorders, spleen problems, strengthening natural immunity

See MILLET AND SWEET VEGETABLE SOUP in the recipe section.

MILLET CROQUETTES

Bone and joint disorders

Croquettes are a delicious, crispy way to prepare leftover grains and beans. Millet sticks together a little better than rice, but both are very tasty.

Boil ½ cup of carrots cut into matchsticks with a pinch of sea salt in about ½ inch of water for 2 to 3 minutes, or until soft. Save the water for a sauce. Strain the carrots and mix them together with 2 cups cooked millet and ½ cup minced parsley. Fashion into balls. Any round or oval shape is fine. If too dry, add a little whole-wheat pastry flour with a little water to keep the shape of the ball. If too wet, roll the ball in dry wheat flour. After shaping, deep-fry the balls in hot oil for a few minutes following the basic tempura technique (but do not dip them into the batter). Please refer to TEMPURA-STYLE VEGETABLES for frying technique. Cook the balls until they are golden brown and crunchy. Croquettes may be served covered with a sauce made from carrots and onions cooked with a little shoyu, grated fresh ginger, and kuzu to thicken, or they may be served with a dip.

- Buckwheat is also excellent prepared in this way.
- Minced and boiled celery and rinsed and boiled arame are also commonly added to grains when making croquettes.
- Normally onions and scallions are not used when deep-frying because they become too watery.
- Leftover beans can also be cooked in this way. Lentils and chickpeas are best. Kidney and adzuki beans usually become too dark when deep-fried.

MISO PLASTER

Infectious disease

Soybeans have a cooling effect on the body. Raw soybeans soaked in water, crushed, and applied on the affected area can take out fever. Miso—the fermented soybean paste used daily in macrobiotic cooking for soup, condiments, and seasoning—also has many medicinal applications. A miso plaster consists of raw miso applied directly on the body. The enzymes in miso neutralize bacteria and help to prevent infection. In the kitchen, nicks and cuts suffered while cutting vegetables can be treated with a dab of miso on the hand or finger.

A miso plaster can also draw out bee stingers,

help relieve itchy skin diseases, and reduce any kind of swelling. It is an essential ingredient in a home first-aid kit. Use regular barley, rice, or hatcho miso for this purpose. It is all right if the miso has been pasteurized. It will still be effective.

Place raw miso over the affected area, about ¼ to ½ inch thick. Wrap with a single layer of cheesecloth.

- When putting miso directly on the skin, do not pack it down firmly, as this can cause scarring.

MISO-SCALLION CONDIMENT

Ankylosing spondylitis and bladder cancer

The pungent taste of scallions goes very well with miso, creating a warm energy. Use on rice, other grains, noodles, boiled vegetables, or as a spread on bread.

Wash 2 to 3 scallions with scallion roots very well. Soak the roots in cold water, if necessary, to loosen any soil. Finely slice the scallions and roots and measure their volume. Pour an equal amount of sesame oil into a frying pan. Layer the roots and then the scallions in the oiled frying pan. Form a little hollow in the center of the scallions. Measure out 3 times the amount of miso as scallions or oil, and purée it in a very small amount of spring water. Pour this mixture into the hollow. Cover and simmer for about 3 minutes. Mix very well when done, and serve.

MISO SOUP

Alzheimer's disease, epilepsy, gastroenteritis, heart disease, hypoglycemia, liver problems, Lyme disease, prostate problems, spleen problems, stress, tuberculosis, valve disorders, varicose veins, and many other conditions and disorders

See MISO SOUP in the recipe section.

MISO SOUP WITH BROWN RICE MOCHI

Anemia, mental conditions, nervous conditions, and spinal cord disorders

See BROWN RICE MOCHI IN MISO SOUP.

MISO SOUP WITH OKARA AND VEGETABLES

Bone cancer

Okara is the coarse soybean pulp left over when tofu is made fresh at home. It is very delicious in soups but should not be cooked too long in order to preserve its taste.

Make mild MISO SOUP with 1 part each of chopped onion, winter squash or pumpkin, cabbage, carrot, daikon and daikon leaves, as well as a small amount of washed, soaked, and chopped wakame seaweed. Cook until all the vegetables are soft. Then reduce the heat to very low and add the okara and puréed miso to the soup stock. Simmer the soup 2 to 3 minutes longer and serve hot.

MISO-ZOSUI (OJIYA)

Anemia, ankylosing spondylitis, dizziness, environmental illness, leukemia, and prostate cancer

Also called BROWN RICE ZOSUI (OJIYA), this porridge consists of soft-cooked brown rice with seaweed, root vegetables, leafy greens, round sweet vegetables, and miso.

Cook brown rice in 3 times the volume of water until it becomes softened and has an almost *kayu*-like creamy texture. Add some chopped vegetables, such as winter squash, pumpkin, onion, daikon, carrot, and cabbage. Simmer until every ingredient becomes soft and it is smooth and creamy. Add a moderate amount of miso, which has been fermented for a long time, and gently stir. Simmer for another 2 to 3 minutes on a low flame and then remove the pot from the flame. Set aside for 5 minutes or more before eating.

- If you use rice that has been already cooked, simmer the cooked rice with 2 times the volume of water in a pot and follow the above directions.

MISO-ZOSUI BROWN RICE AND MILLET

Stomach cancer

Wash and finely chop cabbage (1 part), soaked dried shiitake mushroom (1 part), daikon (1 part), daikon leaves (1 part), and onion (1 part). Wash and drain 3 parts brown rice and 1 part millet. Layer onion, shiitake, daikon leaves, daikon, and cabbage in a pot, and then millet and brown rice on top. Gently pour in 2½

to 3 times the total volume of water. Bring it to a boil, lower the flame, and simmer for 1 hour or more with a heavy lid covering the pot. Season lightly with puréed miso.

MOCHI

Stress and many other conditions

See PAN-FRIED MOCHI in the recipe section and BROWN RICE MOCHI FRIED IN OIL, BROWN RICE MOCHI IN BANCHA, BROWN RICE MOCHI IN MISO SOUP, MISO-ZOSUI WITH BROWN RICE MOCHI, and MISO-ZOSUI WITH SCALLIONS AND MOCHI.

MOXIBUSTION

Multiple sclerosis, sinus problems, and other conditions and disorders

Moxibustion (or *moxa*) is a traditional Far Eastern healing method that employs heat along the meridians and points to activate and supply energy to specific regions, organs, systems, and functions of the body. Moxa can be used for general strengthening, such as on Stomach Meridian 36 on the leg for health and longevity; to help relieve specific symptoms such as constipation or facial problems, e.g., Large Intestine 4 on the hand; or for chronic conditions such as multiple sclerosis on certain points along the spine. It has also been used for helping someone who is dying recover strength, energy, or consciousness.

Traditionally, dried mugwort is used, and long sticks of moxa or small moxa cones are available in acupuncture clinics, Oriental markets, or, occasionally, natural food stores.

To apply, light the moxa stick and approach the point in a slow, gently clockwise spiral. Hold the moxa stick above the point (not touching the skin) for several seconds until the person feels strong heat. Then pull back the stick and after a few seconds apply again in the same way. Usually 5 times is enough for most applications, though emergency treatments may take more time.

- Locations of the points are different for everyone. So you can't just mechanically follow an acupuncture chart or diagram in a book. *A thorough understanding of Far Eastern philosophy and medicine, including the meridian system, is recommended before use of this method. Moxa is generally not used for yang conditions or symptoms characterized by excess energy.* Please consult a text on moxibustion for further information.
- If a moxa stick is not available, an ordinary cigarette may be used.

MU TEA

Bone and joint disorders, bronchitis, kidney problems, sexual vitality, swollen intestines, tiredness, wet mucousy coughs, and respiratory disorders

This tea was developed by George Ohsawa. He modified a traditional herbal remedy called *chujo-to,* "hot drink," which was invented over 300 years ago. It was used to strengthen women's reproductive organs and was very popular. George Ohsawa slightly changed it, and it is good for everyone. *Mu* means "nothing," and the name comes from the phrase "mu cha kui cha." *Mu cha* means "confusion, disorder,

mixed-up theories"; *kui* means "nine." George took the name Mu Tea Nine Herbs and used nine ingredients, including ginseng.

Ordinarily, in the macrobiotic way of eating, we do not use ginseng, because it is very yang and gives constricting effects. Breathing becomes difficult and body temperature becomes cold. However, by blending it with more yin herbs, the effect is neutralized. Still, mu tea is a slightly yang drink, and it is better not to cook it or rewarm it a long time, or strong effects may result. In addition to the mu tea with nine herbs, there is another variety with sixteen herbs that is even slightly more yang.

For healthy persons, boil a tea bag for 10 minutes in 3 cups of water. For persons with yin conditions such as a weak stomach, yin coughing, menstrual cramps or irregular menstruation, boil the bag in 3 cups of water for 5 minutes, then simmer for 25 minutes or until only half the liquid (1½ cups) remains. It may be taken several times a week for 3 to 4 weeks.

MUSTARD PLASTER

Allergies, bronchitis, cystic fibrosis, lung congestion, and pulmonary heart disease

The mustard plaster, a traditional Far Eastern remedy, dissolves stagnation and stimulates circulation, especially in the lungs. It can help relieve mucus accumulation or coughing and is good for muscle stiffness.

While preparing the plaster, warm up 2 towels. Crush enough mustard seeds to obtain a handful of mustard powder. As a substitute, mustard powder or, if unavailable, mustard spread from a jar may be used. Bring some water to a boil and add enough to the mustard to make a moist paste. The consistency should be light and soft, something like mustard from a jar. Spread the paste onto half of a triple layer of paper towels or one layer of waxed paper. (The area should be large enough to cover the chest if it is being used for the lungs or upper back.) Fold in half and cover the paste on both sides. Spread a towel on the area to be treated. Place the mixture in this wrapper of paper towels or waxed paper on top of the towel and cover with the second towel. Leave the plaster on until the heat starts to feel uncomfortable, usually 10 to 15 minutes.

- The skin will become red, which is normal.
- The effects will last as long as the red color remains.
- Do not apply mustard directly on the skin, as it will burn!
- When using this plaster on children, mix in an equal amount of flour.
- If some mustard inadvertently leaks and burns the skin, spread a small amount of olive oil or other light vegetable-quality oil on the affected area.
- For lung troubles, you may apply the plaster on the chest, back, or both.
- In case of an acute condition, you may apply the plaster 2 or 3 times a day, but refrain from too frequent use, as it may burn the skin if repeated too often.

NABE-STYLE VEGETABLES WITH DIPPING SAUCE

Cervical cancer and many other conditions and disorders

Nabe style is a quick light summer style of boiling that is done on a portable burner at the table, usually in a large open ceramic or metal nabe pot. If a special earthenware nabe pot and portable burner are not available, this dish may be prepared quickly on the stovetop in a large stainless-steel skillet. It differs from nishime style since it uses more leafy green than root vegetables, more water, no lid, no seasoning, a higher flame, and much less cooking time.

Ingredients:

- Select among green, upward-growing vegetables and slice several of the following: kale, collard greens, cabbage, Chinese cabbage, red cabbage, leeks, mustard greens, carrot tops, daikon tops, radish tops, turnip tops, scallions, dandelion greens, broccoli, broccoli rabe, fresh or dried shiitake and other mushrooms, string beans, celery, chives, snap peas, snowpeas, sprouts, Brussels sprouts, bamboo shoots, fresh green shiso leaves, onion, etc.
- Select among daikon, carrot, lotus root, and other root vegetables, in smaller amounts (optional)
- Select among fresh or dried tofu, precooked udon noodles, fu, mochi, white meat fish (optional)
- Strip of kombu (about 2 by 3 inches for 4 cups of vegetables)
- Spring or well water.

Slice as many types of the vegetables as desired, and place in sections on a large platter. Pour 1 to 2 inches of water into the nabe pot with a strip of kombu (may be omitted, if necessary) and with soaked and chopped dried shiitake mushrooms, if desired. Bring to a rapid boil on a high flame and cook until the kombu and/or mushrooms soften. You need not add any other seasonings to this dish. Then begin to add the sliced vegetables to the rapidly boiling broth. Add them in separate sections, starting with the harder vegetables which require the longest cooking time. Slowly add all the vegetables: most should require only 1 to 2 minutes of boiling. End with those such as sprouts, scallions, and fresh green shiso leaves, which require only several seconds of cooking. Occasionally, for variety, fresh or dried tofu, precooked udon noodles, soaked fu, mochi, or white meat fish may be added. It may be necessary to add more water during cooking as the bubbling broth evaporates.

When finished, this dish should yield a large pot of bright green, fresh and light vegetables. It should be served immediately. If cooked at the table, vegetables may be eaten continuously and new ones added to the pot. Cook only enough that can be eaten by a family at one meal to get the maximum freshness and lightness. It should be the main dish at this particular meal, ⅔ or more or the total meal volume and with grains ⅓ or less of the total volume.

Dipping broth

Nabe cooking broth
Miso or shoyu or umeboshi paste
Grated ginger (optional)

Chopped scallions
Toasted nori (optional)

The cooking broth is very delicious and refreshing to drink, and it may be used to make a dipping sauce as follows: Heat up a small volume of the broth and add miso or shoyu or umeboshi paste to taste. Simmer for about 3 minutes. Grate a small amount of ginger and squeeze in a few drops of juice, if desired. Add freshly chopped scallions and small pieces of toasted nori. Pour into a small dipping cup and dip in vegetables while eating at the table.

- For cervical cancer, nabe-style vegetables are also nice to eat often. But do not use udon noodles. Cook shiso leaves, Chinese cabbage, cabbage, and other leafy greens together. It is all right to add tofu or yuba. Rather than ginger, use nori and chopped scallions for the dipping sauce. It is all right to add a squeeze of yuzu (a kind of lemon) or lemon juice to the dipping sauce.

NISHIME-STYLE DAIKON WITH MISO FLAVOR

Headaches, vitality, and many other conditions

Use a heavy pot for nishime-style cooking. Soak about a 2-inch strip of kombu for 1 to 2 cups daikon, and slice it into 1-inch squares. Place the kombu on the bottom of the pot and add about 1 inch of water.

Cut daikon into large rounds and place it on top of the kombu. Add only a small amount of water to just cover the bottom of the pot. Cover and bring to a boil on a high flame. You may add a pinch of sea salt to make the daikon sweeter. Reduce the heat to low, and simmer for a long time, at least 15 to 20 minutes. (This period can be shortened. Especially in the summer season, it can be made shorter by chopping the daikon into smaller chunks.) Add a small amount of water to the bottom of the pot if the liquid completely evaporates. It is good that the daikon is cooked in the liquid that comes from daikon, with only a small amount of extra water.

When the daikon becomes soft, season it with a small amount of miso dissolved with water, at the last stage of cooking. Be careful not to make the preparation too salty. Shake the pot up and down with the cover on to distribute the salty taste. Simmer another 3 to 5 minutes on a low flame with the cover on. Finally, remove the cover and turn off the heat. Set aside for 2 minutes before serving. Be sure to serve the daikon with the cooking liquid.

See NISHIME-STYLE VEGETABLES in the recipe section.

NISHIME-STYLE ROOT VEGETABLES

AIDS, allergies, anemia, arthritis, blood disorders, diastolic high blood pressure, hypoglycemia, leukemia, Lyme disease, pancreatic problems, pulmonary heart disease, stroke, and varicose veins

Nishime-style cooking is a method of cooking large chunks of root vegetables for a long time in their own juices. Only a small amount of water is added. Seasoning may be at the beginning or at the end. The cooked vegetables are very juicy and are served along with the cooking liquid. See NISHIME-STYLE VEGETABLES in the recipe section.

Suggested combinations of vegetables include the following (all cooked with kombu): carrot, burdock, onions; carrot, parsnip, cabbage; turnip, shiitake mushroom, cabbage; burdock, leeks, lotus root; daikon or lotus root, carrot, corn; carrot, onion, cabbage; squash, onion, daikon; daikon, squash, cabbage; cabbage, onion. Carrot and daikon or carrot and turnip do not go together very well. Do not use oil or sweeteners in this recipe.

- For leukemia, nishime-style burdock, carrot, daikon, lotus, jinenjo, and kombu, cooked over a low flame, is particularly good.

NISHIME-STYLE SWEET VEGETABLES

Hypoglycemia

Cut an assortment of sweet vegetables in big pieces. Add a small amount of water and cook over a low flame for a long time with the juice, which eventually comes out from the vegetables while cooking. Seasoning may be done at the beginning or the end of cooking. Serve with the juice from the vegetables. See NISHIME-STYLE VEGETABLES in the recipe section.

Suggested vegetables include carrot, winter squash (buttercup, butternut, Hokkaido pumpkin, delicata, sweet dumpling, etc.), pumpkin, onion, cabbage, daikon, dried daikon, carrot, parsnip, sweet corn, and other sweet vegetables.

NOODLES

As a snack for many conditions

See UDON NOODLES IN BROTH and FRIED NOODLES WITH VEGETABLES in the recipe section.

NORI CONDIMENT

Bone and joint disorders and other conditions

Tear or cut 5 to 6 sheets of nori into 1-inch pieces. Put it into a saucepan and cover it with spring water, about ½ cup. Bring to a boil, cover, and reduce the heat to low. Simmer until most of the water evaporates and the nori forms a thick paste, about 30 minutes. Add several drops of shoyu a few minutes before the end of the cooking time. The nori should have a light salt taste. Cool and store in a glass jar.

• For a saltier condiment for those whose condition permits, use 1 to 3 tablespoons of shoyu.

OHAGI

Hypoglycemia, leukemia

Ohagis are soft, dumpling-size balls of brown rice and sweet brown rice filled with or coated with other ingredients. They are a traditional festive dish in the Far East and may be used medicinally as well as for special occasions. Popular types include ohagis with adzuki beans cooked with barley malt or brown rice syrup, ohagis cooked and mashed with winter squash or pumpkin, and ohagis with mashed chestnut.

Cook 2 cups sweet rice with 1½ cups water per cup of rice and a pinch of sea salt, as in the recipe for PRESSURE-COOKED BROWN RICE. Pound the rice in a wooden bowl with a heavy pestle or mallet until all the grains are half crushed and sticky. Wet the pestle occasionally to prevent the rice from sticking to it. This takes about 20 minutes or more of pounding. Form the dough into small balls and roll in various coatings.

For ohagis with adzuki beans, soak adzuki beans overnight and cook them the next morning. Add barley malt or salt several minutes before putting out the flame and mix well. Mash well with a suribachi. Cover the small rice ball with the adzuki paste when the adzuki mixture has cooled. Adzuki paste may be ¼ inch thick.

For ohagis with squash or pumpkin, peel the skin of a medium-size squash or pumpkin and cut it in pieces. Place in a saucepan with a lid and add water to a level of about one-third the vegetable pieces. Cook over a strong flame, reduce when it starts to boil, and cook until tender. Add a pinch of salt and cook another 2–3 minutes. Mash it in a suribachi. When it is cool, cover the small rice ball with the paste to make it about ¼ inch thick.

For ohagis with chestnut, take off the shell of a cup or more of chestnuts and put them in a saucepan with a lid. Add water to a level of about one-third the chestnuts. Cook with a strong flame, reduce when it starts to boil, and cook until the chestnuts become soft. Add a pinch of salt, cook another 3–4 minutes, and mash in the suribachi. When the mixture has cooled, cover the small rice balls with the paste to about ¼ inch thick. Note that dried chestnuts must be soaked overnight.

- For leukemia, ohagis made with black sesame seed gomashio are particularly recommended.

OKARA

Osteoarthritis, osteoporosis

Okara is the residue left over from making tofu. It is traditionally enjoyed in the Far East in a variety of dishes and is high in protein, vitamins, and minerals. In the United States, most commercial okara is sold as animal feed. You can obtain it by making tofu at home or by contacting a local soy dairy and asking them to save you some. It may be steamed, boiled, sautéed, and cooked in other styles and has a light, crumbly consistency and mild taste.

OSTEOARTHRITIS AND OSTEOPOROSIS STEW

Osteoarthritis and osteoporosis

Prepare the following dish: yellow or black soybeans soaked overnight (2 parts), kombu (1 part), dried shiitake mushroom (1 part), carrots (1 part), onions (1 part), squash (1 part), daikon greens or any hard leafy greens (2 parts). Chop all the ingredients finely and cook in 5 times the volume of water for a half hour or longer. Toward the end of cooking, add sweet young miso to taste (or half young miso and half older, 2–3-year aged miso). The liquid from this stew may be taken 3–4 times a week. Otherwise, cook the mixture longer and eat and drink all the ingredients. As a stew, it may be taken a little bit less often, 2–3 times a week.

PALM HEALING

ALS, cerebral palsy, heart problems, kidney cancer, leukemia, nervous conditions, spleen problems, stomach problems, upper digestive cancer, and many other conditions and disorders

Palm healing involves the use of the palms and hands to channel energy to different parts of the body. It is also known as *laying on of hands* and *therapeutic touch*. Simple techniques allow the energies of heaven and earth to circulate through the giver's palms and hands to the head, neck, shoulders, chest, or other region of the recipient. Palm healing is a very powerful type of healing and may succeed in difficult cases where dietary and lifestyle methods are not effective. The standard reference, *Macrobiotic Palm Healing* by Michio Kushi with Olivia Oredsen, presents the principles of palm healing along with hundreds of practical applications and exercises.

POTATO PLASTER

Colon cancer (pain), diverticular disease, enteritis, kidney cancer, liver problems, pancreatic problems, and pneumonia

Peel, grate, and mash an ordinary potato. Add 20 to 30 percent white flour and make into a paste, adding a little water if necessary. Spread the mixture about 1 inch thick on a cotton cloth. Before applying, do a HOT TOWEL COMPRESS on the affected area for about 3 minutes to promote better circulation. Then apply the plaster directly on the skin. Tie it with a cotton strip, cheesecloth, or cotton towel so the plaster does not move. Leave on for 4 hours or the whole night. Repeat every day for 2 weeks or more.

POTATO-CABBAGE PLASTER

Kidney cancer, stomach cancer, and testicular cancer

This plaster has a softening and drawing effect on tumors.

Grate potato. If the potato is too watery, place it in a double layer of cheesecloth and squeeze out the excess water before combining it with the other ingredients. In a suribachi, mash an equal amount of finely chopped raw cabbage leaves. Combine potato (1 part) and cabbage (1 part). Make a plaster by mashing them together. Twenty to 30 percent white flour may be added to make a paste. Spread the mixture about 1 inch thick on a cotton cloth. Before applying, do a HOT TOWEL COMPRESS on the affected area for about 3 minutes to promote better circulation. Then apply the plaster directly on the skin. Tie it with a cotton strip, cheesecloth, or cotton towel so the plaster does not move. Leave on for 4 hours or the whole night. Repeat every day for 2 weeks or more.

POTATO-CABBAGE-HATO-MUGI PLASTER

Pancreatic cancer

Follow the instructions for making a potato-cabbage plaster above, adding 1 part cooked hato mugi.

RAN-SHO

Acute heart weakness including heart attack, stroke, and heart failure.

Ordinarily we do not eat eggs in the standard macrobiotic way of eating. However, for certain medical conditions, egg may be beneficial. *Ran* means "egg" and *sho* means "fermented liquid" or "soy sauce." This preparation is very yang. Eggs as well as soy sauce are very yang foods. The purpose of ran-sho, however, is not to supply egg, but to provide quickly a large amount of shoyu in a form that is harmless and will be easily absorbed by the body. For this reason, it is necessary to add a large amount of protein (in the form of an egg) to the shoyu. This mixture has a very strong effect. Therefore we should use ran-sho only in special, extreme circumstances.

This remedy is prepared from two ingredients: an organic, preferably fertilized egg and shoyu. They are mixed in a proportion of 2 (up to 4) parts egg to 1 part shoyu. Break the egg and beat the yolk and the egg white together. (Sometimes only the yolk is used to prepare ran-sho.) Add about 1 tablespoon of shoyu to the egg. The traditional way to determine how much shoyu should be added was as follows: take the half shell of the broken egg and fill it half full with shoyu. Now mix these ingredients very, very well, beating for several minutes. Give only once the first day, and then, if needed, a second time a half day later, but no more than twice altogether.

- For ordinary, milder use, use the raw egg and shoyu as is. For a stronger effect, use just the egg yolk and shoyu.

- Ran-sho is good for yin conditions—such as someone near death—to make the heart start beating. In this case, give teaspoon by teaspoon, repeating 2 or 3 times a day if necessary. But be very careful; in other cases, such as a drug overdose, which is also caused by extreme yin, giving ran-sho may produce the opposite effect and cause the heart to stop. In the case of drug overdose, yin should be dispersed by giving strong MISO SOUP with ginger. This is much safer. Ideally, give ran-sho under the supervision of an experienced macrobiotic teacher.

- For emergency first aid in case of heart attack or stroke until medical help arrives, press, bite, or apply fire (moxa) to the little finger to activate the heart. The heart meridian ends just below the nail on the inside of the little fingers, and stimulation here will help revive the person. Or put strong pressure on the nails of the little finger with a needle, chopstick, or finger pressure. Press the heart point on the lower inside of the wrists to activate the heart meridian, especially on the left side. Breathe strongly while pressing. Repeat several times for up to several minutes or until the person begins to stabilize.

For Acute Heart Weakness Caused by Yin Products

- During sports competitions in the Orient, mothers traditionally used to give ran-sho to their children to make their hearts strong. But people in those days were not eating much animal food, so they could take this strong combination. For vegetarians it is good, but for people eating animal food, it has such a powerful effect that it is better not given.

- Specifically, it will strengthen the heart when it has become weak by an overintake of yin substances (sugars, sweets, soft drinks, fruits, alcohol, and other extremely expansive foods). It has been used to activate the heart, especially for heart failure.

- You can give ran-sho to people showing signs of acute heart weakness caused by yin products, and who have a rapid and weak pulse. Do not give it in case of mild heart troubles, such as extra systoles or irregular beating.

- Also do not give it to people with heart troubles produced by a yang cause. In that case the cheeks or the ears look red, and usually there is a strong pain in the chest area. For yang heart failure, such as that caused by meat, poultry, eggs, cheese, or too much salt, ran-sho has the opposite effect and makes the condition worse. In such cases give WARM APPLE JUICE instead or put a DAIKON PLASTER on the heart area.

- To tell if a heart attack or stroke is caused by more yin or yang, look at the person's hands after the attack. If open, the cause is more yin and ran-sho can be given. If the hands are closed, it is more yang, and ran-sho should not be given.

- If you cannot decide whether it is yin or yang, put a raw egg in MISO SOUP with plenty of scallions, Chinese cabbage, onions, and a little ginger. That will make the heart beat actively and improve circulation. This is also good for severe anemia.

- Do not give this preparation more than once per day, and not more than 3 days in a row.

For Sanpaku (Yin) Near Death

- You can give ran-sho to yin people in a near-death state. At that time they will usually show a marked yin *sanpaku* condition (the pupils of the eyes are pointing upward, so that much of the sclera, the white part of the eyes, becomes visible under the iris). Give the preparation teaspoon by teaspoon; otherwise its effect may be too sudden.
- Repeat this treatment 2 or 3 times a day. It has a very strengthening effect.

RAW RICE

Bloodshot eyes, eye inflammations, and glaucoma

Raw rice has traditionally been used to treat eye inflammations, bloodshot eyes, glaucoma, and other conditions. The rice is soaked in water so that it becomes slightly soft. Then the water is drained, and the moist rice grains are crushed in a suribachi. Again a little water is added and the mixture is kneaded and further pounded. Without applying heat, this type of uncooked rice is eaten every day for 4 to 5 days. Energetically, if we use fire, a rising upward-type of energy becomes more activated, which would not benefit bloodshot eyes. Rather, we use here the gathering, downward energy created by pounding and kneading.

RICE BRAN (NUKA) PLASTER

Allergies, boils, broken bones, hives, infections, inflammations, and other conditions

Generally, commercial soaps, creams, and lotions clog the meridians, holes, and sweat glands, impeding ki. People who eat dairy food are especially attracted to these products. Dry skin comes from a layer of oil and fat blocking the skin, not from a lack of oil. Rice bran is very helpful for this and many other skin conditions. It is soothing for broken bones and may also be put on the toes for frostbite lesions.

Traditionally, rice bran (known as *nuka* in the East) has been used thousands of years. Rice was traditionally kept unpolished until eaten, and then the polishings, or bran, were kept for pickling and soap. Nuka will make the skin very clean and shiny. It has strong healing power.

To a handful of rice bran, add about ⅓ as much flour, and mix. Use rice flour if available, or hato mugi flour. Otherwise use wheat or white flour. Add cold water as needed to make a thick paste. Put the mixture in a cheesecloth, dip in hot water, and apply on the skin. Rinse the plaster off and apply a fresh one when it becomes warm.

- Nuka water can be applied around the vagina, but do not use as a douche because the bran texture may be irritating in this region. Nuka may also be added to the bath.
- Use wheat or oat bran if rice bran is not available.

ROASTED BROWN RICE PORRIDGE

Rheumatoid arthritis

Lightly roast washed brown rice in a dry skillet without oil. Then make BROWN RICE PORRIDGE (KAYU) by cooking 1 part of rice with 2 to 3 times the amount of water.

- For rheumatoid arthritis, have this with umeboshi, shiso leaf powder, or GOMASHIO several times a week.

ROASTED BROWN RICE PORRIDGE WITH GRATED DAIKON AND SHOYU

Uterine cancer

Roast washed brown rice in dry skillet without oil. Place in a large pot, and add 3 to 4 times the volume of water. Bring to a boil and simmer to make a thin porridge (gruel). Add 1 tablespoon of grated daikon for 1 cup of porridge. Simmer for another 2 to 3 minutes, and then add a little shoyu.

ROASTED BUCKWHEAT AND SCALLION TEA

Liver cancer

Make a tea by mixing lightly roasted buckwheat groats (3 parts) with chopped raw scallion (2 parts), and adding 5 times the total volume of water.

SALMON HEAD–SOYBEAN STEW

Anemia, blood disorders, and impaired vitality

This dish is made from a salmon head cooked together with yellow soybeans and kombu and seasoned with miso or shoyu.

Chop a salmon head into small pieces. Place them in a large pot. Add soaked yellow soybeans that are twice as much as the volume of the salmon head, and add the soaked, softened kombu that is as much as 10 to 15 percent of the total amount. Then add twice the amount of water as the total amount of other ingredients, and cover the pot with a heavy lid.

Bring to a boil on a high flame. Lower the heat and simmer for long time, about 2 to 3 hours. It may take only 1 to 1½ hours using a pressure cooker. When the bone of the salmon head has melted and the soybeans have become soft, add miso and gently stir. Simmer for another 5 minutes with the cover on. After long boiling, the salmon head becomes very tender and it often melts; it can be consumed completely.

- You may add chopped carrot that is as much as 10 percent of the total amount.
- If you have made a large amount, save the remaining in the refrigerator, and eat a bowl of this dish every day for about 3 days, heating it up as needed.
- For anemia, this dish makes the blood stronger.

SALT PACK

Appendicitis, arm and hand problems, bone and joint problems, bursitis, diarrhea (yin), digestive disorders, enteritis, foot and leg problems, pancreatic problems, stomach ulcers, and other conditions

The purpose of the salt pack is to heat and ease tension in various parts of the body, including stiff muscles, the abdominal area in cases of diarrhea, intestinal cramps, and stomach cramps, or under the feet.

Dry-roast 1½ pounds of any kind of sea salt in a stainless steel skillet until it is very hot.

Wrap the hot salt in a thick cotton towel and tie it securely with a string. Apply to the affected area. Change the salt or reheat it when it starts to cool off. Save the salt, as it can be used for a salt pack again. Eventually, discard it when the salt becomes gray and no longer holds heat.

- Sand may be used, if salt is not readily available.

SALT WATER ENEMA

Constipation

As an alternative to commercial enemas, you can mix ½ quart warm water with 1 to 2 tablespoons sea salt. Pour this liquid into a refillable enema bottle and then do the enema. If you have not done an enema before, consult with someone who has experience doing enemas. See also BANCHA TEA AND SEA SALT ENEMA

SAUTÉED KONNYAKU

Constipation

Chop a block of KONNYAKU, a gelatinous cake, into shapes like noodles or matchsticks (or use noodle-like konnyaku). Then sauté it with a little sesame oil. Season with shoyu to taste.

SAUTEED VEGETABLES

Anemia, cardiomyopathy, Lyme disease, spleen problems, valve problems, and varicose veins

See SAUTÉED VEGETABLES in the recipe section.

SCALLION-MISO CONDIMENT

Skin cancer (after surgery), and upper digestive cancers

See MISO-SCALLION CONDIMENT on page 482.

SEEDS

Mad cow disease

Dry-roasted sesame, sunflower, pumpkin, or squash seeds will help strengthen the nucleus of cells and are very delicious. To prepare, first gently rinse the seeds; then place a handful or two (but not too many seeds at a time) in a dry skillet. Adjust the heat to medium-low and gently stir the seeds using a wooden roasting paddle or wooden spoon for 5 to 10 minutes, shaking the pan from time to time. When done, seeds will have darkened in color, become crisp, and will have a fragrant aroma. Seeds may be lightly seasoned with sea salt or soy sauce toward the end or roasted to make them more digestible and tasty.

SEMI-FASTING

Headache

It is helpful to practice SEMI-FASTING or FASTING, but it must be limited to 1 week to 10 days. Take water or tea at that time. You may also take BROWN RICE PORRIDGE, a thick rice gruel. Besides, it is helpful to have a cup of SWEET VEGETABLE DRINK every morning and every evening.

SESAME OIL–GINGER RUB

Bone cancer (after radiation stiffness), bone and joint problems, rheumatoid arthritis, and frontal headache

In the Far East, sesame seeds were considered medicine for longevity. By adding a little ginger oil to the sesame, its effectiveness can be increased. This remedy is good for arthritis, rheumatism, or pain in the joints or to activate blood circulation. It is also good for dandruff and for hair falling out. It can also be put in the ear or eye (see note below). Use toasted dark sesame oil if available. Otherwise, light sesame is suitable.

Mix raw sesame oil (1 part), with the juice squeezed from freshly grated ginger (1 part). Shake well before using, and soak a cotton cloth in the mixture. Rub the stiff area with the cloth to make the muscles relax.

- If a burning sensation results, reduce the ginger.
- If put in the eye, first heat the oil, let it cool, and strain through a handkerchief.
- For radiation stiffness, after radiotherapy, clean the skin with a warm towel after 10 minutes. Do it twice a day.
- To improve circulation in rheumatism and arthritis, rub on the stiff area for 10–15 minutes and wipe the oil out with a warm towel. This may be repeated every day or every other day for 2–3 weeks.

SESAME OIL WITH SHOYU AND GRATED GINGER

Constipation

Lightly simmer 3 to 4 tablespoons of SESAME OIL and add 1 to 2 teaspoons of SHOYU and ⅓ teaspoon of GRATED GINGER. Mix and drink slowly.

SESAME SEED TEA

Constipation, eye problems

Use black sesame seeds if available. Otherwise, use white (tan or brown) seeds.

To 2 tablespoons of slightly crushed sesame seeds, add 1 cup of boiling water and cook 15 minutes. Drink the seeds as well as the liquid.

- A sweet taste, such as barley malt, may be added if desired. Take daily for 2 to 3 weeks.

SHIATSU

Adrenal problems, cerebral palsy, headaches, heart problems, nervous conditions, pancreatic problems, pituitary problems, sinus problems, spleen problems, stomach problems, and many other conditions

Shiatsu is a form of acupressure massage that stimulates energy flow in the body through pressure on points, meridians, and other parts of the body. It can be very effective to treat a wide range of conditions and disorders. It is easy to learn and can be done among family members and friends. For serious conditions, a qualified practitioner is recommended. Please refer to some of the numerous books about doing shiatsu at home or consult with a qualified specialist: *Beginner's Guide to Shiatsu* by Patrick McCarty; *Basic Shiatsu* by Michio Kushi; *Barefoot Shiatsu* by Shizuko Yamamoto and Patrick McCarty; or *Shiatsu Handbook* by Shizuko Yamamoto and Patrick McCarty.

SHIITAKE TEA

Bronchitis, post-traumatic stress disorder, yang heart conditions, and other conditions

Traditionally this tea was known to reduce fever, dissolve animal-quality fat, and relax a contracted or tense condition. Dried shiitake mushrooms are preferred to fresh, whenever possible.

Soak 1 shiitake mushroom in 1 cup of water for 20 to 30 minutes. When the shiitake mushroom is soft, chop it finely. Bring to a boil, reduce the flame, and simmer gently for 10 to 15 minutes. Add a pinch of sea salt or a few drops of shoyu toward the end. Drink while hot.

SHIITAKE-DAIKON TEA

Bone and joint disorders, kidney and bladder problems, and muscle problems

This tea is also good to help eliminate the accumulation of fat and lower fever.

Soak 2 shiitake mushrooms for a half hour. Add ¼ cup grated daikon and 2 cups of water. Bring to a boil and simmer for 20 to 30 minutes. Take only half of this preparation at one time.

SHIO-KOMBU

Bone and joint disorders, brain cancer, food allergies, Lyme disease, and stroke

Shio-kombu means "salty kombu" and is a popular condiment in Japan. It is traditionally made by rinsing the dust off kombu strips, cutting with scissors into small squares, and soaking in shoyu for 1 to 2 days. After soaking, the kombu is put in a pot with just enough shoyu to cover and cooked over a slow heat without a cover. It is cooked until nearly all the juice has evaporated, 1 to 2 hours, and care is taken to prevent burning. At the end, each piece of kombu is mixed very slowly to coat it with the remaining juice. A few roasted sesame seeds are mixed in at the end. The salty kombu will keep unrefrigerated for over a year. Only 1 or 2 small pieces are eaten each time.

For a faster method, soak 5 to 6 strips of kombu, 8 to 12 inches long, for several minutes, or until they are soft enough to cut. Slice into 1-inch squares. Place in a saucepan and cover with a mixture of ½ cup shoyu and ½ cup water. Simmer until all the liquid evaporates, about 30 to 40 minutes. Cool off and store in a glass jar.

For an even faster method, wash and soak 1 ounce of dried kombu for 3 to 5 minutes. Cut with scissors into ½-inch squares. Put the kombu in a pressure cooker and add 3 tablespoons shoyu and ½ cup water. Bring up to pressure and cook for 10 minutes. Let the pressure come down naturally, uncover, and simmer until all the liquid has evaporated.

SHOYU BANCHA TEA

Concussion, fainting, fatigue, frontal head-ache, nausea and vomiting, and other more yin ailments and conditions

This drink is good to strengthen the blood if an overly acidic condition exists, to relieve fatigue, to relieve headaches due to overconsumption of simple sugars and/or fruit juice, and to stimulate good blood circulation.

Place one teaspoon of shoyu into a teacup and pour in hot bancha twig or bancha stem tea that has been made a little stronger than usual. Stir well and drink hot. (You may add one chopped umeboshi into this drink for UME-SHO BANCHA.)

- Be careful to pour the hot tea over the shoyu in a cup, not the other way around (adding the shoyu to the pot).

SMALL INTESTINE DRINK

Small intestine conditions and disorders

Prepare the following special drink: daikon greens or other hard greens (2 parts), dried shiitake mushroom (1 part), corn (including corn products such as grits) or sweet vegetables such as cabbage (2 parts), wakame or nori (1 part). Add 4–5 times the volume of water. Drink 1 cup per day for three weeks.

SOBA WITH GRATED JINENJO

Constipation

Cook soba noodles and pour on broth made from kombu, dried shiitake, and shoyu. Finely grate jinenjo (mountain potato) and spoon it on top of the noodles and broth.

SOUR GREEN APPLE SAUCE

Liver cancer (jaundice)

Grate 2 to 3 cups of sour green (Granny Smith) apples. Add a small amount of water, and simmer for 2 minutes. Take frequently until the jaundice disappears. Be sure to use tart apples.

SOYBEAN SPROUTS WITH LEEKS

Constipation

Choose soybean sprouts on which the beans still remain. Place chopped leeks in a pot, and layer sprouts on top. Cook in a small amount of water until all vegetables are soft. Season the dish lightly with sea salt or shoyu.

STEAMED LEAFY GREENS

Heart attack, high blood pressure

See the recipe section. Use daily as a fresh dish instead of raw salad.

STRETCHING EXERCISES

For many conditions and general good health.

Stretching exercises, as taught by various systems of yoga, tai chi and the martial arts, and aerobics classes are very helpful to stimulate energy flow and harmonize mind, body, and spirit.

SWEET KUZU DRINK (AME KUZU)

Hypoglycemia

This drink helps relax the mind and body. It is especially recommended for children and can bring down fever in small children. It is also good for stomach and intestinal problems, hypoglycemia, premenstrual and menstrual cramps, and tension caused by intake of too much yang such as chips, crackers, and other hard baked goods. In olden days, monks would drink ame kuzu after begging in order to make themselves mellow and relaxed to study.

Dissolve 1 heaping teaspoon of kuzu in 2 or 3 tablespoons of cold water. Add 1 cup of cold water to the dissolved kuzu. Add 1 to 2 teaspoons brown rice syrup, barley malt, amazake; or ½ cup apple juice or apple cider. Bring to a boil over a medium flame, stirring constantly to avoid lumping, until the liquid becomes transluscent. Reduce the flame as low as possible. Drink while hot.

SWEET VEGETABLE DRINK

AIDS, Alzheimer's disease, atopy, bone cancer, brain tumor, breast cancer, diabetes, gout, hypoglycemia, kidney cancer, lung problems, Lyme disease, lymphoma, mental disorders, nervous conditions, ovarian cancer (pain), pancreatic cancer, post-traumatic stress disorder, rheumatoid arthritis, seasonal affective disorder, skin cancer, stomach cancer, stress, testicular problems, thyroid and throat cancer, women's reproductive cancers, and many other conditions

This drink was developed to help offset the effects of chicken, egg, and cheese consumption, leading to hypoglycemia, or chronic low blood sugar, a condition that affects about 75 or 80 percent of everyone in modern society.

Sweet vegetable drink is good for softening tightness caused by heavy animal food consumption and for relaxing the body and muscles. It is especially beneficial for softening the pancreas and helping to stabilize blood sugar levels. A small cup may be taken daily or every other day, especially in the mid- to late afternoon. It will satisfy the desire for a sweet taste and help reduce cravings for simple sugars and other stronger sweets.

Use equal amounts of 4 sweet vegetables, finely chopped (onions, carrots, cabbage, and sweet winter squash). Boil 3 to 4 times the amount of water, add chopped vegetables, and allow to boil uncovered for up to 3 minutes. Reduce the flame to low, cover, and let simmer for 20 minutes.

Strain the vegetables from the broth. (You may occasionally use them later in soups and stews.) Drink the broth, either hot or at room temperature.

- No seasoning is used in this recipe.
- Sweet vegetable drink may be kept in the refrigerator for up to 2 days, but should be warmed again or allowed to return to room temperature before drinking.
- Substitute daikon and lotus root for carrots and squash; prepare according to the recipe above.

TANGERINE JAM

Ovarian Cancer

Finely slice tangerines. (Do not peel them.) Add a small amount of water and a pinch of sea salt, and bring to a boil. Lower the flame and then simmer to make a jam.

TANGERINE TEA

Ovarian cancer

Dissolve TANGERINE JAM in BANCHA TWIG TEA or hot water and drink.

TARO PLASTER

Appendicitis, boils, burns, cysts, fractures and dislocations, gallbladder problems, leprosy, pancreatic problems, sprains and strains, tuberculosis, and yang diarrhea
See contraindications for cancer below

Taro is a small, hairy tuber native to Hawaii, the Caribbean, Southeast Asia, and other tropical and semitropical regions. It is used in cooking in these regions as well as medicinally.

Traditionally, the taro potato plaster has been used to draw out blood, pus, carbon, and excess protein and fat from boils and tumors. Dr. Sagen Ishizuka, the grandfather of modern macrobiotics in Japan, used this remedy for tumors caused by egg, fish, or other animal food consumption; George Ohsawa received the remedy from him. It is good for strong yang conditions such as colon, pancreas, or liver tumors, but for yin type of conditions such as breast cancer it can cause the tumor to spread. It is also better to put the taro plaster on isolated organs and not on the prostate, ovaries, or other organs which (though yang) are located close to other organs and which might cause the tumor to spread.

Before applying the taro potato plaster, you may do a very short-time GINGER COMPRESS (3 to 5 minutes) to warm up the skin and to increase the effectiveness of the plaster.

If the plaster feels too cold, a SALT PACK may be placed on top. If the plaster feels itchy, you may rub sesame oil on the skin before the plaster is applied the next time.

Remove the skin from the taro potato and grate the potato. Add 5 percent grated ginger and mix. (If the paste causes too much itching, you may omit the ginger.) If the paste is very wet, add a little unbleached white flour for finer consistency. The paste, however, should remain moist and have the consistency of wet cement or mud.

Spread the mixture about ½ inch thick on a clean cotton cloth. Apply the mixture directly on the affected area (not the cloth side). Leave the plaster on for about 4 hours. If the plaster has dried and is difficult or painful to remove, apply enough warm water to moisten the paste.

- For cancer or other serious illness, it is recommended that you see a qualified macrobiotic teacher regarding the use of this plaster. It is not recommended for malignancies of the breast, spine, reproductive organs, and other areas of the body.

TEKKA

Bone and joint disorders, drug allergies, epilepsy, gastroenteritis, mental disorders, nervous conditions, and stroke

See TEKKA in the Condiments and Seasonings part of the recipe section.

TEMPURA-STYLE VEGETABLES

Anemia, blood disorders, and other conditions

Food dipped in batter and deep-fried in oil at very high temperatures is called tempura. This unique method makes for a very delicious, crispy meal. The ingredients cook quickly, have a light taste, and produce strong energy. Almost all foods can be prepared tempura-style, including seafood, sea vegetables, vegetables, grains, and beans. The major exception is soft, watery vegetables, which turn soggy. Tempura is traditionally served with a shoyu-ginger sauce. The cooked morsels are dipped into this sauce at the table. A small amount of grated daikon is usually eaten with tempura as a condiment at the table in order to make the oil more digestible. A little mustard or horseradish is also served with fish or seafood tempura.

Tempura Batter

Combine the dry ingredients consisting of 1 cup whole wheat pastry flour, 1 to 2 tablespoons kuzu or arrowroot flour, and a pinch of sea salt. Then stir in 1 cup spring water per cup of flour and kuzu. Do not mix too much. Ideally the batter should be kept cold until it is used. It should be neither too dry nor too wet. If too watery, add a little more flour. If too dry, add a little more water. If the batter sits too long, it tends to thicken, so don't prepare it too far in advance. The more kuzu mixed into the flour, the more transparent and crispy the tempura will be. Small amounts of batter keep their consistency better than large amounts. When cooking large amounts of food, make additional batter as needed.

Tempura oil is traditionally sesame oil. Dark sesame oil is very delicious, but if you find its flavor too strong, use light sesame oil instead. Tempura oil can be saved and reused. It must be allowed to cool and then strained into a glass bottle or jar, and kept in a cool, dark place until needed. Fresh oil is ideal, but oil may be reused several times. Replenishing it each time with some fresh oil will make it last longer, but it should be discarded after 2 to 3 months.

Tempura vegetables include many combinations of vegetables and any style of cutting, including small pieces, large slices, flowerets, and whole leaves. The vegetables need to be dry and should be lightly patted with a cloth if too moist. It is nice to select about 2 vegetables from each group of root vegetables, round and ground vegetables, and green leafy vegetables. For each person, allow 2 to 3 pieces of each vegetable. The exact amount depends on the size and thickness of the pieces, the season of the year, and the freshness of the produce. *Root vegetables,* such as carrots, parsnips, lotus root, and burdock, are often sliced thinly for tempura. They may also be cut into small matchsticks, dipped together in batter, and deep-fried.

A single carrot slice and burdock slice are nice to combine. Watery root vegetables such as daikon, turnip, and rutabaga, are not usually cooked tempura-style. Round and ground vegetables, such as sliced onion rings, thinly sliced winter squashes, cauliflower and broccoli flowerets, finely minced cabbage, and string beans, snow peas, or thinly-sliced zucchini, can be used for tempura. Green leafy vegetables give tempura a beautiful shape. The leaves may be deep-fried whole or sliced. Especially nice are tempura dandelion (roots and flower can be cooked whole along with the greens), celery (the leafy part), and carrot tops. (Carrot stems can be minced and cooked tempura-style with root vegetables.) Also nice are parsley, watercress, kale, collards, milkweed, and lambsquarters, chrysanthemum leaves (with the batter applied on only 1 side and dipped in hot oil only 1 or 2 seconds, so that the other side remains bright green). Watery greens, such as Chinese cabbage, bok choy, and lettuce, are not usually cooked tempura-style.

In tempura cooking, slice all the vegetables first, prepare the batter and let it sit a few minutes, and then heat up the oil. A cast-iron pot, high-sided frying pan, or wok is ideal for making tempura. Cast-iron allows for more even control, and the oil doesn't evaporate as quickly as with other metals. A minimum of 1 inch of oil is needed in the pot, and 2 to 3 inches are often used. The oil needs to be between 345 and 355 degrees Fahrenheit. The ingredients will burn at higher heats or become soggy at lower temperatures. If the oil smokes, the temperature is too high. To check for the right temperature, drop a piece of batter into the hot oil. If the temperature is right, it will sink to the bottom

and then rise quickly to the top. If it stays at the bottom for a minute or so before rising, the temperature of the oil is too low. If the batter stays at the top and doesn't sink, the temperature is too high. Normally the heat is kept within the medium range.

When the correct temperature is attained, coat the sliced ingredients with batter and dip them one by one into the hot oil. It is important not to cover the pieces with too much batter or they will stick together or turn out too soft. Use chopsticks or fingers to dip them in and out of the batter quickly but evenly. Cook only 4 or 5 pieces of food in the pot at a time. More than that lowers the temperature of the oil and makes the tempura soggy. If the batter separates from the morsels while they are cooking, it is too thin, and you must add a little more flour to the batter. Sometimes you can dip the coated vegetables in a little dry flour before dipping them into the oil. This adds extra body and texture.

The ingredients should be deep-fried until golden brown. After a minute in the hot oil, turn them over with chopsticks to cook them evenly on the other side. Altogether the pieces will crisp up in 1 to 3 minutes, depending on the type of vegetable and the way it is cut. When the morsels are finished, allow them to drain off excess oil in a wire mesh tempura rack that fits over one side of the pot, or on paper towels or brown paper shopping bags on the counter. After cooking each piece, also skim the top of the oil with a wire oil skimmer to remove any particles of burnt oil and batter. After the ingredients have cooked and drained, keep them warm on a baking sheet in the oven at low temperature. When everything is ready, arrange the tempura attractively on a large platter, with like ingredients grouped together. The sauces and garnish are usually served individually. Making tempura properly takes time, usually about 30 to 60 minutes altogether for slicing ingredients, preparing the batter and oil, and deep-frying.

Tempura dipping sauce

Each individual serving consists of 1 tablespoon shoyu, 1 tablespoon dashi (kombu stock), a touch of grated ginger, ½ teaspoon grated daikon, and 1 teaspoon mirin (optional). If you do not have dashi stock on hand, use water. Mirin may be added to the basic dipping sauce, if desired, for a slightly sweeter taste. The sauce is served individually in small cups or bowls. At the table, each person dips the tempura in the sauce before eating.

Tempura garnish

In addition to the dipping sauce, a little grated daikon or grated turnip is traditionally served with the meal. To prepare, finely grate raw daikon or turnip and add 1 or 2 drops of shoyu to each serving. One teaspoon to 1 tablespoon of garnish per person is plenty. This helps to make the oil more digestible. (For fish or seafood, a stronger garnish of mustard or horseradish may also be served.)

THYROID DRINK

Graves disease and other thyroid conditions

Prepare the following special drink: carrots (2 parts), burdock (2 parts), daikon (2 parts), lotus root (2 parts), kombu (1 part), and daikon

greens or other hard leafy greens (4 parts). Chop finely, add four times as much water, boil, and simmer for about 15–20 minutes. Add a pinch of sea salt at the end of cooking or 3–4 drops of shoyu. Drink and eat the residue every day, 1 cup, for 10–14 days. Then every other day for an equal period.

TOFU AND LEAFY GREENS PLASTER

Arm and hand problems, bone and joint disorders, foot and leg problems, gout, hemorrhage, and other conditions

This is a milder plaster than the TOFU PLASTER and is especially good for hemorrhages and to relieve pain and inflammation.

Finely chop several leafy green vegetables, such as daikon leaves, kale, collards, Chinese cabbage, etc. Place in a suribachi and mash well. Squeeze out the liquid from an equal volume of tofu and mash tofu in a suribachi. Mix well to take out all lumps. Thoroughly mix the mashed greens and tofu. You may need to add 10 to 20 percent unbleached white flour to make a paste. Mix well. Apply the mixture (which should be moist) directly to the skin and cover with a towel. You may want to secure it in place with a bandage, or tie with a cotton strip. Change the plaster every 2 to 3 hours, or when it becomes hot.

TOFU PLASTER

Ankle problems, appendicitis, arm and hand problems, bone and joint problems, brain disorders, bronchitis, burns, concussion, digestive disorders, fever, foot and leg problems, frontal headache, knee problems, lung problems, muscular dystrophy, myasthenia gravis, muscle problems, nervous conditions, neuralgia, osteoarthritis, peripheral nerve disease, pneumonia, ruptured spleen, spinal cord disorders, stomach ulcers, stroke, and other conditions

Contraindication: high fever from chicken pox or measles (see note below)

The tofu plaster is good to help relieve inflammations, swellings, fevers, burns, dental abscesses, and bruises. The tofu is cold and therefore leads to contraction (a yang effect), serving to neutralize heat or inflammation. It is more effective than ice. The soft, yin quality of the tofu, meanwhile, absorbs fevers far more effectively than ice (which is hard or yang), and does not produce any side effects such as a secondary increase in fever. It extinguishes inflammatory processes and prevents swelling or decreases existing swelling.

This remedy has been successfully used in some cases of paralysis, such as stroke, or for a concussion such as a motorcycle accident in which the person is left unconscious. In such a case, after seeking medical attention and going to the hospital, immediately apply crushed, cold tofu to the affected part of the head, and continuously make and apply tofu plasters. They will help to heal and repair the damage quickly. Apply as soon as possible. Four hours later may be too late.

Squeeze out the liquid from a block of tofu and mash tofu in a suribachi. Mix well to take out all lumps. Add 10 to 20 percent unbleached white flour and 5 percent grated ginger. Mix well. (It is better to peel the ginger before grating for cool plasters, as ginger can irritate the skin.)

Apply the mixture (which should be moist) directly to the skin and cover with a towel. You may want to secure it in place with a bandage, or tie with a cotton strip. Change the plaster every 2 to 3 hours, or when it becomes hot.

- A tofu plaster may be combined with chopped, mashed leafy greens (as in the LEAFY GREENS PLASTER), especially for hemorrhages. (See TOFU AND LEAFY GREENS PLASTER.)
- A tofu and grain plaster may be used as an alternative, especially if the tofu plaster feels too cold. Make by mixing 50 percent cooked and mashed whole grain (rice or barley) which has cooled to room temperature, with 50 percent squeezed and mashed tofu.
- For high fevers, apply the tofu plaster on the head, including the brain area, if affected.
- For inflammatory processes, such as acute pneumonia or bronchitis, when the inflammation is located deeper in the body, first apply a GINGER COMPRESS.
- For bleeding within tissue, including brain hemorrhage, tofu plasters will prevent the clotting and hardening of the blood and will accelerate the reabsorption of the blood.
- Contraindication: do not apply tofu plasters when fever is caused by measles or chicken pox, unless really high (105 degrees Fahrenheit or 40 degrees centigrade, or higher). Temperature should only be kept within a safe range.

TOMATO-MISO SAUCE WITH SCALLIONS AND CHINESE CABBAGE

Prostate cancer

Combine mashed tomatoes (7 parts), chopped scallion (1 part), and chopped Chinese cabbage (1 part). Bring to a boil, and simmer. Add 10 percent miso and simmer for a long time. Take 1 tablespoonful at dinnertime.

UME CONCENTRATE (Bainiku Ekisu)

Headache, intestinal problems including infections, and stomach troubles such as lack of appetite, vomiting, and food toxicity (especially from shellfish, fish, and meat)

Bai means "ume, plum"; *niku* means "meat"; *ekisu* means "condensed extract or essence." Ume concentrate is actually more a medicine than a food, while umeboshi is as much a food as a medicine. The concentrate is prepared in the following way: The meat of raw green ume plums is crushed and pressed, and the juice is then simmered for about 48 hours, until a thick dark syrup is obtained. It takes 1 kilogram of fresh plums to make 20 grams of ume concentrate.

This preparation has an effectiveness similar to umeboshi, but it is much more concentrated and much less yang: salt, sunshine, pressure, and long time (all yang) are not used in its processing. It is therefore more suitable for use by meat-eating people. For yin, pale, tired persons, the umeboshi is preferable.

UMEBOSHI JUICE

Cramps, diarrhea (yin type), and other weakening conditions

Take a small volume of the juice that comes in a jar of umeboshi plums and mix with hot tea. Or you can make a similar juice by boiling the meat of several umeboshi in bancha tea or water. This is very strong so use sparingly.

UMEBOSHI PLUM

AIDS, asthma, dizziness, drug allergies, dysentery, enteritis, epilepsy, fainting, food allergies, gallbladder problems, gastroenteritis, headache (deep inside), influenza, liver problems, Lyme disease, mad cow disease, mental disorders, motion sickness, nausea and vomiting, nervous conditions, ovarian problems, pancreatic problems, stomach problems, stroke, and many other conditions

Umeboshi plum satisfies the desire for a sour taste. It is very strengthening and can help relieve fatigue, neutralize acidity or alkalinity, and improve blood and energy circulation. See UMEBOSHI PLUMS in the recipe section.

UME-KUZU

Anemia, blood disorders, colon cancer (with bleeding), leukemia (constipation or diarrhea), and lymphoma (constipation or sweating)

Dissolve 1 teaspoon of kuzu in 2 to 3 teaspoons of cold water. Add 1 cup of cold water to the dissolved kuzu. In a saucepan, bring this to a boil over a medium flame, stirring constantly with a wooden spoon or wooden chopsticks to avoid lumping, until the liquid becomes translucent. Reduce the flame as low as possible. To this liquid, add the pulp of ½ to 1 umeboshi plum that has had the pit removed and been chopped or ground to a paste. Do not add shoyu for UME-KUZU (this is called UME-SHO KUZU). Simmer for a short time longer, and then drink it hot.

UME-KUZU LOTUS TEA

Hemorrhoids

Dissolve 1 teaspoon of kuzu in 2 to 3 teaspoons of cold water. Add 1 cup of cold water to the dissolved kuzu. In a saucepan, bring this to a boil over a medium flame, stirring constantly with a wooden spoon or chopsticks to avoid lumping, until the liquid becomes translucent. Reduce the flame as low as possible. Grate a small amount of fresh lotus root (several teaspoons). Wrap the grated pulp in cheesecloth and then squeeze out the juice by hand. Add the juice to the kuzu mixture. Simmer for several more minutes and drink hot.

UME-SHISO BANCHA

Uterine cancer

Slightly rinse an umeboshi plum and ume-shiso leaves (that have been pickled with the plum) to remove the surface salt. Chop them and place them in a cup. Pour over the plum and leaves 7 to 8 times the total volume of either BANCHA TWIG TEA or BANCHA STEM TEA.

UME-SHO BANCHA

Alcohol reaction, anemia, anthrax, bladder cancer (bleeding), brain tumor, concussion, constipation, diabetes, diarrhea (yin style), digestive disorders, fainting, fatigue, frontal headache, headache (with constipation), heartburn, hypoglycemia, influenza, leukemia (with constipation or diarrhea, nausea and vomiting), prostate cancer (pain), stomach problems, stress, uterine cancer, and many other conditions

This drink strengthens the blood; regulates digestion and circulation; relieves fatigue and weakness; and is used to obtain relief from over-consumption of simple sugars, fruit, fruit juices, or other acid-forming foods or beverages.

Place ½ to 1 umeboshi plum into a teacup or small coffee cup. Add ½ to 1 teaspoon of shoyu. Pour in hot bancha twig or bancha stem tea that has been made a little stronger than usual. Stir well and then drink hot, eating the plum.

- The strongest, most effective umeboshi plums for medicinal use are aged 5 years or longer.
- For brain tumor, if conscious, give UME-SHO BANCHA using a spoon.

UME-SHO KUZU

Allergies, anemia, ankle problems, atopy, bladder cancer (bleeding), blood disorders, bone and joint disorders, brain cancer, brain tumor, breast cancer (with constipation), chemical allergies, colitis, concussion, constipation, diabetes, diarrhea (yin style), digestive disorders, environmental illness, fatigue, headache (frontal), headache (with constipation), hypoglycemia, insomnia (with constipation), infectious heart disease, irritable bowel syndrome, kidney and bladder problems, liver problems, Lyme disease, mad cow disease, mental disorders, nervous conditions, pulmonary heart disease, schizophrenia, sinus problems, skin cancer, spleen problems, stomach problems, upper digestive cancers, and other conditions

This drink strengthens the blood, promotes good digestion, and restores energy.

Dissolve one teaspoon of pure kuzu in 2 or 3 tablespoons of cold water. Add 1 cup cold water to the dissolved kuzu. Bring to a boil over a very low flame, stirring constantly with a wooden spoon or wooden chopsticks to avoid lumping, until the liquid becomes translucent, for about 2 to 3 minutes. Add the pulp of ½ to 1 umeboshi plum that has been pitted, chopped, and ground to a paste. Reduce the flame as low as possible. Add from several drops to ½ teaspoon of shoyu and gently stir. Simmer for 2 to 3 minutes. Drink and eat while hot.

VISUALIZATION

Cancer, heart disease, irritable bowel syndrome, post-traumatic stress disorder, and many other conditions and disorders

Visualization is a type of meditation in which the person sits quietly for a few minutes, focusing on a visual image or sound. Commonly for healing purposes, some people are encouraged to visualize red-blood cells fighting cancer cells or other diseased parts of the body. From the macrobiotic view, this type of violent, combative visualization is counterproductive

and should be avoided. Disease is not an attack on the body, but the result of living in disharmony with nature. It is actually a beneficial mechanism. Therefore, visualization should be entirely peaceful and harmonious. Visualizing oneself getting better as a result of wholesome food, natural environmental influences, and healthy relationships is strongly encouraged.

WARM APPLE JUICE

Acute heart trouble (caused by yang), intestinal cramping, and other contracted conditions

Grate an apple and press out its juice through cheesecloth. Heat in a saucepan on a low flame until warm, and drink.

- We do not recommend RAN-SHO for people with heart troubles resulting from a yang cause. In that case the cheeks or the ears look red, and usually there is a strong pain in the chest area. In such cases give WARM APPLE JUICE or put a DAIKON PLASTER on the heart area.
- For heart attack caused by yang, if the fists are clenched, give boiled or heated apple juice.
- For a seizure caused by yang, give hot apple juice, 1 to 2 cups. Again, the person will usually have clenched fists in this case.

WATER-SAUTÉED DAIKON AND DAIKON LEAVES

Colon cancer and uterine cancer

Chop daikon and daikon leaves, and water-sauté as in SAUTEED VEGETABLES in the recipe section. Season with a little miso or shoyu for colon cancer and a few drops of shoyu for uterine cancer.

WATER-SAUTÉED DAIKON OR TURNIP LEAVES

Ankylosing spondylitis

Chop daikon leaves or turnip leaves. Water-sauté as in SAUTÉED VEGETABLES and season with a little shoyu.

WHOLE-WHEAT FLOUR AND RICE VINEGAR PLASTER

Broken bones

In a mixing bowl, put enough whole wheat flour to make a plaster to cover the broken bone area. Pour in enough brown rice vinegar (not another type of vinegar) and knead with your hands until you can form a nice paste. Spread about 1 inch thick on a cotton cloth, and apply directly to the broken bone area of the skin. Bandage with cotton gauze or cheesecloth and fasten in place. You may leave this plaster on overnight.

WHOLE-WHEAT FLOUR WITH WILLOW LEAVES

Fractured bones, sprained joints, strained muscles

Mix willow leaves with wheat flour and some water. Apply this paste on fractured bones or on sprained joints or strained muscles.

YOGA

General good health and for many conditions and disorders

Yoga is a traditional system of unifying mind, body, and spirit that originated in India. It is now practiced all around the world. There are many types and styles of yoga. You may acquaint yourself with yoga by reading books or attending a class with a qualified teacher. It is recommended to study with a yoga teacher who is eating macrobiotically or understands the energetics of food. Avoid complicated and inverted postures, as a general practice.

ZOSUI WITH SCALLIONS AND MISO

Anemia

Prepare MISO-ZOSUI, using chopped scallions as the principal vegetable.

ZOSUI WITH SWEET VEGETABLES AND NORI

Bone cancer

Cook a porridge using 70 percent brown rice (barley, millet, or other grains can be mixed 20 to 30 percent) and 30 percent cabbage, onion, winter squash or pumpkin, carrot, daikon, and nori (same amount for each). Season with a small amount of miso, shoyu, or sea salt. See MISO-ZOSUI.

• Seasoning is not necessary for 10 days, in the case of no appetite for salt.

GLOSSARY

Adzuki beans Small red beans, especially beneficial for urinary functions. Also called azuki or aduki.

Agar-agar A white gelatinous sea vegetable product used in cooking as a thickener, in making aspics, and kanten. Comes in bars, flakes, or powder.

Amasake A beverage or sweetener made from fermented sweet rice and koji.

Arame A wiry, dark sea vegetable that turns dark brown when cooked.

Arrowroot A starchy root from a native American plant used as a thickening agent for making sauces, stews, and desserts.

Bancha twig tea Tea prepared from the twigs of the tea bush. High in calcium and other nutrients, it aids digestion and gives a calm, soothing energy. Also known as kukicha.

Barley A traditional grain in Southern Europe, North Africa, the Middle East, Central Asia, and most recently North America. It is used in soup, stews, bread, and beer and gives light, upward energy.

Barley malt A thick, dark brown sweetener made from barley. It is used in desserts, to sweeten beans, and to make medicinal preparations.

Black soybeans Shiny black soybeans, usually smaller and lower in fat than yellow soybeans. Also known as Japanese black beans.

Boiled salad A crisp, colorful salad made by lightly dipping different combinations of sliced vegetables into boiling water for 30 seconds to several minutes.

Bok choy A leafy green vegetable with thick white stems. Also known as *pok choy*.

Brown rice Unpolished rice that retains the germ, bran, and other outer layers of the whole grain. It contains an ideal balance of minerals, protein, and carbohydrates and gives strong, peaceful energy. It is available in three main varieties: short, medium, and long grain.

Brown rice vinegar A mild, delicate vinegar made from fermented brown rice or sweet brown rice. It is used in dressings, sauces, and medicinal drinks.

Buckwheat A cereal plant native to Siberia, Russia, and Eastern Europe. It is eaten in the form of kasha, whole groats, or soba noodles and gives strong, active energy.

Burdock A long, dark root vegetable that grows wild in many regions of the world. It is used in soups, stews, and nishime- and kinpira-style dishes and gives strong, contractive energy.

Chakras Energy centers in the human body extending from the crown of the head to the midbrain, throat, heart, solar plexus, intestines, and reproductive area. The chakras (from the Sanskrit word for "wheel") and the network of meridians extending from them are highly charged with natural electromagnetic energy and together form the human spiritual constitution.

Chinese cabbage A large leafy vegetable with light green leaves and thick white stems. Its mild, juicy flavor goes well in soups, stews, pickles, and other dishes.

Complex carbohydrates The food component that provides the body with a continuous source of energy. Known chemically as polysaccharides, they are found in whole grains, beans, vegetables, and sea vegetables and form the main part of the macrobiotic diet.

Condition A person's current state of health, which changes from day to day, month to month, and year to year. It may also refer to a less serious ailment in contrast to a sickness or disorder.

Constitution A person's physical, mental, and spiritual characteristics and tendencies at birth. It is determined primarily from the health, vitality, and way of eating of the mother during pregnancy, as well as the influence of the father, grandparents, and ancestors.

Couscous A variety of semolina wheat that cooks up quickly and is used in light grain salads and cakes.

Daikon A long white radish that is used in many regular and medicinal preparations. It helps discharge fat and oil from the body. It is cooked fresh or dried and grated raw as a garnish for fish, seafood, and other oily foods.

Discharge The elimination of fat, mucus, toxins, and other excess from the body through normal channels such as urination or bowel movement and abnormal channels such as coughing, sneezing, cysts, and tumors.

Do-in A form of acupressure self-massage in which the points and meridians are gently tapped, pressed, or manipulated with the hands. Also includes stretching exercises for the whole body.

Dulse A red-purple sea vegetable harvested in the North Atlantic Ocean. It is used in soups, salads, and side dishes and has a zesty flavor.

Electromagnetic energy The natural energy of the cosmos and the earth that flows through all things, including the human body. Artificial electromagnetic energy refers to energy and vibration from satellites, high-voltage lines, nuclear reactors, power plants, computers, television, and other modern high-energy sources.

Fermentation The living activity of enzymes and bacteria causes certain foods to change chemically and make them easier to digest. In the macrobiotic diet, fermented foods include miso, shoyu, natto, tempeh, amasake, sourdough bread, sauerkraut, and pickles.

Fiber The indigestible cellulose part of whole foods, especially the bran of whole grains and the outer skin of beans, vegetables, and fruits. Fiber helps cleanse the intestines and protect against cancer and other diseases. Refined, processed, and peeled foods are low in fiber.

Fu A dried wheat gluten product available in thin sheets or thick cakes. It cooks up softly and adds protein and texture to soups, stews, and other dishes.

Ginger A spicy, pungent, gold-colored root used in cooking as a seasoning, as a garnish, and for medicinal applications. It is primarily used fresh and grated with a small hand grater.

Ginger juice The liquid squeezed from grated ginger, used in cooking or medicinal preparations.

Ginger compress A hot compress made from the juice squeezed from hot gingerroot and water. It stimulates circulation, dissolves stagnation, and penetrates deeply into muscles and tissues, easing soreness and tension.

Gluten The sticky substance that remains after the bran has been kneaded and rinsed from whole wheat flour. Gluten is used to make seitan and fu.

Gomashio Sesame salt made from roasted, ground sesame seeds and sea salt. The most popular condiment in macrobiotic cooking, it is sprinkled on brown rice and other whole grains.

Grain coffee A mild beverage made from roasted barley, acorns, chicory, or other plants and sometimes a natural sweetener. It is used like instant coffee and is free of caffeine and stimulating effects.

Green nori flakes A sea vegetable condiment that is sprinkled on grains, vegetables, and salads. It is from a different variety of nori than the packaged variety available in sheets.

Hatcho miso A rich dark miso made from soybeans and sea salt without any grain added during fermentation. It has a mild salt taste and is used in soups, condiments, and other dishes.

Hijiki A dark brown sea vegetable that turns black when dried. It has a strong ocean taste and is rich in protein, calcium, and iron. It is imported from Japan or harvested off the Maine coast.

Hokkaido pumpkin A small round or blocky winter squash that originated in New England, was brought to the cold northern Japanese island of Hokkaido, and is now grown again in North America. One variety has a deep orange color and another has a light green skin similar to Hubbard squash.

Kanten A gelatin dessert made from agar-agar. It may include apples, berries, melons, or other fruits; amasake; adzuki beans; and other foods. After cooking, it is usually served chilled.

Kasha Buckwheat groats that are roasted and boiled.

Kayu Soft, creamy grain made by cooking rice or other whole grain with five to ten times as much water over a low flame for a long time.

Ki Natural electromagnetic energy from heaven and earth, as well as the vitality of food, water, breath, and other substances taken directly by the body. Known as *chi* in China, *prana* in India, and *holy spirit* in the Middle East.

Kinpira Sautéed root vegetables, especially burdock and carrots, cut into matchsticks and seasoned with shoyu. A strengthening, warming dish, it can also be made in the form of soup for additional vitality.

Koji A grain, often polished or semipolished rice, inoculated with the same bacteria that is used to initiate fermentation in miso, amasake, natto, sake, and other foods.

Kokkoh A porridge for babies and infants made from brown rice, sweet brown rice, adzuki beans, sesame seeds, kombu, and usually a little brown rice syrup or barley malt.

Kombu A thick, dark green sea vegetable that is cooked with whole grains, beans, and vegetables. It is also used to make soup stocks.

Kuzu A fine white starch made from the root of

the kuzu or kudzu plant. It is used in making soups, sauces, desserts, and medicinal drinks.

Lotus A water lily whose edible roots have a light brown skin, long hollow chambers, and an off-white inside. The large white seeds are also eaten. Lotus is especially beneficial for the lungs and sinuses.

Meridian A stream of natural electromagnetic energy flowing through the body. Far Eastern medicine and philosophy, including dietetics, acupuncture, shiatsu, do-in, and the martial arts are based on reestablishing the meridian flow, which can be impeded by improper diet and lifestyle.

Millet A small, yellow grain native to China, India, and Africa. It gives strong, balanced energy, has a mild, sweet taste, and is especially good for the pancreas, stomach, spleen, and lymphatic functions.

Mirin A sweet rice wine that may be used as a seasoning in cooking for special dishes.

Miso A nourishing, mildly sweet-tasting paste or purée made from soybeans, sea salt, and usually fermented barley or brown rice. There are many varieties of miso that are used in making miso soup, seasoning other dishes, and preparing sauces and dressings. Miso contains enzymes and other compounds that facilitate digestion, strengthen the blood, and help protect against cancer, heart disease, and radiation sickness. It is used externally as a plaster.

Mochi A dumpling, cube, or cake made from cooked, pounded sweet brown rice. It is especially good for lactating mothers, as it promotes the production of breast milk.

Mucus Heavy fluid normally secreted by the mucous membranes to protect and lubricate many parts of the body. However, excessive intake of fat, sugar, dairy, and flour products can cause the overproduction of mucus and clog the lungs, intestines, and other organs, preventing the body from discharging toxic excess. Pollution, smoking, and other environmental and lifestyle factors may also contribute to mucus buildup.

Natto Soybeans that are cooked, mixed with beneficial enzymes, and allowed to ferment for 24 hours. High in protein and vitamin B_{12}, natto is especially beneficial to digestion and strengthening the intestines.

Natural foods Foods that are traditionally or minimally processed without artificial additives or preservatives.

Nigari The crystallized salt residue from the liquid droppings of dampened sea salt. Used in making tofu.

Nishime A method of cooking in which different combinations of vegetables, sea vegetables, or soy products are cooked slowly with a small amount of water and shoyu. Also called waterless cooking.

Nori Thin black or dark purple sheets of dried sea vegetable. Turns green when toasted over a flame. High in vitamins and minerals, it is used to make sushi, wrap rice balls, and as a condiment. In the West it is also known as *laver*.

Ohagi Small ball or wedge of sweet rice, adzuki beans, or chestnut purée covered with sesame seeds, green nori flakes, or other coating. Ohagis are served on festive occasions.

Palm healing A healing art based on using the palms and hands to stimulate and balance the flow of electromagnetic energy in the body. Similar to the laying on of hands and therapeutic touch.

Polyunsaturated fats Lighter, healthier fats such

as those found in grains, beans, vegetables, and other whole foods, as well as white-meat fish.

Pressed salad Sliced or shredded vegetables combined with sea salt, umeboshi plums, brown rice vinegar, or shoyu and placed in a pickle press for a few hours. The pressing or pickling retains many of the enzymes and vitamins and makes the vegetables more digestible.

Refined oil Salad or cooking oil that has been chemically processed or extracted to maximize yield and extend shelf life. Refining strips the oil of its natural color, flavor, and aroma and reduces its nutritive value.

Rice balls Cooked brown rice shaped into balls, triangles, or wedges, usually containing a piece of umeboshi plum in the center, and covered with a wrapping of toasted nori or occasionally shiso leaves, toasted sesame seeds, or other condiment. Rice balls are eaten as snacks, lunches, and picnics, and are especially good for traveling since they keep for several days and do not require utensils.

Rice syrup A sweet, thick syrup made from brown rice used as a concentrated sweetener for desserts, beverages, and special dishes. High in complex carbohydrates, it metabolizes more gradually than simple sugars and is easier on the pancreas.

Sea salt Salt obtained from evaporated sea water and either sun-baked or kiln-baked. High in trace minerals, it is lower in sodium than ordinary salt and contains no sugar or chemical additives.

Sea vegetables Edible seaweeds. High in minerals and vitamins, sea vegetables strengthen the blood, contribute flexibility to the circulatory system, and calm and soothe the nerves.

Seitan High protein product prepared by cooking wheat gluten with shoyu, kombu, and water. It can be made at home or purchased ready-made at natural foods stores and be fashioned into cutlets and grain burgers or be added to soups and stews.

Sesame Tiny round seeds traditionally eaten in the Far East, Middle East, and other parts of the world. Used to make gomashio, tahini, sesame butter, sesame oil, and medicinal preparations.

Shiatsu A form of massage that releases blockages of electromagnetic energy and harmonizes energy flow in the body.

Shiitake A mushroom native to the Far East and now grown in North America and throughout the world. The dried variety is used in macrobiotic cooking for soup stocks, vegetable dishes, and medicinal preparations. It is very calming and helps discharge excess animal fat from the body.

Shio kombu Pieces of kombu cooked for a long time in shoyu and used as a condiment. *Shio* means "salt," and shio kombu has a strong, salty taste.

Shiso A red pickled leaf used to color umeboshi plums and as a condiment. Known in English as beefsteak plant, it is sometimes spelled chiso.

Shoyu Traditional, naturally made soy sauce made from fermented whole soybeans, wheat, and sea salt. Shoyu is best aged naturally for at least a year and not chemically processed.

Simple sugars Quick-burning carbohydrates such as those in sucrose (table sugar), fructose (fruit sugar), glucose, dextrose, and lactose (milk sugar). They enter the bloodstream rapidly and give a burst of energy but quickly subside.

Soba Noodles made from buckwheat flour or a combination of buckwheat and whole-wheat flour. Soba gives strong, warming energy and may be served in broth, in salads, with vegetables, or lightly chilled in summer.

Somen Very thin Oriental-style wheat or whole wheat noodles.

Suribachi A serrated, glazed clay bowl used with a pestle for grinding and puréeing foods. It is used for making condiments, spreads, dressings, baby foods, nut butters, and medicinal preparations.

Sushi Bite-size pieces of rice containing or topped with vegetables, pickles, fish, or other items. Vegetable sushi is wrapped in nori and sliced in rounds.

Sweet brown rice A glutinous, sweet-tasting variety of brown rice used to make mochi, ohagis, dumplings, baby foods, brown rice vinegar, and amasake.

Tahini A seed butter made by grinding hulled sesame seeds until smooth and creamy.

Tamari The liquid poured off during the process of making soybean miso. It is heavier, stronger, and more flavorful than regular shoyu and does not include wheat. Sold as "original" or "real" tamari, it is used for special occasions.

Taro A small, compact potato with a thick, dark brown, hairy skin. It is eaten in the tropics and used in macrobiotic health care as a plaster. Also known as *albi* and *poi*.

Tekka A condiment made from sautéed hatcho miso, sesame oil, burdock, lotus seed, carrot, and ginger root. It is dark brown or black in color and rich in iron and other minerals.

Tempeh A soy food made from split soybeans, water, and beneficial bacteria that ferments for several hours. Native to Indonesia, Sri Lanka, and Southeast Asia, it has spread around the world. Rich in protein and vitamin B_{12}, it can be made at home or be obtained ready made at natural foods stores and supermarkets. It is used in cutlets, soyburgers, soups, stews, and other hardy dishes.

Tempura A method of cooking in which seasonal vegetables and fish or seafood are coated with batter and deep-fried in vegetable oil. Native to Portugal, it was brought to the Far East and is now used by cooks worldwide.

Tofu Soybean curd made from soybeans cooked with nigari, a crystallized salt residue. High in protein, tofu blends well with many other foods and is enjoyed in soups, vegetable dishes, dressings, and frostings.

Toxin A compound of animal, vegetable, or mineral origin that is harmful to the body.

Udon Oriental-style noodles made from whole wheat or wheat flour. They are served in broth plain or with vegetables, seasoned with shoyu, and garnished with scallions or nori. Leftover udon may be fried.

Umeboshi plum A salty, pickled plum that stimulates the appetite, aids digestion, and strengthens the blood. Shiso leaves impart a bright red color and natural flavoring to the plums (actually a form of apricot) during pickling. They may be taken whole or in pieces as a condiment, used instead of salt as a seasoning in cooking, be added to rice balls or sushi, or used in medicinal teas. The hard pit is not eaten but can be saved and carbonized for use in special healing preparations.

Umeboshi paste A creamy paste made from umeboshi plums. It is used to season corn on the cob and to make sauces and other special dishes. It is not as strong as whole umeboshi, which is preferred for medicinal preparations.

Umeboshi vinegar A salty, sour vinegar made from umeboshi plums. Diluted with water, it is used in sauces, dressings, and as a condiment or seasoning.

Unrefined oil Vegetable oil that has been cold-pressed or solvent-extracted to retain its original color, flavor, aroma, and nutritive value.

Wakame A long, thin sea vegetable that cooks up a beautiful translucent green. High in minerals and vitamins, it has a sweet taste and delicate texture and is used in cooking miso soup and a variety of dishes.

Wheat berries Wheat grains in whole form are called wheat berries. They are used to make whole-wheat flour, noodles, and cracked or cut and processed into couscous and bulgur. Wheat berries are very chewy and are usually cooked together with other grains, beans, or vegetables.

Wild rice A wild grass native to the Great Lakes region that grows in water and is harvested by hand. The long, dark thin grains add taste, texture, and flavor to a variety of dishes.

Yang One of the two complementary/antagonistic tendencies that make up all phenomena. Yang is the energy or force moving in a centripetal, inward, or downward direction. Its qualities include hardness, gathering, and contraction.

Yin One of the two complementary/antagonistic tendencies that make up all phenomena. Yin is the energy or force moving in a centrifugal, outward, or upward direction. Its qualities include softness, dispersion, and expansion.

MACROBIOTIC RESOURCES

PERSONAL GUIDANCE

Office of Michio Kushi, 62 Buckminster Road, Brookline, MA 02446; (617) 232-6876; fax (617) 734-0635. The Kushi office handles Michio Kushi's lecture tour, speaking requests, consultations, and correspondence.

Alex and Gale Jack, 305 Brooker Hill Road, Becket, MA 01223; (413) 623-0012; fax (413) 623-6042; e-mail shenwa@bcn.net. Alex and Gale offer dietary and way of life consultations and private instruction on macrobiotic cooking and health care.

ORGANIZATIONS

Kushi Foundation, Box 7, Becket, MA 01223; (800) 975-8744; (413) 623-5741; fax (413) 623-8827; e-mail programs@kushiinstitute.org, Web site www.kushiinstitute.org. The Kushi Institute was founded in 1979 by Michio and Aveline Kushi and offers year-round programs and seminars, including the Way to Health Program, Macrobiotic Career Training Program, and the annual Summer Conference. It also offers counseling, work-exchange, and meals and accommodations at its 600-acre site in the Berkshire Mountains of western Massachusetts. There is an affiliate in the Netherlands.

Amberwaves, Box 487, Becket, MA 01223; (413) 623-0012; e-mail info@amberwaves.org. Amberwaves was founded by Alex and Gale Jack and their associates in 2001 and is a network devoted to creating planetary health and peace, especially preserving organic rice and other essential foods from the threat of genetic engineering. Amberwaves publishes a magazine and books, sponsors musical concerts and other events, and has branches "from sea to shining sea."

The NOAH Center, 401 Stockbridge Road, Great Barrington, MA 01230; (413) 528-0297. A facility founded by Linda Norris featuring "New Opportunities of Alternative Healing," NOAH offers macrobiotic counseling and support groups by Alex and Gale Jack, cooking classes and lectures, a macrobiotic food service, literature, and other activities.

The Preventive Medicine Center, 1000 Asylum Ave., Hartford, CT 06105; (800) 789-7738. A macrobiotic center founded by Robert Silverstein, M.D., offering a wide range of classes, lectures, and activities.

Strengthening Health Institute, 1223 S. 2nd Street, Philadelphia, PA 19147; (215) 271-0158. A macrobiotic center founded by Denny Waxman, offering weeklong intensive and graduate study weekends.

MAIL-ORDER NATURAL FOODS, COOKWARE, AND BOOKS

Kushi Institute Store, Box 500, Becket, MA 01223; toll-free (800) 645-8744; (413) 623-5741; fax (413) 623-8827; e-mail kushi@macrobiotics.org, Web site www.kushiinstitute.org.

Gold Mine Natural Food Co., 7805 Arjons Drive, San Diego CA 92126; toll-free (800) 475-3663; fax (619) 695-0811; e-mail goldmine@ix. netcom.com.

Natural Lifestyle Supplies, 16 Lookout Drive, Asheville, NC 28804; toll-free (800) 752-2775; fax (828) 252-3386; e-mail debi@natural-lifestyle.com Web site www.natural-lifestyle.com.

Eden Foods, 701 Tecumseh Road, Clinton, MI 49236; (517) 456-7424; fax (517) 456-6075; e-mail info@eden-foods.com; Web site www. edenfoods.com

MACROBIOTICS ON THE INTERNET

www.kushiinstitute.org, the Web site of the Kushi Foundation in Becket, Massachusetts, offers information on programs, classes, and conferences, as well as select information on macrobiotic

philosophy, case histories, and mail order books, foods, and specialty items.

www.macrobiotics.nl, the Web site of the Kushi Institute of Europe in Amsterdam, the Netherlands, offers information in English, French, German, and Dutch on educational programs, as well as research articles on diet and health, recovery stories, and mail order books, foods, and speciality items.

www.amberwaves.org, a Web site offering regular updates on genetically modified rice, wheat, and other grains and organic alternatives, macrobiotic recipes, music and entertainment (including free downloadable MP3s), and other features, hosted by Alex and Gale Jack and Edward and Wendy Esko.

www.cybermacro.com, a Web site offering information, articles, live chats, discussions, and other services, hosted by Gary Miller.

www.9starki.com, a Web site offering guidance in macrobiotics, Eastern cosmology, and other arts, hosted by Wayne Weber.

www.worldmacro.com, the Web site of Non-Credo, provides an online macrobiotic newsletter with articles, interviews, and graphics edited by Yogen Kushi.

A NOTE TO READERS

The authors of this book welcome your comments and suggestions, as well as case histories, experiences with home remedies, and other personal accounts. Communications may be sent to the address below.

For regular updates on macrobiotic health and healing, readers are cordially invited to subscribe to *The Macrobiotic Path*, a new newsletter with information on the international macrobiotic community, including a calendar of events, a summary of new scientific and medical research, recovery stories, new home remedies, seasonal recipes, and other essential information. A yearly subscription is $35.00 and includes discounts on macrobiotic books and study materials, as well as counseling and other services.

> The Macrobiotic Path
> P.O. Box 487
> Becket, MA 01223
> (413) 623-0012
> www.macrobioticpath.com

RECOMMENDED READING

Akizuki, Tatsuichiro, M.D., *Nagasaki 1945* (Quartet Books, U.K., 1981). Absorbing account of how a macrobiotic doctor saved his patients after the atomic bomb of Nagasaki.

Benedict, Dirk, *Confessions of a Kamikaze Cowboy* (Avery, 1991). An actor's recovery from prostate cancer.

Briscoe, David, and Charlotte Mahoney-Briscoe, *A Personal Peace* (Japan Publications, 1989). A mother helps her son recover from schizophrenia with the help of macrobiotics.

Campbell, Don, *The Mozart Effect* (Avon, 1997). The healing power of music. Written with Alex Jack.

Dobic, Mina, *My Beautiful Life* (Findhorn Press, 2000). The story of a Yugoslavian journalist and mother who healed herself of incurable ovarian cancer with macrobiotics.

Esko, Edward, *Healing Planet Earth* (One Peaceful World Press, 1995). The macrobiotic approach to ecology.

———, *Contemporary Macrobiotics* (1stbooks. com, 2000). Essays on health and healing by a leading macrobiotic teacher and counselor.

Esko, Wendy, *Aveline Kushi's Introducing Macrobi-* *otic Cooking* (Japan Publications, 1987). Excellent general cookbook.

———, *Eat Your Veggies* (One Peaceful World Press, 1996). 100 easy-to-make, delicious recipes.

———, *Rice Is Nice* (revised edition, Amberwaves, 2001). 108 delicious brown rice recipes.

———, *Soup du Jour* (One Peaceful World Press, 1995). Over 100 hearty soups, stews, and broths.

Jack, Alex, *Biowisdom: Using Diet and Lifestyle to Strengthen Natural Immunity, Develop Your Intuition, and Radiate Clarity and Peace* (Amberwaves, 2002). A natural approach to bioterrorism, nuclear radiation, GMOs, and other threats.

———, *Imagine a World Without Monarch Butterflies* (One Peaceful World Press, 2000). Awakening to the hazards of genetically altered foods.

———, *Profiles in Oriental Diagnosis*, vol. 1: *The Renaissance;* vol. 2: *Vegetarian Bride of Frankenstein;* vol. 3: *Evolution at the Dinner Table* (One Peaceful World Press, 1995–2000). Case histories of famous artists, scientists, and poets, including Leonardo da Vinci, Shakespeare, Descartes, Newton, Darwin, and Pasteur.

Jack, Alex, and Edward Esko, editors, *Saving Organic Rice* (Amberwaves, 2001). Passionate critique of genetically engineered rice, featuring essays by Vandana Shiva, Mae-Wan Ho, Amory and Hunter Lovins, and other scientists and environmentalists.

Jack, Gale, and Alex Jack, *Amber Waves of Grain* (One Peaceful World Press, 2000). Traditional American whole foods cooking and contemporary vegetarian, vegan, and macrobiotic cuisine.

———, *Promenade Home: Macrobiotics and Women's Health* (Japan Publications, 1988). Autobiography of a Texas schoolteacher.

Harper, Virginia M. and Tom Monte, *Controlling Crohn's Disease: The Natural Way* (Kensington, 2002). A macrobiotic approach to an incurable digestive disorder.

Kushi, Aveline, and Wendy Esko, *Aveline Kushi's Wonderful World of Salads* (Japan Publications, 1989). Complete guide to salads and an in-depth introduction to the art of cutting.

———, *The Changing Seasons Macrobiotic Cookbook* (Avery, 1985). Cooking with the four seasons.

———, *The Complete Whole Grain Cookbook* (Japan Publications, 1997). 250 grain-based recipes for all occasions.

Kushi, Aveline, Wendy Esko, and Maya Tiwari, *Diet for Natural Beauty* (Japan Publications, 1991). Encyclopedia of using food internally and externally for beautiful skin and radiance.

Kushi, Aveline, and Alex Jack, *Aveline: The Life and Dream of the Woman Behind Macrobiotics Today* (Japan Publications, 1988). Aveline's autobiography and history of macrobiotics in America.

———, *Aveline Kushi's Complete Guide to Macrobiotic Cooking for Health, Harmony, and Peace* (Time-Warner Books, 1985). The standard all-purpose macrobiotic cookbook.

Kushi, Michio, *Basic Home Remedies* (One Peaceful World Press, 1994). Guide to the 50 most common macrobiotic home remedies.

———, *How to See Your Health: The Book of Oriental Diagnosis* (Japan Publications, 1980). Standard text on physiognomy.

———, *The Macrobiotic Way* (Avery, 1993). Excellent general introduction to macrobiotics, including recipes and exercises.

Kushi, Michio, and Edward Esko, *Basic Shiatsu* (One Peaceful World Press). How to give a simple, home-style massage.

———, *Dream Diagnosis* (One Peaceful World Press, 1995). How diet affects our dreams, including a dictionary of symbols.

———, *Macrobiotic Seminars of Michio Kushi* (One Peaceful World Press, 1998). Classic lectures on health, diet, and the order of the universe.

Kushi, Michio, and Alex Jack, *The Book of Macrobiotics* (Japan Publications, 1986). Standard text on macrobiotic principles and practice.

———, *The Cancer-Prevention Diet* (revised edition, St. Martin's Press, 1993). Standard text on cancer with chapters on the 20 major types of cancer, including dietary guidelines, recipes, and menus.

———, *Diet for a Strong Heart* (St. Martin's Press, 1985). Standard text on all aspects of cardiovascular health.

———, *The Gospel of Peace: Jesus's Teachings of Eternal Truth* (Japan Publications, 1992). Commentary on the lost Gospel of Thomas and Jesus' macrobiotic approach.

———, *Humanity at the Crossroads* (One Peaceful World Press, 1997). Dietary and lifestyle guidelines for the age of cloning, EMFs, AIDS, mad cow disease, and global warming.

———, *One Peaceful World* (St. Martin's Press, 1986). Michio Kushi's autobiography and standard text on world peace and a macrobiotic approach to social change.

Kushi, Michio, Aveline Kushi, and Alex Jack, *Food Governs Your Destiny: The Teachings of Mizuno Namboku* (Japan Publications, 1986). Insightful observations of an 18th-century physiognomist.

———, *Macrobiotic Diet* (Japan Publications, 1993). Standard text on nutrition and food energy.

Kushi, Michio, and Olivia Oredson Saunders, *Macrobiotic Palm Healing: Energy at Your Fingertips* (Japan Publications, 1988). Standard text on healing directly with heaven and earth's forces.

McKenna, Marlene, with Tom Monte, *When Hope Never Dies* (Kensington Press, 2000). The story of a stockbroker and mother who healed herself of incurable malignant melanoma with the help of macrobiotics.

Monte, Tom, *The Way of Hope: Michio Kushi's Anti-AIDS Program* (Warner Books, 1989). The story of ten men with AIDS-related symptoms who followed a macrobiotic approach.

Nussbaum, Elaine, *Recovery: from Cancer to Health Through Macrobiotics* (Avery, 1992). A mother heals herself of inoperable uterine cancer.

Ohsawa, George, *The Art of Peace* (G.O.M.F., 1990). A meditation on how to achieve universal peace, freedom, and justice.

Pirello, Christina, *Cooking the Whole Foods Way* (Putnam Berkley Group, 1997). 500 natural foods recipes from a noted macrobiotic teacher and host of the PBS show *Christina Cooks!*

Ralston, Norman, D.V.M., with Gale Jack, *Raising Healthy Pets* (One Peaceful World Press, 1996). Keeping dogs and cats healthy, by a macrobiotic vet.

Rogers, Sherry A., M.D., *The Cure Is in the Kitchen* (Prestige, 1991). The story of a macrobiotic physician who healed herself of environmental illness.

Sattilaro, Anthony, M.D., and Tom Monte, *Recalled by Life* (Avon, 1982). A medical doctor and president of a large hospital in Philadelphia overcomes terminal cancer with macrobiotics.

Spear, William, *Feng Shui Made Easy* (Harper Collins, 1995). The art of household siting and arrangement.

Stanchich, Lino, *Power Eating Program* (Healthy Products, 1989). Macrobiotic self-development program emphasizing thorough chewing.

Todd, Alexandra, *Double Vision* (University Press of New England, 1994). A mother helps her son overcome a brain tumor with macrobiotics and modern medicine.

Waxman, Denny, *Strengthening Health* (Strengthening Health Press, 1998). A ten-step program to better health by an experienced macrobiotic teacher and counselor.

———, *The Great Life Handbook* (Denny Waxman Enterprises, 2003). A practical guide to diet and lifestyle.

Yamamoto, Shizuko, and Patrick McCarty, *The Shiatsu Handbook* (Avery, 1996). A comprehensive collection of acupressure techniques.

INDEX

RECIPES

HOME REMEDIES

ABOUT THE AUTHORS

Michio Kushi, leader of the international macrobiotic community, was born in Japan in 1926, studied international law at Tokyo University, became acquainted with macrobiotic philosophy at George Ohsawa's educational center, and came to America in 1949. Influenced by the devastation of World War II, he resolved to dedicate his life to the achievement of world peace and the development of humanity. Sponsored by Norman Cousins, he came to New York and furthered his studies at Columbia University and in personal meetings with Albert Einstein, Thomas Mann, Upton Sinclair, Pitirim Sorokin, and other prominent scientists, authors, and statesmen.

With the help of his future wife, Aveline, who came to the United States in 1951, the Kushis introduced modern macrobiotics and founded Erewhon, the pioneer natural foods company in Boston in the early 1960s that introduced organic brown rice, tofu, tempeh, miso, and dozens of other natural foods to America. The Kushis went on to found the East West Foundation, the *East West Journal,* the Kushi Foundation, and other organizations to spread macrobiotics worldwide. Over the last thirty years, the Kushis have guided thousands of individuals and families to greater health and happiness, lectured to physicians and scientists, advised governments, inspired medical research, and served as consultants to natural foods businesses and industries.

The author of many books, Michio Kushi received the Award of Excellence from the United Nations Writers Society. In recognition of his role in launching the modern health and diet revolution, the Smithsonian Institution opened a permanent Kushi Family Collection on Macrobiotics and Alternative Health Care in 1999. In Washington, D.C., he made a presentation on macrobiotics to the White House Commission on Complementary and Alternative Medicine and has lectured at the United Nations, Harvard Medical School, the World Health Organization, and other institutions.

Michio Kushi lives in Brookline, Massachusetts, and continues a busy international speaking and seminar schedule. He has four children and thirteen grandchildren. His wife, Aveline, died in 2001.

Alex Jack was born in Chicago in 1945, grew up in Evanston, Illinois, and Scarsdale, New York, and received a degree in philosophy from Oberlin College. He served as a reporter in Vietnam and has written for many magazines and publications. Over the last twenty-five years, he has been active in the natural health community as an author, macrobiotic teacher, and dietary counselor. He has served as editor-in-chief of the *East West Journal*, general manager of the Kushi Institute, and director of the One Peaceful World Society. He is founder and president of Amberwaves, a grassroots network devoted to promoting whole grains and protecting rice, wheat, and other essential foods from the threat of genetic engineering.

He is the author, coauthor, or editor of many books, including *The Cancer Prevention Diet* and *Diet for a Strong Heart* with Michio Kushi (both published by St. Martin's Press), *Aveline Kushi's Complete Guide to Macrobiotic Cooking* (Warner Books), *The Book of Macrobiotics* with Michio Kushi (Japan Publications), *The Mozart Effect* with Don Campbell (Avon Books), and *Saving Organic Rice* (Amberwaves).

Alex has traveled and helped introduce macrobiotics in Russia, China, and other countries and lectures on literature, music, and the arts. He lives in western Massachusetts with his wife, Gale, a macrobiotic cooking teacher, and his family.